Health Care Information Systems

Health Care Information Systems

A Practical Approach for Health Care Management

Third Edition

Karen A. Wager

Frances Wickham Lee

John P. Glaser

JB JOSSEY-BASS™

A Wiley Brand

Published by Jossey-Bass
A Wiley Brand
One Montgomery Street, Suite 1200, San Francisco, CA 94104-4594—www.josseybass.com

Jossey-Bass books and products are available through most bookstores. To contact Jossey-Bass directly call our Customer Care Department within the U.S. at 800-956-7739, outside the U.S. at 317-572-3986, or fax 317-572-4002.

Wiley publishes in a variety of print and electronic formats and by print-on-demand. Some material included with standard print versions of this book may not be included in e-books or in print-on-demand. If this book refers to media such as a CD or DVD that is not included in the version you purchased, you may download this material at http://booksupport.wiley.com. For more information about Wiley products, visit www.wiley.com.

Library of Congress Cataloging-in-Publication Data
Wager, Karen A., 1961– author.
   Health care information systems : a practical approach for health care management / Karen A. Wager, Frances W. Lee, John P. Glaser. – Third editon.
       p. ; cm.
   Includes bibliographical references and index.
   ISBN 978-1-118-17353-4 (paperback), ISBN 978-1-118-41936-6 (ePDF), ISBN 978-1-118-42093-5 (ePub)
   I. Lee, Frances Wickham, 1953– author.   II. Glaser, John P. (John Patrick), 1955– author.   III. Title.
   [DNLM: 1. Health Information Systems–organization & administration. W 26.55.I4]
   R858
   610.68–dc23
                                    2013019370

Printed in the United States of America

THIRD EDITION

PB Printing   10 9 8 7 6 5 4 3

Contents

Appendixes

Tables, Figures, and Exhibits

TABLES

FIGURES

EXHIBITS

Foreword

Two pieces of recent federal legislation in the United States—the American Recovery and Reinvestment Act in 2009 and the Patient Protection and Affordable Care Act in 2010—have put health care information technology (IT) on center stage. On the one hand, physicians now have financial incentives to adopt electronic health records (EHRs) and make meaningful use of their capabilities. On the other hand, accountable care organizations have financial incentives to support these and other IT investments (such as computerized physician order entry systems and decision-support systems) to measure, monitor, and achieve defined metrics for the quality of care they deliver.

There is renewed promise that IT investments can help the United States to not only improve the quality of care provided to the population but also lower the cost (or at least moderate the rate of increase in that cost). Recent studies and meta-analyses suggest this promise may be difficult to achieve, especially on the cost side. Mark Pauly and I have summarized the evidence on the cost-reducing potential of various types of information technology and found it wanting (see the November 2012 issue of *Health Affairs*). Moreover, while the impacts of IT on quality are a bit more positive, the results are neither consistent nor overwhelmingly strong. What is going on? Are we all mistaken about IT? Will this ship ever come in?

Information systems (IS) constitute the source of many of the problems in the health care industry. Health care is one of the most transaction-intensive industries (estimated at thirty billion transactions annually), given all the encounters between patients and providers, providers and other providers, providers and insurers, suppliers and providers, and so on. Yet compared to other industries, health care has historically underinvested in IS—and it shows. The transactions between parties in health care take place not so much electronically as through a mixture of telephone, paper, fax, and electronic data exchange (EDI) media. The result is that much information is never captured, is captured incorrectly, is captured inefficiently, or is difficult to retrieve and use. Moreover, the industry relies heavily on legacy systems that cannot communicate with one another, not only between organizations but often within the same organization.

What is required to fix this messy situation? To paraphrase an old adage, the system may be the solution. The U.S. health care industry is in need of a massive infusion of capital to fund the adoption of new IS. Such capital is already being invested right now in EHRs and meeting meaningful use requirements. But money is not enough. In order to work well and live up to its promise, IS must be integrated into clinicians' daily workflow to speed up (rather than slow down) their decision making, as well as to efficiently and conveniently bring greater information to bear at the point of diagnosis and treatment. Scholars call such integration a "sociotechnical system." Finally, to convince all parties to adopt the necessary IS systems, we will need rigorous studies that document the cost and quality returns from these investments and the parties to which these returns accrue. This is not a small task; the value of IS investments still remains a messy discussion.

This book provides an incredibly thorough overview of information systems and their importance in the health care industry. It provides an overview of the health care information industry; a history of health care IS in the United States; a review of the fundamental characteristics of information, the uses to which it is put, and the processes it supports; and a highly detailed discussion of the primary clinical and managerial applications of information (including electronic medical records), the value of information and IS to multiple stakeholders, and, most important, the management of information and IS. This approach is particularly helpful when one considers that the vast majority of health system executives underwent their graduate training at a time when information systems were in their infancy and thus when no such text existed. The second edition of this book also included a dozen minicases documenting the challenges of IT implementation. This is incredibly valuable, since the technology costs are usually outweighed by the process costs of installation and achieving adoption by end users. This new edition is thus a great primer, offering a systematic presentation of a complex, important topic.

The reader will benefit from the collaborative effort that went into this volume. Authors Wager and Lee are academics with considerable experience in teaching health care information management; Glaser is the former chief information officer at one of the most prominent hospital (and integrated) systems in the United States, and is now CEO of Siemens. The combined talents of these two academics and one practitioner (all of whom have doctoral degrees) are reflected in the scope and depth presented here. This book is both systematic and practical, serving the needs of graduate students and current executives in the industry. What I have found particularly helpful is the book's ability to show how information and IS integrate with the other functions of the health care provider organization. The reader comes away from this book with a more profound understanding of how information serves as the lifeblood of the institution and as the real glue that can cement together professionals and departments within a health care organization—and that can also tie the organization more closely to its upstream trading partners (manufacturers, wholesalers, and group purchasing organizations) and downstream trading partners (insurers and managed care organizations). At the end of the day, information and IS construct the real pathway to the utopia sought by providers during the past decade: integrated health care.

This book is required reading for all those who toil in the field of health care management—whether as managers, professionals, consultants, suppliers, customers, students, or scholars. The topic of IS in health care is simply too important, and until recently too often ignored, to be left to haphazard learning. I commend the authors for their great contribution to the field of health care management and information management.

Lawton Robert Burns
James Joo-Jin Kim Professor
The Wharton School
March *2013*

To our students

Preface

Having ready access to timely, complete, accurate, legible, and relevant information is critical to health care organizations, providers, and the patients they serve. Whether it is a nurse administering medication to a comatose patient, a physician advising a patient on the latest research findings for a specific cancer treatment, a billing clerk filing an electronic claim, a chief executive officer justifying to the board the need for building a new emergency department, or a health policy analyst reporting on the cost-effectiveness of a new prevention program to the state's Medicaid program, each individual needs access to high-quality information with which to effectively perform his or her job. The need for quality information in health care has never been greater, particularly as this sector of our society strives to provide quality care, contain costs, and ensure adequate access. Recent health care reform initiatives, including the restructuring of how health care providers are paid, have a profound impact on how health care organizations manage data. Needed are systems that can provide evidence-based information at the point of care and that take into account patient preferences. Being able to manage patients with chronic illness in a cost-effective manner is increasingly important. At the same time as the demand for information has increased, we have seen advances in information technology—such advances have the potential to radically change how health care services are accessed and delivered in the future.

To not only survive but thrive in this new environment, health care executives must have the knowledge, skills, and abilities to effectively manage both clinical and administrative information within their organizations and across the health care sector. Within the next decade the predominant model for maintaining health care information will shift from the current, largely paper-based medical record system, in which information is often incomplete, illegible, or unavailable where and when it is needed, to a system in which the patient's clinical information is integrated, complete, stored electronically, and available to the patient and authorized persons anywhere, anytime—regardless of the setting in which services are provided or the health insurance or coverage the patient carries. Patients and other consumers of health care services will also have a much greater role in the content of and access to their personal health information. Comparative data will be publicly available to consumers on the quality and cost of health care services available within the community. Providers involved in patient care will have immediate access to electronic decision-support tools, the latest relevant research findings on a given topic, and patient-specific reminders and alerts. Moreover, health care executives will be able to devise strategic initiatives that take advantage of access to real-time, relevant administrative and clinical information.

PURPOSE AND ORGANIZATION OF THIS BOOK

The purpose of this book is to prepare future health care executives with the knowledge and skills they need to manage information and information systems technology effectively in this new environment. We wrote this book with the graduate student (or upper-level undergraduate student) enrolled in a health care management program in mind. Our definition of health care management is fairly broad and includes a range of academic programs from health administration, health information management, and public health programs to master of business administration (MBA) programs with an emphasis in health to nursing administration and physician executive educational programs. This book may also serve as an introductory text in health informatics programs. Both the first (2005) and second (2009) editions have been widely used by a variety of health care management and health information systems programs throughout the United States and abroad. We maintain the original organizational structure and chapter order in this third edition, but we have thoroughly revised and updated the content to reflect changes in the health care industry and the renewed focus on health information technology initiatives. We have also added two new chapters, Federal Efforts to Enhance Quality of Patient Care through the Use of Health Information Technology (Chapter Six) and Strategy Considerations (Chapter Fourteen). In addition, given the increased focus on global health, we have included an international perspective on health information technology in Appendix C. We updated the case studies of organizations experiencing management-related information system challenges from the second edition and added several new ones. These reality-based cases are designed to stimulate discussion among students and enable them to apply concepts in the book to real-life scenarios.

The chapters in this book are organized into four major sections:

- Part One: "Health Care Information" (Chapters One through Three)
- Part Two: "Health Care Information Systems" (Chapters Four through Eight)
- Part Three: "Information Technology" (Chapters Nine through Eleven)

- Part Four: "Senior Management IT Challenges" (Chapters Twelve through Eighteen)

Part One, "Health Care Information," is designed to be a health information primer for future health care executives. Often health information system textbooks begin by discussing the technology; they assume that the reader understands the basic clinical and administrative information found in a health care organization and the processes that create and use this information. So they jump into health information system or technology solutions without first examining the fundamental characteristics of the information and processes such solutions are designed to support (Chapter One), data quality (Chapter Two), or the laws, regulations, and standards that govern the management of information (Chapter Three) in health care organizations. It has been our experience that many students aspiring to be health care executives do not have a clinical background and therefore have a limited understanding of patient care processes and the information that is created and used during these processes. The three chapters we have included in Part One are designed to set the stage and provide the requisite background knowledge for the remainder of the book. Students with extensive clinical or health information management backgrounds may choose to skim this section as a refresher.

Part Two, "Health Care Information Systems," provides the reader with an understanding of how health care information systems have evolved and the major clinical and administrative applications in use today (Chapter Four). Special attention is given to the use of clinical information systems, with a focus on electronic health record (EHR) systems. Chapter Five has been entirely revised from the second edition. It provides up-to-date information on the adoption and use of a range of clinical information systems, including systems for electronic health records, computerized provider order entry (CPOE), medication administration using bar coding, telemedicine, and telehealth. It also includes a section on patient portals and personal health records (PHRs).

The last two chapters in Part Two describe the process that a health care organization typically goes through in selecting (Chapter Seven) and implementing (Chapter Eight) a health care information system. Because most health care organizations are not equipped to develop their own applications, we focus on vendor-acquired systems and describe the pros and cons of contracting with an application service provider (ASP). Despite the best-made plans, things can and do go wrong when an organization is selecting or implementing a health care information system. Chapter Seven concludes with a discussion of the issues that can arise during the system acquisition process and strategies for addressing them. We devote a substantial section of Chapter Eight to the organizational and cultural aspects of incorporating information technology (IT) systems into the health care organization. Chapter Eight ends with a discussion of issues that can arise during system implementation and strategies for addressing them.

Part Two focuses on health care information systems and the value they can bring to health care organizations and providers and to the patients they serve. Part Three, "Information Technology," turns to the technology underlying these systems, that is, how they work. The chapters in Part Three are designed to provide a basic understanding of information technology concepts such as architectures and of the core technologies needed to support health care information systems in terms of databases and networks (Chapter Nine), standards (Chapter Ten), and security (Chapter Eleven). The intent is to provide the reader with enough IT knowledge that he or she could carry on a fairly intelligent conversation with a chief information officer (CIO) or a technically savvy clinician, understand the reasons why it is important to have a sound technical infrastructure to support systems, and appreciate the benefits of ensuring system security. New to this edition is an increased focus on cloud computing, mobile technologies, and the use of Web 2.0 tools.

Part Four, "Senior Management IT Challenges," provides a top-level view of what it takes to effectively manage, budget, govern, and evaluate information technology services in a health care organization. Chapter Twelve introduces the reader to the IT function, the services typically found in an IT department in a large health care organization, and the types of professionals and staff generally employed there.

We believe it is critical for health care executives to become involved in discussions and decisions that influence their organization's use of IT. These discussions typically cover such topics as the organization's IT strategy (Chapter Thirteen), strategic considerations (Chapter Fourteen), IT budgeting and governance (Chapter Fifteen), management's role in major IT initiatives (Chapter Sixteen), and methods for evaluating return on investment or the value of health care information systems to the organization, the provider, and the patient (Chapter Seventeen). This part concludes with a series of management-related case studies designed to stimulate discussion and problem solving (Chapter Eighteen). Most of the cases are based on actual events or management situations; three new cases have been added to this edition.

Each chapter in the book (except Chapter Eighteen) begins with a set of chapter learning objectives and an overview and concludes with a summary of the material presented and a set of learning activities. These activities are designed to give students an opportunity to explore more fully the concepts introduced in the chapter and to gain hands-on experience by visiting and talking with IT professionals in a variety of health care settings.

Three appendixes offer supplemental information. Appendix A presents an updated overview of the health care IT industry, the companies that provide

IT hardware, software, and a wide range of services to health care organizations. Appendix B contains an example of a project charter. Appendix C, new to this edition, gives the reader a global perspective on the use of health information technology internationally.

IT CHALLENGES IN HEALTH CARE

The health care industry is one of the most information intensive and technologically advanced in our society. Yet if you asked a roomful of health care executives and providers from a typical health care organization if they have easy access to timely, complete, accurate, reliable, and relevant information when making important strategic or patient-care decisions, most would respond with a resounding no. Despite the need for administrative and clinical information to facilitate the delivery of high-quality, cost-effective services, most organizations still function using insufficient and ineffective information systems. There are many reasons why this situation exists, not the least of which is that the health care industry is complex, both overall and in many of its functions. This complexity poses challenges for both the purchasers and vendors of health care information technology (IT) products and services.

Health care is often accused of being "behind" other industries in applying IT. Statistics, such as percentage of revenue spent on IT, are often used to indict health care for underinvesting in IT. The health care industry spends an average of about 5 percent of its operating expense on IT, while the banking and finance industries spend in excess of 12 percent of their operating expense on IT (Smith & Potter, 2009). The indictment of being behind often carries with it an aspersion that health care executives are not as sharp or "on top of it" as executives in other industries. This is not true.

The complexity and the structure of health care organizations and the industry have historically made it very challenging to implement health care information technology effectively. We emphasize this fact not to excuse health care organizations from having to make thoughtful investments or to claim that all health care executives are world-class but to make it clear those health care executives need to understand the context.

Large Numbers of Small Organizations

The health care industry includes large numbers of very small organizations. A majority of physicians practice in one- or two-physician offices. Thousands of hospitals have fewer than 100 beds. There are over 7,000 home health agencies. Small organizations often find it difficult to fund information system investments. An investment of $25,000 in an electronic health record may be more than a solo practitioner can bear. In addition, these organizations rarely have IT-trained staff members and, hence, are challenged when technology misbehaves—for example, when a printer malfunctions or files are inadvertently deleted.

The small size of these organizations also makes it difficult for software and hardware vendors to make money from them. Often these vendors cannot charge much for their applications, making it challenging for them to recover the costs of selling to small organizations and providing support to them. As a result most major vendors often avoid small organizations. Those vendors that do sell to this market are often small themselves, having perhaps four to six customers. This smallness means that if they have even one bad year—if, for example, they lose two customers—it may put them out of business. Hence, there is significant turnover among small IT vendors. This turnover clearly places the small provider organization at risk of having the vendor of its IT system go out of business.

Incentive Misalignment

Many health care information technology applications have the potential to improve the quality of care. CPOE can reduce adverse drug events. Reminder systems in the electronic medical record can improve the management of the chronically ill patient. Improvements in care are worthy goals, and providers may opt to bear the costs of the systems to gain them. In truth, however, the provider does not always reap a reward for such actions. The insurance payment mechanism may not provide a financial reward for the provider who has fewer medical errors. There may be no direct financial reward for better management of the diabetic.

Because of this misalignment the bearer of the cost may see no financial gain and providers can, rightfully, be hesitant to invest in IT that has care quality improvement as its goal. For them the IT investment reduces their income—with no corresponding financial upside. This misalignment rarely occurs in other industries. For example, if you are in the banking industry and you make IT investments to improve the quality of your service, you expect to be rewarded by having more customers and by having existing customers do more business with you.

Fragmented Care

Most of us, over the course of our lives, will seek care in several health care organizations. At times this care will also occur in various regions of the country. The data about our care are not routinely shared across the organizations we use. And the organizations do not have to be on different sides of this country for this failure to occur; they may be across the street from each other. This failure to share data means that any given provider may not be fully aware of allergies, history, and clinical findings that were recorded in other settings. Medical errors and inefficiencies—for example, unnecessary repeats of tests—can result.

This lack of exchange is due in part to the fact that many providers still use paper-based systems that make exchange more expensive and less likely to happen.

The lack of exchange also occurs because the U.S. health care system is not a single system of care but rather a conglomeration of systems, including organizations in both the public and private sectors. Even within an individual health care organization there may be a number of fragmented systems and processes for managing information.

Thus, another major challenge facing health care is the integration of heterogeneous systems. Some connectivity problems stem from the fact that many health care organizations acquired a variety of departmental clinical systems, with little regard for how they fit together in the larger context of the organization or enterprise. There was little emphasis initially on enterprise-wide systems or on answering such questions as, Will the departmental systems communicate with each other? With the patient registration system? With the patient accounting system? To what degree will these systems support the strategic goals of the organization? As health care organizations merged or were purchased from larger organizations, the problems with integrating systems multiplied.

Integration issues may be less of an issue when a health care organization acquires an enterprise-wide system from a single vendor or when the organization itself is a self-contained system. For example, Hospital Corporation of America (HCA), a for-profit health care system comprising hundreds of hospitals throughout the nation, has adopted an enterprise-wide system from a single vendor that is used across all HCA facilities. However, rarely does a single vendor offer all the applications and functionality needed by a health care organization. Significant progress has been made in terms of interoperability standards, yet much work remains.

Finally, health information exchange is limited because there is no incentive for either the sender or the receiver to make the exchange happen. It may seem odd, perhaps counter to the mission of health care, that organizations need financial incentives to do what is best for the patient. However, it is a harsh reality of health care that organizations do need positive operating margins.

Complexity of the Process of Care

If one views the process of care as a manufacturing process (sick people are inputs, a "bunch of stuff" is done to them, and the outputs are better or well people), it is arguable that medical care is the most complex manufacturing process that exists. This high level of complexity has three major sources: the difficulty of defining the best care, care process variability, and process volatility.

Our current ability to define the best care process for treating a particular disease or problem can be limited. Process algorithms, guidelines, or pathways are often

- Based on heuristics (or rules of thumb), which makes consensus within and between organizations difficult or impossible. Available facts and science are often insufficient to define a consistent, let alone the most effective, approach. As a result, competing guidelines or protocols are being issued by payers, provider organization committees, and provider associations.

- Condition or context specific. The treatment of a particular acute illness, for example, can depend on the severity of the illness and the age and general health of the patient.

- Reliant on outcome measurements with severe limitations. For example, these measures may be insensitive to specific interventions, be proxies for "real" outcomes, or reflect the bias of an organization or researcher.

An organization is unlikely to be able to define or adopt a consistent approach for each type of care. And even a defined approach may permit substantial latitude on the part of the provider. This results in great variability in treatment. In an academic medical center a physician may have at his or her disposal 2,500 medications (each with a range of "allowable" frequencies, doses, and routes of administration), 1,100 clinical laboratory tests, 300 radiology procedures, and large numbers of other tests and procedures. The selection of tests and procedures, their sequence, and the relative timing of their use, along with patient condition and comorbidity, all come together to determine the relative utility of a particular approach to treatment.

There is no simple standard operating procedure the provider can turn to for diagnosing, treating, and managing an individual patient's care. Although there are standards of care and practice guidelines, the individual provider still plays a pivotal role in conducting the physical examination, assessment, and history of the patient. The provider relies on prior knowledge and experience and may order a battery of tests and consult with colleagues before arriving at a diagnosis or an individualized treatment plan.

The variability of approaches to treating a disease is compounded by the diversity of diseases and problems. There are approximately 10,000 diseases, syndromes, and problems, each of which, in theory, requires its own pathway, guideline, or approach, and perhaps multiple approaches.

This variability and opportunity for variability is unparalleled by any other manufacturing process. No automobile manufacturer produces 10,000 models of cars or provides for each model 2,500 different types of paint, 300 different arrangements of wheels, and 1,100 different locations for the driver's seat.

These challenges are exacerbated by the volatility of the medical process. In an average year, over 700,000 articles are added to the base of refereed medical literature, articles that may require us to continually revisit our treatment consensus. In addition, medical technology often induces changes in practice before the studies that measure practice efficacy can be completed.

The complexity of the medical process places unique and tough demands on the design of clinical information systems, the ability to support provider and patient decision making, and the ability to measure the quality of the care that providers deliver.

Complexity of Health and Medical Data

Health care information may include text, images, pictures, and other graphics. Terminologies used to describe health information are also complex and are not used consistently among clinicians.

A patient's health status and medical condition are difficult to describe using comprehensive, coded data. Several factors contribute to this problem:

- Although research is ongoing, well-accepted methods to formally decompose many key components of the patient record—for example, admission history and physical status—into coded concepts have not yet been developed.

- When data models are developed, vocabularies of standardized terms to use in these models are difficult to compile. The condition of a patient is often complex and probabilistic, requiring a nuanced description. Multifactorial and temporal relationships can exist between pieces of data. This complexity makes it inherently difficult to develop codes for many types of medical data.

- Even when a data model is developed and coded terms are defined, the entry of coded data is cumbersome and constraining for the provider compared to using pen and paper.

Health information is highly sensitive and personal. What could be more sensitive than a patient's personal health habits, family history, mental health, and sexual orientation? Yet such information may be relevant to the accurate diagnosis and treatment of the patient. Every patient must feel comfortable sharing such sensitive information with health care providers and confident that the information will be kept confidential and secure. Until the passage of the Health Insurance Portability and Accountability Act (HIPAA), there were no federal laws that protected the confidentiality of *all* patient health information, and the state laws varied considerably. Today's younger generation, however, is very technologically savvy and far more comfortable with using the Internet for managing money, purchasing goods, seeking health information or second opinions, joining electronic support groups, and the like, so among these younger patients the concept of managing their own Personal Health Record may take off if the confidentiality and security of their health information can be assured.

Nature of Provider Organizations

Health care organizations, particularly providers, have attributes that can hinder information technology adoption. Provider organizations are unusual in that they have two parallel power structures: the administrative staff and the medical staff. The medical staff side is often loosely organized and lacks an organizational chart with clear lines of authority. This two-part structure leads to a great deal of negotiating and coalition building. Negotiation is an aspect of any major decision within a provider organization, including decisions about health care information technology. This can result in very long decision-making cycles; reaching an agreement on an IT vendor can take months or years.

RISING TO THE CHALLENGES

The factors cited here have hindered the adoption and effective use of information technology in health care (particularly the electronic health record) for decades.

However, as we will discuss throughout this book, the health care industry in the United States (and globally) is in the early stages of sweeping change. This change is largely driven by changes in provider reimbursement approaches that intend to hold providers accountable for the care that they deliver. For example, there will be fiscal penalties for poor quality care or uncoordinated care.

These changes are in their early stages at the time of the writing of this book (we will discuss these changes in Chapter Six). The changes will evolve over the course of many years, and the mature form and effectiveness of them is unclear. Nonetheless, changes in reimbursement and the expected reactions of the industry will address many of the challenges cited earlier:

Large Numbers of Small Organizations. To effectively participate in the new era of accountability, providers will need to make investments in electronic health records. Moreover, they will need to develop clinical and management mechanisms to measure care quality, safety, and efficiency and change clinical practice to make necessary improvements.

The majority of small physician practices and hospitals will determine that they lack the necessary resources to prosper in the new era. Hence, many of them are seeking to be acquired by, or affiliate with, large provider health systems that do have the necessary resources. According to PwC Health Research Institute (2011), 58 percent of all physicians are interested in aligning with hospitals. The industry is undergoing significant consolidation.

Incentive Misalignment. Recognizing that providers had few financial incentives to make investments in electronic health records, the HITECH legislation (passed in 2009 and discussed in Chapter Six) provided significant financial incentives for providers to adopt and meaningfully use electronic health records. Moreover, the Patient Protection and Affordable Care Act (passed in 2010 and discussed in Chapter Six) unleashed a series of reimbursement changes that reward high quality, coordinated care and punish the lack thereof. In order to capitalize on these changes, providers will need to make investments in electronic health records, health information exchanges, revenue cycle systems, and business intelligence.

Hence, significant direct and indirect financial incentives for health care information technology adoption have been introduced by federal and state governments. Private sector health insurance companies are following suit.

Fragmented Care. Many of the new reimbursement mechanisms emphasize care coordination and the management of populations of patients, particularly those patients with chronic diseases. Hence, investments will be made in health information exchanges to support the integration of care across a health system, regions, states, and the country. These investments are helped by the federal government's development of data standards that enable more effective data exchange and new privacy and security regulations to help ensure that patients are protected as data are exchanged.

Care Process Complexity. It is not possible to routinize care across all diseases in the course of the lifetime of the authors or readers of this book. Nonetheless, an aspect of the changes in reimbursement is the increased development of quality measurement standards and more robust and extensive guidelines for treating patients with specific diseases, conditions, and procedures.

These efforts will narrow the complexity of care provision variability for diseases such as diabetes and asthma and for procedures such as total hip replacements.

Complexity of Health and Medical Data. For care payments to be based on outcomes, quality measures must be well defined and core pieces of data, such as problems and medications, must be standardized. The federal government has several efforts underway to accomplish these tasks. Hence, to ensure that they are reimbursed, providers will adopt these standards.

Nature of Provider Organizations. Provider organizations will not suddenly become politically, managerially, and clinically simple organizations. However, a consequence of the consolidation of the industry, and efforts to reduce care fragmentation, is that many physicians are seeking to become employees of health systems, forgoing the allure of going into private practice as a small business person.

This change will make lines of decision making and authority clearer as providers make decisions about topics such as electronic health records and care practice improvement.

Sweeping (perhaps radical) changes are underway in the U.S. health care industry. Dramatic changes in provider reimbursement are being made in an effort to improve care quality, efficiency, and safety. These changes will reduce many of the barriers that have hindered health care information technology adoption for decades.

These changes have also materially heightened the strategic importance of the technology. It will not be possible to thrive in the new era of care accountability without a foundation of sophisticated information technology.

We hope you will find this book to be a useful resource in ensuring that your health care organization and its information systems are well equipped to handle patients', providers', administrators', and all other stakeholders' health care information needs.

An instructor's supplement is available at www.josseybass.com/go/wager3e. Additional materials to enrich teaching and learning can be found at www.josseybasspublichealth.com.

REFERENCES

PwC Health Research Institute. (2011). *Top health industry issues of 2012: Connecting in uncertainty.* New York: Author.

Smith, M., & Potter, K. (2009). *IT spending and staffing report, 2009.* Report G00164940. Stamford, CT: Gartner.

Acknowledgments

We wish to extend a special thanks to Amy McLeod, a graduate student in the Master of Health Administration Program at the Medical University of South Carolina (MUSC) for her dedication and assistance in preparing the final manuscript for this book. We also wish to thank the following MUSC students in the doctoral-degree program in health administration, who contributed information systems management stories and experiences to us for use as case studies: Penney Burlingame, Barbara Chelton, Stuart Fine, and David Freed.

Ron Black, Robert Chaloner, Jonathan P. DeShazo, Christopher Harle, Michael Hogarth, Sarah Wills-Dubose, David Gehant, Patricia Givens, Victoria Harkins, Randall Jones, Michael Moran, Catrin Jones-Nazar, Ronald Kintz, Lauren Lent, George Mikatarian, Lorie Shoemaker, and Gary Wilde provided valuable feedback in the early stages of the manuscript's development. Bob Garrie, Mark Gaynor, and Jerry "Micky" Trimm provided thoughtful and constructive comments on the complete draft manuscript.

To all of our students whom we have learned from over the years, we thank you. Finally, we wish to thank James B. Getsinger, technology director for Healthcare Simulation South Carolina, for his much appreciated contributions to the revision of Chapter Nine, "Technologies That Support Health Care Information Systems."

The Authors

Karen A. Wager is professor and associate dean for student affairs in the College of Health Professions at the Medical University of South Carolina (MUSC), where she teaches management and health information systems courses to graduate students. She has nearly thirty years of professional and academic experience in the health information management profession and has published numerous articles, case studies, and book chapters. Recognized for her excellence in interprofessional education and in bringing practical research to the classroom, Wager received the 2008 MUSC outstanding teaching award in the educator-lecturer category and the 2008 Governor's Distinguished Professor Award. She currently serves on the Accreditation Council for the Commission on Accreditation of Healthcare Management Education (CAHME) and is a past fellow of CAHME. Wager serves as a member of the HIMSS-AUPHA-CAHME Task Force responsible for the development of a model curriculum in health information systems appropriate for educating graduate students in health administration programs. She is past president of the South Carolina chapter of the Healthcare Information and Management Systems Society (HIMSS) and past president of the South Carolina Health Information Management Association. In her current position Wager spends part of her time working with the clinical leadership team at the MUSC Medical Center to advance the educational mission of the organization's strategic information systems plan. She holds a DBA degree with an emphasis in information systems from the University of Sarasota.

Frances Wickham Lee is professor and director of instructional operations for Healthcare Simulation South Carolina at the Medical University of South Carolina (MUSC). She has over thirty years of professional and academic experience in the health information management profession. She has published numerous articles and book chapters related to health information management. She is past president of the North Carolina Health Information Management Association and South Carolina chapter of the Healthcare Information and Management Systems Society (HIMSS). For the past six years, Lee has broadened her expertise as a health care educator through her membership in a pioneering team charged with bringing health care simulation to students and practicing professionals across the state of South Carolina. She holds a DBA degree with an emphasis in information systems from the University of Sarasota.

John P. Glaser currently serves as chief executive officer (CEO) of the Health Services Business Unit of Siemens Healthcare, where he is responsible for heading Siemens' global health care IT business. Prior to joining Siemens, Glaser was vice president and chief information officer at Partners HealthCare, Inc. Previously, he was vice president, information systems, at Brigham and Women's Hospital.

Glaser was the founding chairman of the College of Healthcare Information Management Executives (CHIME), and is the former chairman of the eHealth Initiative Board and the Board of the National Alliance for Health Information Technology. He is a former senior advisor to the Office of the National Coordinator for Health Information Technology (ONC). He is also past president of the Healthcare Information and Management Systems Society (HIMSS), and is a fellow of HIMSS, CHIME, and the American College of Medical Informatics, where he previously served on the board.

Glaser has published more than one hundred fifty articles and three books on the strategic application of information technology in health care. He also gives approximately one hundred industry speeches each year. Glaser holds a Ph.D. in Healthcare Information Systems from the University of Minnesota.

Health Care Information Systems

PART ONE

Health Care Information

CHAPTER 1

Introduction to Health Care Information

LEARNING OBJECTIVES

- To be able to compare and contrast the various definitions of health care information.
- To be able to describe the major types of health care information (internal and external) that are captured or used or both in health care organizations.
- To be able to cite specific examples of the major types of health care information.
- To be able to understand the content and uses of patient records.
- To be able to follow a patient's or client's health information throughout a typical encounter or process.

Although it may seem self-evident, it is worth stating: *health care information is the reason we need health care information systems*. No study of information systems in health care would be complete without an examination of the data and information they are designed to support. The focus of this chapter will be on the data and information that are unique to health care, such as the clinical information created during patients' health care encounters, the administrative information related to those encounters, and the external information used to improve the clinical care and administrative functions associated with those encounters.

We begin the chapter with a brief discussion of some common definitions of health care information. Then we introduce the framework that will be used for exploring various types of health care information. The first major section of the chapter looks at data and information created internally by health care organizations, discussing this information at both the individual client level and the aggregate level. This section also examines some core processes involved in an inpatient and an ambulatory care clinical encounter to further explain how and when internal health care data and information originate and how they are used. The final section examines health care data and information created, at least in part, externally to the health care organization, and addresses both comparative and knowledge-based data and information.

TYPES OF HEALTH CARE INFORMATION

Different texts and articles define *health care information*, or *health information*, differently. Often it is the use or setting of the health information that drives the definition. For example, the government or an insurance company may have a certain definition of health care information, and the hospital, nursing home, or physician's office may have other definitions. In this book we are primarily interested in the *information generated or used by health care organizations*, such as hospitals, nursing homes, physicians' offices, and other ambulatory care settings. Of course, this same information may be used by governmental agencies or insurance companies as well.

Definitions of Health Care Information

Different definitions of "health information" and "health care information" have been developed by a variety of agencies and organizations. Some of the most well-known definitions of health information apply to identifiable patient information. These definitions ignore the vast amount of nonidentifiable information that is generated in the delivery of health care. This section examines and compares a few of the most well-known definitions of "health care information."

Health Insurance Portability and Accountability Act Definition

The Health Insurance Portability and Accountability Act (HIPAA), the federal legislation that includes provisions to protect patients' health information from unauthorized disclosure, defines *health information* as any information, whether oral or recorded in any form or medium, that—

(A) is created or received by a health care provider, health plan, public health authority, employer, life insurer, school or university, or health care clearinghouse; and

(B) relates to the past, present, or future physical or mental health or condition of an individual, the provision of health care to an individual, or the past, present, or future payment for the provision of health care to an individual.

HIPAA refers to this type of information as *protected health information,* or PHI. To meet the definition of PHI, information must first of all be *identifiable,* that is, it must have an individual patient perspective and the patient's identity must be known. HIPAA-defined PHI may exist outside a traditional health care institution and is therefore not an appropriate definition for an organizational view of information such as ours. HIPAA is certainly an important piece of legislation, and it has a direct impact on how health care organizations create and maintain health information (HIPAA is discussed further in Chapter Three). However, not all the information that must be managed in a health care organization is protected health information. Much of the information used by health care providers and executives is neither patient specific nor identifiable in the HIPAA sense.

National Health Information Technology Definitions

In an attempt to provide consensus definitions of key health care information terms, the National Alliance for Health Information Technology released a report "On Defining Key Health Information Technology Terms" in April 2008. Although the terms defined in this report are specific to health records, the definitions contain descriptions of the health information that is maintained by each type of record. The following are definitions of *electronic medical record, electronic health record,* and *personal health record.* Each of these definitions refers to patient-specific, identifiable health care information that would meet the HIPAA definition of PHI. (Although the alliance ceased to exist in 2009, these definitions continue to be recognized within the health care community.)

Electronic medical record—An electronic record of health-related information on an individual that can be created, gathered, managed, and consulted by authorized clinicians and staff within one healthcare organization.

Electronic health record—An electronic record of health-related information on an individual that conforms to nationally recognized interoperability standards and that can be created, managed, and consulted by authorized clinicians and staff across more than one healthcare organization.

Personal health record—An electronic record of health-related information on an individual that conforms to nationally recognized interoperability standards and that can be drawn from multiple sources while being managed, shared, and controlled by the individual [National Alliance for Health Information Technology, 2008].

The Joint Commission Definitions

The Joint Commission, the major accrediting agency for health care organizations in the United States, has adopted the HIPAA definition of protected health information as the definition of "health information" listed in their accreditation manual glossary of terms (The Joint Commission, 2011). Creating, maintaining, and managing quality health information is a significant factor in a health care organization achieving Joint Commission accreditation. The 2011 accreditation manual contains dozens of standards that are devoted to the creation and management of health information, including two specific chapters, Record of Care, Treatment, and Services (RC) and Information Management (IM). The RC chapter outlines specific standards governing the components of a complete medical record, while the IM chapter outlines standards for managing information as an important organizational resource.

Health Care Data Framework

Our framework for looking at data and information created, maintained, manipulated, stored, and used within health care organizations is shown in Figure 1.1. The first level of categorization divides data and information into two categories: *internal* and *external*.

Figure 1.1. Types of health care information framework

Internal Data and Information
▪ Patient encounter
▪ Patient-specific
▪ Aggregate
▪ Comparative
▪ General operations
External Data and Information
▪ Comparative
▪ Expert or knowledge-based

Table 1.1. Examples of types of patient encounter data information

Type	Primary Purpose	
	Clinical	Administrative
Patient-specific *(items generally included in the patient medical record are in italics)*	*Identification form or information*	*Identification form*
		Consents
	Problem list	*Authorizations*
	Medication record	*Preauthorization*
	History	*Scheduling*
	Physical	*Admission or registration*
	Progress notes	*Insurance eligibility*
	Consultations	*Billing*
	Physicians' orders	*Diagnoses codes*
	Imaging and X-ray results	*Procedure codes*
	Lab results	
	Immunization record	
	Operative report	
	Pathology report	
	Discharge summary	
	Diagnoses codes	
	Procedure codes	
Aggregate	Disease indexes	Cost reports
	Specialized registers	Claims denial analysis
	Outcomes data	Staffing analysis
	Statistical reports	Referral analysis
	Trend analysis	Statistical reports
	Ad hoc reports	Trend analysis
		Ad hoc reports

Within the broad category of data and information created *internally* by the health care organization, we will focus on clinical and administrative information directly related to the activities surrounding the *patient encounter*, both the individual encounter and the collective encounters. We break information related to the patient encounter into the subcategories of *patient-specific, aggregate,* and *comparative.* Our focus is on the clinical and administrative individual and aggregate health care information that is associated with a patient encounter. Table 1.1 lists the various types of data and information that fall into the patient encounter subcategories of patient-specific and aggregate. Information typically found in a patient medical record is shown in italics. (The comparative data and information subcategory is found in both the internal and external categories; we will discuss it when we discuss external data and information.)

The second major component of internal health care information in our framework is *general operations*. Data and information needed for the health care organization's general operations are not a focus of this text. Health care executives do, however, need to be concerned not only with information directly related to the patient encounter but also with information about the organization's general operations. Health care organizations are, after all, businesses that must have revenues exceeding costs to remain viable. The standard administrative activities of any viable organization also take place in health care settings. Health care executives interact with information and information systems in such areas as general accounting, financial planning, personnel administration, and facility planning on a regular if not daily basis. Our decision to focus on the information that is unique to health care and not a part of general business operations is not intended to diminish the importance of general operations but rather is an acknowledgment that a wealth of resources for general business information and information systems already exists.

In addition to using internally generated patient encounter and general operations data and information, health care organizations use information generated *externally* (Figure 1.1). *Comparative data*, as we will explain, combine internal and external data to aid organizations in evaluating their performance. The other major category of external information used in health care organizations is *expert* or *knowledge-based information*, which is generally collected or created by experts who are not part of the organization. Health care providers and executives use this type of information in decision making, both clinical and administrative. A classic example of knowledge-based clinical information is the information contained in a professional health care journal. Other examples are regional or national databases and informational web sites related to health or management issues.

INTERNAL DATA AND INFORMATION: PATIENT SPECIFIC—CLINICAL

The majority of clinical, patient-specific information created and used in health care organizations can be found in or has originated in patients' medical records. This section will introduce some basic components of the patient medical record. It will also examine an inpatient and an ambulatory care patient encounter to show how the patient medical record is typically created. All types of health care organizations—inpatient, outpatient, long-term care, and so forth—have patient medical records. These records may be in electronic format, paper format, or a combination of both formats but the purpose and basic content are similar regardless of record or organizational type.

Purpose of Patient Records

Health care organizations maintain medical records for several key purposes. As we move into the discussion of clinical information systems in subsequent chapters, it will be important to remember these purposes. These purposes remain constant regardless of the format or infrastructure supporting the records.

1. **Patient care.** Patient records provide the documented basis for planning patient care and treatment. This purpose is considered the number-one reason for maintaining patient records. Health care executives need to keep this primary purpose in mind when examining health care information systems. Too often other purposes, particularly billing and reimbursement, may seem to take precedence over patient care.

2. **Communication.** Patient records are an important means by which physicians, nurses, and others can communicate with one another about patient needs. The members of the health care team generally interact with patients at different times during the day, week, or even month. Information from the patient's record plays an important role in facilitating communication among providers across the continuum of care. The patient record may be the only means of communication between various providers. Patients also have a right to access their records and their engagement in their own care is often reflected in today's medical records.

3. **Legal documentation.** Patient records, because they describe and document care and treatment, can also become legal records. In the event of a lawsuit or other legal action involving patient care, the record becomes the primary evidence for what actually took place during the episode of care. An old but absolutely true adage about the legal importance of patient records says, "If it was not documented, it was not done."

4. **Billing and reimbursement.** Patient records provide the documentation patients and payers use to verify billed services. Insurance companies and other third-party payers insist on clear documentation to support any claims submitted. The federal programs Medicare and Medicaid have oversight and review processes in place that use patient records to confirm the accuracy of claims filed. Filing a claim for a service that is not clearly documented in the patient record could be construed as fraud.

5. **Research and quality management.** Patient records are used in many facilities for research purposes and for monitoring the quality of care provided. Patient records can serve as source documents from which information about certain diseases or procedures can be taken, for example. Although research is most prevalent in large academic medical centers, studies are conducted in other types of health care organizations as well.

6. **Population health.** Information from patient records is used to monitor population health, assess health status, measure utilization of services, track quality outcomes, and evaluate adherence to evidence-based practice guidelines. Health care payers and consumers are increasingly demanding to know the cost-effectiveness and efficacy of different treatment options and modalities.

The importance of maintaining complete and accurate patient records cannot be underestimated. They serve not only as a basis for planning patient care but also as the legal record documenting the care that was provided to patients by the organization. Patient medical records provide much of the source data for health care information that is generated within and across health care organizations. The data captured in a patient medical record become a permanent record of that patient's diagnoses, treatments, and response to treatments.

Content of Patient Records

The American Health Information Management Association (AHIMA) maintains the web site www.myPHR.com, which lists the following components as being common to most patient records, regardless of facility type or medical record system (electronic or paper based) (AHIMA, 2012). Medical record content is determined to a large extent by external requirements, standards, and regulations (discussed in Chapter Three). This is not an exhaustive list, but with our expanded definitions it provides a general overview of this content and of the person or persons responsible for the content. It reveals that the patient record is a repository for a variety of clinical data and information that is produced by many different individuals involved in the care of the patient.

- **Identification form.** Information found on the identification form (sometimes called a *face sheet* or *admission* or *discharge record*) originates at the time of registration or admission. The identification form is generally the first report or screen a user will encounter when accessing a patient record. It lists at least the patient name, address, telephone number, insurance carrier, and policy number, as well as the patient's diagnoses and disposition at discharge. These diagnoses are recorded by the physicians and coded by administrative personnel. (Diagnosis coding is discussed later in this chapter.) The identification sheet is used as both a clinical and an administrative document. It provides a quick view of the diagnoses that required care during the encounter. The codes and other demographic information are used for reimbursement and planning purposes.

- **Problem list.** Patient records frequently contain a comprehensive problem list, which lists significant illnesses and operations the patient has experienced. This list is generally maintained over time. It is not specific to a single episode of care and may be maintained by the attending or primary care physician or collectively by all the health care providers involved in the patient's care.

- **Medication record.** Sometimes called a *medication administration record* (MAR), this record lists medicines prescribed for and subsequently administered to the patient. It often also lists any medication allergies the patient may have. Nursing personnel are generally responsible for documenting and maintaining medication information. In an inpatient setting, nurses are responsible for administering medications according to physicians' written or verbal orders.

- **History and physical.** The history component of this report describes any major illnesses and surgeries the patient has had, any significant family history of disease, patient health habits, and current medications. The information for the history is provided by the patient (or someone acting on his or her behalf) and is documented by the attending physician at the beginning of or immediately prior to an encounter or treatment episode. The physical component of this report states what the physician found when he or she performed a hands-on examination of the patient. The history and physical together document the initial assessment of the patient and provide the basis for diagnosis and subsequent treatment. They also provide a framework within which physicians and other care providers can document significant findings. Although obtaining the initial history and physical is a one-time activity during an episode of care, continued reassessment and documentation of that reassessment during the patient's course of treatment is critical. Results of reassessments are generally recorded in progress notes.

- **Progress notes.** Progress notes are made by the physicians, nurses, therapists, social workers, and other clinical staff caring for the patient. Each provider is responsible for the content of his or her notes. Progress notes should reflect the patient's response to treatment along with the provider's observations and plans for continued treatment. There are many formats for progress notes. In some organizations all care providers use the same note format; in others each provider type uses a customized format.

- **Consultation.** A consultation note or report records opinions about the patient's condition made by a health care provider other than the attending physician or primary care provider. Consultation reports may come from physicians and others inside or outside a particular health care organization, but copies are maintained as part of the patient record.

- **Physician's orders.** Physician's orders are a physician's directions, instructions, or prescriptions given to other members of the health care team regarding the patient's medications, tests, diets, treatments, and so forth. In the current U.S. health care system, procedures and treatments must be ordered by the appropriate licensed practitioner; in most cases this will be a physician.

- **Imaging and X-ray reports.** The radiologist is responsible for interpreting images produced through X-rays, mammograms, ultrasounds, scans, and the like and for documenting his or her interpretations or findings in the patient's medical record. These findings should be documented in a timely manner so they are available to the appropriate physician(s) to facilitate the appropriate treatment. The actual films or digital images are generally maintained in the radiology or imaging departments as hard copies or in a specialized computer system. These images are typically not considered part of the patient medical record, but like other reports, they are stored according to state laws and clinical practice guidelines and are important documentation of patient care.

- **Laboratory reports.** Laboratory reports contain the results of tests conducted on body fluids, cells, and tissues. For example, a medical lab might perform a throat culture, urinalysis, cholesterol level, or complete blood count. There are hundreds of specific lab tests that can be run by health care organizations or specialized labs. Lab personnel are responsible for documenting the lab results. Results of the lab work become part of the permanent patient record. However, lab results must also be available during treatment. Health care providers rely on accurate lab results in making clinical decisions, so there is a need for timely reporting of lab results and a system for ensuring that physicians and other appropriate care providers receive the results. Physicians are responsible for documenting any findings and treatment plans based on the lab results.

- **Consent and authorization forms.** Copies of consents to admission, treatment, surgery, and release of information are an important component of the medical record and related to its use as a legal document. The practitioner who actually provides the treatment must obtain informed consent for the treatment. Patients must sign informed consent documents before treatment takes place. Forms authorizing release of information must also be signed by patients before any patient-specific health care information is released to parties not directly involved in the care of the patient.

- **Operative report.** Operative reports describe any surgery performed and list the names of surgeons and assistants. The surgeon is responsible for the operative report.

- **Pathology report.** Pathology reports describe tissue removed during any surgical procedure and the diagnosis based on examination of that tissue. The pathologist is responsible for the pathology report.

- **Discharge summary.** Each hospital medical record contains a discharge summary. The discharge summary summarizes the hospital stay, including the reason for admission, significant findings from tests, procedures performed, therapies provided, responses to treatments, condition at discharge, and instructions for medications, activity, diet, and follow-up care. The attending physician is responsible for documenting the discharge summary at the conclusion of the patient's stay in the hospital.

Figures 1.2 through 1.5 display screens from electronic health records. A patient record may contain some or all of the documentation just listed. Depending on the patient's illness or injury and the type of treatment facility, he or she may need specialized health care services. These services may require specific documentation. For example, long-term care facilities and behavioral health facilities have special documentation requirements. Our list is intended to introduce the common components of patient records, not to provide a comprehensive list of all possible components. As stated before, the patient record components listed here will exist whether the health care organization uses electronic records, paper records, or a combination of both.

Figure 1.2. Sample EHR information screen

Source: Medical University of South Carolina; Epic.

Figure 1.3. Sample EHR problem list

Source: Medical University of South Carolina; Epic.

Organization of Record Content

Information within patient medical records has traditionally been organized in a diary-like, chronological format. The record content is organized by filing like documents together chronologically. In this type of arrangement all nurses notes would be filed in a different section from the physician notes or lab reports, which would be filed in their own sections of the record. Within each record section the notes or reports are organized in chronological order. This type of record arrangement is sometimes referred to as "source-oriented" because the content is organized by the source of the information.

In the late 1960s, Dr. Lawrence Weed challenged the way records were organized. He introduced the concept of patient-oriented medical records

Figure 1.4. Sample EHR progress notes

Source: Medical University of South Carolina; Epic.

(POMR). The POMR is created and organized around the patient's problems, not the source of the information. The goal of the POMR is to improve patient care through a more systematic way of documentation. Dr. Weed envisioned this system to improve communication and facilitate the continuity of care. The main components of the POMR are:

- The database, which includes information such as the patient's history, physical exam finding, and other initial findings. The database is intended to be very detailed with expanded social and family histories, for example.

- The problem list is the first document in the POMR. It is a list of all patient problems. Problems may be medical or social. Each is documented with the beginning date. As problems are resolved, date of resolution is recorded. No problem is actually removed from the problem list. This problem list becomes the index to the remainder of the record.

Figure 1.5. Sample EHR lab report

Procedure	Abnormality	Status
CBC and differential		

CBC and differential

Status: Final result MyChart: Not Released Next appt with me: None Dx: Diabetes Mellitus

	Range	3yr	3yr
HEMOGLOBIN	13.5 - 17.5 g/dL	13.0 (A)	12.0 (A)
HEMATOCRIT	41 - 53 %	36 (A)	44
RED BLOOD CELL COUNT	4.50 - 5.90 10^6/μL	4.60	4.89
MEAN CORPUSCULAR VOLUME	82.0 - 108.0 fL	89.0	91.2
WHITE BLOOD CELL COUNT	10^3/mL	8.4	7.4
LYMPHOCYTES MANUAL		2	2
EOSINOPHILS MANUAL		0	0
PLATELET COUNT	150 - 399 K/μL	350	389
MEAN PLATELET VOLUME	7.5 - 11.5 fL	9.8	9.9

Resulting Agency
Lab Flowsheet

| Order Details | View Encounter | Lab and Collection Details | Routing | Result History |

Last Resulted: 10/22/09 3:38 PM

Source: Medical University of South Carolina; Epic.

- The initial plan is derived from the problems identified in the initial problem list. All health care provider plans are integrated into the same location, organized by the problem.

- Notes are also integrated in the POMR and follow a prescribed format. Each note, whether written by a physician, nurse, or other health care provider, follows the same format, known as SOAP:
  - Subjective data
  - Objective data
  - Assessment of the patient's status
  - Plan

Although there are few examples of "pure" POMRs in use today, the problem list and the SOAP note are commonplace (Miller & O'Toole, 2003).

Overview of a Patient Encounter

Where do medical record data and information come from? How do they originate? In this section we will walk through an inpatient encounter and also take a brief look at a physician's office patient encounter. Along the way we will point out how medical record information is created and used. Figure 1.6 diagrams a reasonably typical nonsurgical inpatient admission. The middle

Figure 1.6. Inpatient encounter flow

Sample Medical Record Information	Inpatient Encounter	Responsible Party
	Scheduling	
	Determine reason for admission	Physician's office staff
	Determine availability of bed and so forth	Hospital scheduling staff
	Preadmission	
Identification sheet	*Collect demographic and insurance information*	Hospital admission staff
	Determine insurance eligibility	
	Precertify inpatient stay	
	Obtain consents, authorizations	
	Admission or Registration	
Identification sheet	*Verify demographic information*	Hospital admission staff
Consent and authorizations	*Verify insurance*	
	Make bed assignment	
	Issue identification bracelet	
	Treatment	
Problem list	*Coordinate care*	Attending physician
	Medical—	Physicians
History and physical	*Initial assessment*	
Physician orders	*Treatment planning*	
Progress notes	*Orders for treatment, lab, and other diagnostic testing, medications*	
Consultations	*Reassessment*	
and so forth	*Discharge planning*	
	Nursing—	
Nursing notes	*Initial assessment*	Nurses
Medication administration record	*Treatment planning*	
and so forth	*Administration of tests, treatment, medication*	
	Discharge planning	
	Ancillary Services (Radiology, Lab, Pharmacy & so forth)—	Lab technicians
X-ray reports	*Assessment*	Radiologist and radiology technicians
Lab results	*Administration of tests, treatment, medication*	Pharmacists and so forth
Pathology		
Pharmacy		
and so forth		
Identification sheet	**Discharge**	Medical record personnel and coders
Discharge instructions	*Code diagnoses and procedures*	Nurses
Discharge summary	*Prepare instructions for continued care and follow-up*	Attending physician
	Summary of hospital course	

column represents the basic patient flow in an inpatient episode of care. It shows some of the core activities and processes the patient will undergo during a hospital stay. The left-hand column lists some of the points along the patient flow process where basic medical record information is added to the medical record database or file. The right-hand column lists the hospital personnel who are generally responsible for a patient flow activity or specific medical record documentation or both. Using Figure 1.6 as a guide we will follow a patient, Marcus Low, through his admission to the hospital for radiation treatments.

CASE STUDY

Marcus Low's Admission

Mr. Low's admission to the hospital is scheduled by his oncologist, Dr. Good, who serves as the admitting and attending physician during Mr. Low's two-day hospital stay. This process involves the administrative staff in Dr. Good's office calling the Admissions Department of the hospital and arranging a time for Mr. Low to be admitted. The preadmission process involves the hospital corresponding or talking with Mr. Low and with Dr. Good's office to gather the demographic and insurance information that will be needed to file a claim with Mr. Low's insurance company. Generally, hospital personnel contact the patient's insurance company to precertify his or her hospital admission, and in this case the hospital checks that the insurance company agrees that Mr. Low's planned admission is medically necessary and will be approved for payment. The patient medical record is started during the preadmission phase. The Admissions Department must check whether Mr. Low has had a previous stay at the hospital and whether he has an existing medical record number or unique identifier. The *identification form* is started at this stage. Mr. Low's hospital has an electronic health record system, so the demographic information needed is put into the computer system.

On the scheduled day of admission, Mr. Low arrives at the hospital's Admissions Department. There he verifies his demographic and insurance information. He is issued an identification (ID) bracelet and escorted to his assigned room by the hospital staff. Bed assignment is an important activity for the Admissions Department. It involves a great deal of coordination among the Admissions Department, nursing staff, and housekeeping staff. Efficient patient flow within a hospital relies on this first step of bed assignment. Clean rooms with adequate staff need to be available not only for elective admissions like Mr.

Low's but also for emergency admissions. Because this hospital has an electronic health record, there is no paper chart to go to the nursing floor with Mr. Low, but the admissions staff verify that all pertinent information is recorded in the system. The admissions staff also have Mr. Low sign a general *consent to treatment* and the *authorization* that allows the hospital to share his health information with the insurance company.

Once on the nursing floor, Mr. Low receives a nursing assessment and a visit from the attending physician. The nursing assessment results in a nursing care plan for Mr. Low while he is in the hospital. Because Mr. Low saw Dr. Good in his office during the previous week, the *history and physical* is already stored in the electronic health record system. Dr. Good records his *orders* in the physician order entry component of the electronic medical record. The nursing staff respond to these orders by giving Mr. Low a mild sedative. The Radiology Department responds to these orders by preparing for Mr. Low's visit to that department later in the day. During his two-day stay Mr. Low receives several medications and three radiation treatments. He receives blood work to monitor his progress. All these treatments are made in response to orders given by Dr. Good and are recorded in the medical record, along with the *progress notes* from each provider. The medical record serves as a primary form of communication among all the providers of care. They check the electronic health record system regularly to look for new orders and to review the updated results of treatments and tests.

When Mr. Low is ready to be discharged, he is once again assessed by the nursing staff. A member of the nursing staff reviews his discharge orders from the physician and goes over instructions that Mr. Low should follow at home. Shortly after discharge, Dr. Good must dictate or record a *discharge summary* that outlines the course of treatment Mr. Low received. Once the record is flagged to indicate that Mr. Low has been discharged, the personnel in the Health Information Management Department assign codes to the diagnoses and procedures. These codes will be used by the Billing Department to file insurance claims.

When the Billing Department receives the final codes for the records, it will submit the appropriate claims to the insurance companies. It is the Billing Department, or Patient Accounting Department, that manages the patient revenue cycle that begins with scheduling and ends when payments are posted. This department works closely with third-party payers and patients in collecting reimbursement for services provided.

Even in this extremely brief outline of a two-day hospital stay, you can see that patient care and the reimbursement for that care involve many individuals who need access to timely and accurate patient information. The coordination of care is essential to quality, and this coordination relies on the availability of information. Other hospital stays are longer; some are emergency admissions; some involve surgery. These stays will need information additional to that discussed in this section. However, the basic components will be essentially the same as those just described.

An ambulatory care encounter is somewhat different from a hospital stay. Let's follow Mr. Low again. This time we will describe his follow-up office visit with Dr. Good two weeks after his discharge from the hospital. Figure 1.7 is an outline of the process that Mr. Low followed during his office visit and the individuals who were responsible for each step in the process.

CASE STUDY
Mr. Low's Physician's Office Visit

During his follow-up visit, Dr. Good and his professional staff will update Mr. Low's health history, conduct a focused physical exam, and draw blood for a laboratory test. As with the hospital encounter, Dr. Good also maintains a medical record to document the care provided during this visit, but his records are still mainly paper-based. He is planning to implement an electronic health record system within his practice in the next two years. Currently, however, there is no direct link between Dr. Good's and the hospital's medical record systems. Fortunately, Dr. Good can access the hospital's electronic health record system from his office. He can view all the lab results, radiology reports, and discharge summaries for his hospitalized patients. He chooses to print out these reports and file them in the patients' paper medical records. Each medical record in Dr. Good's office contains the general patient demographic and insurance information, an ongoing problem list, a summary of visits, and individual visit notes. These notes include entries by both the nursing staff and Dr. Good. The nursing staff record all their notes by hand. Dr. Good dictates his notes, which are subsequently transcribed by a professional medical transcriber. All phone calls and prescription information are also recorded in the record.

One significant difference between an ambulatory care visit, such as a physician's office visit, and a hospital stay is the scope of the episode of care.

During an inpatient stay patients usually receive a course of treatment, with a definite admission point and discharge point. In an ambulatory care setting, particularly primary care physician visits, patients may have multiple problems and treatments that are ongoing. There may not be a definite beginning or end to any one course of treatment. There are likely to be fewer care providers interacting with the patient at any given ambulatory care visit. There may, however, be more consultations over time and a need to coordinate care across organizations. All these characteristics make the clinical information needs of the inpatient setting and the ambulatory care setting somewhat different, but in each setting, this information is equally important to the provision of high-quality care.

Figure 1.7. Physician's office visit patient flow

Check-In *Verify appointment* *Update insurance information* *Update demographic information* *Pull medical record*	Front office staff
Move to Exam Room *Take vital signs* *Review reason for admission* *Document in medical record*	Nursing staff
Examination *Discussion of hospital stay* *Discussion of disease course and* *next steps*	Physician
Check out *Set next appointment* *Receive payment on bill*	Front office staff
Later *Dictate notes*	Physician
Code visit *File insurance*	Billing clerk

Health care information systems and health care processes are closely entwined with one another. Health care processes require the use of data and information and they also produce or create information. Care providers must communicate with one another and often need to share patient information across organizations. The information produced by any one health care process may in turn be used by others. A true web of information sharing is needed.

INTERNAL DATA AND INFORMATION: PATIENT SPECIFIC—ADMINISTRATIVE

As we have seen in the previous section, patient-specific clinical information is captured and stored as a part of the patient medical record. However, there is more to the story—health care organizations need to get paid for the care they provide and to plan for the efficient provision of services to ensure that their operations remain viable. In this section we will examine individual patient data and information used specifically for administrative purposes. Health care organizations need data to effectively perform the tasks associated with the patient revenue cycle, tasks such as scheduling, precertification and insurance eligibility determination, billing, and payment verification. To determine what data are needed, we can look, first, at two standard billing documents, the UB-04 (CMS-1450) and the CMS-1500. In addition, we will discuss the concept of a uniform data set and introduce the Uniform Hospital Discharge Data Set, the Uniform Ambulatory Care Data Set, and the Minimum Data Set for long-term care.

Data Needed to Process Reimbursement Claims

Generally, the health care organization's accounting or billing department is responsible for processing claims, an activity that includes verifying insurance coverage, billing third-party payers (private insurance companies, Medicare, or Medicaid), and processing the payments as they are received. Centers for Medicare and Medicaid Services (CMS) currently requires health care providers to submit claims electronically, unless the provider qualifies for a waiver. Although this section describes forms, the data requirements are the same whether an organization files electronically or with these forms under a waiver from the Administrative Simplification Compliance Act (ASCA) requirement for electronic submission of claims.

Depending on the type of service provided to the patient, one of two standard billing forms or data sets will be submitted to the third-party payer. The UB-04, or CMS-1450, is submitted for inpatient, hospital-based outpatient, home health care, and long-term care services. The CMS-1500 is submitted for health care provider services, such as those provided by a physician's office. It is also used for billing by some Medicaid state agencies.

UB-04

In 1975, the American Hospital Association (AHA) formed the National Uniform Billing Committee (NUBC, 1999), bringing the major national provider and payer organizations together for the purpose of developing a single billing form and standard data set that could be used for processing health care claims by institutions nationwide. The first *uniform bill* was the UB-82. It has since been modified and improved upon, resulting, first, in the UB-92 data set and now in the currently used UB-04 (see Exhibit 1.1). UB-04 is the de facto hospital and other institution claim standard. It is required by the federal government

Exhibit 1.1. Uniform bill: UB-04

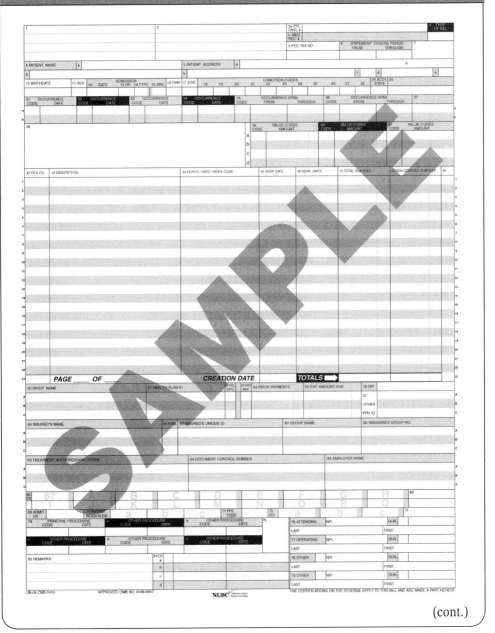

(cont.)

Exhibit 1.1. (*Continued*)

UB-04 NOTICE: THE SUBMITTER OF THIS FORM UNDERSTANDS THAT MISREPRESENTATION OR FALSIFICATION OF ESSENTIAL INFORMATION AS REQUESTED BY THIS FORM, MAY SERVE AS THE BASIS FOR CIVIL MONETARY PENALTIES AND ASSESSMENTS AND MAY UPON CONVICTION INCLUDE FINES AND/OR IMPRISONMENT UNDER FEDERAL AND/OR STATE LAW(S).

Submission of this claim constitutes certification that the billing information as shown on the face hereof is true, accurate and complete. That the submitter did not knowingly or recklessly disregard or misrepresent or conceal material facts. The following certifications or verifications apply where pertinent to this Bill:

1. If third party benefits are indicated, the appropriate assignments by the insured /beneficiary and signature of the patient or parent or a legal guardian covering authorization to release information are on file. Determinations as to the release of medical and financial information should be guided by the patient or the patient's legal representative.

2. If patient occupied a private room or required private nursing for medical necessity, any required certifications are on file.

3. Physician's certifications and re-certifications, if required by contract or Federal regulations, are on file.

4. For Religious Non-Medical facilities, verifications and if necessary re-certifications of the patient's need for services are on file.

5. Signature of patient or his representative on certifications, authorization to release information, and payment request, as required by Federal Law and Regulations (42 USC 1935f, 42 CFR 424.36, 10 USC 1071 through 1086, 32 CFR 199) and any other applicable contract regulations, is on file.

6. The provider of care submitter acknowledges that the bill is in conformance with the Civil Rights Act of 1964 as amended. Records adequately describing services will be maintained and necessary information will be furnished to such governmental agencies as required by applicable law.

7. For Medicare Purposes: If the patient has indicated that other health insurance or a state medical assistance agency will pay part of his/her medical expenses and he/she wants information about his/her medical record released to them upon request, necessary authorization is on file. The patient's signature on the provider's request to bill Medicare medical and non-medical information, including employment status, and whether the person has employer group health insurance which is responsible to pay for the services for which this Medicare claim is made.

8. For Medicaid purposes: The submitter understands that because payment and satisfaction of this claim will be from Federal and State funds, any false statements, documents, or concealment of a material fact are subject to prosecution under applicable Federal or State Laws.

9. For TRICARE Purposes:

   (a) The information on the face of this claim is true, accurate and complete to the best of the submitter's knowledge and belief, and services were medically necessary and appropriate for the health of the patient;

   (b) The patient has represented that by a reported residential address outside a military medical treatment facility catchment area he or she does not live within the catchment area of a U.S. military medical treatment facility, or if the patient resides within a catchment area of such a facility, a copy of Non-Availability Statement (DD Form 1251) is on file, or the physician has certified to a medical emergency in any instance where a copy of a Non-Availability Statement is not on file;

   (c) The patient or the patient's parent or guardian has responded directly to the provider's request to identify all health insurance coverage, and that all such coverage is identified on the face of the claim except that coverage which is exclusively supplemental payments to TRICARE-determined benefits;

   (d) The amount billed to TRICARE has been billed after all such coverage have been billed and paid excluding Medicaid, and the amount billed to TRICARE is that remaining claimed against TRICARE benefits;

   (e) The beneficiary's cost share has not been waived by consent or failure to exercise generally accepted billing and collection efforts; and

   (f) Any hospital-based physician under contract, the cost of whose services are allocated in the charges included in this bill, is not an employee or member of the Uniformed Services. For purposes of this certification, an employee of the Uniformed Services is an employee, appointed in civil service (refer to 5 USC 2105), including part-time or intermittent employees, but excluding contract surgeons or other personal service contracts. Similarly, member of the Uniformed Services does not apply to reserve members of the Uniformed Services not on active duty.

   (g) Based on 42 United States Code 1395cc(a)(1)(j) all providers participating in Medicare must also participate in TRICARE for inpatient hospital services provided pursuant to admissions to hospitals occurring on or after January 1, 1987; and

   (h) If TRICARE benefits are to be paid in a participating status, the submitter of this claim agrees to submit this claim to the appropriate TRICARE claims processor. The provider of care submitter also agrees to accept the TRICARE determined reasonable charge as the total charge for the medical services or supplies listed on the claim form. The provider of care will accept the TRICARE-determined reasonable charge even if it is less than the billed amount, and also agrees to accept the amount paid by TRICARE combined with the cost-share amount and deductible amount, if any, paid by or on behalf of the patient as full payment for the listed medical services or supplies. The provider of care submitter will not attempt to collect from the patient (or his or her parent or guardian) amounts over the TRICARE determined reasonable charge. TRICARE will make any benefits payable directly to the provider of care, if the provider of care is a participating provider.

SEE http://www.nubc.org/ FOR MORE INFORMATION ON UB-04 DATA ELEMENT AND PRINTING SPECIFICATIONS

and state governments in their role as third-party payers and has been adopted across the United States by private third-party payers as well. One important change implemented with the transition from the UB-92 to the UB-04 is the requirement that each claim include a valid National Provider Identifier (NPI) (Centers for Medicare and Medicaid [CMS], 2006). The NPI is a unique identification number for each HIPAA-covered health care provider. Covered health care providers and all health plans and health care clearinghouses use NPIs in the administrative and financial transactions adopted under HIPAA. The NPI is a ten-position, "intelligence-free" numeric identifier, meaning that this ten-digit number does not carry any additional information about the health care provider to which it is assigned, such as the state in which the provider works or the provider's medical specialty (CMS, 2008).

CMS-1500

The National Uniform Claim Committee (NUCC, 2012) was created by the American Medical Association (AMA) to develop a standardized data set for the noninstitutional health care community to use in the submission of claims (much as the NUBC has done for institutional providers). Members of this committee represent key provider and payer organizations, with the AMA appointing the committee chair. The standardized claim form developed and overseen by NUCC is the CMS-1500. This claim form has been adopted by the federal government, and like the UB-04 for institutional care, has become the de facto standard for all types of noninstitutional provider claims, such as those for physician services (see Exhibit 1.2).

It is important to recognize that both the UB-04 and the CMS-1500 claim forms incorporate standardized data sets. Regardless of a health care organization's location or a patient's insurance coverage, the same data elements are collected. In many states UB-04 data and CMS-1500 data must be reported to a central state agency responsible for aggregating and analyzing the state's health data. At the federal level the Centers for Medicare and Medicaid Services (CMS) aggregates the data from these claims forms for analyzing national health care reimbursement, clinical, and population trends. Having uniform data sets means that data can be compared not only within organizations but within states and across the country.

Other Uniform Data Sets

Other uniform data sets have been developed for use in the United States. Three examples are the Uniform Hospital Discharge Data Set (UHDDS), the Uniform Ambulatory Care Data Set (ACDS), and the Minimum Data Set (MDS) used for long-term care. These data sets share two purposes:

1. To identify the data elements that should be collected for each patient, and
2. To provide uniform definitions for common terms and data elements [LaTour, 2002, p. 123].

The UHDDS is the oldest uniform data set used in the United States. The earliest version was developed in 1969 by the National Center for Health

Exhibit 1.2. Claim form: CMS-1500

Exhibit 1.2. (*Continued*)

BECAUSE THIS FORM IS USED BY VARIOUS GOVERNMENT AND PRIVATE HEALTH PROGRAMS, SEE SEPARATE INSTRUCTIONS ISSUED BY APPLICABLE PROGRAMS.

NOTICE: Any person who knowingly files a statement of claim containing any misrepresentation or any false, incomplete or misleading information may be guilty of a criminal act punishable under law and may be subject to civil penalties.

REFERS TO GOVERNMENT PROGRAMS ONLY

MEDICARE AND CHAMPUS PAYMENTS: A patient's signature requests that payment be made and authorizes release of any information necessary to process the claim and certifies that the information provided in Blocks 1 through 12 is true, accurate and complete. In the case of a Medicare claim, the patient's signature authorizes any entity to release to Medicare medical and nonmedical information, including employment status, and whether the person has employer group health insurance, liability, no-fault, worker's compensation or other insurance which is responsible to pay for the services for which the Medicare claim is made. See 42 CFR 411.24(a). If item 9 is completed, the patient's signature authorizes release of the information to the health plan or agency shown. In Medicare assigned or CHAMPUS participation cases, the physician agrees to accept the charge determination of the Medicare carrier or CHAMPUS fiscal intermediary as the full charge, and the patient is responsible only for the deductible, coinsurance and noncovered services. Coinsurance and the deductible are based upon the charge determination of the Medicare carrier or CHAMPUS fiscal intermediary if this is less than the charge submitted. CHAMPUS is not a health insurance program but makes payment for health benefits provided through certain affiliations with the Uniformed Services. Information on the patient's sponsor should be provided in those items captioned in "Insured"; i.e., items 1a, 4, 6, 7, 9, and 11.

BLACK LUNG AND FECA CLAIMS

The provider agrees to accept the amount paid by the Government as payment in full. See Black Lung and FECA instructions regarding required procedure and diagnosis coding systems.

SIGNATURE OF PHYSICIAN OR SUPPLIER (MEDICARE, CHAMPUS, FECA AND BLACK LUNG)

I certify that the services shown on this form were medically indicated and necessary for the health of the patient and were personally furnished by me or were furnished incident to my professional service by my employee under my immediate personal supervision, except as otherwise expressly permitted by Medicare or CHAMPUS regulations.

For services to be considered as "incident" to a physician's professional service, 1) they must be rendered under the physician's immediate personal supervision by his/her employee, 2) they must be an integral, although incidental part of a covered physician's service, 3) they must be of kinds commonly furnished in physician's offices, and 4) the services of nonphysicians must be included on the physician's bills.

For CHAMPUS claims, I further certify that I (or any employee) who rendered services am not an active duty member of the Uniformed Services or a civilian employee of the United States Government or a contract employee of the United States Government, either civilian or military (refer to 5 USC 5536). For Black-Lung claims, I further certify that the services performed were for a Black Lung-related disorder.

No Part B Medicare benefits may be paid unless this form is received as required by existing law and regulations (42 CFR 424.32).

NOTICE: Any one who misrepresents or falsifies essential information to receive payment from Federal funds requested by this form may upon conviction be subject to fine and imprisonment under applicable Federal laws.

NOTICE TO PATIENT ABOUT THE COLLECTION AND USE OF MEDICARE, CHAMPUS, FECA, AND BLACK LUNG INFORMATION
(PRIVACY ACT STATEMENT)

We are authorized by CMS, CHAMPUS and OWCP to ask you for information needed in the administration of the Medicare, CHAMPUS, FECA, and Black Lung programs. Authority to collect information is in section 205(a), 1862, 1872 and 1874 of the Social Security Act as amended, 42 CFR 411.24(a) and 424.5(a) (6), and 44 USC 3101;41 CFR 101 et seq and 10 USC 1079 and 1086; 5 USC 8101 et seq; and 30 USC 901 et seq; 38 USC 613; E.O. 9397.

The information we obtain to complete claims under these programs is used to identify you and to determine your eligibility. It is also used to decide if the services and supplies you received are covered by these programs and to insure that proper payment is made.

The information may also be given to other providers of services, carriers, intermediaries, medical review boards, health plans, and other organizations or Federal agencies, for the effective administration of Federal provisions that require other third parties payers to pay primary to Federal program, and as otherwise necessary to administer these programs. For example, it may be necessary to disclose information about the benefits you have used to a hospital or doctor. Additional disclosures are made through routine uses for information contained in systems of records.

FOR MEDICARE CLAIMS: See the notice modifying system No. 09-70-0501, titled, 'Carrier Medicare Claims Record,' published in the Federal Register, Vol. 55 No. 177, page 37549, Wed. Sept. 12, 1990, or as updated and republished.

FOR OWCP CLAIMS: Department of Labor, Privacy Act of 1974, as amended, Republication of Notice of Systems of Records," Federal Register Vol. 55 No. 40, Wed Feb. 28, 1990, See ESA-5, ESA-6, ESA-12, ESA-13, ESA-30, or as updated and republished.

FOR CHAMPUS CLAIMS: PRINCIPLE PURPOSE(S): To evaluate eligibility for medical care provided by civilian sources and to issue payment upon establishment of eligibility and determination that the services/supplies received are authorized by law.

ROUTINE USE(S): Information from claims and related documents may be given to the Dept. of Veterans Affairs, the Dept. of Health and Human Services and/or the Dept. of Transportation consistent with their statutory administrative responsibilities under CHAMPUS/CHAMPVA; to the Dept. of Justice for representation of the Secretary of Defense in civil actions; to the Internal Revenue Service, private collection agencies, and consumer reporting agencies in connection with recoupment claims; and to Congressional Offices in response to inquiries made at the request of the person to whom a record pertains. Appropriate disclosures may be made to other federal, state, local, foreign government agencies, private business entities, and individual providers of care, on matters relating to entitlement, claims adjudication, fraud, program abuse, utilization review, quality assurance, peer review, program integrity, third-party liability, coordination of benefits, and civil and criminal litigation related to the operation of CHAMPUS.

DISCLOSURES: Voluntary; however, failure to provide information will result in delay in payment or may result in denial of claim. With the one exception discussed below, there are no penalties under these programs for refusing to supply information. However, failure to furnish information regarding the medical services rendered or the amount charged would prevent payment of claims under these programs. Failure to furnish any other information, such as name or claim number, would delay payment of the claim. Failure to provide medical information under FECA could be deemed an obstruction.

It is mandatory that you tell us if you know that another party is responsible for paying for your treatment. Section 1128B of the Social Security Act and 31 USC 3801-3812 provide penalties for withholding this information.

You should be aware that P.L. 100-503, the "Computer Matching and Privacy Protection Act of 1988", permits the government to verify information by way of computer matches.

MEDICAID PAYMENTS (PROVIDER CERTIFICATION)

I hereby agree to keep such records as are necessary to disclose fully the extent of services provided to individuals under the State's Title XIX plan and to furnish information regarding any payments claimed for providing such services as the State Agency or Dept. of Health and Human Services may request.

I further agree to accept, as payment in full, the amount paid by the Medicaid program for those claims submitted for payment under that program, with the exception of authorized deductible, coinsurance, co-payment or similar cost-sharing charge.

SIGNATURE OF PHYSICIAN (OR SUPPLIER): I certify that the services listed above were medically indicated and necessary to the health of this patient and were personally furnished by me or my employee under my personal direction.

NOTICE: This is to certify that the foregoing information is true, accurate and complete. I understand that payment and satisfaction of this claim will be from Federal and State funds, and that any false claims, statements, or documents, or concealment of a material fact, may be prosecuted under applicable Federal or State laws.

According to the Paperwork Reduction Act of 1995, no persons are required to respond to a collection of information unless it displays a valid OMB control number. The valid OMB control number for this information collection is 0938-0999. The time required to complete this information collection is estimated to average 10 minutes per response, including the time to review instructions, search existing data resources, gather the date needed, and complete and review the information collection. If you have any comments concerning the accuracy of the time estimate(s) or suggestions for improving this form, please write to: CMS, Attn: PRA Reports Clearance Officer, 7500 Security Boulevard, Baltimore, Maryland 21244-1850. This address is for comments and/or suggestions only. DO NOT MAIL COMPLETED CLAIM FORMS TO THIS ADDRESS.

Statistics. In 1974, the federal government adopted the UHDDS definitions as the standard for the Medicare and Medicaid programs. The UHDDS has been revised several times. The current version has the following data elements:

1. Personal identification
2. Sex
3. Race
4. Ethnicity
5. Residence
6. Hospital identification
7. Admission date
8. Discharge date
9. Attending physician
10. Operating physician
11. Diagnoses (principal and other)
12. Procedure and date
13. Disposition of patient
14. Expected payer (Dougherty, 2001, p. 72)

The ACDS was approved by the National Committee on Vital and Health Statistics in 1989. The goal of the ACDS is to improve the data collected in ambulatory and outpatient settings. The ACDS has not, however, been incorporated into federal rules or regulations. It remains a recommended rather than a required data set.

The MDS for long-term care is a federally mandated standard assessment tool that is used to collect demographic and clinical information about long-term care facility residents. It is an extensive data set with detailed data elements in twenty major categories. The MDS provides a structured way to organize resident information so that an effective care plan can be developed (LaTour, 2002).

INTERNAL DATA AND INFORMATION: PATIENT SPECIFIC— COMBINING CLINICAL AND ADMINISTRATIVE

As we have discussed in earlier sections of this chapter, diagnostic and procedural information is captured during the patient encounter to track clinical progress and to document care for reimbursement and other administrative purposes. This diagnostic and procedural information is initially captured in narrative form through physicians' and other health care providers' documentation in the patient record. This documentation is subsequently translated into numerical codes. Coding facilitates the classification of diagnoses and procedures not only for reimbursement purposes but also for clinical research and comparative studies.

Two major coding systems are employed by health care providers today:

- ICD-9-CM (International Classification of Diseases, as modified for use in the United States), slated to be replaced by ICD-10 in 2014
- CPT (Current Procedural Terminology), published by the American Medical Association

Use of these systems is required by the federal government for reimbursement, and they are recognized by health care agencies both nationally and internationally.

On January 16, 2009, HHS published a final rule adopting ICD-10-CM (diagnoses codes) and ICD-10-PCS (procedure codes) to replace ICD-9-CM in HIPAA transactions, with the effective implementation date of October 1, 2013. However, the implementation of ICD-10 was delayed from October 1, 2013, to October 1, 2014, by final rule CMS-0040-F, issued on August 24, 2012.

In anticipation of the new system implementation, the discussion in this chapter focuses on the newer ICD-10 coding systems. The primary purpose of the ICD does not change from 9 to 10, but the structure is significantly different.

ICD-10

The U.S. ICD-10 classification system is derived from the International Classification of Diseases, Tenth Revision, which was developed by the World Health Organization to capture disease data. ICD-10-CM, like ICD-9-CM, will be used in the United States to code disease information. Procedure information will be coded using the ICD-10-PCS. Updates to the ICD-10-CM and PCS will be published each year. This publication is considered a federal government document whose contents may be used freely by others. However, multiple companies republish this government document in easier-to-use, annotated, formally copyrighted versions. The precursors to the current ICD system were developed to allow morbidity (illness) and mortality (death) statistics to be compared across nations. ICD-10-CM and PCS coding, like ICD-9-CM, however, has come to play a major role in reimbursement to hospitals. In 1983, ICD-9-CM began being used for determining the *diagnosis related group* (*DRG*) into which a patient is assigned. DRGs are the basis for determining appropriate inpatient reimbursements for Medicare, Medicaid, and many other health care insurance beneficiaries. Accurate ICD coding has as a consequence become vital to accurate institutional reimbursement. Exhibits 1.3 and 1.4 are excerpts from the ICD-10-CM and PCS classification systems. They show the system in its text form, but large health care organizations generally use encoders, computer applications that facilitate accurate coding. Whether a book or text file or encoder is used, the classification system is the same.

The conversion from ICD-9-CM to ICD-10-CM and PCS is a tremendous undertaking for health care organizations. ICD-10 includes substantial increases

---

Exhibit 1.3. ICD 10-CM

Acute upper respiratory infections (J00-J06)

Excludes1: chronic obstructive pulmonary disease with acute lower respiratory infection (J44.0) influenza virus with other respiratory manifestations (J09.X2, J10.1, J11.1)

J00 Acute nasopharyngitis [common cold]
Acute rhinitis
Coryza (acute)
Infective nasopharyngitis NOS
Infective rhinitis
Nasal catarrh, acute
Nasopharyngitis NOS

Excludes1: acute pharyngitis (J02.-)
acute sore throat NOS (J02.9)
pharyngitis NOS (J02.9)
rhinitis NOS (J31.0)
sore throat NOS (J02.9)

Excludes2: allergic rhinitis (J30.1-J30.9)
chronic pharyngitis (J31.2)
chronic rhinitis (J31.0)
chronic sore throat (J31.2)
nasopharyngitis, chronic (J31.1)
vasomotor rhinitis (J30.0)

Source: Centers for Medicare and Medicaid Services, 2012. Retrieved March 2012 from http://www.cdc.gov/nchs/icd/icd10cm.htm.

Exhibit 1.4. ICD 10-PCS

Section	**7**	Osteopathic
Body System	**W**	Anatomical Regions
Operation	**0**	Treatment: Manual treatment to eliminate or alleviate somatic dysfunction and related disorders

Body Region	Approach	Method	Qualifier
0 Head 1 Cervical 2 Thoracic 3 Lumbar 4 Sacrum 5 Pelvis 6 Lower Extremities 7 Upper Extremities 8 Rib Cage 9 Abdomen	X External	0 Articulatory-Raising 1 Fascial Release 2 General Mobilization 3 High Velocity-Low Amplitude 4 Indirect 5 Low Velocity-High Amplitude 6 Lymphatic Pump 7 Muscle Energy-Isometric 8 Muscle Energy-Isotonic 9 Other Method	Z None

Source: Centers for Medicare and Medicaid Services, 2012. Retrieved March 2012 from http://www.cdc.gov/nchs/icd/icd10cm.htm.

in content and many structural changes. When the U.S. modification is released, all health care providers will be required to adjust their systems to handle the conversion.

CPT

The American Medical Association (AMA) publishes an updated Current Procedural Terminology each year. Unlike ICD-9-CM, CPT is copyrighted, with all rights to publication and distribution held by the AMA. CPT was first developed and published in 1966. The stated purpose for developing CPT was to provide a uniform language for describing medical and surgical services. In 1983, however, the government adopted CPT, in its entirety, as the major component (known as Level 1) of the Healthcare Common Procedure Coding System (HCPCS). Since then CPT has become the standard for physician's office, outpatient, and ambulatory care coding for reimbursement purposes. Exhibit 1.5 is a patient encounter form with examples of HCPCS/ CPT codes.

Exhibit 1.5. Patient encounter form coding standards

Pediatric Associates P.A. 123 Children's Avenue, Anytown, USA

Office Visits

99211 Estab Pt—minimal
99212 Estab Pt—focused
99213 Estab Pt—expanded
99214 Estab Pt—detailed
99215 Estab Pt—high complexity

99201 New Pt—problem focused
99202 New Pt—expanded
99203 New Pt—detailed
99204 New Pt—moderate complexity
99205 New Pt—high complexity

99050 After Hours
99052 After Hours—after 10 pm
99054 After Hours—Sundays and Holidays

Outpatient Consult
99241 99242 99243 99244 99245

Preventive Medicine—New
99381 Prev Med 0–1 years
99382 Prev Med 1–4 years
99383 Prev Med 5–11 years
99384 Prev Med 12–17 years
99385 Prev Med 18–39 years

Preventive Medicine—Established
99391 Prev Med 0–1 years
99392 Prev Med 1–4 years
99393 Prev Med 5–11 years
99394 Prev Med 12–17 years
99395 Prev Med 18–39 years

99070 10 Arm Sling
99070 11 Sterile Dressing
99070 45 Cervical Cap

Immunizations, Injections, and Office Laboratory Services

90471 Adm of Vaccine 1
90472 Adm of Vaccine > 1
90648 HIB
90658 Influenza
90669 Prevnar
90701 DTP
90702 DT
90707 MMR
90713 Polio Injection
90720 DTP/HIB
90700 DTaP
90730 Hepatitis A
90733 Meningococcal
90744 Hepatitis B 0–11
90746 Hepatitis B 18+ years

81000 Urinalysis w/ micro
81002 Urinalysis w/o micro
82270 Hemoccult Stool
82948 Dextrostix
83655 Lead Level
84030 PKU
85018 Hemoglobin
87086 Urine Culture
87081 Throat Culture
87205 Gram Stain
87208 Ova Smear (pin worm)
87210 Wet Prep
87880 Rapid Strep

Diagnosis

Patient Name
No.
Date
Time
Address
DOB
Name of Insured   ID
Insurance Company
Return Appointment _____

As coding has become intimately linked to reimbursement, directly determining the amount of money a health care organization can receive for a claim from insurers, the government has increased its scrutiny of coding practices. There are official guidelines for accurate coding, and health care facilities that do not adhere to these guidelines are liable to charges of fraudulent coding practices. In addition, the Office of Inspector General of the Department of Health and Human Services (HHS OIG) publishes compliance guidelines to facilitate health care organizations' adherence to ethical and legal coding practices. The OIG is responsible for (among other duties) investigating fraud involving government health insurance programs. More specific information about compliance guidelines can be found on the OIG web site (www.oig.hhs .gov) (HHS OIG, 2012).

INTERNAL DATA AND INFORMATION: AGGREGATE—CLINICAL

In the previous section we examined different sets of clinical and administrative data that are collected during or in the time closely surrounding the patient encounter. Patient records, uniform billing information, and discharge data sets are the main sources of the data that go into the literally hundreds of aggregate reports or queries that are developed and used by providers and executives in health care organizations. Think of these source data as one or more data repositories, with each data element available to health care providers and executives. What can these data tell you about the organization and the care provided to patients? How can you process these data into meaningful information? The number of aggregate reports that could be developed from patient records or patient accounting information is practically limitless, but there are some common categories of clinical, administrative, and combined reports that the health care executive will likely encounter. We will discuss a few of these in this and the following sections.

On the clinical side, disease indexes and specialized registers are often used.

Disease and Procedure Indexes

Health care organization management often wants to know summary information about a particular disease or treatment. Examples of questions that might be asked are: What is the most common diagnosis in the facility? What percentage of diabetes patients are African American? What is the most common procedure performed on patients admitted with gastritis (or heart attack or any other diagnosis)? Traditionally, such questions have been answered by looking in disease and procedure indexes. Prior to the widespread use of databases and computers, disease and procedure indexes were large card catalogues or books that kept track of the numbers of diseases treated and procedures occurring in a facility by disease and procedure ICD codes. Now that databases and computers are common, the disease and procedure index function is generally handled as a component of the patient medical record system or the registration and discharge system. The retrieval of information related to diseases and procedures is still based on ICD and CPT codes, but the queries are limitless. Users can search the disease and procedure database for general frequency statistics for any number of combinations of data. Figure 1.8 is an example of a screen resulting from a query for a list of diabetes patients.

Specialized Registers

Another type of aggregate information that has benefited tremendously from the use of computerized databases is the specialized register. Registers are lists that generally contain the names, and sometimes other identifying information, of patients seen in a particular area of the health care facility. A health facility might want an accounting of patients seen in the emergency department or operating room, for example. In general, a register allows data retrieval in a particular area of the organization. With the increased availability of large databases, many of these registers can be created on an ad hoc basis.

Trauma and tumor registries are specialized registries that often involve data collection beyond that done for the patient medical record and patient billing process. These registries may be found in facilities with high-level trauma or cancer centers. They are used to track information about patients over time and to collect detailed information for research purposes.

Figure 1.8. Sample diabetes query screen

Source: Partners HealthCare.

Many other types of aggregate clinical reports are used by health care providers and executives. The easy-to-use, ad hoc reporting that is available with databases today gives providers and executives access to any number of summary reports based on the data elements collected during the patient encounter.

INTERNAL DATA AND INFORMATION: AGGREGATE—ADMINISTRATIVE

Just as with clinical aggregate reports, a limitless number of reports can be created for administrative functions from today's databases and data repositories. Commonly used administrative aggregate reports include basic health care statistical reports, claims denial reports, and cost reports. (In keeping with our focus on information unique to health care, we will not discuss traditional income statements, cash flow statements, or other general accounting reports.) Two basic types are described in this section: Medicare cost reports and basic health care statistical reports.

Medicare Cost Reports

Medicare cost reports are filed annually by all hospitals, home health agencies, skilled nursing facilities, and hospices that accept Medicare or Medicaid. These reports must be filed within a specified time after the end of the fiscal year and are subject to scrutiny via compliance audits. The cost report contains such provider information as facility characteristics, utilization data, costs and charges by cost center (in total and for Medicare), Medicare settlement data, and financial statement data. Preparation instructions and the actual forms can be found on the CMS web site (www.cms.gov). Medicare cost reports are used by CMS not only to determine portions of an individual facility's reimbursement but also to determine Medicare rate adjustments, cost limits, and various wage indexes.

Health Care Statistics

The categories of statistics that are routinely gathered for health care executives or others are

- **Census statistics.** These data reveal the number of patients present at any one time in a facility. Several commonly computed rates are based on these census data, including the average daily census and bed occupancy rates.
- **Discharge statistics.** This group of statistics is calculated from data accumulated when patients are discharged. Some commonly computed rates based on discharge statistics are average length of stay, death rates, autopsy rates, infection rates, and consultation rates.

General health care statistics are frequently used to describe the characteristics of the patients within an organization. They may also provide a basis for planning and monitoring patient services.

INTERNAL DATA AND INFORMATION: AGGREGATE— COMBINING CLINICAL AND ADMINISTRATIVE

Health care executives are often interested in aggregate reports that combine clinical and administrative data. Ad hoc statistical reports and trend analyses may draw from both clinical and administrative data sources, for example. These reports may be used for the purpose of improving customer service, quality of patient care, or overall operational efficiency. Examples of aggregate data that relate to customer service are the average time it takes to get an appointment at a clinic and the average referral volume by physician. Quality of care aggregate data take many forms, revealing such things as infection rates and unplanned returns to the operating room. Cost per case, average reimbursement by DRG, and staffing levels by patient acuity are examples of aggregate data that could be used to improve efficiency. These examples represent only a few uses for combined aggregate data. Again, with today's computerized clinical and administrative databases, any number of ad hoc queries, statistical reports, and trend analyses should be readily available to health care executives. Health care executives need to know what source data are collected and must be able to trust in data accuracy. Executives should be creative in designing aggregate reports to meet their decision-making needs.

EXTERNAL DATA AND INFORMATION: COMPARATIVE

Comparative data and information, gathered internally and externally, are used for both clinical and administrative purposes by health care organizations.

Outcome Measures and Balanced Scorecards

Comparative data and information are often aligned with organizations' quality improvement efforts. For example, an organization might collect data on specific outcome measures and then use this information in a benchmarking process. *Outcome measures* are the measurable results of a process. This could be a clinical process, such as a particular treatment, or an administrative process, such as a claim filing. Outcome measures can be applied to individuals or groups. An example of a simple clinical outcome measure is the difference in prescribing practices among providers for patients with the same chronic disease. An example of an administrative outcome measure is the percentage of claims denied by Medicare during one month. Implicit in the idea of measuring outcomes is that they can be usefully compared over time or against a set standard. The process of comparing one or more outcome measures against a standard is called *benchmarking*. Outcome measures and benchmarking may be limited to internally set standards; however, frequently they are involved in comparisons with externally generated benchmarks or standards.

Balanced scorecards are another method for measuring performance in health care organizations. The concept of the balanced scorecard meets executives' need to design measurement systems aligned with their organization's strategy goals (Kelly, 2007). Balanced scorecard systems examine multiple measures, rather than the single set of measures common in traditional benchmarking. Suppose a health care organization uses "lowest-cost service in the region" as an outcome measure for benchmarking its performance against that of like facilities in the region. The organization does very well over time on this measure. However, you can see that it may be ignoring some other important performance indicators. What about patient satisfaction? Employee morale? Patient health outcomes? Balanced scorecards employ multiple measures along several dimensions to ensure that the organization is performing well across the board. The *clinical value compass* is a similar method for measuring clinical process across multiple dimensions (Kelly, 2007).

Comparative Health Care Data Sets

Organizations may select from many publicly and privately available health care data sets for benchmarking. A few of the more commonly accessed data sets are listed in Exhibit 1.6 (along with web addresses). These data sets are divided into five categories: patient satisfaction, practice patterns, health plans, clinical indicators, and population measures. Many of the listed web sites provide examples of the data sets, along with detailed information about their origins and potential uses.

Patient Satisfaction

Patient satisfaction data generally come from survey data. The three organizations listed in Exhibit 1.6, NRC+Picker, Press Ganey, and the health care division of Gallup, provide extensive consulting services to health care organizations across the country. One of these services is to conduct patient satisfaction surveys. There are other private organizations that provide similar services, and some health care organizations undertake patient satisfaction surveys on their own. These private efforts have been significant, but did not facilitate a nationally available system for benchmarking hospital performance. In 2002, CMS partnered with the Agency for Healthcare Research and Quality (AHRQ) to develop the Hospital Consumer Assessment of Healthcare Providers and Systems (HCAHPS), "the first national, standardized, publicly reported survey of patient's perspectives of hospital care" (CMS, 2012). Since 2005, the government has created several financial incentives for hospitals to participate in HCAHPS and it has been widely adopted. Results from HCAHPS are reported through the CMS Hospital Compare program, which is discussed later in this chapter.

Practice Patterns

The Commonwealth Fund Quality Chartbook series and the Dartmouth Atlas of Health Care allow health care organizations to view practice patterns across the United States. The Dartmouth Atlas provides an online interactive tool that allows organizations to customize comparative reports based primarily on Medicare data (Figure 1.9).

Exhibit 1.6. Sources of comparative data for health care managers

Patient Satisfaction

NRC+Picker (National Research Corporation and the Picker Institute): nrcpicker.com

Press Ganey Associates: www.pressganey.com

The Gallup Organization: healthcare.gallup.com

Practice Patterns

Leatherman, S., and McCarthy, D. (2002). *Quality of Healthcare in the United States: A Chartbook.* New York: The Commonwealth Fund. http://www.commonwealthfund.org/publications/publications_show.htm?doc_id=221238

The Center for the Evaluative Clinical Sciences, Dartmouth Medical School. (2008). *The Dartmouth Atlas of Healthcare.* Chicago: American Hospital Publishing. www.dartmouthatlas.org

Health Plans

National Committee for Quality: www.ncqa.org

Clinical Indicators

Joint Commission on Accreditation of Healthcare Organizations

Quality Check: www.qualitycheck.org

Centers for Medicare and Medicaid Services Medicare Clinical Indicators

Hospital Compare: www.hospitalcompare.hhs.gov

Nursing Home Compare: http://www.medicare.gov/NHCompare

Home Health Compare: http://www.medicare.gov/HHCompare

Physician Focused Quality Initiative: http://www.cms.hhs.gov/pqri

Population Measures

State and local health departments

Centers for Disease Control and Prevention, National Center of Health Statistics: www.cdc.gov/nchs

AHRQ—Health Care Innovations Exchange (including Quality and Disparities Reports): http://www.innovations.ahrq.gov

Source: Used with permission from *Applying Quality Management in Healthcare*, 2nd Edition, by Diane Kelly (Chicago: Health Administration Press, 2007), p. 185.

Figure 1.9. Example of Dartmouth Atlas interactive report

Source: Dartmouth Institute for Health Policy & Clinical Practice, 2012.

Health Plans

The mission of the National Committee for Quality Assurance (NCQA) is "to improve the quality of health care." NCQA's efforts are organized around two major activities: accreditation and performance measurement. (We will discuss the accreditation activity in Chapter Three.) To facilitate these activities NCQA developed the Health Plan Employer Data and Information Set (HEDIS) in the late 1980s. HEDIS currently consists of seventy-six measures across five domains of care and is used by more than 90 percent of America's health plans. A few of the health issues measured by HEDIS are (NCQA, 2012a):

- Asthma medication use
- Persistence of beta-blocker treatment after a heart attack
- Controlling high blood pressure

- Comprehensive diabetes care
- Breast cancer screening
- Antidepressant medication management
- Childhood and adolescent immunization status
- Advising smokers to quit

The NCQA web site offers an interactive tool for obtaining *report cards* on specific health plans that have undergone NCQA accreditation. Multiple health plans can be compared to each other and against national averages. The comparison of two South Carolina health plans in Figure 1.10 is an example of an NCQA report card (NCQA, 2012b).

Clinical Indicators

Both the Joint Commission and CMS are committed to the improvement of clinical outcomes. The Joint Commission's Quality Check has evolved since its introduction in 1994 to become a comprehensive guide to health care organizations in the United States. Visitors to www.qualitycheck.org can search for health care organizations by a variety of parameters, identify accreditation

Figure 1.10. Example of NCQA report card

Source: NCQA, 2012b.

status, and download hospital performance measures. In addition, the Joint Commission–accredited organizations can get a summary of their performance measured in terms of the Joint Commission's National Patient Safety Goals and Quality Improvement Goals (The Joint Commission, 2012).

The CMS quality programs are aimed at hospitals, nursing homes, home care, and physicians' practices. The Hospital Compare web site (www .hospitalcompare.hhs.gov) and interactive comparison tool were developed in collaboration with other public and private organizational members of the Hospital Quality Alliance. Comparison reports for hospitals can be created based on location and on specific medical conditions or surgical procedures. The resulting reports provide information on process of care measures, outcome of care measures, use of medical imaging, surveys of patients' hospital experiences from HCAHPS, patient safety measures, and medical payment information (HHS, 2012).

Population Measures

Other comparative data sources that could be useful for the health care manager are those that provide population measures. Most state health

Figure 1.11. Example of hospital compare graphical report

Source: HHS, 2012.

departments collect statewide morbidity and mortality data. These data generally come from a variety of sources, including hospital and provider bills. At the national level both the Centers for Disease Control and Prevention (CDC) and the Agency for Healthcare Research and Quality (AHRQ) provide a wealth of population-based health care data.

EXTERNAL DATA AND INFORMATION: EXPERT OR KNOWLEDGE BASED

The Joint Commission accreditation manual (2011, p. GL-9) defines knowledge-based information as "A collection of stored facts, models, and information that can be used for ongoing staff development, for designing and redesigning processes, and for solving problems. . . . Knowledge-based information is found in the clinical, scientific, and management literature." Health care executives and health care providers rely on knowledge-based information to maintain their professional competence and to discover the latest techniques and procedures. The content of any professional journal falls into the category of knowledge-based information. Other providers of knowledge-based information are the many online health care and health care management references and resources. With the development of rule-based computer systems, the Internet, and push technologies, health care executives and providers are finding that they often have access to vast quantities of expert or knowledge-based information at the time they need it, even at the patient bedside. Most clinical and administrative professional organizations not only publish print journals but also maintain up-to-date web sites where members or other subscribers can get knowledge-based information. Several organizations also provide daily, weekly, or other periodic e-mail notifications of important events that are pushed onto subscribers' personal computers.

Knowledge-based information can also be incorporated into electronic medical records or health care organization web sites. Figure 1.12 is a sample of the knowledge-based information resources available through an electronic medical record interface.

SUMMARY

Without health care data and information, there would be no need for health care information systems. Health care information is a valuable asset in health care organizations, and it must be managed like other assets. To manage information effectively, health care executives should have an understanding of the sources and uses of health care data and information. In this chapter we introduced a framework for discussing types of health care information,

Figure 1.12. Sample electronic knowledge-based information resources

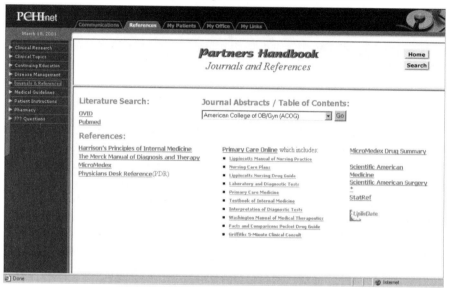

Source: Partners HealthCare.

looked at a wide range of internal data and information whose creation and use must be managed in health care organizations, and also discussed a few associated processes that are typically part of patient encounters. We examined not only patient-specific (individual) internal information but also aggregate information. We addressed both clinical and administrative data and information in our discussions. In addition, we examined several types of external data and information that are available for use by health care organizations, including comparative and knowledge-based data and information. Throughout, our view of data and information was organizational and the focus was on that information that is unique to health care.

KEY TERMS

Aggregate data and information

American Health Information
    Management Association (AHIMA)

American Hospital Association

American Medical Association
    (AMA)

Balanced scorecards

Benchmarking

Centers for Disease Control and
    Prevention (CDC)

Centers for Medicare and Medicaid

CMS-1500

Comparative data and information

Current Procedural Terminology
    (CPT)

Electronic health record

Electronic medical record
External data and information
Health care information
Health care statistics
Health information
Health Insurance Portability and
   Accountability Act (HIPAA)
Health Plan Employer Data and
   Information Set (HEDIS)
Hospital Compare
Internal data and information
International Classification of
   Diseases (ICD-10-CM; ICD-10-PCS)
The Joint Commission
Knowledge-based data and
   information

Minimum Data Set (MDS)
National Provider Identifier (NPI)
National Uniform Billing Committee
Office of the Inspector General (OIG)
Outcomes measures
Patient records
Patient-specific data and information
Personal health record
Protected health information
Quality Check
UB-04 (CMS-1450)
Uniform Ambulatory Care Data Set
   (ACDS)
Uniform Bill
Uniform Hospital Discharge Data Set
   (UHDDS)

LEARNING ACTIVITIES

1. Contact a health care facility (hospital, nursing home, physician's office, or other organization) to ask permission to view a sample of the health records they maintain. These records may be in paper or electronic form. Answer the following questions for each record:

   a. What is the primary reason (or condition) for which the patient was admitted to the hospital?

   b. How long has the patient had this condition?

   c. Did the patient have surgery during this admission? If so, what procedure(s) was (were) done?

   d. Did the patient experience any complications during this admission? If so, what were they?

   e. How does the physician's initial assessment of the patient compare with the nurse's initial assessment? Where in the record would you find this information?

   f. To where was the patient discharged?

   g. What were the patient's discharge orders or instructions? Where in the record should you find this information?

2. Make an appointment to meet with the business manager at a physician's office or health care clinic. Discuss the importance of ICD-10 coding or CPT coding (or both) for that office. Ask to view

the books or encoders that the office uses to assign diagnostic and procedure codes. After the visit, write a brief summary of your findings and impressions.

3. Visit www.oig.hhs.gov. What are the major responsibilities of the Office of Inspector General as they relate to coded health care data? What other responsibilities related to health care fraud and abuse does this office have?

4. List and briefly describe several types of aggregate health care reports that you believe would be commonly used by health care executives in a hospital or other health care setting.

5. Using the Internet sites identified in this chapter or found during your own searches, find a report card for one or more local hospitals. If you were trying to make a decision about which hospital to use for health care for yourself or for a family member, would you find this information useful? Why or why not?

6. Using Microsoft HealthVault (a free Internet-based service), create your own personal health record (PHR).

REFERENCES

American Health Information Management Association. (2012). What is a personal health record? *MyPHR*. Retrieved March 2012 from http://www.myphr.com /StartaPHR/what_is_a_phr.aspx

Centers for Disease Control and Prevention. (2012). *International classification of diseases, tenth revision, clinical modification (ICD-10-CM)*. Retrieved March 2012 from http://www.cdc.gov/nchs/icd/icd10cm.htm

Centers for Medicare and Medicaid Services. (2006, November 3). *CMS manual system* (Pub 100-04 Medicare claims processing). Retrieved February 2008 from http://www.cms.hhs.gov/Transmittals/Downloads/R1104CP.pdf

Centers for Medicare and Medicaid Services. (2008). *National Provider Identifier standard (NPI)—Overview*. Retrieved June 2008 from http://www.cms.hhs.gov /NationalProvIdentStand/01_Overview.asp

Centers for Medicare and Medicaid Services. (2012). HCAHPS: Patients' perspectives of care survey. Retrieved March 2012 from https://www.cms.gov/Hospital QualityInits/30_HospitalHCAHPS.asp

Dartmouth Institute for Health Policy & Clinical Practice. (2012). *Dartmouth atlas of health care*. Retrieved March 2012 from http://www.dartmouthatlas.org

Department of Health and Human Services, Office of Inspector General. (2012). *Compliance guidance*. Retrieved March 2012 from www.oig.hhs.gov

Department of Health and Human Services (HHS). (2012). *Hospital Compare.* Retrieved March 2012 from http://www.hospitalcompare.hhs.gov

Dougherty, M. (2001). On the line: Professional practice solutions. *Journal of AHIMA, 72*(10), 72–73.

The Joint Commission. (2011). *Comprehensive accreditation manual for hospitals* (updated September 2011). Oakbrook Terrace, IL: Author.

The Joint Commission. (2012). *Quality Check.* Retrieved March 2012 from http://www.qualitycheck.org/consumer/searchQCR.aspx

Kelly, D. (2007). *Applying quality management in healthcare: A process improvement* (2nd ed.). Chicago: Health Administration Press.

LaTour, K. (2002). Healthcare information standards. In K. LaTour & S. Eichenwald (Eds.), *Health information management concepts, principles, and practice* (pp. 121–136). Chicago: American Health Information Management Association.

Miller, B. F., & O'Toole, M. T. (2003). *Miller-Keane encyclopedia and dictionary of medicine, nursing, and allied health* (7th ed.) Philadelphia: W. B. Saunders.

National Alliance for Health Information Technology. (2008). *Report to the Office of the National Coordinator for Health Information Technology on defining key health information technology terms.* Department of Health and Human Services. Retrieved August 2008 from http://www.nahit.org/docs/hittermsfinalreport_051508.pdf

National Committee for Quality Assurance. (2012a). *HEDIS and quality measurement.* Retrieved March 2012 from http://www.ncqa.org/tabid/59/Default.aspx

National Committee for Quality Assurance. (2012b). *Health plan report card.* Retrieved March 2012 from http://reportcard.ncqa.org/plan/external/plansearch.aspx

National Uniform Billing Committee. (1999). *The history of the NUBC.* Retrieved January 2013 from http://www.nubc.org/history.html

National Uniform Claim Committee. (2012). *Who are we?* Retrieved June 2008 from http://www.nucc.org/index.php?option=com_frontpage&Itemid=1

CHAPTER 2

Health Care Data Quality

LEARNING OBJECTIVES

- To be able to discuss the relationship between health care data and health care information.
- To be able to identify problems associated with poor-quality health care data.
- To be able to define the characteristics of data quality.
- To be able to discuss the challenges associated with measuring and ensuring health care data quality.

Chapter One provided an overview of the various types of health care data and information that are generated and used by health care organizations. We established the importance of understanding health care data and information in order to reach the goal of having effective health care information systems. There is another fundamental aspect of health care data and information that is central to developing effective health care information systems—data quality. Consider for a moment an organization with sophisticated health care information systems that affect every type of health care information, from patient specific to knowledge based. What if the quality of the documentation going into the systems is poor? What if there is no assurance that the reports generated from the systems are accurate or timely? How would the users of the systems react? Are those information systems beneficial or detrimental to the organization in achieving its goals?

According to the International Standards Organisation (ISO) definition, quality is "the totality of features and characteristics of an entity that bears on its ability to satisfy stated and implied needs" (ISO 8402–1986, Quality-Vocabulary). In this chapter we will examine several aspects of data quality. We begin by distinguishing between health care data and health care information. We then look at some problems associated with poor-quality health care data, both at an organizational level and across organizations. The discussion continues with a presentation of two sets of guidelines that can be used in evaluating data quality and ends with an examination of the major types of health care data errors.

DATA VERSUS INFORMATION

What is the difference between data and information? The simple answer is that *information is processed data.* Therefore, we can say that *health care information* is *processed health care data.* (We interpret *processing* broadly to cover everything from formal analysis to explanations supplied by the individual decision maker's brain.) Health care data are raw health care facts, generally stored as characters, words, symbols, measurements, or statistics. One thing apparent about health care data is that they are generally not very useful for decision making. Health care data may describe a particular event, but alone and unprocessed they are not particularly helpful. Take, for example, this figure: 79 percent. By itself, what does it mean? If we process this datum further by indicating that it represents the average bed occupancy for a hospital for the month of January, it takes on more meaning. With the additional facts attached, is this figure now information? That depends. If all a health care executive wants or needs to know is the bed occupancy rate for January, this could be considered information. However, for the hospital executive who is interested in knowing the trend of the bed occupancy rate over time or how the facility's bed occupancy rate compares to that of other, similar facilities, this is not yet information.

Knowledge is seen by some as the highest level in a hierarchy with data at the bottom and information in the middle (Figure 2.1). *Knowledge* is defined by Johns (1997, 53) as "a combination of rules, relationships, ideas, and experience." Another way of thinking about knowledge is that it is information applied to rules, experiences, and relationships, with the result that it

Figure 2.1. From data to knowledge

can be used for decision making. A journal article that describes the use of bed occupancy rates in decision making or one health care facility's experience with improving its occupancy rates might be an example of knowledge.

Where do health care data end and where does health care information begin? Information is an *extremely* valuable asset at *all* levels of the health care organization. Health care executives, clinical staff, and others rely on information to get their jobs accomplished. An interesting point to think about is that the same data may provide different information to different users. One person's data may be another person's information. Think back to our bed occupancy example. The health care executive needing verification of the rate for January has found her information. The health care executive needing trend analysis that includes this rate has not. In the second case, the rate for January is data needing to be processed further. The goal of this discussion is not to pinpoint where data end and information begins but rather to further an understanding of the relationship between health care data and information— health care data are the beginnings of health care information. You cannot create information without data (Lee, 2002).

PROBLEMS WITH POOR-QUALITY DATA

Now that we have established the relationship between health care data and health care information, we can look at some of the problems associated with having poor-quality data. Health care data are the source of health care information, so it stands to reason that a health care organization cannot have high-quality health care information without first establishing that it has high-quality health care data. Data quality must be established at the most *granular* level. Much health care information is gathered through patient care documentation by clinical providers and administrative staff either through manual or electronic systems. As was discussed in Chapter One, the patient record is the source for most of the clinical information generated by the health care organization. This clinical information is in turn coded for purposes of reimbursement and research. We also saw that medical record information is shared across many providers and payers, aggregated, and used to make comparisons relevant to health care and related issues.

This increased reliance on networked health care data brings new challenges in ensuring and maintaining high-quality data. The Markle Foundation's Connecting for Health Collaborative identifies five negative effects of "dirty" (inaccurate, out-of-date, incomplete, and similar) health care data (Markle Foundation, 2006, p. 1):

- Affects the quality of care
- Introduces privacy and other civil liberty concerns
- Increases costs and inefficiencies
- Creates liability risks
- Undermines the reliability and benefits of information technology (IT) investments

Where do these "dirty" health care data originate? There are two essential components needed to ensure data quality: content and form. First, to ensure quality content, the data must have all of the characteristics outlined in the AHIMA Data Quality Model (discussed later in this chapter). In addition to these characteristics, however, the data must be stored and presented in a manner that makes it usable. This is form.

Problems with health care data content can generally be traced to documentation practices. This is not a problem limited to health care. The Markle Foundation notes that "76 percent of all errors, across sectors and settings, result from data entry" (2006, p 3).

Sharon Schott (2003) has summarized some of the common problems associated with poor-quality medical record documentation (see the following Perspective). She focuses on the medical record used as evidence in court, but the same problems can affect the quality of care, create civil liberty concerns, and increase costs.

PERSPECTIVE
Documentation

In pointing out the serious consequences of documentation problems when records (especially paper-based records) are called into evidence in court cases, Sharon Schott cites several specific examples, including these three:

> Simple things such as misspelled names of common drugs or procedures can have a major effect on jurors' impression of the competency of the clinician documenting in the record. In one recent case, a nurse administered 5,000 units of Heparin when the order was for 2,500 units. The patient became critically ill as a result. When the documentation was reviewed, it was discovered that the nurse committing the error had misspelled Heparin as "Hepirin." This spelling error was presented to the jury as an additional demonstration of incompetence. The plaintiff's attorney argued that Heparin is a commonly used drug and obviously this nurse had no knowledge of it, because she couldn't spell it correctly. Juries will also doubt the competence of a nurse who writes "The wound on the left heal is healed."
>
> The nurse who documented an assessment with a post date was called as a witness. She was asked to explain how she could perform an assessment two days after the patient died. The nurse explained that Friday was the actual due date for the assessment but because she had some extra time on Tuesday, she decided to do it early and put Friday's date on it to be compliant with the due date. The plaintiff's attorney then asked, "Is that the only place in the chart that you lied?" Then the jury was suspicious of the integrity of the entire medical record and the nurse.
>
> The continuity of the record also needs special scrutiny on a regular basis. Some institutions allow the record to be "split," which means placing the progress notes at the bedside while maintaining the rest of the chart documentation at the nurses' station. To avoid having to go back to the bedside to document, a nurse might take a new progress note sheet, document findings, and then put the page in the chart at the nurses' station. This documentation will not be in proper sequence with the progress notes from the bedside when they are entered into the chart.

As you read these vignettes, think about ways that information systems could assist in preventing these problems.

Source: Examples from Schott, 2003, pp. 22–23.

The problems with poor-quality patient care data are not limited to the patient medical record or other data collected and used at the organizational level. The Medical Records Institute (MRI), a professional organization dedicated to the improvement of patient records through technology, has identified five major functions that are negatively affected by poor-quality documentation (MRI, 2004). These problems are found not only at the organizational level but also across organizations and throughout the overall health care environment:

- *Patient safety* is affected by inadequate information, illegible entries, misinterpretations, and insufficient interoperability.
- *Public safety,* a major component of public health, is diminished by the inability to collect information in a coordinated, timely manner at the provider level in response to epidemics and the threat of terrorism.
- *Continuity of patient care* is adversely affected by the lack of shareable information among patient care providers.
- *Health care economics* are adversely affected, with information capture and report generation costs currently estimated to be well over $50 billion annually.
- *Clinical research and outcomes analysis* is adversely affected by a lack of uniform information capture that is needed to facilitate the derivation of data from routine patient care documentation [MRI, 2004, p. 2].

This same report identifies health care documentation as having two parts: information capture and report generation. *Information capture* is "the process of recording representations of human thought, perceptions, or actions in documenting patient care, as well as device-generated information that is gathered and/or computed about a patient as part of health care" (MRI, 2004, p. 2). Some means of information capture in health care organizations are handwriting, speaking, typing, touching a screen or pointing and clicking on words or phrases, videotaping, audio recording, and generating images through X-rays and scans. *Report generation* "consists of the formatting and/or structuring of captured information. It is the process of analyzing, organizing, and presenting recorded patient information for authentication and inclusion in the patient's healthcare record" (MRI, 2004, p. 2). In order to have high-quality documentation resulting in high-quality data, both information capture and report generation must be considered.

ENSURING DATA AND INFORMATION QUALITY

The importance of having quality health care information available to providers and health care executives cannot be overstated. Health care decision makers rely on high-quality information. The issue is not whether quality information is important but rather how it can be achieved. Before an organization can measure the quality of the information it produces and uses, it must establish data standards. That is, data can be identified as high quality only when they conform to a recognized standard. Ensuring this conformance is not as easy as it might seem because, unfortunately, there is no universally recognized set of health care data quality standards in existence today. One reason for this is that the quality of the data needed in any situation is driven by the use to which the data or the information that comes from the data will be put. For example, in a patient care setting the margin of error for critical lab tests must be zero or patient safety is in jeopardy. However, a larger margin of error may be acceptable in census counts or discharge statistics. Health care organizations must establish data quality standards specific to the intended use of the data or resulting information.

Although we have no nationally recognized data quality standards, two organizations have published guidance that can assist a health care organization in establishing its own data quality standards: the Medical Records Institute (MRI) has published a set of "essential principles of healthcare documentation," and the American Health Information Management Association (AHIMA) has published a data quality management tool. These two guides are summarized in the following sections.

MRI Principles of Health Care Documentation

The MRI argues that there are many steps that must be taken to create systems that ensure quality health care documentation. It has developed the following key principles that should be adhered to as these systems (and their accompanying policies) are established:

- Unique patient identification must be assured within and across healthcare documentation systems.
- Healthcare documentation must be
  - Accurate and consistent.
  - Complete.
  - Timely.
  - Interoperable across types of documentation systems.
  - Accessible at any time and at any place where patient care is needed.
  - Auditable.
- Confidential and secure authentication and accountability must be provided [MRI, 2004, p. 3].

The MRI takes the position that when practitioners interact with electronic resources, they have an increased ability to meet these guidelines (MRI, 2004).

AHIMA Data Quality Model

AHIMA (2012) has developed and published a set of health care data quality characteristics. You will note similarities between these characteristics and the MRI principles. The AHIMA data quality characteristics can serve as the basis for establishing data quality standards because they represent common dimensions of health care data that should always be present, regardless of the use of the data or resulting information.

- **Data accuracy.** Data that reflect correct, valid values are accurate. Typographical errors in discharge summaries and misspelled names are examples of inaccurate data.

- **Data accessibility.** Data that are not available to the decision makers needing them are of no use.

- **Data comprehensiveness.** *All* of the data required for a particular use must be present and available to the user. Even relevant data may not be useful when they are incomplete.

- **Data consistency.** Quality data are consistent. Use of an abbreviation that has two different meanings is a good example of how lack of consistency can lead to problems. For example, a nurse may use the abbreviation CPR to mean *cardiopulmonary resuscitation* at one time and use it to mean *computer-based patient record* at another time, leading to confusion.

- **Data currency.** Many types of health care data become obsolete after a period of time. A patient's admitting diagnosis is often not the same as the diagnosis recorded upon discharge. If a health care executive needs a report on the diagnoses treated during a particular time frame, which of these two diagnoses should be included?

- **Data definition.** Clear definitions of data elements must be provided so that both current and future data users will understand what the data mean. One way to supply clear data definitions is to use data dictionaries. A case described by A. M. Shakir (1999) offers an excellent example of the need for clear data definitions. (See the following Perspective.)

A large national health maintenance organization (HMO) was planning to create a disease management program for pediatric care. As part of the planning effort, the HMO decided to conduct a survey of its regional sites to determine the utilization pattern for pediatric care. It sent a questionnaire to each of the twelve regional offices asking these two questions:

1. How many pediatric members were enrolled as of year-end?
2. How many pediatric visits took place during the year?

On the surface, the questions seemed quite simple and appropriate. The HMO would determine the number of pediatric members and the number of pediatric visits by region. It could then compute pediatric utilization by region—and across the program as a whole. This data would then be used to determine a baseline for development of utilization management programs and would assist in comparative analysis of pediatric utilization across regions.

There was only one problem—the absence of common data definitions. Each of the regions operated somewhat autonomously and interpreted the request for information differently. As a result, the regional offices raised a number of questions and revealed numerous discrepancies in their interpretations of data definitions:

What is a pediatric member?

A dependent member under the age of 18

A dependent member under the age of 21

A dependent child member, regardless of age

A patient under the age of 18

What is a pediatric visit?

A visit by a pediatric member

A visit by a patient under the age of 18

Any visit to the pediatric department

A visit with a pediatrician

(cont.)

Attempts to answer these questions only raised more questions. What is a member? What does it mean to be enrolled? What is a dependent? How is patient or member age calculated? What is a visit? What is a patient and how does one differ from a member? What is a department? What are the department types? What is a pediatrician?

This story shows us how important it is that suppliers and consumers of data agree on data definitions before exchanging information. Had the regions not revealed their assumptions, the discrepancies in their interpretations of the data definitions might never have been recognized, and the organization would have unknowingly compared apples to oranges. In the long term, a business strategy with significant implications would have been based upon invalid information.

Source: Shakir, 1999, pp. 48–49.

- **Data granularity.** Data granularity is sometimes referred to as *data atomicity.* That is, individual data elements are "atomic" in the sense that they cannot be further subdivided. For example, a typical patient's name should generally be stored as three data elements (last name, first name, middle name—"Smith" and "John" and "Allen"), not as a single data element ("John Allen Smith"). Again, granularity is related to the purpose for which the data are collected. Although it is possible to subdivide a person's birth date into separate fields for the month, the date, and the year, this is usually not desirable. The birth date is at its lowest practical level of granularity when used as a patient identifier. Values for data should be defined at the correct level for their use.

- **Data precision.** Precision often relates to numerical data. Precision denotes how close to an actual size, weight, or other standard a particular measurement is. Some health care data must be very precise. For example, in figuring a drug dosage it is not all right to round up to the nearest gram when the drug is to be dosed in milligrams.

- **Data relevancy.** Data must be relevant to the purpose for which they are collected. We could collect very accurate, timely data about a patient's color preferences or choice of hairdresser, but are these matters relevant to the care of the patient?

- **Data timeliness.** Timeliness is a critical dimension in the quality of many types of health care data. For example, critical lab values must be available to the health care provider in a timely manner. Producing accurate results after the patient has been discharged may be of little or no value to the patient's care.

Types and Causes of Data Errors

Failures of data to meet established quality standards are called data errors. A data error will have a negative impact on one or more of the characteristics of quality data. For example, if a final diagnosis is coded incorrectly, that datum is no longer accurate. If the same diagnosis is coded in several different ways, those data are not consistent. Both examples represent data errors. Data errors are often discussed in terms of two types of underlying cause—systematic errors and random errors (Table 2.1). *Systematic errors* are errors that can be attributed to a flaw or discrepancy in adherence to standard operating procedures or systems. The diagnosis coding errors just described would be systematic errors if they resulted from incorrect programming of the encoding software or improper training of the individuals assigning the codes. Systematic health care data errors can also be caused by unclear data definitions or a failure to comply with the established data collection protocols, such as leaving out required information. If the diagnosis coding errors were the result of poor handwriting or transcription errors, they would be considered *random errors*. Carelessness rather than lack of training leads to random errors (Arts, DeKeizer, & Scheffer, 2002).

comes up as patterns.

Table 2.1. Some causes of poor health care data quality

Systematic	Random
Unclear data definitions	Illegible handwriting in data source
Unclear data collection guidelines	Typing errors
Poor interface design	Lack of motivation
Programming errors	Frequent personnel turnover
Incomplete data source	Calculation errors (not built into the system)
Unsuitable data format in the source	
Data dictionary is lacking or not available	
Data dictionary is not adhered to	
Guidelines or protocols are not adhered to	
Lack of sufficient data checks	
No system for correcting detected data errors	
No control over adherence to guidelines and data definitions	

Source: Adapted from Arts, DeKeizer, & Scheffer, 2002, p. 604.

Preventing, Detecting, and Fixing Data Errors

Both systematic and random errors lead to poor-quality data and information. Both types need to be prevented to the extent possible. Errors that are not preventable need to be detected so that they can be corrected. There are multiple points during data collection and processing where system design can reduce data errors. The Markle Foundation recommends the following strategies to improve data quality. These combine automated and human strategies (2006, p. 4):

- Standardize data entry fields and processes for entering data
- Institute real-time quality checking, including the use of validation and feedback loops
- Design data elements to avoid errors (for example, use check digits and checking algorithms on numeric identifiers where human entry is involved and use well-designed user interfaces)
- Develop and adhere to guidelines for documenting the care that was provided to the patient
- Review automated billing software
- Build human capacity, including training, awareness building, and organizational change

In addition to these specific recommendations, the group urges the development of a "data quality culture" within health care organizations.

Arts, DeKeizer, and Scheffer (2002) have published a useful framework for ensuring data quality in a centralized health care database (or *medical registry*, as these authors call it). Although the entire framework is not reproduced here, several key aspects are outlined in Figure 2.2. This framework illustrates that there are multiple reasons for data errors and multiple approaches to preventing and correcting these errors.

Using IT to Improve Data Quality

Information technology has tremendous potential as a tool for improving health care data quality. To date some of this potential has been realized, but many opportunities remain that are not commonly employed by health care organiza-tions. Clearly, electronic health records (EHRs) improve legibility and accessibility of health care data and information. But what about the remaining dimensions of health care data quality? As noted in the Perspective that follows, a recent GAO report (2007) found that many of the data in existing EHR systems were recorded in an unstructured format—"in narrative form or other text, rather than in data fields designated to contain specific pieces of information." Physician notes and discharge summaries are often dictated and transcribed. This lack of structure limits the ability of an EHR to be a data quality

Figure 2.2. Activities for improving data quality

Data Error Prevention

Compose a minimum set of necessary data items
Define data and data characteristics in a data dictionary
Develop a data collection protocol
Create user-friendly data entry forms or interface
Compose data checks
Create a quality assurance plan
Train and motivate users

Data Error Detection

Perform automatic data checks
Perform data quality audits
Review data collection protocols and procedures
Check inter- and intraobserver variability (if appropriate)
Visually inspect completed forms (online or otherwise)
Routinely check completeness of data entry

Actions for Data Quality Improvement

Provide data quality reports to users
Correct inaccurate data and fill in incomplete data detected
Control user correction of data errors
Give feedback of data quality results and recommendations
Resolve identified causes of data errors
Implement identified system changes
Communicate with users

Source: Adapted from Arts, DeKeizer, & Scheffer, 2002, p. 605.

improvement tool. In systems requiring structured data input, data comprehensiveness, relevance, and consistency can be improved. When health care providers respond to a series of prompts, rather than dictating a free-form narrative, they are reminded to include all necessary elements of a health record entry. Data precision and accuracy are improved when these systems also incorporate error checking. A clear example of data improvement achieved through information technology is the result seen from incorporating medication administration systems designed to prevent medication error (see Chapter Five). With structured data input and sophisticated error prevention, these systems can significantly reduce medication errors.

PERSPECTIVE
Testing the Use of IT

In April 2007, the U.S. Government Accountability Office (GAO) published a report on the findings from eight hospital case studies that examined the impact of information technology on the collection and submission of required Centers for Medicare and Medicaid (CMS) health care quality data. The study hospitals used six steps to collect and submit the required data:

1. Identify the patients.
2. Locate information in their medical records.
3. Determine appropriate values for the data elements.
4. Transmit the data to CMS.
5. Ensure that the data have been accepted by CMS.
6. Supply copies of medical records to CMS to validate the data.

The case studies demonstrated that the hospitals' existing IT systems helped the data abstractors to gather some of the data but fell short of allowing the hospitals to automate that process. The IT systems improved accessibility to and legibility of the patient medical records. However, multiple limitations were noted:

- Hospitals had a mix of paper and electronic records, requiring abstractors to look in multiple locations for required data elements.
- Most data were recorded as unstructured or narrative text, which made locating information within records time consuming.
- Hospitals had IT systems that were not integrated, requiring abstractors to access multiple IT systems to obtain related data.

The GAO report recommends that the secretary of the U.S. Department of Health and Human Services identify specific plans to promote the use of IT for the collection and submission of data to CMS.

Source: Adapted from GAO, 2007.

SUMMARY

Without health care data and information, there would be no need for health care information systems. Health care information is a valuable asset in health care organizations and it must be managed like other assets. To manage information effectively, health care executives should have an understanding of health care data and information and recognize the importance of ensuring data quality. Health care decisions, both clinical and administrative, are driven by data and information. Data and information are used to provide patient care and to monitor facility performance. It is critical that the data and information be of high quality. After all, the most sophisticated of information systems cannot overcome the inherent problems associated with poor-quality source data and data collection or entry errors. The data characteristics and frameworks presented here can be useful tools in the establishment of mechanisms for ensuring the quality of health care data.

The challenge of health care organizations today is to implement information technology solutions that work to improve the quality of their health care data.

KEY TERMS

Data	Government Accountability Office
Data accessibility	(GAO)
Data accuracy	Information
Data comprehensiveness	Information capture
Data consistency	Knowledge
Data currency	Random errors
Data definition	Report generation
Data errors	Systematic errors
Documentation	Unique patient identifier

LEARNING ACTIVITIES

1. Contact a health care facility (hospital, nursing home, physicians' office, or other facility) to ask permission to view a sample of the health records they maintain. These records may be in paper or electronic form. For each record, answer the following questions about data quality:

   a. How would you assess the quality of the data in the patient's record? Use the MRI's key principles and AHIMA's data characteristics as guides.

b. What proportion of the data in the patient's medical record is captured electronically? What information is recorded manually? Do you think the method of capture affects the quality of the information?

c. How does the data quality compare with what you expected?

2. Visit a health care organization to explore the ways in which the facility monitors or evaluates data quality.

3. Consider the following scenarios and the questions they raise about data quality. What should an organization do? How does one create an environment that promotes data quality? What are some of the problems associated with having poor-quality data?

A late entry is written to supply information that was omitted at the time of the original entry. It should be done only if the person completing it has total recall of the omission. For example, a nurse completed her charting on December 12 and forgot to note that the physician had talked with the patient. When she returned to work on December 13, she wrote a late entry for the day before and documented the physician visit. The clinician must enter the current date and the documentation must be identified as a late entry including the date of the omission. Additionally, a late entry should be added as soon as possible.

A late entry cannot be used to supplement a record because of a negative clinical outcome that occurs after the original entry. For example, while a patient received an antibiotic for two days, the nurse charted nothing unusual. Yet, on the third day, the patient had an acute episode of shortness of breath and chest pain and died later that same day. At the time of death, documentation revealed that the patient had a dark red rash on his chest.

An investigation into the cause of death was conducted and all the nurses who provided care during the three days were interviewed and asked whether they had seen the rash prior to the patient's death. None of the nurses remembered the rash. However, one nurse wrote a late entry for each of the first two days that the patient was receiving the antibiotic stating that there was no rash on those days. This is an incorrect late entry. Her statement is part of the investigation conducted after the fact and was not an omission from her original entry [Schott, 2003, pp. 23–24].

REFERENCES

American Health Information Management Association. (2012). Data quality management mode (updated). *Journal of AHIM, 83*(7), 62–67. Retrieved August 2012 from http://library.ahima.org

Arts, D., DeKeizer, N., & Scheffer, G. (2002). Defining and improving data quality in medical registries: A literature review, case study, and generic framework. *Journal of the American Medical Informatics Association, 9*(6), 600–611.

Government Accountability Office. (2007, April). *Hospital data quality: HHS should specify steps and time frame for using information technology to collect and submit data* (GOA-07-320). Retrieved July 2008 from www.gao.gov/cgi-bin /getrpt?GAO-07-320

Johns, M. (1997). *Information management for health professionals.* Albany, NY: Delmar.

Lee, F. W. (2002). Data and information management. In K. LaTour & S. Eichenwald (Eds.), *Health information management concepts, principles, and practice* (pp. 83–100). Chicago: American Health Information Management Association.

Markle Foundation. (2006). T5 background issues on data quality. *Connecting for Health Common Framework.* Retrieved March 2012 from http://www.policy archive.org/handle/10207/bitstreams/15515.pdf

Medical Records Institute. (2004). *Healthcare documentation: A report on information capture and report generation.* Boston: Author.

Schott, S. (2003, April). How poor documentation does damage in the courtroom. *Journal of AHIMA, 74*(4), 20–24.

Shakir, A. (1999). Tools for defining data. *Journal of AHIMA, 70*(8), 48–53.

CHAPTER 3

Health Care Information Regulations, Laws, and Standards

LEARNING OBJECTIVES

- To be able to discuss how accreditation, facility licensure, and certification influence the information needs of health care facilities.
- To be able to identify and differentiate among major health care accrediting bodies.
- To be able to discuss Patient Safety Organizations and their relevance to health care organizations and consumers.
- To be able to understand and manage the impact of the health record as a legal document.
- To be able to discuss the HIPAA privacy regulations and their relevance to health care organizations and consumers.
- To be able to describe the laws, regulations, and standards that govern patient confidentiality.

Chapters One and Two focused on the health care information and data that are available to, used by, and managed by health care organizations. We mentioned that there are external drivers that affect and in some cases dictate the types of health care information that health care organizations maintain and to a certain extent the ways in which those types are maintained. These external forces take the form of laws and regulations mandated at both the state and federal levels. Voluntary accreditation standards are additional external forces. In this chapter we will examine more closely the most important of these laws, regulations, and standards and the external organizations that promulgate them. We will do this under two main headings.

In the section titled "Licensure, Certification, and Accreditation," we define these processes and examine some of the missions and general functions of two of the major accrediting organizations in the United States, the Joint Commission and the National Committee for Quality Assurance (NCQA), and introduce several other accrediting bodies. These discussions focus on how the licensure, certification, and accreditation processes affect health care information and, as a consequence, health care information systems.

Then, in the section titled "Legal Aspects of Managing Health Information," we look at state and federal laws that address the use of the patient medical record as a legal document, and current laws and regulations that govern patient privacy and confidentiality. These legal requirements have a significant impact on how patient-specific health care information is maintained and secured in health care information systems.

LICENSURE, CERTIFICATION, AND ACCREDITATION

Health care organizations, such as hospitals, nursing homes, home health agencies, and the like, must be licensed to operate. If they wish to file Medicare or Medicaid claims, they must also be certified, and if they wish to demonstrate excellence, they will undergo an accreditation process. What are these processes, and how are they related? If a health care organization is licensed, certified, and accredited, how will this affect the health care information that it creates, uses, and maintains? In this section we will examine each of these processes and their impact on the health care organizations. We will also discuss their relationships with one another.

Licensure

Licensure is the process that gives a facility legal approval to operate. As a rule, state governments oversee the licensure of health care facilities, and each state sets its own licensure laws and regulations. All facilities must have a license to operate, and it is generally the state department of health or a similar agency that carries out the licensure function. Licensure regulations tend to emphasize areas such as physical plant standards, fire safety, space allocations, and sanitation. They may also contain minimum standards for equipment and personnel. A few states tie licensure to professional standards and quality of care. In their licensure regulations, most states set minimum standards for the content, retention, and authentication of patient medical records. Exhibit 3.1 is an excerpt from the South Carolina licensure regulations for hospitals. This excerpt governs patient medical record content (with the exception of newborn patient records, which are addressed in a separate section of the regulations). Although each state has its own set of licensure standards, these are fairly typical in scope and content.

Exhibit 3.1. Medical record content: Excerpt from South Carolina Standards for Licensing Hospitals and Institutional General Infirmaries

601.5 Contents:
A. Adequate and complete medical records shall be written for all patients admitted to the hospital and newborns delivered in the hospital.
egibly written or typed and signed. Although use of
censed nurses' signatures is not encouraged, initials
(ec   ovided such initials can be readily identified within
A minimum medical record shall include the follow-

rd: An admission record must be prepared for each
st contain the following information, when obtain-
ldress, including county; occupation; age; date of
· ɒ   tal status; religion; county of birth; father's name;
n name; husband's or wife's name; dates of military
insurance number; provisional diagnosis; case
care; social security number; the name of the person
nation; name, address and telephone number of
ns to be notified in the event of emergency; name
referring physician; name, address and telephone
· aʲ   ding physician; date and hour of admission;
sical within 48 hours after admission;
.orking diagnosis;

(cont.)

Exhibit 3.1. (*Continued*)

4. Pre-operative diagnosis;

5. Medical treatment;

6. Complete surgical record, if any, including technique of operation and findings, statement of tissue and organs removed and post-operative diagnosis;

7. Report of anesthesia;

8. Nurses' notes;

9. Progress notes;

10. Gross pathological findings and microscopic;

11. Temperature chart, including pulse and respiration;

12. Medication Administration Record or similar document for recording of medications, treatments and other pertinent data. Nurses shall sign this record after each medication administered or treatment rendered;

13. Final diagnosis and discharge summary;

14. Date and hour of discharge summary;

15. In case of death, cause and autopsy findings, if autopsy is performed;

16. Special examinations, if any, e.g., consultations, clinical laboratory, x-ray and other examinations.

Source: South Carolina Department of Health and Environmental Control, Standards for Licensing Hospitals and Institutional General Infirmaries, Regulation 61-16 § 601.5, 2010.

An initial license is required before a facility opens its doors, and this license to operate must generally be renewed annually. Some states allow organizations with the Joint Commission accreditation to forgo a formal licensure survey conducted by the state; others require the state survey regardless of accreditation status. As we will see in the section on accreditation, the Joint Commission standards are more detailed and generally more stringent than the state licensure regulations. Also, the Joint Commission standards are updated annually; most licensure standards are not.

Certification

Certification gives a health care organization the authority to participate in the federal Medicare and Medicaid programs. In other words, an organization must be certified to receive reimbursement from the Centers for Medicare and Medicaid Services (CMS). Legislation passed in 1972 mandated that hospitals had to be reviewed and certified in order to participate in the Medicare and Medicaid programs. At that time the Health Care Financing Administration (now the Centers for Medicare and Medicaid Services) developed a set of minimum standards known as the Conditions of Participation (CoPs). The federal government is required to inspect facilities to make sure they meet these minimum standards; however, this survey process is generally contracted out to the states to perform. In the case of hospitals, those accredited by the Joint Commission are *deemed* to have met the federal certification standards. One interesting historical fact is that the original CoPs were essentially the same as the then existing Joint Commission standards. The Joint Commission standards, however, have undergone tremendous change over the past forty years whereas the CoPs have not. Exhibit 3.2 displays the section of the current Medicare and Medicaid Conditions of Participation for Hospitals that governs the content of hospital medical records.

Accreditation

Accreditation is an external review process that an organization elects to undergo. The accrediting agency grants recognition to organizations that meet its predetermined performance and outcome standards. The review process and standards are devised and regulated by the accrediting agency. By far the best-known health care accrediting agency in the United States is the Joint Commission. A few other notable accrediting agencies are the National Committee for Quality Assurance (NCQA), the Commission on Accreditation of Rehabilitation Facilities (CARF), and the Accreditation Association for Ambulatory Health Care (AAAHC).

Although accreditation is voluntary, there are financial and legal incentives for health care organizations to seek accreditation. As we stated earlier, the Joint Commission accreditation can lead to deemed status for CMS programs, and many states recognize accreditation in lieu of their own licensure surveys. Other benefits for an organization are that accreditation

- Is required for reimbursement from certain payers
- Validates the quality of care within the organization
- May favorably influence liability insurance premiums
- May enhance access to managed care contracts
- Gives the organization a competitive edge over nonaccredited organizations

Exhibit 3.2. Medical record content: Excerpt from the Conditions of Participation for hospitals

Sec. 482.24 Condition of participation: Medical record services.

(c) Standard: Content of record. The medical record must contain information to justify admission and continued hospitalization, support the diagnosis, and describe the patient's progress and response to medications and services.

(1) All entries must be legible and complete, and must be authenticated and dated promptly by the person (identified by name and discipline) who is responsible for ordering, providing, or evaluating the service furnished.

(i) The author of each entry must be identified and must authenticate his or her entry.

(ii) Authentication may include signatures, written initials or computer entry.

(2) All records must document the following, as appropriate:

(i) Evidence of a physical examination, including a health history, performed no more than 7 days prior to admission or within 48 hours after admission.

(ii) Admitting diagnosis.

(iii) Results of all consultative evaluations of the patient and appropriate findings by clinical and other staff involved in the care of the patient.

(iv) Documentation of complications, hospital acquired infections, and unfavorable reactions to drugs and anesthesia.

(v) Properly executed informed consent forms for procedures and treatments specified by the medical staff, or by Federal or State law if applicable, to require written patient consent.

(vi) All practitioners' orders, nursing notes, reports of treatment, medication records, radiology, and laboratory reports, and vital signs and other information necessary to monitor the patient's condition.

(vii) Discharge summary with outcome of hospitalization, disposition of case, and provisions for follow-up care.

(viii) Final diagnosis with completion of medical records within 30 days following discharge.

Source: Conditions of Participation: Medical Record Services, 42 C.F.R. §§ 482.24c et seq., 2007.

The Joint Commission

The Joint Commission's stated mission is "To continuously improve health care for the public, in collaboration with other stakeholders, by evaluating health care organizations and inspiring them to excel in providing safe and effective care of the highest quality and value" (The Joint Commission, 2012a).

The Joint Commission on Accreditation of Hospitals (as the Joint Commission was first called) was formed as an independent, not-for-profit organization in 1951, as a joint effort of the American College of Surgeons, American College of Physicians, American Medical Association, and American Hospital Association. The Joint Commission has grown and evolved to set standards for and accredit more than 19,000 health care organizations and programs in the United States. Approximately 82 percent of U.S. hospitals are currently accredited by the Joint Commission. In addition to hospitals, the Joint Commission has accreditation programs for health care organizations that offer ambulatory care, behavioral health care, home care, long-term care, and office-based surgery. They also offer an accreditation program for organizations that offer laboratory services (The Joint Commission, 2011).

In order to maintain accreditation, a health care organization must undergo an on-site survey by a Joint Commission survey team every three years. Laboratories must be surveyed every two years. This survey is conducted to ensure that the organization continues to meet the established standards. The standards themselves are the result of an ongoing, dynamic process that incorporates the experience and perspectives of health care professionals and others throughout the country. New standards manuals are published annually and health care organizations are responsible for knowing and incorporating any changes as they occur.

Categories of accreditation (The Joint Commission, 2011) that an organization can achieve are the following:

- *Preliminary accreditation:* for organizations that demonstrate compliance with selected standards under the "Early Survey Policy." The Early Survey Policy allows organizations to undergo a survey prior to having the ability to demonstrate full compliance. Organizations that receive preliminary accreditation will be required to undergo a second on-site survey.

- *Accredited:* for organizations that demonstrate compliance with all standards.

- *Accreditation with follow-up survey:* for organizations that are not in compliance with specific standards and require a follow-up survey within thirty days to six months.

- *Contingent accreditation:* for organizations that fail to address all requirements in an Accreditation with Follow-up Survey decision or for organizations that do not have the proper license or other similar issue at the time of the initial survey. A follow-up survey is generally required within thirty days.

- *Preliminary denial of accreditation:* for organizations for which there is justification for denying accreditation. This decision is subject to appeal.

- *Denial of accreditation:* for organizations that fail to meet standards and that have exhausted all appeals.

In addition to the survey process, the Joint Commission (2011) requires accredited organizations to

- Complete a self-directed Periodic Performance Review (PPR) on an annual basis (except the survey years) and submit a specific Plan of Action (POA). PPR is a process "whereby an organization reviews its compliance with all applicable Joint Commission accreditation requirements." The POA is subsequently submitted for any requirements that are not in full compliance.

- Select and use core performance measures to meet ORYX (National Hospital Quality Measures) requirements. Currently Joint Commission–accredited hospitals are required to collect and submit data on a minimum of four core measures or a combination of core and noncore measures (up to nine noncore measures). Organizations may choose their core measure sets from among several that are currently available. Examples of currently available sets are

  Acute myocardial infarction (AMI)

  Children's asthma care (CAC)

  Heart failure (HF)

  Surgical Care Improvement Project (SCIP)

  Pneumonia (PN)

  Hospital outpatient measures (HOP)

  Perinatal care (PC)

  Venous thromboembolism (VTE)

  Hospital-based inpatient psychiatric services (HBIPS)

  Stroke (STK)

Data for all applicable measures must be submitted through performance measurement vendor(s) that have been evaluated and listed by the Joint Commission (The Joint Commission, 2012b).

- Participate in the Joint Commission Quality Report process. Quality Reports can include the following information (The Joint Commission, 2012c):

  Accreditation and certification decision

  National Patient Safety Goal compliance

  National Quality Improvement Goals performance

  Patient satisfaction data

  Centers for Medicare and Medicaid Services mortality measures

  Special quality awards

  As discussed in Chapter One, this information can be publicly searched and viewed on the Joint Commission's Quality Check web site (www.qualitycheck.org).

- Comply with currently identified National Patient Safety Goals. Effective January 1, 2012, the Joint Commission National Patient Safety Goals included (among others):

  Use at least two patient identifiers when providing care, treatment, and services.

  Eliminate transfusion errors related to patient misidentification.

  Report critical results of tests and diagnostic procedures on a timely basis.

  Label all medications, medication containers, and other solutions on and off the sterile field in perioperative and other procedural settings.

  Maintain and communicate accurate patient medication information.

The Joint Commission focus on quality of care provided in health care facilities dates back to the early 1900s, when the American College of Surgeons began surveying hospitals and established a hospital standardization program. With the program came the question, How is quality of care measured? One of the early concerns of the standardization program was the lack of documentation in patient records. The early surveyors found that documentation was so poor that they had no way to judge the quality of care provided. The Joint Commission's emphasis on health care information and the documentation of care has continued to the present. Not only do the Joint Commission reporting requirements rely heavily on patient information, but the current survey process also uses "tracer methodology," through which the surveyors analyze the organization's systems by tracing the care provided to individual patients. Patient records provide the road maps for the tracer methodology. The absence of quality health records would have a direct impact on the accreditation process. The following sections discuss Joint Commission standards that directly influence the creation, maintenance, and use of health care information. These sections further illustrate how the overall accreditation process relies on the availability of high-quality health care information.

The Joint Commission Record of Care, Treatment, and Services Standards

In 2009, the Joint Commission introduced a "new and improved" hospital accreditation manual and survey process. One significant aspect of the new manual was the creation of the Record of Care, Treatment and Services (RC) chapter of standards. This chapter defines the components of the medical record. The content of health records is greatly influenced, if not determined, by these standards. Although the RC chapter is new, the standards within it are not. The standards were found within the Information Management (IM) chapter prior to 2009. By splitting the RC standards out of the overall IM chapter and creating a stand-alone chapter, the Joint Commission clearly defined and distinguished standards governing patient record content from standards governing the management of information. The RC standards require hospitals to

- Maintain complete and accurate medical records for each individual patient
- Ensure medical record entries are authenticated appropriately by authorized persons
- Ensure documentation in medical records is timely
- Audit their medical records
- Retain their medical records according to relevant laws and regulations
- Ensure medical records contain specific information that "reflects the patient's care, treatment and services"
- Ensure medical records accurately reflect operative and high-risk procedures and use of sedation and anesthesia
- Ensure documentation of proper use of restraints and/or seclusion
- Ensure ambulatory care records contain a summary list
- Ensure qualified staff receive and record verbal orders
- Document specific discharge information for each patient

Each RC standard has specific elements that must be addressed. For more information refer to the most recent edition of the *Comprehensive Accreditation Manual (CAMH) for Hospitals*. All Joint Commission–accredited hospitals have access to the complete manual in electronic and paper form.

In the introduction of the RC chapter, the Joint Commission explicitly states that the same standards apply whether the organization uses electronic, paper, or combination health records. A further caution is directed at hospitals transitioning from paper to electronic systems, "as the period of transition can present increased opportunity for errors in recordkeeping that can affect the delivery of safe quality care" (The Joint Commission, 2011, RC-1).

The Joint Commission Information Management Standards

The Information Management (IM) standards reflect the Joint Commission's belief that quality information management influences quality care. In the overview of the IM standards, the Joint Commission states, "Every episode of care generates health information *that must be managed systematically*" (emphasis is the authors'). Information is a resource that must be managed like any other resource within the organization. Whether the information management systems employed by the organization are basic or sophisticated, the functions should include features that allow for:

- Categorizing, filing, and maintaining all data and information used by the organization
- Accurately capturing health information generated by delivery of care, treatment, and services
- Accessing information by those authorized users who need the information to provide safe, quality care

The IM standards apply to both noncomputerized systems and systems employing the latest technologies. The first standard within the IM chapter focuses on information planning. The organization's plan for information management should consider the "full spectrum of data" generated and used by the organization as well as the flow of information within and to and from external organizations. Identifying and understanding the flow of information is critical to meeting the organization's needs for data collection and distribution, while maintaining the appropriate level of security (The Joint Commission, 2011, IM-3).

The remaining IM standards address the requirements for health care organizations to

- Provide continuity of the information management process, including managing system interruptions and maintaining backup systems
- Ensure the privacy, security, and integrity of health information
- Manage data collection, including use of standardized data sets and terminology, and limiting the use of abbreviations
- Manage health information retrieval, dissemination, and transmission
- Provide knowledge-based information resources twenty-four hours a day, seven days a week
- Ensure the accuracy of the health information (The Joint Commission, 2011)

National Committee for Quality Assurance

The National Committee for Quality Assurance (NCQA) was discussed in Chapter One as the developer and overseer of the Health Plan Employer Data and Information Set (HEDIS) and for its work in providing quality measures for health plans. In addition to these programs, the NCQA also serves as an accrediting body for health plans, including health maintenance organizations (HMOs), Preferred Provider Organizations (PPOs), and Point of Service (POS) plans. NCQA began accrediting MCOs in 1991 "to meet increasing demand for objective, standardized plan performance information" (NCQA, 2012). Although the NCQA accreditation process is voluntary, many large employers, including American Airlines, IBM, AT&T, and Federal Express, will not do business with a health plan that is not NCQA accredited. Many states recognize NCQA accreditation, eliminating the need for accredited plans to undergo separate state review.

The full list of NCQA Health Plan Accreditation Requirements are published on their web site at www.ncqa.org. The 2011 requirements include specific criteria divided into the following sections:

- Quality management and improvement (QI)
- Utilization management (UM)
- Credentialing and recredentialing (CR)
- Members' rights and responsibilities (RR)
- Standards for member connections (MEM)
- Medicaid benefits and services (MED)
- HEDIS and Consumer Assessment of Healthcare Providers and Systems (CAHPS) performance measures

NCQA accreditation surveys are conducted by teams of physicians and other health care providers. These surveys rely heavily on health care data and information, including the HEDIS measures. The results of the surveys are evaluated by a national oversight committee that assigns one of five accreditation levels:

- Excellent
- Commendable
- Accredited
- Provisional
- Denied

The NCQA accreditation process is viewed as rigorous. A health plan must be aggressively managing quality in order to achieve accreditation at the excellent level. NCQA provides a free, online *health plan report card* that shows the accreditation status of all plans that it has surveyed (NCQA, 2012).

Other Accrediting Organizations

Although the Joint Commission and NCQA are arguably the most visible and well-known accrediting bodies in the U.S. health care system, there are others. The Commission on Accreditation of Rehabilitation Facilities (CARF) accredits health and human services programs, including aging services, behavioral health, business and services management networks, child and youth services, employment and community services, and medical rehabilitation. There are currently over 47,000 CARF-accredited programs and services. (CARF, 2012). The Accreditation Association for Ambulatory Health Care (AAAHC) accredits ambulatory care organizations based on a set of core and adjunct standards. There are currently over five thousand ambulatory care organizations with AAAHC accreditation (AAAHC, 2012). These accreditation processes have several features in common. They are based on preestablished standards aimed at improving the quality of health care, they require an on-site survey, they make health care information and documentation critical components of the process, and they award a level of accreditation or approval. All have standards that affect organizations' health care information and health care information systems.

PATIENT SAFETY ORGANIZATIONS

In 2000, the landmark report "To Err Is Human: Building a Safer Health System" was published by the Institute of Medicine. This report outlined serious concerns about and the need to improve the safety and quality of health care in the United States. In spite of the ongoing efforts by voluntary accrediting bodies to ensure high-quality care, this report identified (among other things) a critical need for reporting and analyzing individual facility and aggregate data related to adverse events. To address this need to capture information to improve health care quality and prevent harm to patients, the Patient Safety and Quality Improvement Act of 2005 (Patient Safety Act) was passed by Congress. The goals of the Patient Safety Act are "to encourage the expansion of voluntary, provider-driven initiatives to improve the quality and safety of health care; to promote rapid learning about the underlying causes of risks and harms in the delivery of health care; and to share those findings widely, thus speeding the pace of improvement" (AHRQ, 2012).

The Patient Safety Act

- Encourages the development of Patient Safety Organizations (PSOs)— organizations that can work with clinicians and health care organizations to identify, analyze, and reduce the risks and hazards associated with patient care.
- Fosters a culture of safety by establishing strong federal confidentiality and privilege protections for information assembled and developed by provider organizations, physicians, and other clinicians for deliberations and analyses regarding quality and safety.
- Accelerates the speed with which solutions can be identified for the risks and hazards associated with patient care by facilitating the aggregation of a sufficient number of events in a protected legal environment.

To implement the act, the Department of Health and Human Services issued the Patient Safety Rule (effective January 2009), which authorizes PSOs to

- Offer health care providers a secure environment—protected by legal privilege and confidentiality—to conduct patient safety activities so that health care providers can analyze quality and safety issues to improve care and reduce risk to patients.
- Encourage health care providers to voluntarily submit and share information, which will be deidentified and used to track patient safety trends nationwide.
- Give feedback to health care providers on ways to reduce risk and improve patient quality and safety.

PSOs are responsible for the collection and analysis of health information that is referred to in the final rule as "patient safety work product" (PSWP). The PSWP contains identifiable patient information that is covered by specific privilege and confidentiality protections. Currently there are over seventy-five PSOs listed as operating in the United States; however, this list is updated on a weekly basis at www.pso.ahrq.gov.

In the first half of this chapter, we have taken a brief overview of licensure, certification, and accreditation, as well as patient safety organization reporting. Each of these processes is designed to have a positive impact on health care quality, with health care data and information as integral components. The accreditation processes and standards provide guidance to organizations for the development of information planning, retention, and retrieval and to a great extent determine the content of patient records. Health care executives must be familiar with the processes and standards that apply to their health care organizations to ensure that their information management plans and information systems will facilitate compliance, whether voluntary or mandatory.

LEGAL ASPECTS OF MANAGING HEALTH INFORMATION

Health care information, particularly patient-specific information, is governed by multiple state and federal laws and regulations in addition to those for licensure and certification. Laws and regulations governing the privacy and confidentiality of patient information and also record retention and authentication have existed for many years. When all patient records were on paper, it was fairly easy to identify what constituted a patient record and what did not. Authentication was a signature on a document, and destruction of records involved burning or shredding. As patient records are increasingly stored in electronic form and involve multiple types of media from paper to digital images, implementation of the regulations governing health care information has had to change. In some cases the laws and regulations themselves have been rewritten.

At this juncture it is worth emphasizing that laws governing patient information and medical records vary from state to state and a full discussion of them is beyond the scope of this text. The complexity of the U.S. legal system makes it very important for health care organizations to employ personnel who are knowledgeable about all state and federal laws and regulations that govern their patients' information and to have legal counsel available who can provide specific guidance. With that caveat, in this section we will look at several legal aspects of managing health care information, including a brief discussion of some of the significant laws and regulations related to each aspect and a discussion of legal compliance in an increasingly multimedia environment. Specifically, we will address the medical record as a legal document, including the issues of retention and authentication of health care information, and selected federal regulations governing patient and health information privacy and confidentiality, including an overview of the Health Insurance Portability and Accountability Act (HIPAA) and the HIPAA Privacy Rule.

The Health Record as a Legal Document

When the patient medical record is a file folder full of paper housed in the health information management department of the hospital, identifying the *legal* record is fairly straightforward. Records kept in the normal course of business (in this case, providing care to patients) represent an exception to the hearsay rule, are generally admissible in a court, and therefore can be subpoenaed—they are legal documentation of the care provided to the patients. The health care organization might struggle with which documents to file in an individual's medical record, because of varying and changing state and federal laws and regulations, but once those decisions are made, the entire legal record for any given patient can be found on the file shelf when it is needed. Only one "official," original copy exits.

When the patient record is a hybrid of electronic and paper documents or when it is totally computer based, how does that change the definition of the legal record? There is no simple, one-paragraph answer to this question, as state governments and the federal government are modifying laws and regulations to reflect the change from paper to digital documentation. The *legal health record* (LHR) purpose is to provide the information that is recognized as the official business record of the health care organization for evidentiary purposes. As such it represents a subset of the health care organization's patient database. The organization, therefore, has an obligation to clearly define the elements of the patient database that make up the LHR. This is not a simple undertaking. The documents and data that could potentially be a part of the LHR may exist in several physically separate paper-based and electronic systems. An organization might have stored within its overall patient database, not only the organization's records, but also outpatient test results, other care provider records, or even the patients' own personal health records. Multiple types of media could also be stored, such as images, videos, audio files, and e-mails. Clearly, the organization's LHR definition must include not only the sources of the data it contains, but also the storage media and location (AHIMA, 2011a).

An approach recommended by the American Health Information Management Association (AHIMA) is to develop a "health record matrix" outlining the type and name of the components of the record, primary source, system start date, location for legal purposes, and whether or not the record is part of the LHR. (For more information, see "Fundamentals of the Legal Health

Record and Designated Record Set: Appendix A," available online in the AHIMA Body of Knowledge at www.ahima.org.) The matrix helps identify and track the components of the organization's entire patient database. From this, the organization must determine which components constitute the LHR.

In defining their LHR, organizations should also consider issues such as these (AHIMA, 2011a):

- The available functions in the EHR system—for example, will information sent by the patient through a web-based portal be considered part of the LHR?

- The storage capacity and cost for the required retention period of the health record—for example, what is the organization's image storage capacity?

- The data's importance for long-term use—some raw data might be considered useful only until the final report is created.

- Whether or not the EHR system is able to provide both readable electronic and paper copies of all components of the LHR.

Examples of information that will generally be found in an organization's LHR are all components of the clinical record and patient-identifiable source clinical data such as X-rays, fetal strips, and images. Health care records from other providers may or may not be included. Administrative records such as committee reports and encounter forms will generally not be included in the LHR.

Retention of Health Records

The majority of states have specific retention requirements for health care information. These state requirements should be the basis for the health care organization's formal retention policy. (The Joint Commission and other accrediting agencies also address retention but generally refer organizations back to their own state regulations for specifics.) When no specific retention requirement is made by the state, all patient information that is a part of the LHR should be maintained for at least as long as the state's statute of limitations or other regulation requires. In the case of minor children the LHR should be retained until the child reaches the age of majority as defined by state law, usually eighteen or twenty-one. Health care executives should be aware that statutes of limitations may allow a patient to bring a case as long as ten years after the patient learns that his or her care caused an injury. AHIMA (2011b) currently recommends that patient health records for adults should be retained for ten years after the most recent encounter and patient health records for children should be retained until the time the person reaches the age of majority plus the time stated in the relevant statute of limitations.

Although some specific retention requirements and general guidelines exist, it is becoming increasingly popular for health care organizations to keep all LHR information indefinitely, particularly if the information is stored in an electronic format. If an organization does decide to destroy LHR information, this destruction must be carried out in accordance with all applicable laws and regulations. Some states require that health care organizations create an abstract of the patient record prior to its destruction. Others specify methods of destruction that can be used. If specific methods of destruction are not specified, the health care organization can follow general guidelines such as those in the following list (AHIMA, 2011b). These destruction guidelines apply to any patient-identifiable health care information, whether or not that information is identified as part of the LHR.

- Destroy the records so there is no possibility of reconstruction:
  - Burn, shred, pulp, or pulverize paper.
  - Recycle or pulverize microfilm or microfiche.
  - Pulverize write-once read-many laser disks.
  - Degauss computerized data stored on internal or external magnetic media (that is, alter the magnetic alignment of the storage media, making it impossible to recover previously recorded data).
  - Shred or cut DVDs.
  - Demagnetize magnetic tapes.
- Document the destruction:
  - Date of destruction.
  - Method of destruction.
  - Description of destroyed records.
  - Inclusive dates of destroyed records.
  - A statement that the records were destroyed in the normal course of business.
  - Signatures of individuals supervising and witnessing the destruction.
- Maintain the destruction documentation indefinitely.

Under the HIPAA privacy rule, when destruction services are outsourced, the contract with the business associate must include the following measures to protect patient privacy (AHIMA, 2011b):

- The method of destruction or disposal.
- The time that will elapse between acquisition and destruction or disposal.
- Safeguards against breaches.
- Indemnification for the organization to provide for loss due to unauthorized disclosure.
- Requirement that the business associate maintain liability insurance in specified amounts at all times.

Authentication of Health Record Information

State and federal laws and accreditation standards require that health record entries be authenticated to ensure that the legal document identifies the person or persons responsible for the care provided. Generally, authentication of an LHR entry is accomplished when the physician or other health care professional signs it, either with a handwritten signature or an electronic signature.

Electronic signatures are created when the provider enters a unique code, biometric, or password that verifies his or her identity. The term *electronic signature* is used to describe a broad range of technologies and methods, ranging from an agreement button following a written statement to a digitally encrypted ID or certificate. Often electronic signatures show up on the computer screen or printout in this form: "Electronically authenticated by Jane H. Doe, M.D., on 4/1/2012 at 12:50pm" (AHIMA, 2009). Electronic signatures are now accepted by both the Joint Commission and CMS. State laws and regulations vary on the acceptability of electronic signatures, so it is important that health care organizations know what their respective state laws and regulations are before implementing such signatures. Most states do allow for electronic signatures in some fashion or are silent on the subject.

Regardless of the state laws and regulations, policies and procedures must be adopted by the health care organization to ensure that providers do not share any codes or passwords that are used to produce electronic signatures. Generally, a provider is required to sign a statement that he or she is the only person who has possession of the signature "key" and that he or she will be the only one to use it (AHIMA, 2009).

Privacy and Confidentiality

Privacy is an individual's constitutional right to be left alone, to be free from unwarranted publicity, and to conduct his or her life without its being made public. In the health care environment, *privacy* is the individual's right to limit access to his or her health care information. *Confidentiality* is the expectation that information shared with a health care provider during the course of treatment will be used only for its intended purpose and not disclosed otherwise. Confidentiality relies on trust.

There are many sources for the legal and ethical requirement that health care professionals maintain the confidentiality of patient information and protect patient privacy. Ethical and professional standards, such as those published by the American Medical Association and other organizations, address professional conduct and the need to hold patient information in confidence. Accrediting bodies, such as those mentioned in the previous section (the Joint Commission, NCQA, and so forth), and the CMS CoPs dictate that health care organizations follow standard practice, state, and federal laws to ensure the confidentiality of patient information. State regulations, as a component of state facility licensure or other statutes, also address confidentiality and privacy.

However, the regulations and statutes vary widely from state to state. Protections offered by the states also vary according to the holder of the information and the type of information. For example, state regulations may address the confidentiality of AIDS or sexually transmitted disease (STD) information but remain silent on all other types of health care information. Few states specifically address the redisclosure of information, and the lack of uniformity among states causes difficulty when interstate health care transactions are necessary. In today's environment it is not uncommon for a preferred provider of a technical medical procedure to be out of state. Telemedicine also often requires interstate communication of patient information.

Federal Privacy Laws

The federal laws governing patient privacy have evolved over the past several decades. In this section we will describe the following key privacy laws, rules, and regulations that affect health care information management today:

- The Privacy Act of 1974 (5 U.S.C. §552a; 45 C.F.R. Part 5b; OMB Circular No. A-108 [1975])
- Confidentiality of Substance Abuse Patient Records (42 U.S.C. §290dd-2, 42 C.F.R. Part 2)
- Health Insurance Portability and Accountability Act (HIPAA); Privacy Rule (45 C.F.R. Part 160 and Subparts A and E of Part 164)
- Health Information and Technology for Economic and Clinical Health (HITECH) Act expansion of HIPAA Rules

The Privacy Act of 1974

In 1966, the Freedom of Information Act (FOIA) was passed. This legislation provides the American public with the right to obtain information from federal agencies. The Act covers all records created by the federal government, with nine exceptions. The sixth exception is for personnel and medical information "the disclosure of which would constitute a clearly unwarranted invasion of personal privacy." There was, however, concern that this exception to the FOIA was not strong enough to protect federally created patient records and other health information. Consequently, Congress enacted the Privacy Act of 1974. This Act was written specifically to protect patient confidentiality only in *federally operated* health care facilities, such as Veterans Administration hospitals, Indian Health Service facilities, and military health care organizations. Because the protection was limited to those facilities operated by the federal government, most general hospitals and other nongovernment health care organizations did not have to comply. Nevertheless, the Privacy Act of 1974 was an important piece of legislation, not only because it addressed the FOIA exception for patient information but also because it explicitly stated that patients had a right to access and amend their medical records. It also required facilities to maintain documentation of all disclosures. Neither of these things was standard practice at the time.

Confidentiality of Substance Abuse Patient Records

During the 1970s, people became increasingly aware of the extrasensitive nature of drug and alcohol treatment records. This led to the regulations currently found in 42 C.F.R. (Code of Federal Regulations) Part 2, Confidentiality of Substance Abuse Patient Records. These regulations have been amended twice, with the latest version published in 1999. They offer specific guidance to federally assisted health care organizations that provide referral, diagnosis, and treatment services to patients with alcohol or drug problems. Not surprisingly, they set stringent release of information standards, designed to protect the confidentiality of patients seeking alcohol or drug treatment.

HIPAA

The HIPAA Privacy Rule is an important federal regulation. It is the first comprehensive federal regulation that offers specific protection to private health information. Prior to the HIPAA Privacy Rule there was no single federal regulation governing the privacy and confidentiality of patient-specific information.

To put the Privacy Rule in context, we will begin our discussion by briefly outlining the content of the entire Act that authorized this regulation. We will then discuss the specifics of the Privacy Rule and its impact on the maintenance, use, and release of health care information.

The Health Insurance Portability and Accountability Act of 1996 has two main parts:

- Title I addresses health care access, portability, and renewability, offering protection for individuals who change jobs or health insurance policies. Although Title I is an important piece of legislation, it does not address health care information specifically and will therefore not be addressed in this chapter.

- Title II includes a section titled Administrative Simplification. It is in a subsection to this section that the requirement to establish privacy regulations for individually identifiable health information is found. Two additional subsections under Administration Simplification are particularly relevant to health care information: Transaction and Code Sets, standards for which were finalized in 2000, and Security, standards for which were finalized in 2002. (HIPAA security regulations are discussed at length in Chapter Ten.)

HIPAA Privacy Rule

Although the HIPAA Privacy Rule is a comprehensive set of federal standards, it permits the enforcement of existing state laws that are more protective of individual privacy, and states are also free to pass more stringent laws in the future. Therefore, health care organizations must still be familiar with their own state laws and regulations related to privacy and confidentiality.

The HIPAA Privacy Rule defines *covered entities*, that is, those individuals and organizations that must comply. This definition is broad and includes

- Health plans, which pay or provide for the cost of medical care.
- Health care clearinghouses, which process health information (for example, billing services).
- Health care providers who conduct certain financial and administrative transactions electronically. (These transactions are defined broadly, so that the reality of the HIPAA Privacy Rule is that it governs nearly all health care providers who receive any type of third-party reimbursement.)

If any of these covered entities shares information with others, it must establish contracts to protect the shared information.

HIPAA-protected information is also defined broadly under the Privacy Rule. *Protected health information* (PHI) is information that

- Relates to a person's physical or mental health, the provision of health care, or the payment for health care
- Identifies the person who is the subject of the information
- Is created or *received* by a covered entity
- Is transmitted or maintained in *any* form (paper, electronic, or oral)

There are five major components to the HIPAA Privacy Rule:

1. **Boundaries.** PHI may be disclosed for health purposes only, with very limited exceptions.
2. **Security.** PHI should not be distributed without patient authorization, unless there is a clear basis for doing so, and the individuals who receive the information must safeguard it.
3. **Consumer control.** Individuals are entitled to access and control their health records and are to be informed of the purposes for which information is being disclosed and used.
4. **Accountability.** Entities that improperly handle PHI can be charged under criminal law and punished and are subject to civil recourse as well.
5. **Public responsibility.** Individual interests must not override national priorities in public health, medical research, preventing health care fraud, and law enforcement in general.

HITECH Expansion of HIPAA Privacy Rules

A portion of the American Recovery and Reinvestment Act of 2009 known as the Health Information Technology for Economic and Clinical Health (HITECH) Act was enacted to provide substantial Medicare and Medicaid incentives for hospitals and physicians to adopt electronic health records and provide grants to develop health information exchanges. (See Chapter Six for a complete discussion of these aspects of HITECH.) The HITECH Act also substantially expands the HIPAA Privacy and Security Rules (Coppersmith, Gordon, Schermer, & Brokelman, PLC, 2012).

This expansion has four main components:

- Application of the HIPAA privacy and security requirements directly to business associates. The Act also clarifies that certain entities, such as Health Information Exchange Organizations, Regional Health Information Organizations, e-prescribing gateways, or a vendor that contracts with a covered entity to allow the covered entity to offer a personal health record as a part of its EHR, are business associates if they require access to PHI on a routine basis.

- Establishment of mandatory federal security breach reporting requirements for covered entities and business associates. (See Chapter Eleven for a complete discussion of this expansion to the HIPAA Security Rule.)

- Establishment of new criminal and civil penalties for noncompliance and new enforcement responsibilities. The new penalties are applied using a tiered schedule that ranges from $100 for a single violation where the individual did not know he was not in compliance to $1,500,000 for multiple violations due to willful neglect. State attorney generals now have enforcement authority.

- Creation of new privacy requirements for HIPAA-covered entities and business associates. There are several areas of expansion to the HIPAA privacy requirements. In general the rights of individuals to request and obtain their PHI are strengthened, as is the right of the individual to prevent a health care organization from disclosing PHI to a health plan if the individual paid in full out of pocket for the related services. There are also some new provisions for accounting of disclosures made through an EHR for treatment, payment, and operations.

The federal privacy laws, rules, and regulations create a tension within health care organizations between the need to *protect* patient information and the need to *use* patient information. Thinking back to Chapter One, remember the purposes for maintaining patient-specific health information. The number-one reason is patient care; however, there are other legitimate reasons for sharing or "releasing" identifiable health information.

Release of Information

Because of the various state and federal laws and regulations that exist to protect patient-specific information, health care organizations must have comprehensive release of information policies and procedures in place that ensure compliance. Exhibits 3.3 and 3.4 are samples of release of information forms

PERSPECTIVE
*Examples of Recently Published
HIPAA Privacy Violations*

From HHS.gov on July 2, 2011 (HHS, 2011a):

University of California at Los Angeles Health System (UCLAHS) agrees to settle for $865,500 and has committed to a corrective action plan aimed at remedying gaps in its compliance with the HIPAA rules. The settlement came after two separate complaints filed on behalf of two celebrity patients alleging that UCLAHS employees repeatedly and without permissible reason looked at their electronic protected health information.

From HealthData Management on June 14, 2011 (Woman Faces Criminal Charges, 2011):

A woman under investigation for credit card fraud was charged in U.S. District Court for "wrongful disclosure of individually identifiable health information." She faced up to ten years in prison and a fine up to $250,000. She was charged with taking schedules from a patient registration area on multiple occasions between March 22 and April 8, 2011.

From HHS.gov on Feb. 22, 2011 (HHS, 2011b):

The Office of Civil Rights (OCR) found that Cignet Health violated forty-one patients' rights by denying them access to their medical records between September 2008 and October 2009. These patients individually filed complaints with OCR, initiating investigations of each complaint. The penalty for these violations was $1.3 million. OCR also found that Cignet failed to cooperate with investigations and that the failure to cooperate was due to willful neglect to comply with the Privacy Rule. The penalty for these violations was $3 million.

From HHS.gov on Feb. 24, 2011 (HHS, 2011c):

Mass General has agreed to pay the U.S. government $1 million to settle potential violations of the Privacy Rule. The violation involved the loss of documents consisting of a patient schedule containing names and medical record numbers for a group of 192 patients, and billing

(cont.)

encounter forms containing the name, date of birth, medical record number, health insurer and policy number, diagnosis, and name of providers for 66 of those patients. These documents were lost on March 9, 2009, when an employee, while commuting to work, left the documents on the subway train.

From HHS.gov on July 27, 2010 (HHS, 2011d):

Rite Aid Corporation and its forty affiliated entities agreed to pay $1 million to settle potential violations of the Privacy Rule. The investigation began after television media videotaped incidents in which pharmacies were shown to have disposed of prescriptions and labeled pill bottles containing individuals' identifiable information in industrial trash containers that were accessible to the public. These incidents were reported as occurring in a variety of cities across the United States. Rite Aid pharmacy stores in several of the cities were highlighted in media reports.

From UC San Diego Health Sciences in Aug. 2009 (UC San Diego, 2009):

A physician and two former hospital employees pled guilty to HIPAA violations in Arkansas. Both were charged with a misdemeanor violation based on their accessing a patient's record without any legitimate purpose. Each faced a maximum penalty of one year imprisonment, a fine of not more than $50,000, or both.

From the *Milwaukee Journal Sentinel* on May 9, 2002 (Sink, 2002):

A jury in Waukesha, Wisconsin, found that an emergency medical technician (EMT) invaded the privacy of an overdose patient when she told the patient's co-worker about the overdose. The EMT claimed that she called the patient's co-worker out of concern for the patient. The jury, however, found that regardless of her intentions the EMT had no right to disclose confidential and sensitive medical information and directed the EMT and her employer to pay $3,000 for the invasion of privacy.

Exhibit 3.3. Annual permission by patient to access protected health information

SEND TO:
Health
Information
Services

MUSC Health

PERMPATPHA

ANNUAL PERMISSION BY PATIENT TO ACCESS PROTECTED HEALTH INFORMATION

(Not a Healthcare Power of Attorney)

Page 1 of 1

ANNUAL PATIENT ACCESS	
(Please Initial)	(Internal Use)
_____ All PHI (records)	HPF
_____ Communication Only	AOD
	PP
Expires: _____	

PATIENT NAME:

_____

Date of Birth:_____

MRN:_____

Social Security (last 4): _____

Purpose of this disclosure is to grant access only and must be completed in its entirety to be considered valid.

Unless otherwise canceled / revoked, this authorization will expire / end one year from this date or _____ .

➡ I authorize the exchange of ANY AND ALL MEDICAL RECORDS VIA (check all preferred methods):

☐ mail ☐ fax ☐ e-mail ☐ phone ☐ in person ☐ electronic view

To the following Individual / Organization:_____

Street Address:_____ City: _____ State: _____ Zip Code: _____

Phone Number:_____ Fax Number: _____ E-mail Address: _____

I understand this information may include reference to psychiatric / psychological care*, sexual assault, drug abuse, results of tests for all infectious diseases including HIV / AIDS and / or alcohol abuse.

I understand that I have a right to cancel / revoke this authorization at any time. I understand that if I cancel / revoke this authorization I must do so in writing and present my written cancellation / revocation to the Health Information Services Department (Medical Records). I understand that the cancellation / revocation will not apply to information that has already been released in response to this authorization, as stated in the Notice of Privacy Practice.

I understand that authorizing the disclosure of protected health information is voluntary. I can refuse to sign this authorization. I do not need to sign this form to receive treatment. I understand I may review and / or copy the information to be disclosed, as provided in 45 CFR §164.524. I understand that any disclosure of information carries with it the possibility of unauthorized disclosure by the person / organization receiving the information. I understand I will be given a copy of this authorization.

A copy of my identification will be made and attached to this authorization.

_____   _____
Signature of Patient or Legal Guardian / Representative   Date / Time

_____
Printed Name of Patient or Legal Guardian / Representative

_____   _____
Relationship to Patient, if signed by Legal Guardian / Representative   Witness Signature

Description of patient representative's authority: _____
* DOES NOT INCLUDE PSYCHOTHERAPY   (The reason the patient is not signing)

To contact Health Information Services (Medical Records) in writing, the address is: 169 Ashley Avenue / MSC 349 / Attention: Release of Information / Charleston, South Carolina 29425-3490; the phone number is (843) 792-3881; FAX NUMBER 843-792-7292.

Original to medical record   **Copy to patient**
all_all_consent_authtorelease_ptannualaccess   OTE 700732 Rev. 8/11

Source: © 2012 Medical University Hospital Authority. All Rights Reserved. This form is provided "as is" without any warranty, express or implied, as to its legal effect or completeness. Forms should be used as a guide and modified to meet the laws of your state. Use at your own risk.

Exhibit 3.4. Authorization to disclose protected health information

MUSC Health

AUTHRELSE
AUTHORIZATION TO DISCLOSE PROTECTED HEALTH INFORMATION
Page 1 of 1
This form must be completed in its entirety in order to be considered valid.

Patient Name:_____ Date of Birth:_____

Medical Record Number:_____ Last 4 digits Social Security Number:_____

☐ I authorize MUSC Medical Center to disclose / release information to:
☐ I authorize MUSC Medical Center to obtain information from:
Name of Individual / Organization: _____

Street Address: _____ City: _____ State: _____ Zip Code: _____

Phone Number:_____ Fax Number:_____ E-mail Address: _____
The purpose of the disclosure is: ☐ Continued care ☐ Legal ☐ Insurance ☐ Disability ☐ Patient Request
☐ Other_____ **Date(s) of service** : _____

☐ An **"abstract"** of the medical record is provided as the first level of release of information (comprehensive overview of entire record). This includes: history and physical, consults, lab and radiology reports, discharge summary, operative / procedure reports, Emergency Department reports, Occupational Therapy / Physical Therapy reports.

In addition to the "abstract" information, the following information may be requested:

☐ Films / images	☐ Immunization records	☐ Medication list	☐ Physician progress / visit notes
☐ Physician orders	☐ Nurses notes	☐ Entire record	☐ Other:

I understand this information may include reference to psychiatric / psychological care, sexual assault, drug abuse, results of tests for all infectious diseases including HIV / AIDS and / or alcohol abuse.

I authorize the exchange of this information via (check all preferred methods): ☐ mail ☐ fax ☐ e-mail ☐ other_____

I understand that I have a right to cancel / revoke this authorization at any time. I understand that if I cancel / revoke this authorization I must do so in writing and present my written cancellation / revocation to the Health Information Services Department (Medical Records). I understand that the cancellation / revocation will not apply to information that has already been released in response to this authorization, as stated in the Notice of Privacy Practice. Unless otherwise canceled / revoked, this authorization will expire / end one year from this date or _____

I understand that fees for copies of medical records and postage fees may be charged.

I understand that authorizing the disclosure of protected health information is voluntary. I can refuse to sign this authorization. I do not need to sign this form to receive treatment. I understand I may review and / or copy the information to be disclosed, as provided in 45 CFR §164.524. I understand that any disclosure of information carries with it the possibility of unauthorized disclosure by the person / organization receiving the information. I understand I will be given a copy of this authorization.

A copy of my identification will be made and attached to this authorization.

_____   _____
Signature of Patient or Legal Guardian / Representative   Date

_____
Printed Name of Patient or Legal Guardian / Representative

_____   _____
Relationship to Patient, if signed by Legal Guardian / Representative   Witness Signature
Description of patient representative's authority: _____
(The reason the patient is not signing)

To contact Health Information Services (Medical Records) in writing, the address is: 169 Ashley Avenue / MSC 349 / Attention: Release of Information / Charleston, South Carolina 29425-3490; the phone number is (843) 792-3881.

Original to medical record   Copy to patient
all_all_consent_authtorelease   OTE 700078 Rev. 5/10

Source: © 2012 Medical University Hospital Authority. All Rights Reserved. This form is provided "as is" without any warranty, express or implied, as to its legal effect or completeness. Forms should be used as a guide and modified to meet the laws of your state. Use at your own risk.

used by a hospital, showing the elements that should be present on a valid release form:

- Patient identification (name and date of birth)
- Name of the person or entity to whom the information is being released
- Description of the specific health information authorized for disclosure
- Statement of the reason for or purpose of the disclosure
- Date, event, or condition on which the authorization will expire, unless it is revoked earlier
- Statement that the authorization is subject to revocation by the patient or the patient's legal representative
- Patient's or legal representative's signature
- Signature date, which must be *after the date of the encounter that produced the information to be released*

Health care organizations need clear policies and procedures for releasing patient-identifiable information. There should be a central point of control through which all nonroutine requests for information pass, and all of these disclosures should be well documented.

In some instances patient-specific health care information can be released without the patient's authorization. For example, some state laws require disclosing certain health information. It is always good practice to obtain a patient authorization prior to releasing information when feasible, but in state-mandated cases it is not required. Some examples of situations in which information might need to be disclosed to authorized recipients without the patient's consent are the presence of a communicable disease, such as AIDS and STDs, that must be reported to the state or county department of health; suspected child abuse or adult abuse that must be reported to designated authorities; situations in which there is a legal duty to warn another person of a clear and imminent danger from a patient; bona fide medical emergencies; and the existence of a valid court order.

In addition to situations mandated by law, there are other instances in which patient information can be released without an authorization. In general, health information can be released to another health care provider who is directly involved in the care of the patient, but the regulations governing this may vary from state to state. Information can also be released to other authorized persons within a health care organization to facilitate patient care. Information can also be used by the organization for billing or reimbursement purposes once a patient signs a proper consent form for treatment. It may be released for medical research purposes provided all patient identifiers have been removed.

The HIPAA rule attempts to sort out the routine and nonroutine use of health information by distinguishing between patient *consent* to use PHI and patient *authorization* to release PHI. Health care providers and others must obtain a patient's written consent prior to disclosure of health information for routine uses of treatment, payment, and health care operations. There are some exceptions to this in emergency situations, and the patient has a right to request restrictions on the disclosure. However, health care providers can deny treatment if they feel that limiting the disclosure would be detrimental. Health care providers and others *must* obtain the patient's written authorization for nonroutine uses or disclosures of PHI.

SUMMARY

In this chapter we examined a number of external drivers that dictate not only the types of health care information that health care organizations maintain but also the way in which they are maintained. These external forces include federal and state laws and regulations and voluntary accreditation standards. Specifically, this chapter was divided into two main sections. In the first section we defined licensure, certification, and accreditation and examined some of the missions and the general functions of several major accrediting organizations, including the Joint Commission and the NCQA. Patient Safety Organizations were also discussed. In the second major section we looked at a variety of legal issues in managing health care information, including state and federal laws that address the use of the patient medical record as a legal document and current laws and regulations that govern patient privacy and confidentiality. This chapter concluded with an in-depth discussion of the HIPAA Privacy Rule, including the HITECH expansion, and release of information practices. Current examples of privacy violations were presented.

KEY TERMS

Accreditation
Accreditation Association for Ambulatory Health Care (AAAHC)
Authentication
Centers for Medicare and Medicaid Services (CMS)
Certification

Commission on Accreditation of Rehabilitation Facilities (CARF)
Conditions of Participation
Confidentiality
Confidentiality of Substance Abuse Patient Records
Covered entities

Freedom of Information Act (FOIA)

Health Insurance Portability and
   Accountability Act (HIPAA)

HIPAA Privacy Rule

Laws

Legal health record (LHR)

Licensure

National Committee for Quality
   Assurance (NCQA)

Patient Safety and Quality
   Improvement Act of 2005

Patient Safety Organizations

Privacy

Privacy Act of 1974

Protected health information (PHI)

Record retention

Regulations

Release of information

Standards

U.S. Department of Health and
   Human Services (DHHS)

LEARNING ACTIVITIES

1. Visit a health care organization to find out about its current licensure, accreditation, and certification status. How are these processes related to one another in your state?

2. Visit the CMS web site at www.cms.gov. Find the Conditions of Participation for a particular type of health care facility (hospital, nursing home, or other). Review this document and comment on the standards. Are they minimal or optimal standards? Support your answer.

3. Visit the Joint Commission web site at www.jointcommission.org. What accreditation programs other than the Hospital Accreditation Program does the Joint Commission have? List the programs and their respective missions.

4. Visit the NCQA web site at www.ncqa.org. Look up a health care plan with which you are familiar. What does the report card tell you about this plan?

5. Do an Internet or library search for a recent article discussing the impact of the HIPAA privacy regulations on health care practice. Write a summary of the article.

6. Visit the patient safety organization web site at www.pso.ahrq.gov. Does your state currently have a PSO? If so, do a search to find out how long the PSO has been in operation and its number of current clients.

7. Contact a health care facility (hospital, nursing home, physician's office, or other organization) to talk with the person responsible for maintaining patient records. Ask about the organization's release of information, retention, and destruction policies.

REFERENCES

Accreditation Association for Ambulatory Health Care. (2012). *About AAAHC*. Retrieved March 2012 from http://www.aaahc.org/eweb/dynamicpage.aspx ?site=aaahc_site&webcode=about_aaahc

Agency for Healthcare Research and Quality. (2012). *Patient safety organizations*. Retrieved March 2012 from http://www.pso.ahrq.gov

American Health Information Management Association. (2009). Electronic signature, attestation, and authorship (updated). *Journal of AHIMA*, *80*(11), expanded online edition. Retrieved March 2012 from http://library.ahima.org

American Health Information Management Association. (2011a). Fundamentals of the legal health record and designated record set. *Journal of AHIMA*, *82*(2), expanded online version. Retrieved March 2012 from http://library.ahima.org

American Health Information Management Association. (2011b). *Retention and destruction of health information* (updated August 2011). Retrieved March 2012 from http://library.ahima.org

Commission on Accreditation of Rehabilitation Facilities. (2012). *Who we are*. Retrieved March 2012 from http://www.carf.org/About/WhoWeAre

Coppersmith, Gordon, Schermer, and Brokelman, PLC. (2012). HITECH act expands HIPAA privacy and security rules. Retrieved March 2012 from http://www.azhha .org/member_and_media_resources/documents/HITECHAct.pdf

Department of Health and Human Services (HHS). (2011a). News release. Retrieved March 2012 from http://www.hhs.gov/news/press/2010pres/07/20100727a .html

Department of Health and Human Services (HHS). (2011b). News release. Retrieved March 2012 from http://www.hhs.gov/news/press/2011pres/02/20110222a.html

Department of Health and Human Services (HHS). (2011c). Health information privacy. Retrieved March 2012 from http://www.hhs.gov/ocr/privacy/hipaa /news/uclahs.html

Department of Health and Human Services (HHS). (2011d). News release. Retrieved March 2012 from http://www.hhs.gov/news/press/2011pres/02/20110224b.html

Institute of Medicine. (2000). *To err is human: Building a safer health system*. Washington, DC: National Academies Press.

The Joint Commission. (2011). *Comprehensive accreditation manual for hospitals* (updated September 2011). Oakbrook Terrace, IL: Author.

The Joint Commission. (2012a). About the Joint Commission. Retrieved March 2012 from http://www.jointcommission.org/about_us/about_the_joint_commission _main.aspx

The Joint Commission. (2012b). Facts about ORYX® for hospitals (National Hospital Quality Measures). Retrieved March 2012 from http://www.jointcommission.org /assets/1/18/ORYX_for_Hospitals_8_22_11.pdf

The Joint Commission. (2012c). Facts about Quality Check® and Quality Reports®. Retrieved March 2012 from http://www.qualitycheck.org/help_qc_facts.aspx

National Committee for Quality Assurance. (2012). *2011 NCQA health plan accreditation requirements*. Retrieved March 2012 from http://www.ncqa.org

Sink, L. (2002, May 9). Jurors decide patient privacy was invaded. *Milwaukee Journal Sentinel*. Retrieved March 2011 from http://nl.newsbank.com/nl-search /we/Archives

UC San Diego. (2009). HIPAA privacy rule violations. *HealthSpan*, *1*(2). Retrieved March 2012 from http://healthspan.ucsd.edu/2009/08/Pages/mc-hipaa.aspx

Woman faces criminal charges for HIPAA privacy violations. (2011, June 14). *HealthData Management*. Retrieved March 2012 from http://www .healthdatamanagement.com/news/criminal-charges-hipaa-privacy -violations-42622-1.html

PART TWO

Health Care Information Systems

CHAPTER 4

History and Evolution of Health Care Information Systems

- To be able to describe the history and evolution of health care information systems from the 1960s to the present.

- To be able to identify the major advances in information technology and significant federal initiatives that influenced the adoption of health care information systems.

- To be able to identify the major types of administrative and clinical information systems used in health care.

- To be able to discuss why information technology (IT) adoption rates are lower in health care compared with other industries.

- To be able to discuss the relationship between incentives and health care IT adoption and use.

After reading Chapters One, Two, and Three (or from your own previous experience), you should have an understanding of the nature of health care information and the processes and regulations that influence the management of information in health care organizations. In this chapter we build upon these fundamental concepts and introduce *health care information systems*, a broad category that includes both administrative and clinical applications. We describe how health care information systems have evolved during the past fifty years. Much of this evolution can be attributed to environmental factors, changes in reimbursement practices, and major advances in information technology. Over the years the health care executive's role and involvement in making information systems–related decisions have also changed considerably. We discuss these changes and conclude by describing the opportunities that abound in using health care information technology in new and innovative ways to engage patients and to deliver high-quality, cost-effective care.

DEFINITION OF TERMS

Health care executives interact frequently with professionals from a variety of disciplines and may find the terminology used confusing or intimidating. It's no wonder. Most professional disciplines have their own terminology to describe concepts related to their normal course of business. Even professionals within a single discipline often use different terms to describe the same concepts and the same terms to describe different concepts! Throughout the remainder of this book we will use a variety of terms related to information systems. Our goal is to expose you to many of the information technology–related terms you are likely to encounter in discussions with your organization's chief information officer, information technology (IT) staff, and IT-savvy health care professionals.

An *information system (IS)* is an arrangement of information (data), processes, people, and information technology that interact to collect, process, store, and provide as output the information needed to support the organization (Whitten & Bentley, 2007). Note that information technology is a component of every information system. *Information technology (IT)* is a contemporary term that describes the combination of computer technology (hardware and software) with data and telecommunications technology (data, image, and voice networks). Often in current management literature the terms *information system (IS)* and *information technology (IT)* are used interchangeably.

Within the health care industry, health care IS and IT include a broad range of applications and products and are used by a wide range of constituent groups such as payers, government, life sciences, and patients, as well as providers and provider organizations. For our purpose, however, we have chosen to focus on health care information systems from the provider organization's perspective. The provider *organization* is the hospital, the physician practice, the integrated delivery system, the nursing home, or the rural health clinic. That is, it is any setting where health-related services are delivered. We also examine the use of patient engagement tools such as personal health record and secure patient portals, and health information exchanges. Yet our focus is from an organization or provider perspective.

Thus, a *health care information system (HCIS)* is an arrangement of information (data), processes, people, and information technology that interact to collect, process, store, and provide as output the information needed to support the *health care* organization. The organization (namely, the capacity, decisions about how health IT is applied, and incentives) and the external environment (regulations and public opinion) are important elements in how systems are used by clinicians and other users (IOM, 2011). We use the term *health care IT* interchangeably with health care information systems, particularly since "health care IT" has become more mainstream in both the literature and in practice in recent years.

This definition of an HCIS is congruent with the definitions of *data* and *information* provided in Chapter Two. Data are raw facts about people, places, events, and things that are of importance in an organization. Information is data that have been processed or reorganized into a more meaningful form for the user; information can lead to knowledge and facilitate decision making. To simplify, we will assume that the information in a health care information system is made up of both raw and processed data.

There are two primary classes of health care information systems: *administrative* and *clinical*. A simple way to distinguish them is by purpose and the type of data they contain. An *administrative information system* (or an *administrative application*) contains primarily administrative or financial data and is generally used to support the management functions and general operations of the health care organization. For example, an administrative information system might contain information used to manage personnel, finances, materials, supplies, or equipment. It might be a system for human resource management, materials management, patient accounting or billing, or staff scheduling. Revenue cycle management is increasingly important to health care organizations and generally includes:

- Charge capture
- Coding and documentation review
- Claims processing
- Managed care contracting
- Denial management of claims
- Payment posting
- Accounts receivable follow-up

- Patient collections
- Reporting and benchmarking

In contrast, a *clinical information system* (or *clinical application*) contains clinical or health-related information used by providers in diagnosing and treating a patient and monitoring that patient's care. Clinical information systems may be departmental systems—such as radiology, pharmacy, or laboratory systems—or clinical decision-support, medication administration, computerized provider order entry, or electronic health record systems, to name a few. They may be limited in their scope to a single area of clinical information (for example, radiology, pharmacy, or laboratory), or they may be comprehensive and cover virtually all aspects of patient care (as an electronic medical record system does, for example). Clinical information systems will be discussed more fully in Chapter Five. They are presented here in the context of their role in the history and evolution of health care information systems. Table 4.1 lists common types of clinical and administrative health care information systems.

Table 4.1. Common types of administrative and clinical information systems

Administrative Applications	Clinical Applications
Patient administration systems	**Ancillary information systems**
Admission, discharge, transfer (ADT) tracks the patient's movement of care in an inpatient setting	Laboratory information supports collection, verification, and reporting of laboratory tests
Registration may be coupled with ADT system; includes patient demographic and insurance information as well as date of visit(s), provider information	Radiology information supports digital image generation (picture archiving and communication systems [PACS]), image analysis, image management
Scheduling aids in the scheduling of patient visits; includes information on patients, providers, date and time of visit, rooms, equipment, other resources	Pharmacy information supports medication ordering, dispensing, and inventory control; drug compatibility checks; allergy screening; medication administration
Patient billing or accounts receivable includes all information needed to submit claims and monitor submission and reimbursement status	**Other clinical information systems**
Utilization management tracks use and appropriateness of care	Nursing documentation facilitates nursing documentation from assessment to evaluation, patient care decision support (care planning, assessment, flow-sheet charting, patient acuity, patient education)
Other administrative and financial systems	
Accounts payable monitors money owed to other organizations for purchased products and services	Electronic health record (EHR) facilitates electronic capture and reporting of patient's health history, problem lists, treatment and outcomes; allows clinicians to document clinical findings, progress notes, and other patient information; provides decision-support tools and reminders and alerts
General ledger monitors general financial management and reporting	

Table 4.1. (*Continued*)

Administrative Applications	Clinical Applications
Personnel management manages human resource information for staff, including salaries, benefits, education, and training	**Computerized provider order entry (CPOE)** enables clinicians to directly enter orders electronically and access decision-support tools and clinical care guidelines and protocols
Materials management monitors ordering and inventory of supplies, equipment needs, and maintenance	**Telemedicine and telehealth** supports remote delivery of care; common features include image capture and transmission, voice and video conferencing, text messaging
Payroll manages information about staff salaries, payroll deductions, tax withholding, and pay status	**Rehabilitation service documentation** supports the capturing and reporting of occupational therapy, physical therapy, and speech pathology services
Staff scheduling assists in scheduling and monitoring staffing needs	**Medication administration** is typically used by nurses to document medication given, dose, and time
Staff time and attendance tracks employee work schedules and attendance	
Revenue cycle management monitors the entire flow of revenue generation from charge capture to patient collection; generally relies on integration of a host of administrative and financial applications	

HISTORY AND EVOLUTION

The history of the development and implementation of information systems in health care is most meaningful when considered in the context of a chronology of major health care sector and information technology events. In this section we explore the history and evolution of health care information systems in each of the past five decades and in the present era by asking several key questions:

- What was happening in the health care environment and at the federal level that influenced organizations to adopt or use computerized systems?
- What was the state of information technology at the time?
- How did the environmental factors, coupled with advances in information technology, affect the adoption and use of health care information systems?

We start with the 1960s and move forward to the current day (see Table 4.2).

Table 4.2. Timeline of major events + advances in information technology = HCIS

Decade	Health Care Environment	State of Information Technology	Use of Health Care Information Systems
1960s	Enactment of Medicare and Medicaid Cost-based reimbursement "Building" mode Focus on financial needs and capturing revenues	Large mainframe computers Centralized processing Few vendor-developed products	Administrative or financial information systems used primarily in large hospitals and academic medical centers Developed and maintained in-house Shared systems available to smaller hospitals Centralized data processing
1970s	Still time of growth Medicare and Medicaid expenditures rising Late in decade, recognition of need to contain health care costs	Mainframes still in use Minicomputers become available, smaller, more affordable	Turnkey systems available through vendor community Increased interest in clinical applications (for example, laboratory, radiology, and pharmacy) Shared systems still used
1980s	Medicare introduces prospective payment system for hospitals Medicaid and private insurers follow suit Need for financial and clinical information	Microcomputer or personal computer (PC) becomes available—far more powerful, affordable; brings computing power to desktop; revolutionizes how companies process data and do business Advent of local area networks	Distributed data processing Expansion of clinical information systems in hospitals Physician practices introduce billing systems Integrating financial and administrative information becomes important
1990s	Medicare changes physician reimbursement to a resource-based relative value scale (RBRVS) Health care reform efforts of Clinton era (HIPAA) Growth of managed care and integrated delivery systems Institute of Medicine (IOM) calls for computer-based patient record (CPR) adoption	Unveiling of the Internet and World Wide Web—revolutionizes how organizations communicate with each other, market services, conduct business	Growth of Internet has profound effect on health care organizations' business Vendor community explodes Products more widely available and affordable Enterprise-wide systems Increased interest in clinical application Relatively small percentage of health care organizations adopt CPR

2000s	IOM report on patient safety and medical errors Both President Bush and President Obama call for electronic health record (EHR) adoption HIPAA privacy and security regulations in effect Leapfrog Group Medicare Modernization Act Transparency on quality and price; consumer empowerment Funding for health information technology (HIT) initiatives Reimbursement practices changing to include telehealth Personalized medicine Late 2000s ARRA and HITECH Act passed	Internet expansion continues Broadband access in rural areas Portable devices become more widespread (including multipurpose cell phones) Bar coding Advances in voice and handwriting recognition Wireless technology Podcasts, wikis, Web 2.0 technologies Standards and connectivity Radio-frequency identification devices (RFIDs)	Focus on EHR systems Health care organizations invest in information systems that promote safety (for example, CPOE, medication administration, e-prescribing, and other decision-support systems) Personal health record (offered by insurers, Google, and Microsoft) Health information exchange activities promulgated
2010+	Meaningful use of EHR Medicare and Medicaid EHR Incentive Programs in effect Affordable Care Act goes into effect New models of care and payment reform (such as accountable care organizations and bundled payment) IOM Report on Patient Safety and Health IT Implementation of ICD-10 Personalized medicine	iPads and hand-held readers more widely used Smart phones become ubiquitous "Cloud" computing Web 2.0 and social media used in innovative ways in health care Home monitoring devices and web apps Huge databases compiled by health information exchanges (HIE)	Expansion in the adoption and meaningful use of EHR systems Certification of EHR products State-supported HIEs Home as the new medical home—growth in telehealth Mobile health apps

1960s: Billing Is the Center of the Universe; Managing the Money; Mainframes Roam the Planet

It was in the mid-1960s that President Lyndon Johnson signed into law Medicare and Medicaid. These two federal programs provided, for the first time, guaranteed health care insurance benefits to the elderly and the poor. Initially, Medicare provided health care benefits primarily to individuals sixty-five and older. The program has since been expanded to provide health care coverage to individuals with long-term disabilities. Through a combination of federal and state funds, the Medicaid program provides health care coverage to the poor. Initially, both of these programs reimbursed hospitals for services using a cost-based reimbursement methodology. Basically, this meant hospitals were reimbursed for services based on their financial cost reports; in other words, they received a percentage above what they reported it cost them to render the services. Hospitals at that time were also still benefiting from the funds made available through the Hospital Survey and Construction Act (also known as the Hill-Burton Act) of 1946, which had provided them with easier access to capital to build new facilities and expand their services. In these cost-based reimbursement times, the more a hospital built, the more patients it served, and the longer the patients stayed, the more revenue the hospital generated.

Health care executives realized that to capitalize on these sources of funds, their organizations needed information systems that could automate the patient billing process and facilitate accurate cost reporting. Most of the early information systems in health care were therefore administrative applications almost exclusively driven by financial needs. The primary focus was to collect and process patient demographic data and insurance information and merge it with charge data to produce patient bills. The sooner the hospital could bill Medicare or Medicaid, the sooner it could get paid for services. Patient accounting systems also enabled hospitals to keep better records of all activities, reducing the amounts of *lost charges* and *unbilled services*. Revenue reports and volume of service statistics were needed to justify new capital equipment, just as billing, accounts receivable, and general ledger data were needed for reimbursement. Few clinical data were captured by these information systems.

The administrative applications that existed in the 1960s were generally found in large hospitals, such as those affiliated with academic medical centers. These larger facilities were often the only ones with the resources and staff available to develop, implement, and support such systems. These facilities often developed their own administrative or financial information systems in-house, in what were then known as "data processing" departments. Reflecting its primary purpose, the data processing department was generally under the direction of the finance department or chief financial officer. The data

Figure 4.1. Typical mainframe computer

Source: Medical University of South Carolina.

processing department got its name from the fact that the systems were transaction based, with the primary function of processing billing data.

These early administrative and financial applications ran on large *mainframe computers* (Figure 4.1), which had to be housed in large rooms, with sufficient environmental controls and staff to support them. Because the IS focus at the time was on automating manual administrative processes and computers were so expensive, only the largest, most complex tasks were candidates for mainframe computing. The high cost limited the development of departmental or clinical systems, although there were notable efforts in this direction, such as the Technicon system at El Camino Hospital. The mainframe was also associated with centralized rather than distributed computing. Centralized computing meant that end users entered data through *dumb* terminals, which were connected to a remote computer, the mainframe, where the data were processed. A dumb terminal had no processing power itself but was simply a device for entering data and viewing results.

Recognizing that small, community-based hospitals could not bear the high cost of an in-house, mainframe system, leading vendors began to offer *shared systems*, so called because they allowed hospitals to share the use of a mainframe with other hospitals. A hospital using a shared system captured billing data manually or electronically and sent them in *batch* form to a company that then processed the claims for the hospital. Most shared systems processed data in a central or regional data center. Shared Medical Systems (now known as Siemens), located in Malvern, Pennsylvania, was one of the first vendors to offer data processing services to hospitals. These vendors charged participating hospitals for computer time and storage, for the number of terminals connected, and for reports. Like many of the in-house systems, most shared systems began with financial and patient accounting functions and gradually migrated toward clinical functions, or applications.

1970s: Clinical Departments Wake Up; Debut of the Minicomputer

By the 1970s, health care costs were escalating rapidly, partially due to high Medicare and Medicaid expenditures. Rapid inflation in the economy, expansion of hospital expenses and profits, and changes in medical care, including greater use of technology, medications, and conservative approaches to treatment, also contributed to the spiraling health care costs. Health care organizations began to recognize the need for better access to clinical information for specific departments and for the facility as a whole. Departmental systems began to emerge as a way to improve productivity and capture charges and thereby maximize revenues.

The development of departmental systems coincided with the availability of *minicomputers*. Minicomputers were smaller and also more powerful than some mainframe computers and available at a cost that could be justified by a clinical department such as laboratory or pharmacy. At the same time, improvements in handling clinical data and specimens often showed a direct impact on the quality of patient care because of faster turnaround of tests, more accurate results, and a reduction in the number of repeat procedures (Kennedy, Davis, & Heda, 1992). The increased demand for patient-specific data coupled with the availability of relatively low-cost minicomputers opened a market for a host of new companies that wanted to develop applications for clinical departments, particularly *turnkey systems*. These software systems, which were developed by a vendor and installed on a hospital's computers, were known as turnkey systems because all a health care organization had to do was turn the system on and it was fully operational. Rarely could a turnkey system be modified to meet the unique information needs of an organization, however. What you saw was essentially what you got.

As in the 1960s, the health care executive's involvement in information system–related decisions was generally limited to working to secure the funds needed to acquire new information systems, although now executives were working with individual clinical as well as administrative departments on this issue. Most systems were still stand-alone and did not interface well with other administrative or clinical information systems in the organization.

1980s: Computers for the Masses; Age of the Cheap Machine; Arrival of the Computer Utility

Although the use of health care information systems in the 1970s could be considered an extension of the applications used in the 1960s with a slight increase in the use of clinical applications, the 1980s saw an entirely different story. Sweeping changes in how Medicare reimbursed hospitals and others for services, coupled with the advent of the microcomputer, radically changed how health care information systems were viewed and used. In 1982, Medicare shifted from a cost-based reimbursement system for hospitals to a prospective payment system based on *diagnosis related groups (DRGs)*. This new payment system had a profound effect on hospital billing practices. Reimbursement amounts were now dependent on the patient's diagnosis, and the accuracy of the ICD-9-CM codes used for each patient and his or her subsequent DRG assignment became critical. Hospitals received a predetermined amount based on the patient's DRG, regardless of the cost to treat that patient. The building and revenue enhancement mode of the 1960s and 1970s was no longer always the best strategy for a hospital financially. The incentives were now directed at ordering fewer diagnostic tests, performing fewer therapeutic procedures, and planning for the patient's discharge at the time of admission. Health care executives knew they needed to reduce expenses and maximize reimbursement. Services that had once been available only in hospitals now became more widespread in less resource-intensive outpatient settings and ambulatory surgery centers. As Medicare and many state Medicaid programs began to reimburse hospitals under the DRG-based system, many private insurance plans quickly followed suit.

Hospitals were not the only ones singled out to contain health care costs. Overall health care costs in the 1980s rose by double the rate of inflation. Health insurance companies argued that the traditional *fee-for-service* method of payment to physicians failed to promote cost containment. Managed care plans began to emerge in parts of the nation, and they reimbursed physicians based on *capitated* or fixed rates.

At the same time, as changes were made in reimbursement practices, large corporations began to integrate the organizations making up the hospital system (previously a decentralized industry), enter many other health care–related businesses, and consolidate control. Overall there was a shift toward privatization and corporatization of health care. The integrated delivery system began to emerge, whereby health care organizations offered a spectrum of health care services, from ambulatory care to acute hospital care to long-term care and rehabilitation.

With these environmental changes happening in health care, the development of the *microcomputer* in the mid-1980s could not have been more timely. The microcomputer, or personal computer (PC), was smaller, often as or more powerful, and far more affordable than a mainframe computer. Health care information system vendors were developing administrative and clinical applications for a variety of health care settings and touting the possibilities available in bringing "real computing power" to the user at his or her workstation. Health care executives viewed this as an enormous opportunity for health care organizations, particularly hospitals, to acquire and implement needed clinical information systems. Again, the major focus was on revenue-generating departments.

Although most organizations had patient demographic and insurance information available in their administrative applications, rarely were they able to integrate the clinical and the financial information needed to evaluate care and the cost of delivering that care in this new environment. Most of the clinical information systems or applications were being acquired piecemeal. For example, it was not uncommon for the director of laboratory services to go out and purchase from the vendor community the "best" laboratory information system, the pharmacy director to select the "best" pharmacy system, and so forth. This concept of selecting the "best of breed" among vendors and systems became prevalent in the 1980s and still exists to some extent today. Organizations that adopted the best-of-breed approach then faced a challenge when they tried to build interfaces or integrate data so that the different systems could interoperate or communicate with each other. Even today, system integration remains a challenge for many health care organizations despite progress in the use of interoperability standards.

The use of microcomputers was not confined to large hospitals. During this era a computer market opened among home health organizations, small hospital departments, and physician practices. These health care settings had historically lacked the financial and personnel resources to support information systems. The advent of the microcomputer brought computing capabilities to a host of these smaller organizations. It also led to users' being more demanding of information systems, asking the information system function to be more responsive.

Sharing information among microcomputers also became possible with the development of *local area networks (LAN)*. A local area network is a group of computers and associated devices that share a common communications line or wireless link and are controlled by a single organization. Typically, connected devices share the resources of a single processor or server within a small geographic area (for example, within an office building) or within a certain geographic location. One or more *servers* house applications and data storage that are then shared by multiple PC users. A LAN may serve as few as two or three users (for example, in a home network) or as many as thousands of users (for example, in a large academic medical center).

1990s: Round One of Health Care Reform; Advent of the Internet

The 1990s marked another time of great change in health care. It also marked the evolution and widespread use of the Internet along with a new focus on electronic medical records. In 1992, owing partly to the success of the DRG-based reimbursement system for hospitals, Medicare introduced a new method for reimbursing physicians. Formerly paid under a customary, prevailing, and reasonable rate methodology, physicians treating Medicare patients were now reimbursed for services under the *resource-based relative value scale (RBRVS)*. The RBRVS payment method factored provider time, effort, and degree of clinical decision making into relative value units. RBRVS was initially designed to redistribute funds from specialty providers to primary care providers. That is, the system would reward financially the physicians who spent time educating patients but would discourage or limit reimbursement to highly skilled specialists who tended to perform invasive procedures and order an extensive number of diagnostic and therapeutic tests.

Under the RBRVS system, primary care physicians such as family medicine, internal medicine, and pediatric physicians began to see slight increases in reimbursement for their services, and specialty physicians such as ophthalmologists, surgeons, and radiologists experienced decreases in payments. In addition to this new payment scheme for physicians, health care organizations and communities promoted preventive medicine with the goal of promoting health and well-being and preventing disease. Much of this preventive medicine and health promotion occurred in the primary care physician's practice. The emphasis on preventive medicine was the foundation on which the concept of managed care was built. The thought was that if we educate and help keep patients well, the overall cost of providing health care services will be lower in the long run. The primary care provider was viewed as the *gatekeeper* and assumed a pivotal role in the management of the patient's care.

Under this managed care model, physicians were reimbursed on a capitated or fixed rate (for example, per member per month) or some type of discounted rate (for example, preferred provider).

The changes in physician reimbursement and the increased focus on prevention guidelines and disease management in the 1990s had implications for the community-based physician practice and its use of information systems. Up until this time, most of the major information systems development had occurred in hospitals. Some administrative information systems were used in physician practices for billing purposes, but as physician payment relied increasingly on documentation substantiated in the patient's record and as computers became more affordable, physicians began to recognize the need for timely, accurate, and complete financial *and* clinical information. Early adopters of clinical information systems also found electronic prompts and preventive health reminders helpful in managing patient care more effectively and efficiently. Likewise, more vendor products designed specifically with the physician practice setting in mind were becoming available.

Health plans, particularly those with a managed care focus, began encouraging health care providers to manage the care of patients differently, particularly patients with chronic diseases. Practice guidelines and standards of care were developed and made available to physicians to use in caring for these patients. Subsequently, several vendors developed electronic *disease management programs* that facilitated the management of chronic diseases and were incorporated into clinical applications. Patients could assume a more active role in monitoring their own care. For example, clinicians at Partners Community Healthcare introduced a disease management program called Matrix that enables providers to plan, deliver, monitor, and improve the quality and outcomes of the treatment and care delivered to patients with diabetes. This program gives clinicians the tools to automate the planning and delivery of patient care as well as monitor and analyze clinical results on an ongoing basis. Disease management programs had also proven in these early years to be effective in helping providers and patients manage mental health issues and conditions such as hypertension, asthma, and unstable angina (Raymond & Dold, 2002).

In 1991, the Institute of Medicine (IOM) published its landmark report *The Computer-Based Patient Record: An Essential Technology for Health Care*. This report brought international attention to the numerous problems inherent in paper-based medical records and called for the adoption of the computer-based patient record (CPR) as the standard by the year 2001. The IOM defined the CPR as "an electronic patient record that resides in a system specifically designed to support users by providing accessibility to complete and accurate data, alerts, reminders, clinical decision support systems, links to medical knowledge, and other aids" (IOM, 1991, p. 11). This vision of a patient's record offered far more than an electronic version of existing paper records—the IOM report viewed the CPR as a tool to assist the clinician in caring for the patient by providing him or her with reminders, alerts, clinical decision-support capabilities, and access to the latest research findings on a particular diagnosis or treatment modality. We will discuss the status of CPR systems and related concepts (for example, the electronic health record) in the next chapter. At this point in the history and evolution of health care information systems, it is important to understand the IOM report's impact on the vendor community and health care organizations. Leading vendors and health care organizations saw this report as an impetus toward radically changing the ways in which patient information is managed and patient care is delivered. During the 1990s, a number of vendors developed CPR systems. Yet only 10 percent of hospitals and less than 15 percent of physician practices had implemented them by the end of the decade (Goldsmith, 2003). These percentages are particularly low when one considers the fact that by the late 1990s, CPR systems had reached the stage of reliability and technical maturity needed for widespread adoption in health care.

Five years after the IOM report advocating computer-based patient records was published, President Clinton signed into law the Health Insurance Portability and Accountability Act (HIPAA) of 1996. HIPAA was designed to make health insurance more affordable and accessible, but it also included important provisions to simplify administrative processes and to protect the confidentiality of personal health information. All of these initiatives were part of a larger health care reform effort and a federal interest in health care IT for purposes beyond reimbursement. Before HIPAA, it was not uncommon for health care organizations and health plans to use an array of systems to process and track patient bills and other information. Health care organizations provided services to patients with many different types of health insurance and had to spend considerable time and resources to make sure each claim contained the proper format, codes, and other details required by the insurer. Likewise, health plans spent time and resources to ensure their systems could handle transactions from a host of different health care organizations, providers, and clearinghouses. The adoption of electronic transaction and code set standards and the greater use of standardized electronic transactions is expected to produce significant savings to the health care sector. In addition, the administrative simplification provisions led to the establishment of health privacy and security standards that went into effect in 2001 and 2003, respectively. The full impact of the initial HIPAA legislation on the health care sector is still being realized years later.

HIPAA also brought national attention to the issues surrounding the use of personal health information in electronic form. During the first half of the

1990s, microcomputers had become smaller and less expensive and were to be found not only in the workplace but in the homes of middle-class America. The Internet, historically used primarily by the U.S. Department of Defense and academic researchers, was now widely available, through the World Wide Web, to consumers, businesses, and virtually anyone with a microcomputer and a modem. Health care organizations, providers, and patients could connect to the Internet and have access to a worldwide library of resources—and at times to patient-specific health information. In the early years of its use in health care, many health care organizations and vendors used the Internet to market their services, provide health information resources to consumers, and give clinicians access to the latest research and treatment findings. Other health care organizations saw Internet use as a strategy for changing how, where, and when they delivered health care services. The Internet provided affordable and nearly universal connectivity, enabling health care organizations, providers, and patients to connect to each other and the rest of the health care system. Along with the microcomputer, the Internet is perhaps the single greatest technological advancement in this era. It revolutionized the way that consumers, providers, and health care organizations access health information, communicate with each other, and conduct business.

With the advent of the Internet and the availability of microcomputers came *electronic mail* (e-mail). Consumers began to use e-mail to communicate with colleagues, businesses, family, and friends. It substantially reduced or eliminated needs for telephone calls and regular mail. E-mail is fast, easy to use, and widespread. Consumers soon discovered that they could not only search the Internet for the latest information on a particular condition but could then also e-mail that information or questions to their physicians. Currently, more than two-thirds of American adults want e-mail access to their physicians to ask questions and discuss their health (Sarasohn-Kahn, 2011).

The use of *telemedicine* and *telehealth* has also become more prevalent during the past few decades, particularly during the 1990s with its major advancements in telecommunications. Telemedicine is the use of telecommunications for the clinical care of patients and may involve various types of electronic delivery mechanisms. It is a tool that enables providers to deliver health care services to patients at distant locations. Most telemedicine programs have been pilot programs or demonstration projects that have not endured beyond the life of specific research and development funding initiatives.

Reimbursement policies for these services vary, and that has been a significant limiting factor. The Balanced Budget Act of 1997 authorized Medicare to reimburse for telemedicine services, but with a very limited focus. In 2003, federal legislation allowed health care organizations to be reimbursed for professional consultations via telecommunication systems with specific clinicians when patients are seen at qualifying sites. More recently, Medicare expanded the telemedicine services covered, but in the 1990s, reimbursement for telemedicine services was a significant limiting issue. State reimbursement policies for telemedicine for Medicaid patients vary from state to state. Most states do not have a single, central organization responsible for telemedicine issues or a complete data repository containing all relevant rules, regulations, and policies for all payers and programs, so it is difficult to gain a comprehensive view of the reimbursement issues nationally (Hall & Hall, 2009). In many states, the physician providing the telemedicine services must be licensed in the state where the patient is located, making licensure an issue as well.

2000 to 2010: Health Care IT Arrives; Patients Take Center Stage

Health care quality and patient safety emerged as top priorities at the start of the millennium. In 2000, the IOM published the report *To Err Is Human: Building a Safer Health Care System*, which brought national attention to research estimating that 44,000 to 98,000 patients die each year due to medical errors. A subsequent report by the Institute of Medicine Committee on Data Standards for Patient Safety—*Patient Safety: Achieving a New Standard for Care* (2004)—called for health care organizations to adopt information technology capable of collecting and sharing essential health information on patients and their care. This IOM committee examined the status of standards, including standards for health data interchange, terminologies, and medical knowledge representation. Here is an example of the committee's conclusions:

> As concerns about patient safety have grown, the health care sector has looked to other industries that have confronted similar challenges, in particular, to the airline industry. This industry learned long ago that information and clear communications are critical to the safe navigation of an airplane. To perform their jobs well and guide their plane safely to its destination, pilots must communicate with the airport controller concerning their destination and current circumstances (e.g., mechanical or other problems), their flight plan, and environmental factors (e.g., weather conditions) that could necessitate a change in course. Information must also pass seamlessly from one controller to another to ensure a safe and smooth journey for planes flying long distances; provide notification of airport delays or closures due to weather conditions; and enable rapid alert and response to extenuating circumstance, such as a terrorist attack.
>
> Information is as critical to the provision of safe health care—care that is free of errors of both commission and omission—as it is to the safe operation of aircraft. To develop a treatment plan, a doctor must have access to complete

patient information (e.g., diagnoses, medications, current test results, and available social supports) and to the most current science base [IOM Committee on Data Standards for Patient Safety, 2004].

Whereas *To Err Is Human* focused primarily on errors that occur in hospitals, the 2004 report examined the incidence of serious safety issues in other settings as well, including ambulatory care facilities and nursing homes. Its authors point out that earlier research on patient safety focused on errors of commission, such as prescribing a medication that has a potentially fatal interaction with another medication the patient is taking, and they argue that errors of omission are equally important. An example of an error of omission is failing to prescribe a medication from which the patient would likely have benefited (IOM Committee on Data Standards for Patient Safety, 2003). A significant contributing factor to the unacceptably high rate of medical errors reported in these two reports and many others is poor information management practices. Illegible prescriptions, unconfirmed verbal orders, unanswered telephone calls, and lost medical records can all place patients at risk.

Since the time the first IOM report was published, major purchasers of health care have taken a stand on improving the quality of care delivered in health care organizations across the nation by promoting the use of health care IT. The Leapfrog Group, for example, an initiative of public and private organizations that provide health care benefits to their employees, works to improve patient safety by identifying problems and proposing solutions for hospital systems. It has developed a list of criteria by which health care organizations should be judged in the future. One of the Leapfrog Group's many recommendations to improve patient safety is the widespread adoption of computerized provider order entry (CPOE) systems among health care organizations. CPOE systems will be discussed more fully in the next chapter, but in the context of today's health care information systems, they are a significant tool for decreasing errors made in the ordering and administration of medications and diagnostic and therapeutic tests.

The federal government has also responded to quality concerns by promoting health care transparency (for example, making quality and price information available to consumers) and furthering the adoption of health care IT. In 2003, the Medicare Modernization Act was passed, which expanded the program to include prescription drugs and mandated the use of electronic prescribing (*e-prescribing*) among health plans providing prescription drug coverage to Medicare beneficiaries. A year later (2004), President Bush called for the widespread adoption of electronic health record systems within the decade to improve efficiency, reduce medical errors, and improve quality of care. By 2006 he had issued an executive order directing federal agencies that administer or sponsor health insurance programs to make information about prices paid to health care providers for procedures and information on the quality of services provided by physicians, hospitals, and other health care providers publicly available. This executive order also encouraged adoption of health information technology (HIT) standards to facilitate the rapid exchange of health information (The White House, 2006).

During this period significant proposed changes in reimbursement practices also materialized in an effort to address patient safety and health care quality and cost concerns. Historically, health care providers and organizations have been paid for services rendered regardless of patient quality or outcome. Nearing the end of the decade, payment reform became a hot item. For example, *pay for performance* (P4P) or *value-based purchasing* pilot programs became more widespread. P4P reimburses providers based on meeting predefined quality measures and thus is intended to promote and reward quality. The Centers for Medicare and Medicaid Services (CMS) notified hospitals and physicians that future increases in payment will be linked to improvements in clinical performance. Medicare also announced it would no longer pay hospitals for the costs of treating certain conditions that could reasonably have been prevented—such as bedsores, injuries caused by falls, and infections resulting from the prolonged use of catheters in blood vessels or the bladder—or for treating "serious preventable" events—such as leaving a sponge or other object in a patient during surgery or providing the patient with incompatible blood or blood products. Private health plans have followed Medicare's lead and are also denying payment for such mishaps.

In addition to the considerable activity that has occurred at the national level in promoting adoption of health care IT and making price and quality information publicly available, significant technological advances occurred in information technology between 2000 and 2010. Electronic devices became smaller, more portable, less expensive, and multipurpose. Broadband access to the Internet became widely available, even in remote, rural communities; wireless technology and portable devices (personal digital assistants, multipurpose cell phones, and so forth) are ubiquitous; significant progress has been made in the area of standards (which will be discussed in Chapter Ten); podcasts, wikis, and Web 2.0 technologies have emerged; and radio-frequency identification devices (RFIDs), used more widely in other industries, have found their way into the health care marketplace.

Some consumers have also assumed a much more active role in managing their health and health information by maintaining their own personal health records (PHRs) or in accessing their personal health information electronically via a secure patient portal. Unlike an EHR, which contains data collected and managed by a health care provider or organization, a PHR is consumer controlled. It is envisioned as a lifelong and comprehensive health record that is accessible from any place at any time (Tang, Ash, Bates, Overhage, & Sands, 2006). A patient portal is generally a Web-based access to administrative or clinical information, giving patients the opportunity to schedule appointments online, view or pay bills, view test results, and send secure messages to their health care provider. Health plans, insurance companies, and companies such as Google and Microsoft made PHRs available to consumers, via secure Web sites, to store their personal health information. Google discontinued its PHR in 2011 after finding most consumers either did not know what a PHR is or did not trust sharing personal health information with a third party. Those that do have a PHR tend to use physician, hospital, or health plan portals to keep track of their records (McGee, 2011). PHRs are described more fully in the next chapter, but they are introduced here as an important development in the evolution of health care information systems.

As progress was being made on a number of fronts nationally, a substantial amount of activity occurred at regional and local levels as well. Regional health information organizations (RHIOs) and health information exchange (HIE) initiatives have emerged that bring multiple stakeholders such as provider organizations (hospitals, physicians, community health clinics, local public health departments, and emergency departments, for example), health plans, payers, and consumer groups into formal partnerships to exchange health data electronically. The purpose of the exchange is to improve quality and patient safety and to address inefficiencies and rising costs in the health care system. A recent national survey reported that 255 HIE initiatives in various stages of development exist today, while in 2004 there were a few dozen (eHealth Initiative, 2011). Some of the early RHIOs have not been able to sustain operations financially (Adler-Milstein, McAfee, Bates, & Jha, 2007). For the most part, RHIO and HIE initiatives have migrated to a model whereby multiple, diverse stakeholders participate in the effort and share costs and governance.

At the institution level, hospitals and health system organizations continue to move forward with the adoption and implementation of systems that promote patient safety, including clinical documentation systems and bar-coding medication administration, CPOE, and electronic health record (EHR) systems. Physicians had also begun to invest in health care information systems, including EHRs, but most are in large practices of fifty or more providers. By the end of the decade, approximately 25 percent of physician practices had implemented "basic" EHR systems (Hsiao, Hing, Socey, & Cai, 2011) and 12 percent of hospitals (Jha, DesRoches, Kralovec, & Joshi, 2010). The vast majority of solo and small physician practices continue to use paper-based medical record systems. Studies have shown that the relatively low adoption rates among solo and small physician practices is due to the cost of health care IT and the misalignment of incentives (Burt, Hing, & Woodwell, 2005; DesRoches et al., 2008). Patients, payers, and purchasers have the most to gain from physician use of EHR systems, yet it is the physician who generally bears the total cost. To address this misalignment of incentives and provide health care organizations and providers with some funding for EHR adoption and meaningful use, the HITECH Act (part of the American Recovery and Reinvestment Act of 2009) passed, creating funding opportunities through the establishment of Medicare and Medicaid EHR Incentive Programs. Realizing that financial resources are not all that is needed to support hospitals and practitioners in becoming meaningful users of EHRs systems, HITECH also funded a number of projects that led to the establishment of health IT workforce training programs, regional extension centers, statewide HIE initiatives, and other programs that would foster health IT research and further development.

2010 to Today: The Era of Accountability, Transparency, and Change; Affordable Care Act, Meaningful Use, and ICD-10 All Kick in

We are in a time of extraordinary change and increased accountability as the federal government, in partnership with the private sector and public agencies, strives to transform our nation's health care system to one where health care providers, hospitals, and consumers use electronic health record (EHR) systems in meaningful ways to improve quality and safety and reduce costs and inefficiencies. Health care IT is viewed as a central component of a safe, high-quality health care system. Two significant pieces of legislation that helped drive these efforts include the HITECH Act and the Patient Protection and Affordable Care Act signed into law by President Obama in March 2010. Combined, these two laws are perhaps the most significant pieces of health care legislation since the enactment of the Medicare and Medicaid programs in 1965. In fact, we devote Chapter Six (new to this edition) in its entirety to discussing the important aspects of the HITECH Act and the Affordable Care Act as they pertain to health care IT and information and knowledge management.

In short, the HITECH Act made available incentive money through the Medicare and Medicaid EHR Incentive Programs for eligible professionals and hospitals to adopt and become "meaningful users" of EHR systems. Health care provider organizations must meet certain meaningful use criteria, unveiled in three stages over the course of the next few years, or risk reductions in Medicare payments. In addition, through the support of HITECH grant funds, a range of HIT workforce training programs and regional extension centers were established to provide the people, skills, resources, and infrastructure needed to assist providers in the selection and implementation process. Seventeen Beacon Communities were identified from around the United States that could serve as model sites for other communities. State and regional health information exchanges (HIEs) became more widespread, with plans established in all areas to facilitate electronic communication and connectivity across communities. The combined efforts of these HITECH initiatives were intended to achieve the overall arching goals of

- Improved individual and population health outcomes
- Increased transparency and efficiency
- Improved ability to study and improve care delivery through the widespread adoption and use of health information technology

Concurrent with the movement to further the adoption and use of health care IT, the Affordable Care Act aims to reform certain aspects of private and public health insurance programs, increases coverage for individuals with preexisting conditions, expands access to insurance to over thirty million Americans, and requires U.S. citizens to have health care insurance. The Act also has provisions that compel health care executives and clinicians to explore new models of delivery care, such as accountable care organizations (ACOs) and patient-centered medical homes (PCMHs), and prepare their organizations for alternative payment methods. The trend is to move away from the traditional fee-for-service model that tends to promote overutilization with little, if any, regard for quality or outcome and to move toward paying providers bundled payments for an episode of care. In the new models, providers and health care organizations are held accountable for managing the quality and cost of care. Incentives would be aligned to provide coordinated, integrated, and team-based care in which the patient assumes an active role in managing his or her own health. Consequently, the IT implications of health care reform are significant. They include, but are not limited to

- Implementing and using in meaningful ways certified EHR technology
- Participating in health information exchange
- Engaging patients in monitoring their own care
- Establishing systems that help to coordinate care
- Ensuring that systems track cost and quality performance

In the midst of a flurry of activity to further the rapid adoption of health IT, the Office of the National Coordinator for Health Information Technology asked the Institute of Medicine to establish a committee to examine how private and public sectors could work together to ensure that health IT–assisted care was safe care. Instances of harm from health care information systems such as CPOE have been reported in the literature (Del Beccaro, Jeffries, Eisenberg, & Harry, 2006; Han et al., 2005), and the concern is that if health IT is designed and applied inappropriately, it can add an additional layer to an already complex system of care, which could lead to unintended adverse consequences such as dosing errors or delaying treatment due to poor human-computer interface or loss of data (IOM, 2011). The IOM (2011) recently published a report titled *Health IT and Patient Safety: Building Safer Systems for Better Care*, in which they offer a number of recommendations to ensure health IT systems are safe. In brief, they suggest that safety is a shared responsibility between vendors and health care organizations and requires

- Building systems using user-centered design principles with adequate testing and simulation
- Embedding safety considerations throughout implementation process
- Developing and publishing best practices
- Having accreditation agencies (such as the Joint Commission) assume a significant role in testing as part of their accreditation criteria
- Focusing on shared learning and transparency
- Creating a nonpunitive environment for reporting (IOM, 2011)

We discuss some of the IOM safety recommendations more fully, particularly as they pertain to the system implementation process, in Chapter Eight. The systems that are being implemented to help promote and ensure patient safety must also cause no harm. As EHR, PHRs, and other health IT systems become more widely deployed and used, it will be critical to develop best practices based upon research and ongoing quality improvement activities.

At the same time as health care provider organizations are grappling with meaningful use, health care reform, and payment reform, the long awaited ICD-10-CM is slated for implementation in 2014. At the time of this writing, organizations are still in the preparation and planning stages. There are actually two separate codes. ICD-10-CM (clinical modification) is a set of diagnosis codes used by insurance companies, health plans, hospitals, and providers. ICD-10-PCS is the procedure coding system. The number of codes increases significantly, from approximately 17,000 in ICD-9 to 155,000 in ICD-10, providing much more granularity and detail. Converting from the old system to the new one is no small task. It involves everything from reeducating coders and physicians to upgrading coding and billing systems (Diamond, 2008).

What does this decade hold for us in terms of the use of health care IT? First, we need to look at a few technological advances and trends in recent years, as well as those predicted by Gartner (2011) to have a significant impact on organizations in the next few years.

- **"Cloud" computing** is a broad term that is often used to describe hosted services delivered over the Internet. A cloud can be private or public. A private cloud is a closed or proprietary network that supplies services to a limited number of people. A public cloud sells services to anyone on the Internet, such as Amazon Web Services or Google Docs. The goal of cloud computing is to provide easy, scalable access to computing resources and IT services. The three broad categories of cloud computing services are

  - Infrastructure as a service: provides virtual server space and storage

  - Platform as a service: a set of software and product development tools where developers create applications on the provider's platform over the Internet (such as Google Apps)

  - Software as a service: a vendor supplies the hardware infrastructure and the software product and interacts with the user through a front-end portal (such as web-based e-mail and inventory management)

- **Mobile Applications and Media Tablets.** More people have mobile phones than those who have access to the Internet. Mobile devices including smart phones have available thousands of applications for platforms like the Apple iPhone and iPad or Kindle Fire.

- **Social Communications and Collaborations.** Social media include social networking (such as Facebook and LinkedIn); social collaboration technologies (such as wikis, blogs, instant messages, and collaborative office); social publishing (such as YouTube); and social feedback—seeing opinions from the community on items as witnessed on YouTube, Flickr, Amazon, and the like. Nearly one third of Americans who go online to research their health currently use social networks to find fellow patients and discuss their conditions before making health care decisions (Elkins, 2008). Social networking has also been used by organizations to provide information to consumers and seek their input. For example, during the 2009 flu season, H1N1 YouTube videos were viewed 2.6 million times, podcasts were downloaded 1.5 million times, and the CDC Facebook page had over fifty thousand followers (CDC, 2009).

- **Next Generation Analytics.** These tools enable users to run simulations or models to predict future outcomes in real time to support decision making. Organizations need to have analytical tools to make data-driven care decisions based on real-time data. Drug interactions, recommended treatments, and evidence-based medicine appropriate to the patient will need to be available at the point of care (Taylor, 2010).

These trends in information technology suggest that during this decade we will continue to see the growth of telehealth and remote monitoring, mobile applications for promoting health and monitoring chronic disease, and engaging patients more fully in their own care (Hall & Hall, 2009). Personalized medicine is also likely to be enabled through advancements in health information technology and the integration of information (West, 2011). It is possible to envision a future where treatments are specifically "tailored to an individual's genetic structures, prescriptions are analyzed in advance for likely effectiveness, and researchers study clinical data in real time to learn what works" (West, 2011). Through social networking sites like PatientsLikeMe, over 120,000 patients have already signed up to share information regarding a variety of different diagnoses and conditions including everything from breast cancer to rheumatoid arthritis (http://www.patientslikeme.com). Furthermore, health care provider organizations will need to have electronic health record systems and data mining tools and expertise with predicting modeling available to assist in ensuring the patient receives the right care, at the right time, in the right setting by the right care provider.

SUMMARY

Health care information system is a broad term that includes both administrative and clinical information systems. An information system is an arrangement of information (derived from data), processes, people, and information technology that interact to collect, process, store, and provide as output the information needed to support the health care organization. Administrative information systems contain primarily administrative or financial data and are used to support the management functions and general operations of the health care organization. Clinical information systems contain clinical, or health-related, data and are typically used by clinicians in diagnosing, treating, and managing the patient's care.

This chapter provided an overview of the history and evolution of health care information systems, including administrative and clinical applications, since the early 1960s. The information was presented in the context of the major events and issues that have been pertinent to health care, changes in reimbursement practices, advances in information technology, and the federal government's growing interest in IT.

Although it is still too early to tell what the next decade holds for health care information systems, if the past is any indication health care executives should keep abreast of major health issues and concerns, proposed changes to reimbursement practices, federal IT initiatives, and advances in IT. The challenge health care organizations face is to overcome the barriers to the widespread adoption of information technology. To that end, the following chapter describes a variety of clinical information systems, the major barriers to their widespread use, and the strategies health care organizations have employed to overcome these barriers.

KEY TERMS

Administrative applications (or
  administrative information
  systems)
Capitation
Clinical applications (or clinical
  information systems)
Cloud computing
Computerized provider order entry
  (CPOE)
Diagnosis related groups (DRGs)
Dumb terminals
Electronic health record (EHR)
Electronic mail (e-mail)
Electronic medical record (EMR)
E-prescribing
Fee for service
Health care information systems
Health information exchange (HIE)
Information systems

Information technology (IT)
Local area network (LAN)
Mainframe computer
Microcomputer
Minicomputer
Pay for performance (P4P)
Personal health record (PHR)
Portable devices
Regional health information
  organization (RHIO)
Resource-based relative value system
  (RBRVS)
Shared systems
Smart phones
Social media and social networking
Telehealth
Telemedicine
Turnkey system

LEARNING ACTIVITIES

1. Visit at least two different types of health care organizations, and compare and contrast the history and evolution of the information systems they use. What administrative information systems does each organization use? What clinical information systems? What factors led to the adoption or implementation of these systems? What role, if

any, do health care executives appear to have in decisions about today's information systems (for example, the planning, selection, implementation, or evaluation of these systems)? Has this role changed over time? Explain.

2. Explore the history and evolution of at least one of the following information technologies. Create a timeline that includes the technology's date of inception, major milestones, and use inside and outside the field of health care.

   a. Bar coding

   b. Voice recognition

   c. Wireless networks

   d. Portable devices (for example, smart phones and iPads)

   e. Digital imaging

   f. Artificial intelligence

   g. The Internet

   h. Electronic mail (e-mail)

   i. Wikis, blogs, tweets, and other Web 2.0 technologies

   j. Radio-frequency identification devices (RFID)

3. Interview a health care provider or executive to explore the extent to which his or her organization is using social media. What types of social media are being used? For what purposes? Are patients using social media for health care purposes? If so, to what extent? What have the patients' experiences or reactions been?

4. Conduct a literature search on a recent health information technology innovation or application of the innovation. Investigate the extent to which the innovation contributed to improved access to care, improved quality of care, reduced costs, and/or the promotion of health or wellness. Share a summary of your findings with the class. Facilitate a class discussion on other possible uses of the innovation in your community and/or state.

REFERENCES

Adler-Milstein, J., McAfee, A., Bates, D., & Jha, A. (2007). The state of Regional Health Information Organizations: Current activities and financing. *Health Affairs, Web Exclusives, 27*(1), w60.

Burt, H., Hing, E., & Woodwell, D. (2005). Electronic medical record use by office-based physicians and their practices: United States, 2006. Retrieved April 19, 2013 from http://www.cdc.gov/nchs/data/ad/ad393.pdf

Centers for Disease Control and Prevention. (2009). 2009 H1N1 flu. Retrieved February 2013 from http://www.cdc.gov/h1n1flu

Del Beccaro, M. A., Jeffries, H. E., Eisenberg, M. A., & Harry, E. D. (2006). Computerized provider order entry implementation: No association with increased mortality rates in an intensive care unit. *Pediatrics*, *118*(1), 290–295.

DesRoches, C. M., Campbell, E. G., Rao, S. R., Donelan, K., Ferris, T. G., Jha, A., . . . & Blumenthal, D. (2008). Electronic health records in ambulatory care: A national survey of physicians. *New England Journal of Medicine*, *359*(1), 50–60.

Diamond, F. (2008). Countdown nears for launch of ICD-10. *Managed Care*. Retrieved February 2013 from http://ftp.managedcaremag.com/archives/0812/0812.icd10.html

eHealth Initiative. (2011). *Report on health information exchange: Sustainable HIE in a changing landscape*. Washington, DC: Author. Retrieved February 2013 from http://www.ehealthinitiative.org/resources/viewdownload/54-annual-surveys/219-2011-report-on-health-information-exchange-sustainable-hie-in-a-changing-landscape-.html

Elkins, N. (2008). How American searches: Health and wellness. *iCrossing*. Retrieved February 2013 from http://www.icrossing.com/sites/default/files/how-america-searches-health-and-wellness.pdf

Gartner. (2011). Gartner identifies the top ten strategic technologies for 2011. Retrieved November 2011 from http://www.gartner.com/it/page.jsp?id=1454221

Goldsmith, J. (2003). *Digital medicine implications for healthcare leaders*. Chicago: Health Administration Press.

Hall, M., & Hall, P. (2009). *Telemedicine reimbursement: A national scan of current policies and emerging initiatives*. Sacramento, CA: California Telemedicine and eHealth Center.

Han, Y. Y., Carcillo, J. A., Venkataraman, S. T., Clark, R., Watson, R. S., Nguyen, T. C., . . . & Orr, R. A. (2005). Unexpected increased mortality after implementation of a commercially sold computerized physician order entry system. *Pediatrics*, *116*(6), 1506–1512.

Hsiao, C., Hing, E., Socey, T. C., & Cai, B. (2011). Electronic health record systems and intent to apply for meaningful user incentives among office-based physician practices: United States, 2001–2011. NCHS Data Brief. Retrieved February 2013 from www.nchs/data/databriefs/DB79

Institute of Medicine. (1991). *The computer-based patient record: An essential technology for health care*. Washington, DC: National Academies Press.

Institute of Medicine. (2000). *To err is human: Building a safer health system*. Washington, DC: National Academies Press.

Institute of Medicine. (2011). *Health IT and Patient Safety: Building Safer Systems for Better Care*. Washington, DC: National Academies Press.

Institute of Medicine, Committee on Data Standards for Patient Safety. (2003). *Reducing medical errors requires national computerized information systems:*

Data standards are crucial to improving patient safety. Retrieved November 2003 from http://www4.nationalacademies.org

Institute of Medicine, Committee on Data Standards for Patient Safety. (2004). *Patient safety: Achieving a new standard for care.* Washington, DC: National Academies Press.

Jha, A. K., DesRoches, C. M., Kralovec, P. D., & Joshi, M. S. (2010, Aug. 26). A progress report on electronic health records in U.S. hospitals. *Health Affairs (Millwood)*, *29*(10), 1951–1957.

Kennedy, O., Davis, G., & Heda, S. (1992). Clinical information systems: 25-year history and the future. *Journal of the Society for Health Systems*, *3*(4), 49–60.

McGee, M. K. (2011). Five reasons why Google Health failed. *Information Week Healthcare.* Retrieved February 2013 from http://www.informationweek.com /news/healthcare/EMR/231000697

Raymond, B., & Dold, C. (2002). *Clinical information systems: Achieving the vision.* Oakland, CA: Kaiser Permanente Institute for Health Policy.

Sarasohn-Kahn, J. (2011). *Primary care, everywhere: Connecting the dots across the emerging health landscape.* California HealthCare Foundation. Retrieved February 2013 from http://www.chcf.org/publications/2011/11/primary-care-everywhere

Tang, P. C., Ash, J. S., Bates, D. W., Overhage, J. M., & Sands, D. Z. (2006). Personal health records: Definitions, benefits, and strategies for overcoming barriers to adoption. *Journal of the American Medical Informatics Association*, *13*(2), 121–126.

Taylor, J. (2010). Transforming healthcare delivery with analytics: Improving outcomes and point-of-care decision making. *Decision Management Solutions.* Retrieved February 2013 from www.decisionmanagementsolutions.com

West, D. M. (2011). *Enabling personalized medicine through health information technology: Advancing the integration of information.* Washington, DC: The Brookings Institution. Retrieved February 2013 from http://www.brookings.edu /research/papers/2011/01/28-personalized-medicine-west

The White House. (2006, August). *Fact sheet: Health care transparency: Empowering consumers to save on quality care.* Retrieved February 2013 from http://www .whitehouse.gov/news/releases/2006/08/20060822.html

Whitten, J., & Bentley, L. (2007). *Systems analysis and design methods* (7th ed.). New York: McGraw-Hill/Irwin.

CHAPTER 5

Clinical Information Systems

Clinical applications such as pharmacy, radiology, and laboratory information systems have been used in health care settings for decades, yet many health care organizations and providers have been slow to adopt electronic health record (EHR) systems and computerized provider order entry (CPOE). The tide, however, is shifting. In 2009, the U.S. government launched an "unprecedented effort to reengineer" the way we capture, store, and use health information (Blumenthal, 2011, p. 2323). This effort was realized in the Health Information Technology for Economic and Clinical Health (HITECH) Act, which was part of the American Recovery and Reinvestment Act (ARRA), or stimulus bill. Nearly $30 billion has been set aside over the next ten years to support the adoption and meaningful use of EHRs and other types of health information technology with the goal of improving health and health care. Rarely, if ever, have we seen public investments in the advancement of health information technology of this magnitude (Blumenthal, 2011).

To help readers appreciate the broad spectrum of clinical information system capabilities, this chapter begins by providing a conceptual framework for understanding the major components and functions of an EHR system. We view the EHR as the hub of the organization's clinical information and as an important tool in improving patient care quality, safety, and efficiency. Our discussion centers on the value of the EHR to the patient, the provider, the health care organization, and the health care community at large. We focus on two key functions that are particularly important to patient safety: CPOE and medication administration using bar-coding technology. We also explore the applications used to deliver patient care services and to interact with patients at a distance (telemedicine and telehealth), as well as tools to engage the patient more fully in monitoring his or her own health including the personal health record and the use of patient portals.

Implementing an EHR or any other health care information system in an organization does not happen overnight. It is a process that generally occurs over a number of years. Health care organizations today are at many different stages of adoption and implementation. We conclude this chapter by discussing primary barriers to the adoption of clinical information systems, particularly EHR systems, along with the strategies being employed to overcome them.

THE ELECTRONIC HEALTH RECORD

As previously discussed, patient medical records are used by health care organizations for documenting patient care, as a communication tool for those involved in the patient's care, and to support reimbursement and research. Historically most patient records have been kept in paper form. Numerous studies have revealed the problems with paper-based medical records (Burnum, 1989; Hershey, McAloon, & Bertram, 1989; Institute of Medicine, 1991). These records are often illegible, incomplete, or unavailable when and where they are needed. They lack any type of *active* decision-support capability and make data collection and analysis very cumbersome. This passive role for the medical record is no longer sufficient in today's health care environment. Health care providers need access to active tools that afford them clinical decision-support capabilities and access to the latest relevant research findings, reminders, alerts, and other knowledge aids. Along with patients, they need access to systems that will support the integration of care across the continuum. The health record of the future will likely become as critical to the accurate diagnosis and treatment of patients as the physician's stethoscope has been to detecting heart murmurs and respiratory problems.

EHR Definition and Functions

What are electronic health records, and how do they differ from merely automating the paper record? In Chapter Four we introduced the concept of the EHR when we described the Institute of Medicine's definition of the computer-based patient record (CPR) in its 1991 report titled *The Computer-Based Patient Record: An Essential Technology for Health Care*. Since this Institute of Medicine (IOM) report was first published, a variety of terms have been used in the literature to describe EHR-related systems. By the late 1990s, the term CPR had been generally replaced with the terms *electronic medical record* (EMR) or *electronic health record* (EHR). In 2008, after having sought widespread input and consensus, the National Alliance for Health Information Technology proposed standard definitions for the electronic medical record, the electronic health record, and the personal health record. Table 5.1 displays these definitions. It is common to find the terms EMR and EHR used interchangeably. The IOM defines the EHR as a system that can perform eight electronic functions (Table 5.2); the first four functions are considered the core of an EHR, although all are important elements to achieving meaningful use.

An EHR can electronically collect and store patient data, supply that information to providers on request, permit clinicians to enter orders directly into a computerized provider order entry (CPOE) system, and advise health care practitioners by providing decision-support tools such as reminders, alerts, and access to the latest research findings or appropriate evidence-based guidelines. These decision-support capabilities make the EHR far more robust than a digital version of the paper medical record.

Figure 5.1 illustrates an EHR alert reminding the clinician that the patient is allergic to certain medication or that two medications should not be taken in combination with each other. Reminders might also show that the patient is due for a health maintenance test such as a mammography or a cholesterol test or for influenza vaccine (Figure 5.2).

Table 5.1. Health information technology definitions

Electronic Medical Record	Electronic Health Record	Personal Health Record
An electronic record of health-related information on an individual that can be created, gathered, managed, and consulted by authorized clinicians and staff in *one* health care organization.	An electronic record of health-related information on an individual that conforms to nationally recognized interoperability standards and that can be created, managed, and consulted by authorized clinicians and staff across *more than one* health care organization.	An electronic record of health-related information on an individual that conforms to nationally recognized interoperability standards and that can be drawn from multiple sources while being managed, shared, and controlled by the individual.

Source: National Alliance for Health Information Technology, 2008.

Table 5.2. Functions of an EHR system as defined by the IOM

Core Functions	Other Functions
Health information and data: includes medical and nursing diagnoses, a medication list, allergies, demographics, clinical narratives, and laboratory test results.	*Electronic communication and connectivity:* enables those involved in patient care to communicate effectively with each other and with the patient; technologies to facilitate communication and connectivity may include e-mail, Web messaging, and telemedicine.
Results management: manages all types of results (for example, laboratory test results and radiology procedure results) electronically.	
Order entry and support: incorporates use of computerized provider order entry, particularly in ordering medications.	*Patient support:* includes everything from patient education materials to home monitoring to telehealth.
Decision support: employs computerized clinical decision-support capabilities such as reminders, alerts, and computer-assisted diagnosing.	*Reporting and population health management:* establishes standardized terminology and data formats for public and private sector reporting requirements.

Source: Adapted from IOM, 2003.

Figure 5.1. Sample drug alert screen

Source: Partners HealthCare.

Figure 5.2. Sample EHR screen

Source: Partners HealthCare.

EHR Current Adoption and Use

How widely are EHR systems used in hospitals, physician practices, and other health care organizations? Up until most recently there have been few national studies to provide reliable estimates on the adoption rates of EHRs by U.S. physicians and hospitals, and estimates varied considerably. A number of professional organizations and researchers have attempted to estimate EHR adoption rates, yet accurately measuring adoption has been difficult for several reasons. First, no one definition for the EHR has been used consistently among researchers, and often convenience samples are used. Second, organizations may be in different stages of adoption. EHR adoption does not occur at a single moment in time, but rather evolves in stages over time. Further, the degree of usage and functionality can differ greatly from one organization to the next or even among divisions or departments in a single organization. It may not be clear whether health care providers use specific EHR functions such as decision support, even if they report having an EHR fully deployed.

The latest national survey of U.S. hospitals found that approximately 12 percent had either a basic or comprehensive EHR system (Jha, DesRoches, Campbell et al., 2009). A "basic system" was defined as including clinical documentation (demographics, physician notes, nursing assessments, problem lists, medication lists, and discharge summaries); lab, radiology, and diagnostic test results; as well as electronic ordering of medications. The comprehensive system included all of the basic system components in addition to advance directives, diagnostic images, consultant reports, computerized provider order entry, and decision-support functions such as drug alerts and clinical reminders. Larger hospitals, teaching facilities, and those located in urban regions are more likely to have EHRs than their small, public, and rural hospital counterparts (Jha, DesRoches, Campbell et al., 2009; Jha, DesRoches, Kralovec, & Joshi, 2010).

The adoption rates in physician practices range from an estimated 17 percent (DesRoches, Campbell, Rao et al., 2008) to 56.9 percent (Hsiao, Hing, Socey, & Cai, 2011), depending on the source and definitions used. As with hospitals, the larger the physician practice, the more likely the practice is to use an EHR system (DesRoches et al., 2008). A 2008 national survey of physicians found 4 percent of physicians report having an extensive, fully functional EHR, and 13 percent reported having a basic system (DesRoches, Campbell, Rao et al., 2008). Table 5.3 lists the differences between a basic system and a fully functional system as defined by these researchers.

Less than 7 percent of solo or two-physician practices reported having either a basic or fully functional EHR (Rao, DesRoches, Donelan et al., 2011). Even among those who have adopted EHR systems, physicians from

Table 5.3. Functions defining the use of EHRs

	Basic System	Fully Functional System
Health Information Data		
Patient demographics	X	X
Patient problem lists	X	X
Electronic lists of medications taken by patients	X	X
Clinical notes	X	X
Notes including medical history and follow-up		X
Order Entry Management		
Orders for prescriptions	X	X
Orders for laboratory tests		X
Orders for radiology tests		X
Prescriptions sent electronically		X
Orders sent electronically		X
Results Management		
Viewing laboratory results	X	X
Viewing imaging results	X	X
Electronic images returned		X
Clinical Decision Support		
Warnings of drug interactions or contraindications provided		X
Out-of-range test levels highlighted		X
Reminders regarding guidelines-based interventions or screening		X

small practices are less likely to use certain features such as viewing and ordering radiologic tests, electronic prescribing, and maintaining clinical notes electronically.

Less is known about EHR adoption rates in settings other than hospitals and physician practices. The first and only study found of home health and hospice agencies reported that approximately 32 percent of home health agencies and 18 percent of hospice agencies are estimated to use computerized systems for record keeping, although it is not clear if these systems offer the level of functionality defined by the IOM (Pearson & Bercovitz, 2006). Data used in estimating these adoption rates come from the 2000 National Home and Hospice Care Survey, conducted before the latest IOM definition existed. Some states, such as California, have attempted to assess health information technology use in nursing homes and long-term care facilities (Hudak & Sharkey, 2007), but again, EHR functions can differ in these settings, and national estimates are nearly nonexistent. Most are qualitative studies examining the barriers to adoption in long-term care facilities (Cherry, Carter, Owen, & Lockhart, 2008) and experiences of early adopters (Cherry, Ford, & Peterson, 2011).

Factors Influencing EHR Adoption

Despite the relatively low rates of EHR use historically, a number of factors are driving demand. The extraordinary focus in recent years on health information technology at the federal level is a major factor. One of the primary goals of the HITECH part of the American Recovery and Reinvestment Act (ARRA) of 2009 is to improve the quality and value of health care through meaningful use of EHR systems. The law specifies that meaningful use includes electronic prescribing, health information exchange, and the reporting of quality measures. Providers participating in Medicare and Medicaid programs have the opportunity to receive incentive dollars for achieving meaningful use of EHR, or risk Medicare payment reductions if they fail to achieve meaningful use of EHR within a specified period of time. Health care payment reform initiatives require that health care providers and organizations are able to provide high-quality, coordinated, cost-effective care and report on quality indicators and outcomes. Trying to achieve these goals in a paper-driven environment, often laden with inefficient processes and duplicate tests, is nearly impossible.

In addition, over the years a number of empirical studies suggest that there is growing evidence that EHR-type systems help improve the quality and efficiency of care. Examples of this include the Veterans Health Administration (VA), which uses an EHR systemwide, so that any veteran treated at any VA hospital throughout the nation will have electronic access to his or her medical record. The VA has also been able to transform its health care system to one of the best in the world based upon quality measures (Jha, Perlin, Kizer, & Dudley, 2003). The Kaiser Permanente Health Plan is another example of an EHR adopter that has made significant improvements in the management and treatment of patients with chronic conditions through their systemwide EHR (Chen, Garrido, Chock, Okawa, & Liang, 2009). Since the early 1990s, Institute of Medicine has called repeatedly for the increased use of EHR systems in health care (1991, 2000, 2001), provided systems are safe and implemented appropriately (2011).

Health care leaders are becoming increasingly aware of the value of EHR systems to the patient, the provider, the organization, and the health care community at large in improving quality, managing population health, addressing patient safety concerns, and decreasing administrative costs. It is no longer a matter of *if* a health care organization will adopt and implement an EHR system; it is now a matter of when and how.

Value of EHR Systems

A number of studies over the past thirty years have demonstrated the value of using EHR systems and other types of clinical information systems within organizations. The potential benefits fall into three major categories: (1) quality, outcomes, and safety; (2) efficiency, productivity, and cost reduction; and (3) service and satisfaction. Following is a discussion of each of these major categories, along with several examples illustrating the value of EHR systems to the health care process. It is important to note, however, that not all studies have demonstrated positive outcomes. Some have shown no effect and others have shown possible safety issues associated with the introduction and use of features such as CPOE (Han et al., 2005; Koppel, Metlay, Cohen, Kimmel, & Storm, 2005) and other types of health information technology (Koppel & Kreda, 2009; Sittig & Singh, 2011; Sittig, Teich, Osheroff, & Singh, 2009). With the increased interest in and adoption of health IT, the Office of the National Coordinator for Health Information Technology (ONC) asked the IOM to establish a committee to investigate how private and public participants can make health IT–assisted care safer. In 2011, the IOM published its report *Health IT and Patient Safety* and outlined a number of key recommendations that are discussed more fully in Chapter Seven.

Quality, Outcomes, and Safety

Clinical information systems, including EHRs, can have a significant impact on patient quality, outcomes, and safety. Three major effects on quality are increased adherence to guideline-based care, enhanced surveillance and monitoring, and decreased medication errors. For example, several early studies have shown that physicians who had access to clinical practice guidelines and features such as computerized reminders and alerts were far more likely to provide preventive care than were physicians who did not (Balas et al., 2000; Bates et al., 1999; Kuperman, Teich, Gandhi, & Bates, 2001; Ornstein, Garr, Jenkins, Rust, & Arnon, 1991; Teich et al., 2000). Other studies have found that computerized reminders used in an outpatient setting can have a significant effect on cancer prevention activities such as the performance of stool occult-blood tests, rectal examinations, breast examinations, smoking cessation counseling, and dietary counseling (Landis, Hulkower, & Pierson, 1992; McPhee, Bird, Fordham, Rodnick, & Osborn, 1991; McPhee, Bird, Jenkins, & Fordham, 1989; Yarnall et al., 1998). EHR-related systems have also been shown to improve drug prescribing and administration by providing clinicians with information on the appropriate use of antibiotics at the point of care (Berman, Zaran, & Rybak, 1992), to reduce adverse drug reactions (Bates & Gawande, 2003; Burke & Pestotnik, 1999), to improve the accuracy of drug dosing (Duxbury, 1982), and to reduce errors of omission such as failing to act on results or to carry out indicated tests (Bates & Gawande, 2003; Overhage, Tierney, Zhou, & McDonald, 1997). Bates and Gawande (2003) suggest that information technology can reduce the rate of medical errors by (1) preventing errors and adverse effects, (2) facilitating a more rapid response after an adverse event has occurred, and (3) tracking and providing feedback about adverse effects. Likewise, EHR systems can improve communication, make knowledge more readily available, require key pieces of information (such as the dose of the drug), assist with calculations, perform checks in real time, assist with monitoring, and provide decision support. If effectively incorporated into the care process, all of these features have the potential to improve quality, outcomes, and patient safety.

Efficiency, Productivity, and Cost Reduction

In addition to improving the quality of care the patient receives, some studies have shown that the EHR can improve efficiency, increase productivity, and lead to cost reductions (S. Barlow, Johnson, & Steck, 2004; Grieger, Cohen, & Krusch, 2007; Tierney, Miller, Overhage, & McDonald, 1993). It is not uncommon for clinicians who do not have EHR access to order a second set of tests because the results from the first set are unavailable, so one way EMR systems improve efficiency is by making test results readily available to clinicians (Bates, Kuperman et al., 1999; Tierney, McDonald, Hui, & Martin, 1988; Tierney, Miller, & McDonald, 1990). In addition, EHR features such as computerized reminders and alerts can reduce pharmaceutical costs by prompting physicians to use generic and formulary drugs (Bates & Gawande, 2003; Donald, 1989; Garrett, Hammond, & Stead, 1986; Karson et al., 1999; Levit et al., 2000). EHRs can also provide the infrastructure necessary to measure care processes and aid in continuous quality improvement efforts (Edwards, Huang, Metcalfe, & Sainfort, 2008).

The cost of EHR implementations can range from $15,000 to $50,000 per provider. A network of twenty-six primary care practices in north Texas recently conducted a study evaluating the hardware and software costs, as well as the time and effort invested in EHR implementation. The average cost per physician of implementing an EHR through the first sixty days of launch was $32,409 with an estimated 134.2 hours of staff time expended per physician (Fleming, Culler, McCorkle, Becker, & Ballard, 2011). Several studies have shown that the use of EHR systems can reduce costs related to the retrieval and storage of medical records. For instance, the Memorial Sloan-Kettering Cancer Center estimated that it realized space savings of two thousand square feet after implementing an EMR, equating to a savings of approximately $100,000 a year (Evans & Hayashi, 1994). Twenty-eight ambulatory care providers affiliated with the University of Rochester Medical Center found initial EHR costs were recaptured within sixteen months of implementation, with ongoing annual savings of $9,983 per provider (Grieger et al., 2007). Much of their savings was due to reductions in storage and retrieval costs. Savings have also been realized through the decreased use or elimination of transcription services (Zlabek, Wickus, & Mathiason, 2011). Others have reported that an EHR system has led to higher-quality documentation, resulting in improved coding practices and subsequently higher reimbursement (Barlow et al., 2004; Bleich, Safran, & Slack, 1989; Wager, Lee, White, Ward, & Ornstein, 2000) and also in savings from lower drug expenditures, reduced laboratory and radiology tests (Zlabek, Wickus, & Mathiason, 2011), and decreased billing errors (Wang et al., 2003). As to the impact of EHRs on clinician time, results are mixed. Nurses are more likely to realize time savings in using computer systems to document patient information than their physician counterparts are (Poissant, Pereira, Tamblyn, & Kawasumi, 2005). This may be due in part to the fact that nurses often document using standardized forms or care plans, whereas physicians rarely use standardized templates to document their notes. One recent time-motion study found it took twenty-five seconds longer to enter a prescription order using CPOE than to handwrite the order (Devine, Hollingworth, Hansen et al., 2010). However, the study did not examine time spent in interpreting the legibility of the handwritten orders or time spent in processing the orders. Investments in patient safety and quality of care may well be worth the investment in time.

Service and Satisfaction

The third category of potential benefits to be realized as a result of using EHR systems is improved service and satisfaction, from both the patient's and the user's perspectives. Patients whose physicians use EHR systems like the fact that their health information (health history, allergies, medications, and test results) is readily available when and where it is needed. Several early qualitative studies have shown that patients' response to physicians using an EMR in the examination room is quite positive (Ornstein & Bearden, 1994; Ridsdale & Hudd, 1994). Patients in practices that use an EHR system view their physicians as being innovative and progressive. And even though some physicians initially expressed concern that using the EHR in the examination room might distance them from patients or impede the physician-patient relationship, the majority by far of the studies in this area have shown that EMR use has had no negative impact on the physician-patient relationship (Gadd & Penrod, 2000; Legler & Oates, 1993; Shield, Goldman, Anthony, Wang, Doyle, & Borkan, 2010; Solomon & Dechter, 1995; Wager, Ward et al., 2005) and can enhance it by involving patients more fully in their own care (Marshall & Chin, 1998). Both physicians and patients at Kaiser Permanente found the EHR can expand and strengthen the physician-patient relationship (Cochran, 2010).

In fact, a recent national study of U.S. hospitals found that those with EHRs had significantly higher patient satisfaction scores on items such as "staff always giving patients information about what to do for recovery at home," "patients rating the hospital as a 9 or a 10 overall," and "patients would definitely recommend the hospital to others" than hospitals that did not (Kazley, Diana, Ford, & Menachemi, 2011, p. 26). Yet the same study found that EHR use was not significantly associated with other patient satisfaction measures (such as having clean rooms) that one would not expect to be affected by EHR use. The patient's perception of his experience and care is important, and EHRs may play an increasing role in facilitating communication.

EHR systems can also positively affect provider and support staff satisfaction. In a 2008 national survey of physicians, 90 percent of providers using EHRs reported that they were satisfied or very satisfied with them, and large majorities could point to specific quality benefits (DesRoches, Campbell, Rao et al., 2008). Those who have had systems in place for two or more years are more likely to be satisfied (Menachemi, Powers, Au, & Brooks, 2010). Physicians who have successfully implemented an EHR system in their practice have also reported that it has improved the quality of documentation, efficiency, and had a positive impact on their job satisfaction and stress levels (Wager et al., 2000, 2005, 2008). They are proud of the quality of their records and believe that their documentation is now more complete, accurate, and available and more useful in substantiating the diagnostic and procedural codes assigned for billing purposes. EHR users such as nurses and support staff have reported that the EHR has enhanced their ability to respond to patient questions promptly. Support staff who have historically been responsible for filing paper reports, pulling paper records, and processing bills tout the many benefits of having easy access to patient information through the use of an EHR system (Wager et al., 2000).

Limitations and Need for Future Research

Despite the promising work that has been done to date in evaluating EHRs, much more work is needed, particularly in studying the impact of such systems on organizations or communities that share patient data *across* organizational boundaries through a health information exchange. Until most recently, the majority of research on EHRs has been limited to four academic institutions that implemented internally developed systems over many years (Chaudhry et al., 2006). In addition, studies that have examined the impact of EHR systems on efficiency have tended to focus on the user level instead of the organizational level or, ultimately, the health system level (Poissant et al., 2005). Thus, an EHR might not save an individual physician time in documenting patient information, yet that information may be more complete and therefore may reduce unnecessary tests or improve the coordination of care, and so the process may save time or money in the long run. The "system-" level benefits such as impact on quality and cost reductions over time will be increasingly important to measure with health care reform. Some experts argue that to improve quality of care, merely implementing an EHR is not sufficient (Zhou et al., 2009). Long-term users are more likely to have relatively mature EHRs with well-designed clinical decision support and order entry management, and they may be more willing to use these features. Use of decision-support features has historically been quite low among EHR users, despite its availability (DesRoches, Campbell, Vogeli et al., 2010; Zhou et al., 2009).

Noteworthy EHR Implementations

There are many examples of health care organizations that have successfully implemented EHR systems and have realized the value that comes from using them. The following examples profile the 2011 Nicholas E. Davies Award recipients in the ambulatory care category and the community health organization category. The Nicholas E. Davies Award was established in 1994 by the Computer-Based Patient Record Institute (CPRI) to recognize organizations that have carried out exemplary implementations of EMR systems. (The Healthcare Information and Management Systems Society [HIMSS] has administered the Davies Award since 2002, the year that CPRI merged with HIMSS.)

OTHER MAJOR HCIS TYPES

In addition to EHR systems, several other clinical information systems or applications warrant discussion. The five we have selected to discuss are computerized provider order entry, medication administration, telemedicine, telehealth, and the personal health record (PHR), including providing patients with access to their health information through patient portals. We selected these systems because they have an enormous potential to improve quality, decrease costs, and improve patient safety or because they are being widely debated

2011 Davies Award Recipients: Ambulatory Care Category

The Reliant Medical Group (formerly known as the Fallon Clinic) was one of two winners in the ambulatory care category. Reliant Medical Group is a multispecialty group practice made up of 265 physicians and 92 advanced practitioners representing over 30 specialties that provides care for approximately 200,000 active patients. Their EHR journey began in 2001 when the CIO and medical director of informatics began discussing with staff at various sites which types of challenges they were facing, and a consensus emerged that an EHR would solve many of their problems. A multidisciplinary team was formed and the committee and organization identified the financial and nonfinancial benefits of EHR implementation, established a vision with objectives, and selected a vendor. They decided to use Epic and implemented the system in phases with breaks of time in between so all users could become comfortable with one change before tackling another.

The organization was also meticulous in the conversion from paper records to electronic, a lengthy process which included extensive mapping of terms and the utilization and creation of necessary interfaces. The result was a system that providers could log into and then immediately access all of the information on a patient for up to the past fifteen years. Reliant Medical Group supported their physicians by supplying them with typing courses, a note creation software for physicians who wanted to continue dictating notes, as well as demonstrations during Documentation Summits and Live Lunches. Extensive planning and coordination efforts, physician and nurse champions, thorough communication and training, and periodic EHR marketing to maintain positive momentum were some of the organization's keys to success. The organization now utilizes almost every function offered by Epic and over the course of six years saw cost savings of nearly $20 million. Reliant Medical Group is now offering a level of quality care even higher than before and has also seen increases in physician, employee, and patient satisfaction.

2011 Davies Award Recipient: Community Health Organization Category

Hudson River Healthcare, Inc., (HRHCare) was the only winner in the community health organization category. The organization provides care to the underserved, uninsured, and underinsured population of Peekskill, New York, seeing nearly 64,000 patients through over 275,000 visits each year. HRHCare's journey toward full EHR implementation was full of partnerships and collaborations with other organizations. Already valuing a robust clinical information system and data-driven decision making, the organization's first EHR implementation in 1999–2000 was spurred by the desire to capture clinical information at the point of service. In 1999, HRHCare became a beta test site for a Windows-based EHR called Cliniflow and later changed vendors in order to better meet community needs. Over the years HRHCare found that the small size of their vendor company became a barrier and they found themselves doing a lot of double entry. The need for a system with greater capability became even clearer after they participated in Preventative Pilot Collaborative in 2004. In 2006, HRHCare developed a set of Strategic Aims and Measures to guide the organization that were based on the Institute of Medicine's STEEP model and input from all levels of staff, from front-line caregivers to the Executive Team. These Strategic Aims and Measures provided the framework the organization uses to measure strategic planning success, and it was with that framework in mind that HRHCare decided to move to a new system, eClinicalWorks, in 2007. The organization has seen meaningful clinical, financial, and operational improvements and found that their ROI yield was approximately 5.23 to 1.

Source: Adapted from HIMSS, 2011.

and are likely to be hot topics for the next few years—or because they possess both these qualities. In addition, we believe no respectable health information systems text would be complete without a discussion of them!

The first two, computerized provider order entry and medication administration systems, are applications used primarily in health care settings where tests and medications are ordered, performed, or administered. Telemedicine and telehealth are means of delivering services or communicating with patients at a distance. A personal health record is a record the patient creates, maintains, and controls. Its intent is to bring together the data and information that patients need to manage their health. The record can be maintained in paper or electronic form. Each of these information systems is described in the sections that follow, along with their current use and value to the patient care delivery process.

Computerized Provider Order Entry

One of the biggest concerns facing health care organizations today is how to keep patients safe. Several Institute of Medicine studies have brought to the forefront of people's attention the fact that an estimated 98,000 patients die each year in U.S. hospitals due to medical errors (IOM, 2000, 2001). Medication errors and adverse drug events (ADEs) top the list and are common, costly, and clinically important issues to address. A *medication error* is an error in the process of ordering, dispensing, or administering a medication, whether or not an injury occurs and whether or not the potential for injury is present. An *adverse drug event* is an injury resulting from the use of a drug, a use that may or may not have involved a medication error. Thus, a medication error may lead to an adverse drug event but does not necessarily do so (Bates et al., 1999). Studies have shown that computerized provider order entry (CPOE) has the potential to reduce medication errors and adverse drug events (Bates et al., 1999; Bates & Gawande, 2003). In fact the Leapfrog Group has identified CPOE as one of three changes that it believes would most improve patient safety.

Many health care executives have taken steps to implement CPOE or are planning to do so in the near future. What is CPOE? How might it improve patient safety? How widely used are CPOE systems? We begin by defining CPOE and its major functions and then move on to discuss its current use and its potential value in improving patient safety and preventing medical errors.

Definition and Primary Functions of CPOE Systems

During a patient encounter the physician generally orders a number of diagnostic tests and therapeutic plans for the patient. In fact virtually every intervention in patient care—performing diagnostic tests, administering medications, drawing blood—is initiated by a physician's order. Historically, physicians have handwritten these orders or called them in as verbal orders for a nurse or other health care professional to document. The ordering process itself is a critical step in the patient care process and represents a point where intervention can often prevent medication errors and improve adherence to clinical practice guidelines.

CPOE at its most basic level is a computer application that accepts physician orders electronically, replacing handwritten or verbal orders and prescriptions. Most CPOE systems provide physicians with decision-support capabilities at the point of ordering. For example, an order for a laboratory test might trigger an alert to the physician that the test has already been ordered and the results are pending. An order for a drug to which the patient is allergic might

Figure 5.3. Sample CPOE screen

Source: Partners HealthCare.

trigger an alert warning the physician of the patient's allergy and possibly recommending an alternative drug. If a physician orders an expensive test or medication, the CPOE system might show the cost and offer alternative tests or drugs. CPOE systems can also provide other types of clinical decision support to the physician. For instance, if the physician is ordering a series of tests and medications for a common diagnosis, the computer can offer the use of a preprogrammed, institutionally approved set of orders to facilitate the process and can recommend drug therapy to aid the physician in following accepted protocols for that diagnosis (Metzger & Turisco, 2001) (Figure 5.3). The scope of CPOE functions and capabilities can vary considerably. The most advanced systems have sophisticated decision-support capabilities and can aid the provider in diagnosing and treating the patient by supplying information derived from knowledge-based rules and the latest research.

Current Use of CPOE

Estimating the current use of CPOE systems is almost as difficult as assessing the use of EHR systems. A CPOE system is typically an integral part of a comprehensive clinical information system or EHR system and not a stand-alone application. It is estimated that only 8 percent of hospitals have fully implemented CPOE systems (Yu et al., 2009), although approximately 17 percent of hospitals report using CPOE to order medications and 20 percent to order laboratory tests (Jha, DesRoches, Campbell et al., 2009). Hospitals that use CPOE tend to be larger, nonprofit, teaching hospitals.

Why the relatively low usage rate? Part of it may be due to the fact that historically health care executives and vendors did not believe that physicians would be interested in computerized order entry, and consequently CPOE development lagged behind the development of other clinical information system components. Even among hospitals that have implemented a full or partial CPOE system, relatively few require physicians to use the system. We anticipate that this will change in the coming years as hospitals and physicians strive to achieve meaningful use of EHR systems (described more fully in Chapter Six).

Electronic prescribing (e-prescribing) has also surged in popularity since the passage of the Medicare Prescription Drug, Improvement, and Modernization Act (MMA) of 2003, which established a prescription drug benefit for Medicare beneficiaries (Part D) and required that Part D plans support an e-prescribing program should any of their providers or pharmacies choose to prescribe electronically (Friedman, Schueth, & Bell, 2009). Since then, payers, employers, pharmacies, state governments, and others are working to promote e-prescribing adoption through incentive payments and addressing standardization issues.

Value of CPOE

Despite the relatively low usage rates, CPOE systems can provide patient care, financial, and organizational benefits. Clearly, one of the fundamental reasons that CPOE has received so much attention in recent years is its potential to improve patient safety and, more specifically, reduce medication errors (Holdsworth et al., 2007; Kazley & Diana, 2011; Walsh et al., 2008). A review of CPOE studies found that 80 percent of studies report significant reductions in total prescribing errors, 43 percent in dosing errors, and 37.5 percent in adverse drug events when CPOE rather than handwritten orders is used (Shamliyan, Duval, Jing, & Kane, 2008). The use of CPOE is also associated with a 66 percent reduction in total prescribing errors for adults and a positive tendency in children. Niazkhani and colleagues (2009) examined the impact of CPOE on clinical workflow by developing a conceptual framework and conducting a literature review of CPOE evaluations between 1990 and 2007. The most frequently reported workflow advantages cited in fifty-one studies included legibility of orders, remote access, and shorter turnaround times. Disadvantages included time-consuming and problematic user-system interactions, and the enforcement of a predefined relationship between clinical tasks and providers (Niazkhani, Pirnejad, Berg, & Aarts, 2009).

Using CPOE systems in outpatient settings shows promise as well, but not as much research has been done in this area. Authors of two studies have found that CPOE can lead to better adherence to clinical protocols and improvements in the stages of clinical decision making—that is, initiation, diagnosing, monitoring and tracking, and acting (D. Johnston, Pan, Walker, Bates, & Middleton, 2003, 2004). They also found that CPOE can lead to improved patient outcomes by reducing medical errors, decreasing morbidity and mortality, and expediting recovery times. A report from the Agency for Healthcare Research and Quality (2001) substantiates the notion that CPOE systems can significantly reduce medication errors in outpatient settings and estimates that such systems may prevent 28 to 95 percent of adverse drug events.

Besides clinical benefits, CPOE systems can also provide financial benefits to a health care organization. For example, organizations that use CPOE systems may require fewer administrative clinical staff, improve the accuracy and timeliness of billing, and increase transaction processing rates (D. Johnston et al., 2004). Studies have also showed reductions in medication turnaround times, elimination of transcription errors, and improvements in countersigning orders (Ahmad et al., 2002; Jensen, 2006).

Despite growing evidence that CPOE systems have positive effects on patient safety, there have been studies that raised concerns. In 2005, researchers from an academic children's hospital observed an unexpected increase in mortality after implementation of a vendor-acquired CPOE system (Han et al., 2005). Although some have challenged the methods used in this particular study, most would agree that CPOE technology is still evolving and requires ongoing assessment of systems integration and the effectiveness of the human-computer interface (Ash et al., 2007; Kilbridge, Classen, Bates, & Denham, 2006). A CPOE system does not operate in isolation. To function properly, it requires seamless integration within a strong and dynamic health information architecture (Han et al., 2005). Issues such as alert fatigue and the need for ongoing system enhancements are real, and without proper management, unintended consequences can occur. User training conducted by organizations should caution against providers blindly following or unreasonably ignoring alerts and should instead recommend that they use their best judgment in assessing the evidence; otherwise, there are real legal risks (Kesselheim, Cresswell, Phansalkar, Bates, & Sheikh, 2011).

In the late 1980s, the University of Virginia experienced a great deal of resistance to its CPOE initiative. Organizational leaders underestimated the impact of CPOE on clinical workflow as well as on physicians' and nurses' time and, in retrospect, did not invest sufficient resources in the effort. Many physicians, including residents, perceived the CPOE as an Information Systems Department initiative rather than as a clinician-led effort and felt it was forced upon them and offered little flexibility. Physicians complained that administration was trying to "turn them into clerks to save money." Cumbersome interfaces and time-consuming ordering processes, along with the fact that the clinical care processes were never fully redesigned, contributed to the problems encountered (Massaro, 1993a, 1993b). In 2003, Cedars-Sinai Medical Center in Los Angeles experienced some of the same problems with its CPOE system implementation and ended up "pulling the plug" on the system, as the following case study describes. It is one of the most cited cases of all time. Since then, Cedars-Sinai has implemented a different CPOE system.

PERSPECTIVE
CPOE Implementation

Cedars-Sinai Medical Center developed and implemented a computer system known as Patient Care Expert (PCX) several years ago as part of a larger project to modernize the medical center's computing infrastructure. The PCX system included a CPOE component and used browser-based technology, making the system accessible through any browser-enabled computer anytime, anywhere. Other performance criteria specified that

- "The system needed to be highly flexible, allowing for rapid modifications of content and functionality."

- "The system needed to be fully integrated with all ancillary services, patient registration, and patient accounting."

- "The system needed to be user-friendly for large groups of users with a diverse range of familiarity and experience with computers" (Langberg, 2004).

After conducting an extensive review of existing products and obtaining broad input from administration, clinicians, and information technology experts, the Cedars-Sinai board of directors decided the organization should develop an in-house product in collaboration with Perot Systems. In August 2002, after nearly three years of development and testing, Cedars-Sinai launched a pilot program of the PCX system. This pilot involved obstetrical patients over a two-week period, during which approximately 400 patients were entered into the system. As part of the pilot, more than 140 physicians and 200 department staff members used the system to care for all obstetrical patients. Clinical staff tested the system with more than 20,000 orders. By October, more than 2,000 physicians had been trained and certified to use PCX. The pilot was felt to have been very successful, and minor changes were made to the PCX before rolling it out to other areas of the medical center. By January 2003, 700,000 orders had been placed for more than 7,000 patients—more than 10,000 orders per day. The system was operational for more than two-thirds of the medical center's inpatients. However, in late January 2003, the system was suspended after hundreds of physicians complained that the system slowed down the ordering process and said they feared that orders were getting lost in the system. The medical center had worked with a forty-physician medical executive committee throughout the development and implementation process, and the administration believed that physicians were sufficiently involved throughout the project. However, rank-and-file physicians argued that the committee did not represent their views (Chin, 2003). One physician, for example, argued that the CPOE was very cumbersome and didn't follow physician workflow. This same physician complained that to order an antibiotic, doctors had to go through three or four computer screens and wait six to eight seconds between screens (Chin, 2003). After receiving such complaints, the administration made the decision to take down the CPOE system. Those involved in the implementation reported that they found themselves managing two complex processes:

1. *"Physician change management:* Four months into 'go-live' physicians remained deeply concerned about the added time they reported in entering orders and their negative perception of the system's ease of use. Further, [it was] believed that too many physicians . . . did not have an optimal working knowledge of the system's functionality.

2. *"Workflow change management:* The procedures involved in hospital-based patient care are complex in any environment and need to be carefully and thoroughly understood in advance of automation. Additionally, CPOE will affect the workflow of all caregivers. [It was found that] far more operational workflow analysis and adjustment needed [to occur] after the 'go-live' than was initially anticipated" (Langberg, 2004).

(cont.)

> Besides managing these two processes, the management team has instituted a number of system enhancements and has aggregated input from all users to enhance PCX and improve the implementation and workflow procedures. By intensifying training and support resources, and accelerating the system response time, management expects to improve physicians' experiences.
>
> *Source:* Adapted from Langberg, 2004.

We will discuss a host of issues related to the implementation of CPOE and other applications more fully in Chapter Eight. At this point, however, it is important to understand that CPOE systems can have a dramatic impact on physicians—how they spend their time, their work patterns, and the functions they perform. CPOE is an expensive and complex project that touches almost all aspects of the health care operation. It is not simply a niche computer system to replace handwritten orders. Rather, CPOE is a tool to aid the provider in order management. It can directly affect not only physician ordering but also physician decision making (through the decision-support features) and care planning, pharmacist decision making and workflow, nursing workflow and documentation, and communication with ancillary services. Just as automating the paper medical record is not the same as implementing an EHR system, automating the ordering process is not the same as implementing a CPOE system. Like an EHR system, a CPOE system provides decision support and can be a useful tool to the provider in managing the patient's care more effectively.

Medication Administration Systems Using Bar-Coding Technology

Another clinical application that is being widely discussed in terms of its potential to improve patient safety is medication administration that uses bar-code verification technology within an electronic medication administration system, or *bar-code e-mar*. Like EHR and CPOE systems, bar-code e-mar systems have the potential to address many patient safety issues, particularly those relating to correctly identifying patients and medications.

Bar-coding technology is nothing new. It has infiltrated our lives, and we find it in grocery stores, hospitals, department stores, airports, and even in our own homes. In health care, bar-coding technology has been employed in areas such as materials management, supply inventory, and document management.

However, medication administration using bar-coding, which has the potential to enhance productivity, improve patient safety, and ultimately improve quality of care, is still a relatively new area of emphasis. To be effective, medication administration bar-coding systems must be combined with decision-support capabilities and enable alerts and warnings designed to prevent errors. The goal is to ensure that the five "rights" of drug administration are met, meaning getting the right drug to the right patient through the right route at the right dose at the right time (Sakowski et al., 2005).

Most e-mar systems operate in essentially the same way. At the time of admission the patient receives an identification wristband with a bar code. This wristband correctly identifies the patient by name, date of birth, medical record number, and any other important identifying information. Correctly identifying the patient is the first step in seeing that the right patient gets the right medication. Next, the provider scans his or her own bar-coded identification band in order to log into the medication administration system. Bar-coding the provider or employee gives positive identification of the caregiver and ensures secure access to various information systems, according to the individual user's privileges. It also produces an audit trail showing who has accessed what systems at what time and for what information. When the provider scans the patient's bar-coded wristband, he or she has access to the physician's orders and can view what currently needs to be done for the patient. When the caregiver scans a bar-coded item or medication, that code is compared with the order profile. If it does not match, the caregiver is alerted to the discrepancy, and a potential error is averted. The scanning process might also trigger real-time documentation and billing.

Studies have shown that about half of medication errors occur during the ordering process (Hatoum, Catizone, Hutchinson, & Purohit, 1986), but errors also occur in dispensing, administering, and monitoring medications (Kaushal & Bates, 2002; Poon, Cina et al., 2006). Medication administration systems that use bar coding can be highly effective in reducing all types of medication errors, wherever in the treatment cycle they occur (Paoletti et al., 2007; Poon, Cina et al., 2006; Sakowski et al., 2005). A recent prospective, before-and-after, quasi-experimental study compared transcription and medication error rates in units of a 735-bed academic medical center that were using bar-code e-mar technology with the rates in units that had not implemented it (Poon, Keohane et al., 2010). They found a 41.4 percent relative reduction in errors among units that used bar-coding e-mar systems.

A number of resources exist to aid health care organizations in implementing bar-coding systems. HIMSS (2003) developed a resource guide that outlines how bar coding works, describes clinical and administrative applications that can employ bar-coding technology, and offers strategies and tips for successfully implementing bar coding in health care organizations. The University HealthSystem Consortium (UHC) Bar-Coding Task Group has published recommendations for hospitals ranging from general recommendations to technology recommendations and implementation strategies (Cummings, Bush, Smith, & Matuszewski, 2005). In addition, the Department of Veterans Affairs (VA) has implemented bar coding in conjunction with its electronic medical record system used throughout its 163 medical centers. The VA has found that although bar-coding systems can lower medication administration errors, introducing bar coding also presents new challenges (Mills, Neily, Mims, Burkhardt, & Bagian, 2006). To address these challenges, it has employed a series of quality improvement strategies, using multidisciplinary teams to improve the safety and efficiency of the e-mar system. Others have found that it is important to identify and address the barriers to implementation by ensuring adequate training, providing continuous improvement, making certain of ample vendor involvement, acknowledging technology limitations, and providing clear channels of communication (Nanji et al., 2009).

Telemedicine and Telehealth

"Telemedicine is the use of medical information exchanged from one site to another via electronic communications to improve patients' health status" (American Telemedicine Association, n.d.). It is a tool that enables providers to deliver health care services to patients at distant locations, and it is often promoted as a means of addressing the imbalances in the distribution of health care resources. Telemedicine systems have evolved over the past few decades, becoming most prevalent during the 1990s owing to major advancements in telecommunications technology and decreases in equipment and transmission costs. Telemedicine may be as simple as two health care providers discussing a case over the telephone or as sophisticated as using satellite technology and videoconferencing equipment to broadcast a consultation between providers at facilities in two countries. The first method is used daily by most health professionals, and the second is used by the military and some large medical centers. Telemedicine can also include the use of e-mail, smart phones, wireless tools, and other forms of telecommunications technology.

Health care literature often uses the terms *telemedicine* and *telehealth* interchangeably. We use *telehealth* to refer to a broader view of remote health care, one that does not always involve the provision of clinical services, which is generally the province of telemedicine. Telehealth includes the use of technology to access remote health information, diagnostic images, and education.

Current Status and Primary Delivery Methods

Most recent estimates suggest that there are over two hundred telemedicine programs throughout the nation, involving over 3,500 health care institutions (Eron, 2010). The types of telemedicine services may include everything from specialist referral services to patient consultations to remote patient monitoring. Two delivery methods can be used to connect providers to providers or providers to patients. The first is called *store and forward*. This technology is used primarily for transferring digital images from one location to another. For example, a digital image might be taken with a digital camera, stored on a server, and then sent (or forwarded) to a health care provider at another location upon request. *Teleradiology* and *teledermatology* are two telemedicine services that use store-and-forward technology. In the case of teleradiology, one provider might send radiological images such as X-rays, CT scans, or magnetic resonance imaging (MRI) results to another provider to review. In the case of teledermatology, a digital image of the patient's skin might be sent to a dermatologist for diagnosis or consultation. Store-and-forward technology is generally used in nonemergency situations. These images can be sent using private point-to-point networks.

The second major delivery method is known as *two-way interactive video-conferencing* and is used when a face-to-face consultation is necessary. For example, a specialty physician in an urban tertiary care hospital might consult with a primary care physician in a rural community, using high-speed or dedicated Internet lines and real-time videoconferencing capabilities. This gives patients and providers in rural communities access to providers, particularly specialists, in urban areas without having to travel. In addition, a number of peripheral devices can be linked to computers to aid in interactive examination. For example, a stethoscope can be linked to a computer, allowing the consulting physician to hear the patient's heartbeat from a distance. Remote monitoring of patients is also possible through closed-circuit television systems, and electronic monitoring of physiological vital signs can be done through electronic intensive care unit (eICU) patient monitoring systems.

A recent study by Berenson and colleagues examined the reasons hospitals chose either to adopt or not adopt telemedicine to support delivery of their intensive care units (Berenson, Grossman, & November, 2009), also known as eICUs. Some ICU directors felt it was a viable alternative to staffing given the shortage of intensivists and provided the backup and additional patient safety needed for continuous monitoring 24/7, while others preferred to have on-site staff and questioned its return on investment (Berenson, Grossman, & November, 2009). Approximately 10 percent of ICU beds in the United States are now part of eICUs.

Other uses of telemedicine can be found in the military and in university research centers. Robotic equipment is being used for *telesurgery* applications. Telesurgery can enable a surgeon in one location to remotely control a robotic arm to perform surgery in another location. The military have been developing and deploying this technology particularly for battlefield use, although some academic medical centers are also piloting telesurgery technology.

Telehealth is being used to capture and monitor data from patients at home. Examples of early telehealth efforts include capturing cardiac data from congestive heart failure patients at home, monitoring patient blood sugar levels through glucometers attached to cell phones, and conducting teledermatology visits with the aid of cell phone cameras. Home monitoring devices that transmit physiological data electronically to care providers are also being used in a variety of different ways (LeRouge, Hevner, & Collins, 2007; Shea et al., 2006).

Value of Telemedicine and Telehealth

Telemedicine can make specialty care more accessible to rural and medically underserved communities and can easily connect providers at distance locations. Kaiser Permanente conducted a study examining the impact of remote video technology on quality, use, patient satisfaction, and cost savings in the home health care setting. It found that the technology was well received by patients, capable of maintaining quality of care, and had the potential for cost savings if used as a substitute for some in-person caregiver visits (B. Johnston, Wheeler, Deuser, & Sousa, 2000).

Telemedicine has also shown promising results in improving access to care, quality, and outcomes for patients with chronic diseases (J. Barlow, Singh, Bayer, & Curry, 2007; Gambetta, Dunn, Nelson, Herron, & Arena, 2007). Researchers have found that videoconferencing can enhance the availability and use of psychiatric services for patients living in rural or remote communities (Modai et al., 2006; Spaulding, Belz, DeLurgio, & Williams, 2010). Remote surgery also has value. It could bring to local communities access to the top specialists in the world.

Electronic consultation (e-consultation) is another emerging use of technology that primary care clinicians may use to communicate with specialists about patients asynchronously instead of the typical pager, telephone call, or hallway conversation (Horner, Wagner, & Tufano, 2011). The process for conducting an e-consultation can vary depending on the technology but generally includes (1) requesting clinician poses a clinical question to a consultant electronically, (2) consultant reviews questions and accesses patient's EHR or other clinical information systems, (3) consultant replies to the requesting clinician or they may correspond back and forth in consulting mode. The system may be web-based or available through a secure server. Since fewer primary care physicians are providing care in hospital settings where they used to interact frequently with specialists, e-consultations have been found to offer clinicians a number of benefits, including

- Greater satisfaction owing to convenience and timely and helpful advice
- Education transfer from specialist to primary care provider
- Information exchange that does not interrupt workflow (it is less disruptive)
- More appropriate specialty referrals
- Improved information transfer between providers (Horner et al., 2011, p. 5)

Dr. Kendrick, a practicing physician at the University of Oklahoma School of Community Medicine, uses a Web-based e-consultation system called Doc2Doc that was designed to simulate the physician's lounge culture when providers gathered, developed relationships, and discussed patient cases together (Horner et al., 2011). The Oklahoma Department of Corrections implemented the Doc2Doc system using the University of Oklahoma's Medical School faculty for specialty referrals. To defray the overall cost of medical care by eliminating unnecessary referrals, the Department of Corrections paid $50 per e-consultation. Since implementing the e-consult system, they have reduced specialty visits by 50 percent and reduced costs (Horner et al., 2011). They have also conducted over 100,000 e-consultations and expanded the use of the system to Louisiana and Kentucky.

These are a few examples of the value of telemedicine. The possibilities for using telemedicine are endless. However, several major barriers must be addressed if telemedicine is to be more widely used and available. Concerns about provider acceptance, interstate licensure, overall confidentiality and liability, data standards, and lack of universal reimbursement for telemedicine services from private payers are barriers to the widespread use of telemedicine. Furthermore, its cost-effectiveness has yet to be fully demonstrated.

Personal Health Record and Patient Portals

With the advent of the Internet, including e-mail, web logs (blogs), and other web-based technologies, patients or consumers have assumed a much more active role in managing their own health care. To empower consumers in recent years, the concept of a personal health record (PHR) has emerged.

Although a PHR could be in paper or electronic format, the vision is that the electronic PHR would enable individuals to keep their own health records, and they could share information electronically with their physicians or other health care professionals and receive advice, reminders, test results, and alerts from them. Unlike the EHR, which is managed by health care provider organizations, the PHR is managed by the consumer. It may include both health information and wellness information, such as an individual's exercise and diet. The consumer decides who has access to the information and controls the content of the record. A patient portal is a secure web site through which patients can access their PHR or EHR. Portals often allow users to complete forms online, schedule appointments, communicate with providers, request refills on prescriptions, review test results, or pay bills (Emont, 2011). See Figure 5.4.

What is the value of the PHR, and how does it relate to the EHR? Tang and Lansky (2005) believe the PHR enables individuals to serve as "copilots" in their own care. Patients can receive customized content based on their

Figure 5.4. Sample patient portal

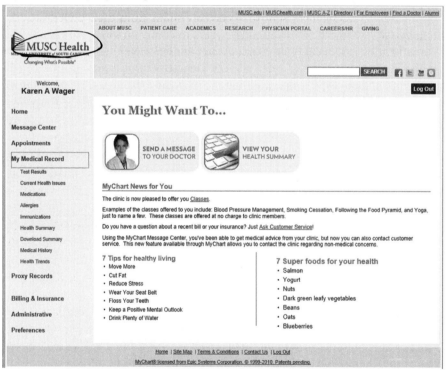

Source: Medical University of South Carolina. Used with permission.

needs, values, and preferences. PHRs should be lifelong and comprehensive and should support information exchange and portability. Patients are often seen by multiple health care providers in different settings and locations over the course of a lifetime. In our fragmented health care system, this means patients are often left to consolidate information from the various participants in their care. A PHR that brings together important health information across an individual's lifetime and that is safe, secure, portable, and easily accessible can reduce costs by avoiding unnecessary duplicate tests and improving health care communications.

PHRs may be particularly helpful to patients with chronic illnesses in enabling them to track their diseases in conjunction with their providers, prompting earlier intervention when they encounter a deviation or problem (Tang, Ash, Bates, Overhage, & Sands, 2006). In addition, PHRs may make it easier for caregivers to care for their loved ones by providing those caregivers with access to complete information. Research in this area is in its early stages; however, experts agree that the value of the PHR is greatest when the PHR is integrated with the provider's EHR (Tang et al., 2006).

Currently, only 7 percent of adults in the United States report having a PHR (Undem, 2010). Six percent indicate they have looked at test results online and 8 percent have sent or received e-mails from their physicians. As EHRs are more widely deployed in the years to come, providing patient access to information will create many policy and technical challenges for health care organizations, payers, and employers, as well as great opportunity. Early adopters have found that a number of important considerations need to be addressed, such as what information (for example, problem lists, medications, laboratory and diagnostic test results, and clinical notes) should be shared with patients, how patients should be authenticated to access their records, what access minors should have, and whether the record should include secure clinician and patient messaging (Halamka, Mandl, & Tang, 2008; Wiljer, Urowitz, Apatu, Leonard, Quartey, & Catton, 2010). Kaiser Permanente's patient portal and PHR, My Health Manager, is used by more than three million of its eight million members (Emont, 2011). A recent review of the literature on the use of patient portals suggests that they offer a number of potential benefits to providers including administrative efficiencies (such as reduced call volume), improved patient satisfaction, decreased utilization of health services, more effective care, and cost savings (Emont, 2011). In the future, demand for PHR and patient portal functionality will likely increase due to the need to meet meaningful use requirements, a greater emphasis on patient-centered care, and patients' demand for access to information. Health care leaders will need to examine the extent to which they are equipped to meet consumer expectations.

FITTING APPLICATIONS TOGETHER

How are the clinical information systems and applications discussed in this chapter related? How can they fit together? We view the patient's electronic health record as the hub of all the clinical information gathered by a health care organization (Figure 5.5). The data that eventually make up each patient's record originate from a variety of sources, both paper and electronic. In an electronic environment, the data are typically captured by a host of different applications, including but not limited to

- **Registration systems:** patient demographic information, health insurance or payer, provider's name, date, reason for visit or encounter, and so forth

- **Accounting systems:** patient billing information such as final diagnosis and procedure codes, charges, dates of services provided, and so forth

- **Ancillary services:** laboratory, radiology, pharmacy, and so forth

- **CPOE systems:** provider's orders, date, time, status, and so forth

- **Medication administration systems:** medications ordered, dispensed, administered, and so forth

- **Other clinical and administrative systems:** nursing, physical therapy, and nutrition education documentation; scheduling information; and so forth

- **Knowledge-based reference systems:** access to Medline, the latest research findings, practice guidelines, and so forth

- **Telemedicine and telehealth systems:** documentation of provision of health care services, online communication with patients and providers, and so forth

Sometimes these applications are all components of a single vendor package. More commonly, however, these applications have been acquired or developed over the many years from multiple vendors. The challenge many health care organizations now face is how to bring the patient's clinical data and administrative data together—how to make all the systems containing these data function as a single, seamless, integrated application. If we are to realize the goal of the electronic health record (EHR)—that is, capturing patient information throughout the patient's lifetime and sharing relevant health information among providers and key stakeholders when and where it is needed—we must implement systems that meet interoperability standards and figure out the numerous workflow and privacy challenges. Electronic health

Figure 5.5. Clinical information schematic

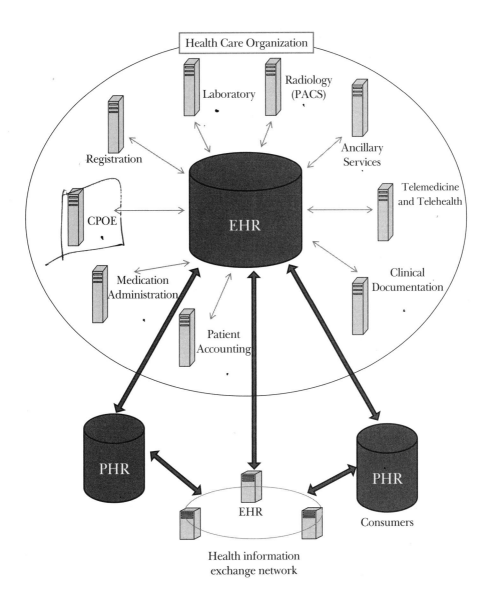

information exchange will be vital to this effort. Its role is further discussed in the next chapter.

OVERCOMING BARRIERS TO ADOPTION

What do the EHR, CPOE, e-mar, telemedicine, and many other clinical applications have in common? They all affect the ways providers deliver care to or communicate with patients, and they all confront the same barriers impeding their widespread adoption and use. Most of these barriers can be categorized as (1) financial, (2) organizational or behavioral, (3) technical, or (4) privacy and security. Financial barriers include lack of the capital or other financial resources needed to develop, acquire, implement, and support a health care information system. Organizational and behavioral barriers relate to provider use and acceptance of such systems and the workflow challenges associated with the introduction of new technology. And technical barriers include everything from the work needed to build system interfaces to a lack of adequate definitions and standards for data interchange. Privacy and security involve ensuring the confidentiality of the patient's personal health information. Although all four types of barriers typically affect all clinical applications, the actual impact of any one barrier may vary considerably. For example, historically the lack of financial resources or of reimbursement for EHR systems has slowed their implementation but not stopped it. Conversely, the lack of financial resources or of reimbursement for telemedicine services has been devastating to telemedicine programs, and many programs have not survived these financial difficulties.

Financial Barriers

EHRs and related systems can be expensive to develop, implement, and support, and even with the EHR incentive funds now available through the Medicare and Medicaid programs, some providers are reluctant to invest in a system when they are unsure of the return on investment and uncertain about the future. Our fee-for-service payment system also does not currently financially reward the improved quality and efficiency that health information technology enables. The up-front investment necessary to acquire an EHR for the small physician practice is substantial. Seventy-eight percent of physicians in the United States practice in groups of eight or fewer, yet it is the small practice that is least likely to adopt an EHR system. As mentioned earlier, estimates of the cost of acquiring and installing an EHR system range from $15,000 to $50,000 (Baron, Fabens, Schiffman, & Wolf, 2005; Miller, West, Brown, Sim, & Ganchoff, 2005), with another amount equal to 15 to 20 percent of the acquisition cost needed to support the system. Physicians and hospitals have historically borne the cost of the EHR system, but the majority of the benefits are realized by patients, payers, and purchasers. Second, EHRs can negatively affect productivity, particularly during the initial months after implementation. One study found that practices experienced a 10 to 15 percent reduction in productivity for at least several months following EHR adoption (Gans, Kralewski, Hammons, & Dowd, 2005). Small physician practices tend to be highly risk averse and are fearful about the possibility of implementation failures. Thus, the misalignment of incentives is a huge barrier.

Beyond changes in reimbursement, in August 2006, the Centers for Medicare and Medicaid Services (CMS) and the U.S. Department of Health and Human Services (HHS) Office of the Inspector General expanded exceptions to the Stark and antikickback regulations, permitting hospitals to offer computerized health information systems (or access to such systems) to physician practices, potentially at a significantly greater discount than the practices could obtain if they purchased the systems individually. To meet requirements, any donated system must be "necessary and used predominately" to create, maintain, transmit, and receive electronic health record information (HHS, 2006).

Organizational and Behavioral Barriers

In addition to the financial barriers, many behavioral or organizational barriers impede the adoption of EHR systems and other clinical applications. These barriers can be equally difficult to overcome as the financial barriers. They include everything from lack of physician acceptance to changes in workflow to differences in state licensing regulations.

EHR and other clinical information systems may alter the way providers interact with patients and other team members and render patient care services. They often require that providers enter visit notes directly into the system, respond to system reminders and alerts, and give complete documentation. Studies have shown that the EHR, CPOE, and other clinical information applications can be difficult to incorporate into existing workflow processes and may require additional time (Devine et al., 2010; Poissant et al., 2005; Poon et al., 2004). When a system is initially implemented, it invariably adds time to the physician's day. This may seem contrary to one of the reasons for implementing EHR systems, to save time. In truth, EHR systems require that physicians respond to reminders, alerts, and other knowledge aids—all of which can lead to better patient care but may also require more time. For instance, suppose a physician is treating a patient with diabetes mellitus. The EHR might remind the physician to follow clinical practice guidelines for treating diabetes, which include conducting an eye exam and checking the patient's hemoglobin A1C levels—both of which take time. Without the EHR reminder, these tasks might have been forgotten.

This is not to say that all health care organizations have been unable to gain physician acceptance. Strong leadership support, initial and ongoing training, sufficient time to learn the intricacies of the system, and evidence that the system is well integrated with patient care workflow are all important factors in gaining physician acceptance and use. Physicians need to realize the value that comes from using the clinical application—or they simply won't use it. This value may be improved patient services, improved quality of care, more highly satisfied patients, happier staff, or something more personal to the physician such as improved quality of documentation, less stress, and more leisure time. Factors leading to physician acceptance of clinical information systems will be discussed further in Chapter Seven.

When it comes to telemedicine and telehealth systems, things such as differences in state laws and in standard medical practice can affect physicians' attitudes and impede adoption. Many states will not permit out-of-state physicians to practice in their state unless licensed by them. Some physicians are concerned about medical liability issues and the lack of hands-on interaction with patients. Many physicians still prefer to meet with the patient and conduct the examination in person for fear of litigation or of missing important information.

Technical Barriers

The third broad category of barriers to adopting EHR systems involves technology; health care organizations must implement the technologies necessary to support and sustain these systems. They must choose these technologies wisely—understanding how emerging technologies fit with existing technologies, and engaging in continuing development and refinement of standards and data definitions.

Getting your arms around health care information standards is not an easy task. Many of the standards issues in health care also exist for the general business community; others are specific to health care. One thing is clear—standards are what enable different computer systems from different vendors and different health care organizations to share data. We discuss standards that affect health care information systems and how these standards are developed in greater detail in Chapter Ten. In the context of the present discussion, what is important to understand is that inadequate standards combined with rapidly changing technologies can be a barrier to widespread EHR adoption and use. Standards, implementation specifications, and certification criteria for EHR technology have been adopted by the Secretary of the Department of

Health and Human Services. EHR technology must be tested and certified by an Office of the National Coordinator (ONC) Authorized Testing and Certification Body (ATCB) in order for a provider to qualify for EHR incentive payments through the Medicare and Medicaid programs (ONC). The certified EHR product list is updated continuously on the ONC web site: http://onc-chpl .force.com/ehrcert. Preparing to exchange data electronically with other providers is not a simple task.

Significant work in standards development has occurred nationally in recent years. The Healthcare Information Technology Standards Panel (HITSP), established in 2005, has brought together experts from across the health care community—from consumers to physicians, nurses, and hospitals; from those who develop health care IT products to those who use them; and from the governmental agencies that monitor the U.S. health care system to those organizations that actually write the standards (http://www.hitsp.org). Although widespread interoperability remains a goal, all the right players seem to be working together toward its achievement.

Privacy and Security Barriers

The fourth major challenge impeding the widespread adoption and use of health IT stems from our concern about privacy and security of health information. Privacy and security have always been important issues, and they become increasingly important when we see examples of identity theft, health care fraud, and other breaches of personal information occurring far more often than we would expect. Personal health records (PHR) are not currently regulated or protected under the Health Insurance Portability and Accountability Act (HIPAA), which is an added concern.

Strategies for Overcoming Barriers

Despite these and other barriers to the widespread adoption of interoperable EHR systems, the desire to overcome them is extraordinarily strong. The biggest remedy to the financial barrier has been the federal government's investment providing $27 billion in extra Medicare and Medicaid incentive dollars to health care professionals and hospitals that become meaningful users of EHRs (Blumenthal, 2011). Through public-private collaborations, vendors, researchers, educators, policymakers, clinicians, and industry leaders have been involved in various aspects of ensuring that providers and hospitals have the local technical assistance and resources they need to assist them on their journey, standards development is progressing, and privacy and security regulations and issues remain a priority. With collaboration between public and private sectors, the federal initiatives successfully implemented, and strong leadership, we expect that interoperable EHRs are achievable in the years to come.

SUMMARY

This chapter provided an overview of five clinical information applications: EHR, CPOE, medication administration, telemedicine and telehealth, and the PHR. We described each application and discussed its current use and its value to the patient, the provider, the health care organization, and the community at large. Special attention was given to the electronic health record at the organizational level and the benefits it offers. These benefits are (1) improved quality, outcomes, and safety; (2) improved efficiency, productivity, and cost reduction; and (3) improved service and satisfaction. Despite the many benefits and advantages found in using EHR systems, the reality is that they are not widely used in health care today—particularly in exchanging health information electronically across organizations. The financial, behavioral, technical, and privacy and security barriers to their use were discussed here, along with some of the current strategies employed to overcome these barriers. Included was a brief discussion of the CMS EHR Incentive Programs available to eligible hospitals and health professionals and advances in standards development and interoperability.

KEY TERMS

Computerized provider order entry (CPOE)

Electronic health record (EHR)

Electronic medical record (EMR)

E-prescribing

Health information exchange (HIE)

Medication administration systems using bar-coding (e-mar)

Patient portal

Personal health record (PHR)

Telehealth

Telemedicine

LEARNING ACTIVITIES

1. Search the Internet and find five health care information system vendors that offer EHR products. Compare and contrast the functions and features of each product. How do these systems compare with the IOM's definitions of the EHR?

2. Search the clinical management literature and find at least one article describing the adoption or use of (a) an EHR system, (b) a CPOE system, (c) a medication administration system using bar-coding

technology, (d) a telemedicine system or telehealth system, (e) a PHR, or (f) another clinical information system or application. Summarize the article for your classmates and discuss it with them. What are the key points of the article? What lessons learned does it describe?

3. Visit a health care organization that uses one of the clinical applications described in this chapter. Find out how the application's value is measured or assessed. What do providers think about it? Health care executives? Nurses? Support staff? What impact has it had on patient care?

4. Investigate what efforts are being made nationally and in your state (in both the public and private sectors) to further the adoption of EHR systems. How likely are these efforts to work? What concerns do you have about them? What else do you think is needed to further the adoption of EHR systems?

5. Four broad categories of barriers to health information technology are discussed in this chapter. Of these, which do you think is the greatest barrier and why? What other barriers do you see? What strategies are being employed to overcome these other barriers? Conduct a search of the literature to support your answers.

REFERENCES

Agency for Healthcare Research and Quality. (2001). *Reducing and preventing adverse drug events to decrease hospital costs*. Retrieved May 2004 from http://www.ahrq .gov/qual/aderia/aderia.htm

Ahmad, A., Teater, P., Bentley, T., Kuehn, L., Kumar, R., Thomas, A., & Mekhjian, H. S. (2002). Key attributes of a successful physician order entry system implementation in a multi-hospital environment. *Journal of the American Medical Informatics Association, 9*, 16–24.

American Telemedicine Association. (n.d.). What is telemedicine? Retrieved February 2013 from http://www.americantelemed.org/learn/what-is-telemedicine

Ash, J. S., Sittig, D. F., Poon, E. G., Guappone, K., Campbell, E., & Dykstra, R. (2007). The extent and importance of unintended consequences related to computerized provider order entry. *Journal of the American Medical Informatics Association, 14*(4), 415–423.

Balas, D., Weingarten, S., Garb, C., Blumenthal, D., Boren, S., & Brown, G. (2000). Improving preventive care by prompting physicians. *Archives of Internal Medicine, 160*(3), 301–308.

Barlow, J., Singh, D., Bayer, S., & Curry, R. (2007). A systematic review of the benefits of home telecare for frail elderly people and those with long-term conditions. *Journal of Telemedicine & Telecare, 13*(4), 172–179.

Barlow, S., Johnson, J., & Steck, J. (2004). The economic effect of implementing an EMR in an outpatient clinical setting. *Journal of Healthcare Information Management, 18*(1), 46–51.

Baron, R. J., Fabens, E. L., Schiffman, M., & Wolf, E. (2005). Electronic health records: Just around the corner? Or over the cliff? *Annals of Internal Medicine, 143*(3), 222–226.

Bates, D., & Gawande, A. (2003). Improving safety with information technology. *New England Journal of Medicine, 348*(25), 2526–2534.

Bates, D., Kuperman, G., Rittenberg, J., Teich, J., Fiskio, J., Ma'luf, N., . . . & Tanasijevic, M. (1999). A randomized trial of a computer-based intervention to reduce utilization of redundant laboratory tests. *American Journal of Medicine, 106*(2), 144–150.

Berenson, R. A., Grossman, J. M., & November, E. A. (2009). Does telemonitoring of patients—The eICU—improve intensive care? *Health Affairs, 28*(5), w937–w947.

Berman, J., Zaran, F., & Rybak, M. (1992). Pharmacy-based antimicrobial-monitoring service. *American Journal of Hospital Pharmacy, 49*, 1701–1706.

Bleich, H., Safran, C., & Slack, W. (1989). Departmental and laboratory computing in two hospitals. *M.D. Computing, 6*(3), 149–155.

Blumenthal, D. (2011). Wiring the health system—origins and provisions of a new federal program: Part one of two. *New England Journal of Medicine, 365*(24), 2323–2329.

Burke, J., & Pestotnik, S. (1999). Antibiotic use and microbial resistance in intensive care units: Impact of computer-assisted decision support. *Journal of Chemotherapy, 11*(6), 530–535.

Burnum, J. (1989). The misinformation era: The fall of the medical record. *Annals of Internal Medicine, 110*, 482–484.

Chaudhry, B., Wang, J., Wu, S., Maglione, M., Mojica, W., Roth, E., . . . & Shekelle, P. G. (2006). Systematic review: Impact of health information technology on quality, efficiency, and costs of medical care. *Annals of Internal Medicine, 144*(10), 742–752.

Chen, C., Garrido, T., Chock, D., Okawa, G., & Liang, L. (2009). The Kaiser Permanente electronic health record: Transforming and streamlining modalities of care. *Health Affairs, 28*(2), 323–333.

Cherry, B., Carter, M., Owen, D., & Lockhart, C. (2008). Factors affecting electronic health record adoption in long-term care facilities. *Journal of Healthcare Quality, 30*(2), 37–47.

Cherry, B. J., Ford, E. W., & Peterson, L. T. (2011). Experiences with electronic health records: Early adopters in long-term care facilities. *Health Care Management Review, 36*(3), 265–274.

Chin, T. (2003). Doctors pull plug on paperless systems. Retrieved February 2003 from http://www.ama-assn.org/amednews/2003/02/17/bil20217.htm

Cochran, J. H. (2010). Continuous healing relationships through connectivity. *Journal of Healthcare Information Management*, *24*(3), 19–20.

Cummings, J., Bush, P., Smith, D., & Matuszewski, K. (2005). Bar-coding medication overview and consensus recommendations. *American Journal of Health-Systems Pharmacy*, *62*, 2626–2629.

Department of Health and Human Services. (HHS) (2006). New regulations to facilitate adoption of health information technology. Retrieved November 2008 from http://www.hhs.gov/news/press/2006pres/20060801.html

DesRoches, C. M., Campbell, E. G., Rao, S. R., Donelan, K., Ferris, T. G., Jha, A., . . . & Blumenthal, D. (2008). Electronic health records in ambulatory care: A national survey of physicians. *New England Journal of Medicine*, *359*(1), 50–60.

DesRoches, C. M., Campbell, E. G., Vogeli, C., Zheng, J., Rao, S., Shields, A. E., . . . & Jha, A. (2010). Electronic health records' limited successes suggest more targeted uses. *Health Affairs*, *29*(4), 639–646.

Devine, E. B., Hollingworth, W., Hansen, R. N., Lawless, N. M., Wilson-Norton, J. L., Martin, D. P., . . . & Sullivan, S. D. (2010). Electronic prescribing at the point of care: A time-motion study in the primary care setting. *Health Services Research*, *45*(1), 152–171.

Donald, J. (1989). Prescribing costs when computers are used to issue all prescriptions. *British Medical Journal*, *299*, 28–30.

Duxbury, B. (1982). Therapeutic control of anticoagulant treatment. *British Medical Journal*, *284*, 702.

Edwards, P. J., Huang, D. T., Metcalfe, L. N., & Sainfort, F. (2008). Maximizing your investment in EHR: Utilizing EHRs to inform continuous quality improvement. *Journal of Healthcare Information Management*, *22*(1), 32–37.

Emont, S. (2011). *Measuring the impact of patient portals: What the literature tells us*. Oakland: California HealthCare Foundation.

Eron, L. (2010). Telemedicine: The future of outpatient therapy? *Clinical Infectious Diseases*, *51*(Suppl. 2), S224–S230.

Evans, J., & Hayashi, A. (1994, September–October). Implementing on-line medical records. *Document Management*, pp. 12–17.

Fleming, N. S., Culler, S. D., McCorkle, R., Becker, E. R., & Ballard, D. J. (2011). The financial and nonfinancial costs of implementing electronic health records in primary care practices. *Health Affairs* (Millwood), *30*(3), 481–489.

Friedman, M. A., Schueth, A., & Bell, D. S. (2009). Interoperable electronic prescribing in the US: A progress report. *Health Affairs*, *28*(2), 393–403.

Gadd, C., & Penrod, L. (2000, November). Dichotomy between physicians' and patients' attitudes regarding EMR use during outpatient encounters. *AMIA 2000 Annual Symposium*, pp. 275–279.

Gambetta, M., Dunn, P., Nelson, D., Herron, B., & Arena, R. (2007). Impact of the implementation of telemanagement on a disease management program in an elderly heart failure cohort. *Progress in Cardiovascular Nursing, 22*(4), 196–200.

Gans, D., Kralewski, J., Hammons, T., & Dowd, B. (2005). Medical groups' adoption of electronic health records and information systems. *Health Affairs, 24*(5), 1323–1333.

Garrett, L., Jr., Hammond, W., & Stead, W. (1986). The effects of computerized medical records on provider efficiency and quality of care. *Methods of Information in Medicine, 25*(3), 151–157.

Grieger, D. L., Cohen, S. H., & Krusch, D. A. (2007). A pilot study to document the return on investment for implementing an ambulatory electronic health record at an academic medical center. *Journal of the American College of Surgeons, 205*(1), 89–96.

Halamka, J. D., Mandl, K. D., & Tang, P. C. (2008). Early experiences with personal health records. *Journal of the American Medical Informatics Association, 15*(1), 1–7.

Han, Y. Y., Carcillo, J. A., Venkataraman, S. T., Clark, R., Watson, R. S., Nguyen, T. C., . . . & Orr, R. A. (2005). Unexpected increased mortality after implementation of a commercially sold computerized physician order entry system. *Pediatrics, 116*(6), 1506–1512.

Hatoum, H., Catizone, C., Hutchinson, R., & Purohit, A. (1986). An eleven-year review of the pharmacy literature: Documentation of the value and acceptance of clinical pharmacy. *Drug Intelligence and Clinical Pharmacy, 20*, 33–48.

Healthcare Information and Management Systems Society. (2003). *Implementation guide for the use of bar code technology in healthcare.* Chicago: Author.

Health Information Management and Systems Society. (2011). Davies Award winners. Retrieved February 2013 from http://www.himss.org/davies/pastRecipients_org.asp

Hershey, C., McAloon, M., & Bertram, D. (1989). The new medical practice environment: Internists' view of the future. *Archives of Internal Medicine, 149*, 1745–1749.

Holdsworth, M. T., Fichtl, R., Raisch, D., Hewryk, A., Behta, M., Mendez-Rico, E., . . . & Greenwald, B. M. (2007). Impact of computerized prescriber order entry on the incidence of adverse drug events in pediatric inpatients. *Pediatrics, 120*(5), 1058–1066.

Horner, K., Wagner, E., & Tufano, J. (2011, October). *Electronic consultations between primary and specialty care clinicians: Early insights.* New York: The Commonwealth Fund.

Hsiao, C., Hing, E., Socey, T. C., & Cai, B. (2011). Electronic health record systems and intent to apply for meaningful user incentives among office-based physician practices: United States, 2001–2011. *NCHS Data Brief.* Retrieved February 2013 from http://www.cdc.gov/nchs/data/databriefs/db79.htm

Hudak, S., & Sharkey, S. (2007). *Health information technology: Are long term care providers ready?* Oakland: California HealthCare Foundation.

Institute of Medicine. (1991). *The computer-based patient record: An essential technology for health care*. Washington, DC: National Academies Press.

Institute of Medicine. (2000). *To err is human: Building a safer health system*. Washington, DC: National Academies Press.

Institute of Medicine. (2001). *Crossing the quality chasm: A new health system for the 21st century*. Washington, DC: National Academies Press.

Institute of Medicine, Committee on Data Standards for Patient Safety. (2003). *Key capabilities of an electronic health record system*. Washington, DC: Institute of Medicine.

Institute of Medicine. (2011). *Health IT and patient safety: Building safer systems for better care*. Washington, DC: National Academies Press.

Jensen, J. (2006). The effects of computerized provider order entry on medication turn-around time: A time-to-first-dose study at the Providence Portland Medical Center. *AMIA 2006 Annual Symposium*, pp. 384–388.

Jha, A. K., DesRoches, C. M., Campbell, E. G., Donelan, K., Rao, S. R., Ferris, T. G., . . . & Blumenthal, D. (2009). Use of electronic health records in US hospitals. *New England Journal of Medicine*, 360, 1628–1638.

Jha, A. K., DesRoches, C. M., Kralovec, P. D., & Joshi, M. S. (2010). A progress report on electronic health records in U.S. hospitals. *Health Affairs* (Millwood), *29*(10), 1951–1957.

Jha, A. K., Perlin, J. B., Kizer, K. W., & Dudley, R. A. (2003). Effect of the transformation of the Veterans Affairs health care system on the quality of care. *New England Journal of Medicine, 348*, 2218–2227.

Johnston, B., Wheeler, L., Deuser, J., & Sousa, K. (2000). Outcomes of the Kaiser Permanente tele-home health research project. *Archives of Family Medicine, 9*(1), 40–45.

Johnston, D., Pan, E., Walker, J., Bates, D., & Middleton, B. (2003). *The value of computerized provider order entry in ambulatory settings*. Chicago: Healthcare Information and Management Systems Society.

Johnston, D., Pan, E., Walker, J., Bates, D., & Middleton, B. (2004). *Patient safety in the physician's office: Assessing the value of ambulatory CPOE*. Oakland: California HealthCare Foundation.

Kaushal, R., & Bates, D. (2002). Information technology and medication safety: What is the benefit? *Quality and Safety in Health Care, 11*, 261–265.

Kazley, A. S., & Diana, M. D. (2011). Does hospital CPOE use mean better quality? A national study. *Health Care Management Review, 36*(1), 86–94.

Kazley, A. S., Diana, M. D., Ford, E., & Menachemi, N. (2011). Is EHR use associated with patient satisfaction in hospitals? *Health Care Management Review, 37*(1).

Kesselheim, A. S., Cresswell, K., Phansalkar, S., Bates, D. W., & Sheikh, A. (2011). Clinical decision support systems could be modified to reduce "alert fatigue" while still minimizing the risk of litigation. *Health Affairs, 30*(12), 2310–2317.

Kilbridge, P. M., Classen, D., Bates, D. W., & Denham, C. R. (2006). The National Quality Forum safe practice standard for computerized physician order entry: Updating a critical patient safety practice. *Journal of Patient Safety, 2*(4), 183–190.

Koppel, R., & Kreda, D. (2009). Health care information technology vendors' "hold harmless" clause: Implications for patients and clinicians. *Journal of the American Medical Association, 301*(12), 1276–1277.

Koppel, R., Metlay, J. P., Cohen, A., Kimmel, S. E., & Storm, B. L. (2005). Role of computerized provider order entry systems in facilitating medication errors. *Journal of the American Medical Association, 293*(10), 1197–1203.

Kuperman, G., Teich, J., Gandhi, T., & Bates, D. (2001). Patient safety and computerized medication ordering at Brigham and Women's Hospital. *Joint Commission Journal on Quality Improvement, 27*(10), 509–521.

Landis, S., Hulkower, S., & Pierson, S. (1992). Enhancing adherence with mammography through patient letters and physician prompts: A pilot study. *North Carolina Medical Journal, 53*(11), 575–578.

Langberg, M. (2004). *Challenges to implementing CPOE: A case study of a work in progress at Cedars-Sinai.* Retrieved April 2004 from http://www .modernphysician.com/page.cms?pageId=216

Legler, J., & Oates, R. (1993). Patients' reactions to physician use of a computerized medical record system during clinical encounters. *Journal of Family Practice, 37*(3), 241–244.

LeRouge, C., Hevner, A., & Collins, R. (2007). It's more than just use: An exploration of telemedicine use quality. *Decision Support Systems, 43*, 1287–1304.

Levit, K., Cowan, C., Lazenby, H., Sensenig, A., McDonnell, P., Stiller, J., et al. (2000). Health spending in 1998: Signals of change. *Health Affairs, 19*(1), 124–132.

Marshall, P., & Chin, H. (1998). *The effects of an electronic medical record on patient care: Clinician attitudes in a large HMO.* Paper presented at the AMIA Annual Symposium, Portland, OR.

Massaro, T. (1993a). Introducing physician order entry at a major academic medical center: I. Impact on organizational culture and behavior. *Academic Medicine, 68*(1), 20–25.

Massaro, T. (1993b). Introducing physician order entry at a major academic medical center: II. Impact on medical education. *Academic Medicine, 68*(1), 25–30.

McPhee, S., Bird, J. A., Fordham, D., Rodnick, J., & Osborn, E. (1991). Promoting cancer prevention activities by primary care physicians: Results of a randomized, controlled trial. *Journal of the American Medical Association, 266*(4), 538–544.

McPhee, S., Bird, J. A., Jenkins, C. N., & Fordham, D. (1989). Promoting cancer screening: A randomized, controlled trial of three interventions. *Archives of Internal Medicine, 149*, 1866–1872.

Menachemi, N., Powers, T., Au, D. W., & Brooks, R. G. (2010). Predictors of physician satisfaction among electronic health record system users. *Journal of Healthcare Quality*, *32*(1), 35–41.

Metzger, J., & Turisco, F. (2001). *Computerized physician order entry: A look at the marketplace and getting started.* Washington, DC, and New York: Leapfrog Group and First Consulting Group.

Miller, R. H., West, C., Brown, T., Sim, I., & Ganchoff, C. (2005). The value of electronic health records in solo or small group practices. *Health Affairs*, *24*(5), 1127–1137.

Mills, P. D., Neily, J., Mims, E., Burkhardt, M. E., & Bagian, J. (2006). Improving the bar-coded medication administration system at the Department of Veterans Affairs. *American Journal of Health-Systems Pharmacy*, *63*, 1442–1447.

Modai, I., Jabarin, M., Kurs, R., Barak, P., Hanan, I., & Kitain, L. (2006). Cost effectiveness, safety, and satisfaction with video telepsychiatry versus face-to-face care in ambulatory settings. *Telemedicine & E-Health*, *12*(5), 515–520.

Nanji, K. C., Cina, J., Patel, N., Churchill, W., Gandhi, T. K., & Poon, E. G. (2009). Overcoming barriers to the implementation of a pharmacy bar code scanning system for medication dispensing: A case study. *Journal of the American Medical Informatics Association*, *16*(5), 645–650.

National Alliance for Health Information Technology. (2008, April 28). *Report to the Office of the National Coordinator for Health Information Technology on defining key health information technology terms.* Department of Health and Human Services. Retrieved February 2013 from http://www.nahit.org/docs/hitterms finalreport_051508.pdf

Niazkhani, Z., Pirnejad, H., Berg, M., & Aarts, J. (2009). The impact of computerized provider order entry systems on inpatient clinical workflow: A literature review. *Journal of the American Medical Informatics Association*, *16*(4), 539–549.

Ornstein, S., & Bearden, A. (1994). Patient perspectives on computer-based medical records. *Journal of Family Practice*, *38*(6), 606–610.

Ornstein, S., Garr, D., Jenkins, R., Rust, P., & Arnon, A. (1991). Computer-generated physician and patient reminders: Tools to improve population adherence to selected preventive services. *Journal of Family Practice*, *32*(1), 82–90.

Overhage, J., Tierney, W., Zhou, X., & McDonald, C. (1997). A randomized trial of "corollary orders" to prevent errors of omission. *Journal of the American Medical Informatics Association*, *4*(5), 364–375.

Paoletti, R. D., Suess, T. M., Lesko, M. G., Feroli, A. A., Kennel, J. A., Mahler, J. M., & Sauders, T. (2007). Using bar-code technology and medication observation methodology for safer medication administration. *American Journal of Health-Systems Pharmacy*, *64*, 536–543.

Pearson, W. S., & Bercovitz, A. R. (2006). Use of computerized medical records in home health and hospice agencies. *Vital Health Statistics*, *13*(161), 1–14.

Poissant, L., Pereira, J., Tamblyn, R., & Kawasumi, Y. (2005). The impact of electronic health records on time efficiency of physicians and nurses: A systematic review. *Journal of the American Medical Informatics Association, 12*(5), 505–516.

Poon, E. G., Blumenthal, D., Jaggi, T., Honour, M., Balas, D., & Kaushal, R. (2004). Overcoming barriers to adopting and implementing computerized physician order entry systems in U.S. hospitals. *Health Affairs, 23*(4), 184–190.

Poon, E. G., Cina, J. L., Churchill, W., Patel, N., Featherstone, E., Rothschild, J. M., . . . & Gandhi, T. K. (2006). Medication dispensing errors and potential adverse drug events before and after implementing bar code technology in the pharmacy. *Annals of Internal Medicine, 145*, 426–434.

Poon, E. G., Keohane, C. A., Yoon, C. S., Ditmore, M., Bane, A., . . . & Gandhi, T. K. (2010). Effect of bar-code technology on the safety of medication administration. *New England Journal of Medicine, 362*(18), 1698–1707.

Rao, S. R., DesRoches, C. M., Donelan, K., Campbell, E. G., Miralles, P. D., & Jha, A. K. (2011). Electronic health records in small physician practices: Availability, use, and perceived benefits. *Journal of the American Medical Informatics Association, 18*(3), 271–275.

Ridsdale, L., & Hudd, S. (1994). Computers in the consultation: The patient's view. *British Journal of General Practice, 44*, 367–369.

Sakowski, J., Leonard, T., Colburn, S., Michaelsen, B., Schiro, T., Schneider, J., & Newman, J. M. (2005). Using a bar-coded medication administration system to prevent medication errors in a community hospital network. *American Journal of Health-Systems Pharmacy, 62*, 2619–2625.

Shamliyan, T., Duval, S., Jing, D., & Kane, R. (2008). Just what the doctor ordered: Review of the evidence of the impact of computerized provider order entry on medication errors. *Health Services Research, 43*(1), 32–53.

Shea, S., Weinstock, R. S., Starren, J., Teresi, J., Palmas, W., Field, L., . . . & Lantigua, R. A. (2006). A randomized trial comparing telemedicine case management with usual care in older, ethnically diverse, medically underserved patients with diabetes mellitus. *Journal of the American Medical Informatics Association, 13*(1), 40–51.

Shield, R. R., Goldman, R. A., Anthony, D. A., Wang, N., Doyle, R. J., & Borkan, J. (2010). Gradual electronic health record implementation: New insights on physician and patient adaptation. *Annals of Family Medicine, 8*(4), 316–326.

Sittig, D. F., & Singh, H. (2011). Defining health information technology-related errors: New developments since *To Err Is Human. Archives of Internal Medicine, 171*(14), 1281–1284.

Sittig, D. F., Teich, J. M., Osheroff, J. A., & Singh, H. (2009) Improving clinical quality indicators through electronic health records: It takes more than just a reminder. *Pediatrics, 124*(1), 375–377.

Solomon, G., & Dechter, M. (1995). Are patients pleased with computer use in the examination room? *Journal of Family Practice, 41*(3), 241–244.

Spaulding, R., Belz, N., DeLurgio, S., & Williams, A. R. (2010). Cost savings of telemedicine utilization for child psychiatry in a rural Kansas community. *Telemedicine and e-Health, 16*(8), 1–6.

Tang, P. C., Ash, J. S., Bates, D. W., Overhage, J. M., & Sands, D. Z. (2006). Personal health records: Definitions, benefits, and strategies for overcoming barriers to adoption. *Journal of the American Medical Informatics Association, 13*(2), 121–126.

Tang, P. C., & Lansky, D. (2005). The missing link: Bridging the patient-provider health information gap. *Health Affairs, 24*(5), 1290–1295.

Teich, J., Merchia, P., Schmiz, J., Kuperman, G., Spurr, C., & Bates, D. (2000). Effects of computerized physician order entry on prescribing practices. *Archives of Internal Medicine, 160*, 2741–2747.

Tierney, W., McDonald, C., Hui, S., & Martin, D. (1988). Computer predictions of abnormal test results. *Journal of the American Medical Association, 259*, 1194–1198.

Tierney, W., Miller, M., & McDonald, C. (1990). The effect on test ordering of informing physicians of the charges for outpatient diagnostic tests. *New England Journal of Medicine, 322*, 1499–1504.

Tierney, W., Miller, M., Overhage, J. M., & McDonald, C. (1993). Physician inpatient order writing on microcomputer workstations: Effects on resource utilization. *Journal of the American Medical Association, 269*, 379–383.

Undem, T. (2010). *Consumers and health information technology: A national survey.* Oakland: California HealthCare Foundation, Lake Research Partners. Retrieved February 2013 from http://www.chcf.org/publications/2010/04/consumers-and-health-information-technology-a-national-survey

Wager, K. A., Lee, F., White, A., Ward, D., & Ornstein, S. (2000). Impact of an electronic medical record system on community-based primary care practices. *Journal of the American Board of Family Practice, 13*(5), 338–348.

Wager, K. A., Ward, D. M., Lee, F. W., White, A. W., Davis, K. S., & Clancy, D. (2005). Physicians, patients and EHRs: When it comes to a consultation, is three a crowd? *Journal of the American Health Information Management Association, 76*(4), 38–41.

Wager, K. A., Zoller, J. S., Soper, D. E., Smith, J. B., Waller, J. L., & Clark, F. C. (2008). Assessing physician and nurse satisfaction with an ambulatory care EMR: One facility's approach. *International Journal of Healthcare Information Systems and Informatics, 3*(1), 63–74.

Walsh, K., Landrigan, C., Adams, W., Vinci, R., Chessare, J., Cooper, M., . . . & Bauchner, H. (2008). Effect of computer order entry on prevention of serious medication errors in hospitalized children. *Pediatrics, 121*(3), e421–e427.

Wang, S., Middleton, B., Prosser, L., Bardon, C., Spurr, C., & Carchidi, P. (2003). A cost-benefit analysis of the electronic medical record in primary care. *American Journal of Medicine, 114*, 397–403.

Wiljer, D., Urowitz, S., Apatu, E., Leonard, K., Quartey, N., & Catton, P. (2010) Understanding the support needs of patients accessing test results online: PHRs offer great promise, but support issues need to be addressed. *Journal of Healthcare Information Management, 24*(1), 57–63.

Yarnall, K., Rimer, B., Hynes, D., Watson, G., Lyna, P., Woods-Powell, C., . . . & Barber, L. T. (1998). Computerized prompts for cancer screening in a community health center. *Journal of the American Board of Family Practice, 11*(2), 96–104.

Yu, F. B., Menachemi, N., Berner, E. S., Allison, J. J., Weissman, N., & Houston, T. K. (2009). Full implementation of computerized physician order entry and medication-related quality outcomes: A study of 3364 hospitals. *American Journal of Medical Quality, 24*(4), 278–286.

Zhou, L., Soran, C., Jenter, C., Volk, L., Orav, E., Bates, D., & Simon, S. (2009). The relationship between electronic health record use and quality of care over time. *Journal of the American Medical Informatics Association, 16*(4), 457–464.

Zlabek, J. A., Wickus, J. W., & Mathiason, M. A. (2011). Early cost and safety benefits of an inpatient electronic health record. *Journal of the American Medical Informatics Association, 18*(2), 169–172.

CHAPTER 6

Federal Efforts to Enhance Quality of Patient Care through the Use of Health Information Technology

LEARNING OBJECTIVES

- To gain a broad understanding of the major federal legislation that has passed in recent years to promote the adoption and meaningful use of electronic health record (EHR) systems.

- To describe the Medicare and Medicaid EHR Incentive Programs for eligible professionals and hospitals.

- To discuss implications of health care reform legislation and new models of care (such as accountable care organizations and patient-centered medical homes) on the health information management needs of the various stakeholders.

- To define health information exchange (HIE) and discuss the efforts that are underway nationally and regionally to promote the exchange of health data across organizations.

- To discuss the health care IT ramifications of payment reform.

From the late 2000s through the early 2010s, the degree of federal legislation that was passed affecting the need for, and effective use of, health information technology has never been greater. The legislative changes are driven by the growing demand to transform the health care delivery system into one that facilitates new methods for improving the quality, efficiency, and patient-centeredness of care. The time for action has come. In the late 2000s, our economy had experienced a major financial crisis and spiraled into a deep recession; health care costs were at an all-time high, with quality uneven and forty-six million Americans uninsured. Unemployment rates hovered around 9 percent. In an effort to stimulate the job market, the *American Recovery and Reinvestment Act (ARRA)* passed in 2009, pouring nearly $787 billion of federal funds into the economy. Although its primary aim was to save and create jobs, its secondary aims were to invest in infrastructure, health, and education. Specifically, the Health Information Technology for Economic and Clinical Health Act (HITECH), a provision of ARRA, outlined a multifaceted approach to improving health care quality and efficiency by encouraging hospitals and clinicians to use electronic health records (EHRs). Both parties of Congress agreed our current health care system could not sustain itself on the antiquated paper-based medical record systems that have prevailed for decades. The ultimate goal is not that health care organizations and providers will merely install EHR systems, although implementing them is an important first step. Rather, the goal is to incentivize clinicians to become "meaningful users" of EHRs, leading to improved quality and efficiencies of care (Blumenthal, 2010). With nearly $30 billion in incentives available to clinicians and hospitals through the Medicare and Medicaid EHR Incentive Programs and the risk of reduced reimbursement payments for those who fail to comply, "meaningful use" likely represents the "single most potent" federal effort to change health care delivery over these two decades (Jha et al., 2009).

Equally as significant for its potential impact on the health care delivery system and the ways in which we manage health information was the passage of the Patient Protection and Affordable Care Act (PPACA), later known as the Affordable Care Act. It builds on the HITECH Act and recognizes health information technology as a critical enabler to broad transformation in health care. The law has multiple objectives, including increasing access to affordable care and extending coverage, investing in research that will help providers, patients, and payers make informed decisions about effective treatment costs by introducing new models of care coordination and delivery, as well as payment reform (Buntin, Jain, & Blumenthal, 2010). To achieve these broad objectives, health care providers must have the tools to easily capture, analyze, and act on patient- and population-level health information.

In this chapter, we will examine the federal legislation and initiatives that have occurred in recent years to further the adoption and meaningful use of electronic health records. Focus is given to the timeline and resources available to assist hospitals and eligible health professionals in achieving meaningful use. We discuss key elements of new models of care including accountable care organizations and patient-centered medical homes. We also introduce the concept of health information exchange (HIE), the Nationwide Health Information Network (NwHIN), and give examples of several successful HIEs to date. Being able to exchange health information across organizations is critical to achieving meaningful use. The chapter concludes with an overview of some of the health care information technology (IT) ramifications of integrated care models and payment reform.

Clearly, we are in a new era of increased accountability for the provision and delivery of high-quality, cost-effective care. To effectively lead in this environment, health care executives and providers will need ready access to information and knowledge-based decision-making tools. Patients, consumers, and payers will expect no less.

HITECH ACT

The *Health Information Technology Economic and Clinical Health (HITECH) Act* established programs and authorized funding to support the widespread, rapid adoption and meaningful use of electronic health records (EHR) by hospitals, physicians, and other health care practitioners.

An Overview of the Legislation

An important component of HITECH was the establishment of the *Medicare and Medicaid EHR Incentive Programs,* both of which enable eligible practitioners and hospitals to qualify for incentive payments for adopting, implementing, upgrading, or demonstrating *meaningful use* of certified EHR technology. Through the Medicare EHR Incentive Program, each eligible professional who adopted and achieved meaningful EHR in 2011 or 2012 was able to earn up to $44,000 over a five-year period. The amount decreased over the five-year period, with the incentive to providers to start sooner rather than later. Eligible hospitals could earn over $2 million through the Medicare EHR Incentive Program. The Medicaid EHR Incentive Program made available up to $63,500 for each eligible professional (through 2021) and over $2 million to each eligible hospital. See Table 6.1 for primary differences between the two incentive programs.

Table 6.1. Differences between Medicare and Medicaid EHR Incentive Programs

Medicare EHR Incentive Program	Medicaid EHR Incentive Program
Federally implemented and available nationally	Implemented voluntarily by states
Medicare Advantage professionals have special eligibility accommodations	Medicaid managed care professionals must meet regular eligibility requirements
Open to physicians, subsection (d) hospitals, and Critical Access Hospitals	Open to five types of professionals and three types of hospitals
Same definition of "meaningful use" applied to all participants nationally	States can adopt a more rigorous definition of "meaningful use"
Must demonstrate meaningful use in first year	Adopt, implement, or upgrade option in first year
Maximum incentive for eligible professionals is $44,000; 10 percent bonus for HPSA (Health Professional Shortage Area)	Maximum incentive for eligible professionals is $63,750
2014 is the last year in which a professional can initiate participation	2016 is the last year in which a professional can initiate participation
Payments over five years	Payments over six years
In 2015 fee reductions (penalties) begin for those who do not demonstrate meaningful use of a certified EHR	No fee reductions (penalties)
2016 is the last incentive payment year	2021 is the last incentive payment year
No Medicare patient population minimum is required	Eligible professionals must have a 30 percent Medicaid population (20 percent for pediatricians) to participate; this must be demonstrated annually

Source: Carson, Garr, Goforth, & Forkner, 2010.

The incentive payments were designed to offset some of the up-front costs of switching from paper to electronic records, or of upgrading from noncertified to certified EHR systems. EHR-certified systems must meet certain minimum capabilities, functionality, and security standards. Implementing a certified EHR, however, is not all that is needed to qualify for the incentive payments. Hospitals and health care providers must also demonstrate that they are using EHR systems in meaningful ways to improve quality of care and efficiency. In addition to the incentives for EHR use, the legislation includes penalties in the form of reduction in Medicare payments for those who fail to initiate meaningful EHR use within a designated time frame.

HITECH goes beyond providing financial incentives for providers to adopt EHR systems. Many small physician practices and rural hospitals do not have the in-house expertise to select, implement, and support EHR systems. To address these needs, HITECH funded sixty-two *Regional Extension Centers (RECs)* throughout the nation to support providers in adopting and becoming meaningful users of EHRs. The RECs are primarily intended to provide advice and technical assistance to primary care providers, especially those in small practices, and to small rural hospitals, which often do not have IT expertise. Furthermore, HITECH provided funding for various *health IT workforce training programs* to support the education of HIT professionals. The education-based programs included curriculum development, community college consortia, competency examination, and university-based training programs, with the overarching goal of training an additional 45,000 health information technology professionals. Funding was also made available to seventeen *Beacon Communities* and *Strategic Health IT Advanced Research Projects (SHARPs)* across the nation. The Beacon programs are leading organizations that are demonstrating how health information technology can be used in innovative ways to target specific health problems within communities (Office of the National Coordinator for Health Information Technology, 2010a). These programs are illustrating health IT's role in improving individual and population health outcomes, and in overcoming barriers such as coordination of care, which plagues our nation's health care system (McKethan et al., 2011).

PERSPECTIVE
Delta Health Alliance BLUES Beacon Community

"It's really going to help the patients make a better decision because they're getting better information," says Karen Fox of the Delta Health Alliance BLUES (Better Living Utilizing Electronic Systems) Beacon Community. Located in the Mississippi Delta, the Delta Health Alliance BLUES Beacon Community was selected and awarded over $14.6 million to be a part of the Beacon Community Program. The Mississippi Delta region includes eighteen counties between the Mississippi and Yazoo rivers. With more than one-third of the population living in poverty and around 13 percent of the population suffering from diabetes, the area is challenged by the lack of a sufficient number of health care providers to address the situation. The goal of the community is to "to improve access to care for diabetic patients through the meaningful use of electronic

(cont.)

health records (EHRs) and health information exchange (HIE) by primary care providers in the Mississippi Delta." The community also hopes to utilize EHR-related interventions to increase efficiency and reduce excess cost. Exchanging patients' health information with their pharmacists who then provide telephonic support to patients on managing their medications and adhering to their regimen, electronically sharing patients' hospital visit information with primary care providers who can then actively follow up with patients when they return home, and implementing evidence-based computerized clinical decision-support systems in primary care clinics are just some of the interventions that have been put in place. As of May 2011, these health IT enhanced interventions were underway in five of the eighteen counties within the Delta region and a spread strategy was in place to reach additional areas.

Four SHARP centers have been funded to develop breakthrough research in areas such as the security of health IT, patient-centered cognitive support, health care application and network platform architectures, and secondary use of EHR data (Office of the National Coordinator for Health Information Technology, 2010b).

Achieving meaningful use requires that health care providers are able to share health information electronically with others using a secure network for *health information exchange (HIE)*. To this end, HITECH provided state grants to help build the HIE infrastructure for exchange of electronic health information among providers and between providers and consumers. Nearly all states have approved strategic and operational plans for moving forward with implementation of their HIE cooperative agreement programs. Further, HITECH has supported the Nationwide Health Information Network (NwHIN), a set of standards, services, and policies that enable secure health information exchange over the Internet (NwHIN, n.d.). The network provides a foundation for the exchange of health information across diverse entities, within communities, and across the nation.

Another key component of HITECH was the establishment of the *EHR certification program*. Within the Office of the National Coordinator for Health IT (ONC), the Office of Interoperability and Standards oversees certification programs for health information technology. The purpose of certification is to provide assurance to EHR purchasers and other users that their EHR system has the technological capability, functionality, and security needed to assist them in meeting meaningful use criteria. Eligible providers who apply for the Medicare and Medicaid EHR Incentive Programs are required to use certified

EHR technology. The ONC has authorized certain organizations to perform the actual testing and certification of EHR systems. A current listing of certified ambulatory care and inpatient EHR systems and modules may be found on the ONC web site (http://onc-chpl.force.com/ehrcert).

Success of all of these HITECH-sponsored initiatives is predicated on patients, consumers, and health care providers trusting that their health information is private and secure. Without trust, patients and providers will not use EHRs to their fullest potential. HITECH imposed several new significant *privacy and security requirements* beyond HIPAA. For example, when an individual's unsecured protected health information is believed to be disclosed because of a breach, HITECH requires the provider to notify the individuals whose information was breached. If the breach involves more than five hundred individuals, it must be reported to Health and Human Services Office of Civil Rights and the media. The HITECH Act also ensures that entities such as personal health record vendors and health information exchanges (HIEs) are subject to the same privacy and security rules as covered entities, by treating these as Business Associates under HIPAA (Kolkman & Brown, 2011). New restrictions on using personal health information (PHI) for marketing purposes have also been included. Other security standards specifically designed to detect and prevent breaches are described in Chapter Ten.

Figure 6.1 illustrates the major components of the HITECH Act. The pathway toward improved health system performance is believed to be achieved through

- Improved individual and population health outcomes
- Increased transparency and efficiency
- Improved ability to study and improve care delivery

It is too early to predict the long-term impact of HITECH on the widespread adoption and meaningful use of EHR systems, but indications such as the number of organizations and providers who have registered for EHR Incentive Programs, growth in HIT venture capital, and the number of organizations involved in EHR system implementations all suggest the momentum is as strong as ever.

Meaningful Use: Definition and Criteria

The HITECH Act specifies three main components of meaningful use:

1. The use of a certified EHR in a meaningful manner, such as e-prescribing

Figure 6.1. Overview of HITECH Act

2. The use of certified EHR technology for electronic exchange of health information to improve quality of health care

3. The use of certified EHR technology to submit clinical quality and other measures to CMS (CMS, n.d.)

"Meaningful use" essentially means that providers need to be able to demonstrate that they are using *certified* EHR technology in significant ways that can be measured in both quality and quantity to achieve health and efficiency goals.

The criteria for meaningful use are to be implemented in three stages from 2011 through 2015. Stage 1 criteria set the baseline for electronically capturing health information in a structured format and using that information to track key clinical conditions, as well as communicating that information for care coordination purposes. Examples of core objectives in Stage 1 are:

- Capture key parts of the patient's health record (detailed demographics, vital signs, active medication and problem lists, and smoking status)
- Create care summary documents
- Provide patients with an electronic copy of their health information
- Have the *capability* to exchange key clinical information electronically
- Implement at least one clinical decision-support tool

There are also optional objectives known as the "menu" set, for which providers must choose five. Examples of optional menu set functions include sending patient reminders for preventive or follow-up care, using EHRs to provide patient-specific education materials, and performing medication reconciliation.

Stage 2 proposed criteria were published in 2012. They build on Stage 1 criteria and require patients to have electronic access to their health record. Stage 3 of the meaningful use criteria build further upon these criteria and are expected to require practitioners and hospitals to demonstrate improved outcomes. Stages 2 and 3 have estimated implementation dates of 2013 and 2015, respectively.

All meaningful use criteria are to be linked and aligned with the nation's health outcome policy priorities:

- Improve health care quality, safety, and efficiency and reduce health disparities
- Engage patients and families in their health care
- Improve care coordination
- Improve population and public health
- Ensure adequate privacy and security of personal health information

The CMS web site is the best source for the latest meaningful use criteria, including those for hospitals (www.cms.gov).

Stage 1 of the meaningful use provisions is expected to improve legibility of patient records, reduce prescription errors, improve adherence to clinical practice guidelines, improve patient access to their records, and ensure that clinicians and hospitals are capable of exchanging clinical data. But until our payment system is reformed to incentivize integration and coordinated care, experts in the field expect the true effect of meaningful use to be modest (Jha, 2010).

Role of Office of the National Coordinator for Health Information Technology and CMS

The *Office of the National Coordinator for Health Information Technology (ONC)* is the entity responsible for developing policies that implement the overall HITECH Act. In this role, the ONC works closely with the *Center for Medicare and Medicaid Services (CMS)*, which is responsible for promulgating policies that relate to Medicare and Medicaid payment for meaningful use of EHRs under HITECH (ONC, 2011). The ONC specifies the standards, implementation specifications, and other criteria for EHR systems to be certified under HITECH, while the CMS rule specifies how hospitals and eligible professionals must demonstrate their meaningful use of these technologies in order to receive Medicare and Medicaid payment incentives (Department of Health and Human Services, 2011). Both sets of rules strongly indicate that standards and criteria for achieving meaningful use of EHRs will grow and become more rigorous in future years as the technology evolves and providers gain experience and sophistication in its use. See Figure 6.2.

Figure 6.2. Federal health IT strategic map

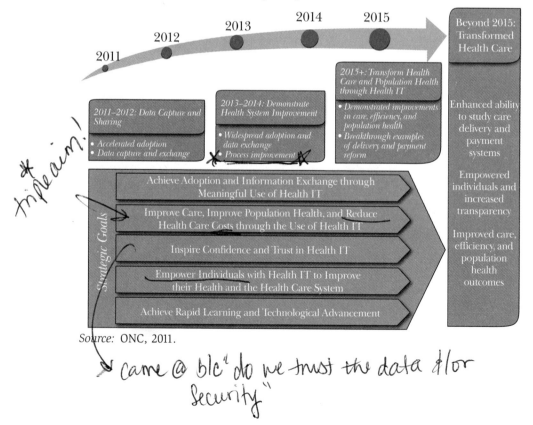

Source: ONC, 2011.

HEALTH CARE REFORM: NEW MODES OF CARE AND PAYMENT REFORM

Along with the widespread effort to promote the use and adoption of health information technology, the early 2010s brought dramatic change to the health care sector with the passage of health care reform legislation. With U.S. health care costs at 17 percent of the gross national product and rising and forty-six million Americans uninsured, President Obama signed into law on March 23, 2010, the *Patient Protection and Affordable Care Act (PPACA)*. For the first time in our nation's history, the federal government mandated that individuals have health insurance—although its constitutionality was challenged by several states and eventually brought forth to the U.S. Supreme Court. The Medicaid Program was expanded to include all non-Medicaid eligible individuals under age sixty-five with incomes up to 133 percent of the federal poverty level. The Act also created the structure for health insurance exchanges, including a greater role for states, and imposed changes to private insurance, such as prohibiting health plans from placing lifetime limits on the dollar value of coverage and prohibiting preexisting condition exclusions. Numerous changes were to be made to the Medicare program including continued reductions in Medicare payments to certain hospitals for hospital-acquired conditions and excessive preventable hospital readmissions (Kaiser Family Foundation, 2011).

Additionally, the Centers for Medicare and Medicaid Services (CMS) established an Innovation Center to test, evaluate, and expand different payment structures and methodologies to reduce program expenditures while maintaining or improving quality of care. Different payment models and modes of care delivery that foster coordinated, patient-centered care in a cost-effective environment are being encouraged and eventually rewarded. Much of the interest in exploring new modes of delivery and payment are due to the facts that U.S. health care is fragmented and that inadequate communication among providers—and between providers and patients and their families—is common (Guterman & Drake, 2010). Historically, there has been a lack of accountability for the total care of patients, the outcomes of their treatment, and the efficiency with which health resources are used. The fact that health care services are paid primarily on a fee-for-service basis has contributed to the fragmentation and lack of accountability. Fee-for-service emphasizes the provision of health services by individual hospitals or providers, rather than care that is coordinated across providers to address the patient's needs. Providers are rewarded for volume and for conducting procedures that are often more complex, when simpler, lower-cost, better methods may be more appropriate (Guterman & Drake, 2010).

It has more than a decade since the Institute of Medicine published its landmark reports, *To Err Is Human: Building a Safer Health System* (2000) and *Crossing the Quality Chasm: A New Health System for the 21st Century* (2001), yet the quality of health care in the United States remains uneven and suboptimal (Schuster, McGlynn, & Brook, 2005). These shortcomings can have a tremendous impact on people with chronic illnesses, who experience frequent changes in health status, as well as multiple transitions between care settings and care providers. Naylor and colleagues conducted a systematic review of the literature and found that these transitions, or "handoffs," have been associated with increased rates of avoidable hospitalizations (Naylor, Aiken, Kurtzman, Olds, & Hirshman, 2011). The movement of patients from hospitals to the community and back again also accounts for approximately $15 billion in annual Medicare spending (Medicare Payment Advisory Commission, as cited in Naylor et al., 2011). Consequently, the Affordable Care Act includes provisions that support transitional care interventions to high-risk Medicare beneficiaries. Examples of interventions include timely postdischarge follow-up services to patients and their caregivers, comprehensive medication review and management, and assistance to ensure timely interactions between patients and postacute and outpatient providers (Naylor et al., 2011).

Although no one knows for certain what the "ideal" care model or models will look like in the future, two proposed frameworks that have received a great deal of consideration are accountable care organizations (ACOs) and patient-centered medical homes (PCMHs). Both rely on health care organizations and physicians providing coordinated and integrated care, which has significant implications for an organization's ability to manage information effectively. We discuss both in the following section.

Accountable Care Organizations

The Affordable Care Act authorizes the Medicare program to contract with *accountable care organizations (ACOs),* which are networks of physicians and other providers who work together to improve the quality of health care services and reduce costs for a defined patient population (Merlis, 2010). Specific provisions of the Act require that the ACO include a sufficient number of primary care professionals to provide services to at least five thousand beneficiaries for a three-year period and demonstrate the ability to report data on cost, quality, and overall patient experience for Medicare beneficiaries (Shortell, Casalino, & Fisher, 2010). The intent is to allow providers organized as ACOs that voluntarily meet quality thresholds to share in the cost savings they achieve for the Medicare program. The shared savings would be realized when the ACO provides care to Medicare beneficiaries for less than a Medicare benchmark cost, while meeting predefined criteria for quality of care and patient service. Each ACO must have a formal legal structure that enables it to receive shared payments and distribute them among providers. The ACO must also show that it can meet the quality and reporting standards.

The concept of the ACO emerged as a means of promoting integration and collaboration between physicians and hospitals. Physicians who are tied to a particular hospital often already function as part of an informal network, and their patients tend to stay within the network for the majority of their care (Merlis, 2010). These facts suggested that groups consisting of one or more hospitals—and the physicians who use them—might be brought together in organized systems. Payers could then hold these "systems" accountable for providing high-quality, cost-effective care to their defined patient population. Organizations that assume a leadership role to improve their performance would be financially rewarded for providing patient-centered, coordinated care (Merlis, 2010).

There is a host of reasons why a health care organization or provider (or even patient) might decide to pursue an ACO arrangement. First, an ACO has the potential to provide more cost-effective, coordinated care to a growing number of individuals with chronic illnesses, who often see multiple health care providers in different locations. Second, ACOs can promote interprofessional collaboration and teamwork among all clinicians involved in the patient's care and can provide rewards for keeping people well (Shortell et al., 2010). They also provide the foundation for implementing EHR systems and encourage patients to be involved in their own care by providing them access to their records, test results, and online patient education materials. Some experts believe ACOs may help address the primary care physician shortage by providing a more positive work environment to recruit graduates into primary care and promote team-based practice (Shortell et al., 2010). CMS is moving toward a bundled payment system, whereby a single payment will be made to hospitals and physicians jointly for a given condition, episode of care, or procedure. Therefore, it will become important to be able to manage the overall care to the patient effectively across the continuum, not just when the patient is in the hospital.

Patient-Centered Medical Homes

A second model that is receiving increased attention as a means to improve quality and reduce costs is the _patient-centered medical home (PCMH)._ The PCMH is an approach to providing comprehensive primary care through an individual's life by facilitating partnerships between the patient, his or her providers, and if appropriate, the patient's family. In 2007, a team of four physician societies published a joint statement of principles calling for accessible, continuous team-based care that focuses on the whole person, with the PCMH taking responsibility for care coordination (Patient-Centered Primary Care Collaborative, 2007). The principles include

- Providing each patient with a personal physician trained to provide first contact, continuous, and comprehensive care
- Ensuring that a personal physician–led team coordinates care
- Viewing the patient as a whole person and providing care appropriate for all stages of life
- Coordinating and integrating care across multiple providers and settings; using appropriate health information technology to share information among providers and patient
- Adhering to evidence-based guidelines that ensure quality and safety; involving patients in decision making
- Providing patients with easy access to care, appointments, and communication with providers
- Paying according to added value to patients who have a PCMH

Integral to the PCMH model is the use of health information technology for sharing information among the team of health care providers involved in the patient's care. Patients are also active participants in their own care, and therefore information technology should be used to support performance improvement, patient education, and enhanced communication (Patient-Centered Primary Care Collaborative, 2007).

A recent national study of PCMHs in the United States identified 447 practices representing 2,274 physicians that have achieved recognition by the National Committee on Quality Assurance (Scholle, Saunders, Tirodkar, Torda, & Pawlson, 2011). Both small and large practices demonstrated achievement of goals related to accessible, coordinated, and patient-centered care. However, practices affiliated with larger organizations achieved higher levels of PCMH recognition compared to unaffiliated smaller practices. The researchers found that smaller practices needed additional assistance with the use of data for population management and patient self-management (Scholle et al., 2011).

Both ACOs and PCMHs require that health IT support the organization and its providers in carrying out the following functions:

- Managing and coordinating integrated care
- Identifying, managing, and reducing or containing costs

- Adhering to evidence-based practice guidelines and standards of care; ensuring quality and safety
- Managing population health
- Engaging patients and their families and caregivers in their own care
- Reporting on quality outcomes

The better equipped organizations are to perform these tasks, the better their position will be in the future. Health care leaders need to ensure that their organizations have the health IT infrastructure and systems to easily support these functions.

New Forms of Payment for Health Services Delivery

In consort with new models of care are new or modified forms of payment for health care services. Different methods are being piloted in various communities around the nation. These are bundled payments, pay for performance, shared savings programs, capitation or global payment, and episode-of-care payments. *Bundled payments* may take different forms such as making a single payment for both hospital and physician services instead of separate payments; bundling payments for inpatient and post-acute care; or paying based on diagnosis instead of treatment. *Pay for performance (P4P)* programs reward hospitals, physician practices, and other providers with both financial and nonfinancial incentives based on performance on select measures. These performance measures can cover various aspects of health care delivery: clinical quality and safety, efficiency, patient experience, and health information technology adoption. Most P4P programs, however, are still a bonus to a fee-for-service model (Miller, 2011). *Shared savings programs* are intended to reward providers by paying them a bonus that is explicitly connected to the amount by which they reduce the total cost of care compared to expected levels. Shared savings is an integral part of the Affordable Care Act. *Capitation or global payment* places full risk with the provider organization. An *episode-of-care payment* system would pay the provider organization a single payment for all of the services associated with a hospitalization or other episode of acute care, including both inpatient and postacute care (Miller, 2011).

These new payment models are being considered because the current fee-for-service payment system contributes to cost and quality problems. Hospitals, physicians, and other providers receive more revenue for delivering more services, not for delivering higher quality or services that are more effective in improving a patient's health. Furthermore, health care providers often make less money if a patient stays healthy. Separate payments are made to each physician, hospital, and other health care provider involved in a patient's care, often leading to duplicate tests and services for the same patient (Miller, 2011). In addition, no financial incentive exists for individual providers to coordinate their services. Harold Miller, the executive director of the Center for Healthcare Quality and Payment Reform, argues that some of the proposed payment reforms do too little to address the problems caused by current payment systems or change payment too drastically for providers to easily implement (2011). He suggests that there is a need for "middle-ground" options—payment systems that provide greater flexibility and accountability for care, while enabling health care providers to deliver some improvements in cost and quality for payers and patients as the providers build the capacity to transition to more comprehensive payment reforms. Although an in-depth discussion of these and other proposed payment reform systems is beyond the scope of this book, the changing payment systems have enormous implications for health IT professionals.

HEALTH INFORMATION EXCHANGE

Essential to successful implementation of new models of care and payment reform is the exchange of clinical and administration information among different health care entities and between providers and patients. The concept of health information exchange (HIE) is not new. For nearly two decades organizations and collaborators have tried to facilitate HIE, but unfortunately a number of HIE initiatives have failed to be sustainable over the long term (Vest & Gamm, 2010). The HITECH Act places renewed interest in the success of HIE by providing incentive payments to eligible providers for meaningful use of electronic health records, which includes having the ability to exchange information electronically with others in order to have a comprehensive view of the patient's health and care (Rudin et al., 2011).

The verb phrase "health information exchange" refers to the "electronic movement of health related information among organizations according to nationally recognized standards" (National Alliance for Health Information Technology, 2008). The noun phrase "health information exchange" refers to "a health information organization that brings together health care stakeholders within a defined geographic area and governs health information exchange among them for the purpose of improving health and care in that community" (National Alliance for Health Information, 2008). These may also be referred to as health information exchange organizations or regional health information organizations (RHIOs).

By participating in an HIE or sharing health information, a number of potential important benefits may be realized:

- Serves as a building block for improved patient care, quality, and safety
- Makes relevant health care information readily available when and where it is needed
- Provides the means to reduce duplication of services that can lead to reduced health care costs
- Enables automation of administrative tasks
- Provides governance and management over the data exchange process
- Facilitates achievement of meaningful use requirements (Health Information Management and Systems Society, 2010)

Nationwide Health Information Network

Most successful health information exchange (HIE) initiatives to date have occurred within a geographical region, community, or state (National eHealth Collaborative, 2011). There have also been coordinated efforts by public and private stakeholders at the national level to develop a *nationwide health information network (NwHIN)*. The NwHIN is "a set of standards, services and policies that enable secure health information exchange over the Internet" (NwHIN, n.d.). The intent is to be able to securely link regional and state HIEs to create a national interoperable "network of networks" for sharing health care data across the nation (Dixon, Zafar, & Overhage, 2010). Connections between individual HIEs will enable health care providers participating in the HIE to access relevant health information when caring for a patient regardless of where that data may be stored.

Two major initiatives affiliated with NwHIN include the Direct Project and the CONNECT Open Source Solution. The Direct Project was launched in March 2010 and was established to specify a simple, secure, scalable, standards-based way for participants to send authenticated, encrypted data over the Internet. Several pilot programs are using the specifications developed by the Direct Project in their exchange of information for patient care and public health reporting and other purposes. Details of these pilot efforts may be found at http://directproject.org.

The CONNECT is an open source software solution that permits HIE, both locally and nationally. CONNECT uses NwHIN standards and services.

It was developed collaboratively by more than twenty federal agencies in 2007 and initially used primarily among federal agencies. Currently, over two thousand organizations, including federal agencies, states, health care providers, insurers, and health IT vendors, are working together to improve the CONNECT Open Source Solution. Additional information and resources that are publicly available to providers, organizations, or HIEs that are interested in learning more about CONNECT should visit their web site at http://www .connectopensource.org.

State and Regional Health Information Exchange (HIE) Efforts

In 2010, the ONC granted fifty-six awards totaling $548 million to assist states in facilitating the electronic exchange of health information among providers within their region (ONC, 2010a). The effort is known as the State HIE Cooperative Agreement Program, and it aims to ensure that every eligible health care provider has at least one option for HIE that meets the requirements of the Medicare and Medicaid EHR Incentive Programs. The following year, eHealth Initiative conducted the 2011 nationwide survey on HIE initiatives and the vendors supporting them; 127 participants responded to the survey (eHealth Initiative, 2011). HIEs are generally structured into one of three different frameworks:

- *Centralized:* health information and data reside in one central location
- *Federated:* health information is stored at the local or regional level with the HIE services acting as a conduit for exchange between other entities
- *Hybrid:* a combination of centralized and federated; central repository may be maintained with "edge servers" used for data storage

The most common architecture is hybrid (52 percent), followed by federated HIEs (27 percent), and centralized (21 percent) (eHealth Initiative, 2011).

The HIE Lessons

Despite the fact that the environment for building and creating and developing an HIE organization has never been better, the concerns about long-term sustainability and the impact and value of exchanging health information persist. The National eHealth Collaborative (NeHC) recently conducted a comprehensive study of twelve fully operationally HIEs across the nation to find out from their leaders what factors have led to their success (NeHC, 2011). In-depth structured interviews were conducted with senior executives representing the business, clinical, and technical areas of each HIE. Key critical success factors these leaders identified in sustaining an HIE are

- *Aligning stakeholders with HIE priorities in an intensive and ongoing effort.* Create a shared vision that all stakeholders can embrace and that serves as the cornerstone to success. Foster an environment that is built on trust and that promotes learning and resolves differences when they arise. Make ongoing and effective stakeholder engagement a priority.

- *Establishing and maintaining consistent brand identity and role as a trusted, neutral entity dedicated to protecting the interests of participants.* Data use and data integrity are two critical elements. The culture, policies, and procedures regarding the use of data must assure that no entity will gain competitive advantage at the expense of others. Consent and security policies must meet the requirements of various stakeholders and regions or states. The HIE infrastructure must ensure that patient data are accurate, reliable, and trustworthy.

- *Ensuring alignment with vision in making strategic choices.* Assess the stakeholders' alignment with the initiative and congruence with the vision before deciding to pursue them. Regardless of how promising a source of funding may have initially appeared, some HIEs chose not to pursue it because the funding source did not have the full support of all stakeholders.

- *Considering structural characteristics and dynamics of the HIE market.* The geographic location, composition of stakeholders, and resource capabilities are all factors to consider.

- *Understanding clinical workflow and managing change.* The implementation of an HIE requires that clinicians and administrative staff understand the impact of HIE applications on workflow and identify opportunities to improve efficiencies (NeHC, 2011).

Different business models, governance structures, and strategies may be used to create value for the HIE participants.

HealthBridge formed an HIE in 1997 as a community effort to share health information electronically in the Greater Cincinnati–Northern Kentucky area. Currently, the network joins over fifty hospitals and 7,500 physicians in three states. The network transmits three million electronic clinical messages each month including laboratory results, radiology reports, operative notes, and discharge summaries. HealthBridge serves over 80 percent of physicians and acute care hospitals within its service area and is estimated to have reduced health care costs by $20 million annually (NeHC, 2011).

Although HealthBridge was formerly funded primarily by fees, in 2010 it received three large federal grants to support its operations. Pricing fees and approaches differ depending on the communities in which they serve. For example, lab fees are based on the number of specimens processed. Fees for EHR data exchange are paid by both the sender and the recipient of data, since both sides benefit from the transaction.

Several of the strategic initiatives for which HealthBridge has been involved to drive value creation are

- Consumer and patient engagement: piloting a PHR under the Indiana HIE Challenge Grant
- New care delivery models: serving as an online data analytical service for aggregating and synthesizing raw data for ACOs
- Serve as HIE for 1,700 clinicians using electronic health records in community (NeHC, 2011)

INFORMATION TECHNOLOGY RAMIFICATIONS OF NEW MODELS OF CARE AND PAYMENT REFORM

What are the information technology ramifications of integrated care models and payment reform? Integrated care generally requires health care professionals from different organizations to work together as a team to provide high-quality, cost-effective care. If the goal is to provide continuity of care, shared care, and seamless care, members of the health care team must be able to share information about, and with, patients at appropriate points in the care process (Protti, 2009). Effective health information exchange (HIE) among primary care providers, specialists, therapists, hospitals, and other care providers is vital to coordinate care and provide clinical integration. Care coordination is providing the *right care in the right place at the right time by the right provider,* all of the time. Clinical integration requires that provider organizations (including ACOs and PCMHs) achieve efficiencies by monitoring and controlling quality, service, and costs; using evidence-based practice guidelines; and providing tools to improve compliance.

To effectively manage costs, health care executives will need tools and data to support different types of financial modeling. For example, an ACO will need actuarial cost and utilization predictors to effectively manage the care of a defined population. Ensuring that adequate cost accounting systems are in place (along with EHR and PHR systems) is critical to effective management under the various payment models. In addition, some IT capability such as home care support or patient engagement tools may be needed to monitor vital patient information and actively involve patients in the management of their own care (Rossignol, 2011). Health IT clearly plays a vital role in the success of new models of care and payment reform and should be an integral part of the organization's planning process.

Accurately Identify and Link Patient Data

An important first step in connecting patient data across different care settings is to establish *master patient indices* (Glaser & Salzberg, 2011). Patient indices can serve as a crosswalk among the different medical record numbers and identifiers that may be used by various provider organizations to correctly identify patients. In addition, a record locator service may be used to determine which patient records exist for a member and where the source data is located. The key concept behind having a record locator service is that a patient's health information is housed on computers at the various sites of his or her care and this information is queried and aggregated from these sites at the time of a request. Functions to look for in a record locator service include the ability to

- Manage participating provider identities
- Maintain and publish a patient index
- Match patients using defined algorithms
- Look up patient record locations (but not the records themselves)
- Communicate securely and maintain an audit log
- Manage patient consent to record sharing (under state laws and HITECH) (Glaser & Salzberg, 2011)

A record locator service would be common in a federated HIE. This differs from a centralized HIE model whereby all known data on the patient is brought together in a single logical database or repository and that database is accessed when data are needed. Besides linking patient data, it is important to have in place a security infrastructure that authenticates users of the health information exchange and ensures data integrity (Glaser & Salzberg, 2011).

Other Important IT Considerations

Beyond identifying and linking patient data across systems, under new payment models it will be important for health care provider organizations to consider the following IT functionality:

1. *Share patient information in standardized format.* Through the HIE, health care providers should be able to send and retrieve continuity of care documents (CCDs) or continuity of care records (CCR). The CCR data set includes a summary of the patient's health status (for example, problems, medications, and allergies) and basic information about insurance, advance directives, care documentation, and the patient's care plan. These documents ideally should be pushed directly into the EHR systems for the providers' use daily; otherwise, the workflow may be cumbersome for the clinician-user and the information may never get to the clinician (Rossignol, 2011).

2. *Establish care coordination systems.* Providers will need systems that allow them to coordinate care for a given patient in multiple care settings. To do so, different types of IT systems are available with different levels of maturity:

   a. *Referral management systems.* These systems are mature and generally a component of the HIE. They automate the referral process, including the request for referral and accompanying required patient documentation (Rossignol, 2011).

   b. *Patient navigation systems.* These systems provide a longitudinal view of patient encounters (including appointments, events such as ED visits or hospitalizations, interactions with members of health care team, patient education, self-monitoring, and so forth) (Rossignol, 2011).

3. *Explore patient engagement systems.* A critical member of the health care team under these new models of care is the patient. To actively involve the patient in his or her own care, health care provider organizations should examine the extent to which their IT

systems enable patients to monitor their health at home. Examples of patient engagement systems include personal health records (PHRs) that provide context-specific alerts, reminders, and medical content when patient vital signs or values are out of range (Rossignol, 2011) and home monitoring devices including mobile applications that can aid in promoting wellness or managing chronic diseases more effectively. Apps like iTriage, which are web-based and mobile, help patients to "self-triage" when they answer select questions and determine whether ED care is needed; they can also report the wait time at local EDs and provide directions to the closest one (Sarasohn-Kahn, 2011).

4. *Participate in disease registries.* Providers may enroll their patients into one or more disease populations and add them to disease registries based on data extracts from the EHR. As consolidated disease registries, the EHRs may track key clinical markers for each patient across all the patient's conditions. For example, one of the tools Kaiser Permanente uses to operate their population-based care is the case management process, whereby a case manager is assigned to monitor patients to see that they stay on track with their disease protocol across care settings, including their home (Kwo & Irani, 2008).

5. *Monitor performance and report quality.* Having the capacity to effectively monitor performance and report on quality measures will be critical under payment reform. Organizations will need to have in place systems that can provide analytical information such as:

   a. Identifying at-risk populations

   b. Monitoring physician performance

   c. Reporting on quality outcomes

   d. Assessing comparative clinical effectiveness by monitoring cost and performance measures (Rossignol, 2011)

Other questions health care executives should ask themselves in assessing their organization's IT capability to effectively manage under new payment models of care:

- To what extent do our providers embrace and adhere to evidence-based practice guidelines?
- How are our systems and incentives designed and aligned to deliver the desired outcome?

- How do we coordinate care resources, engage patients, measure feedback, and improve the patient experience?
- To what extent do our patients trust that their health information is private and secure?

Protti (2009) argues that integrated care calls for integrated information systems to support it. This entails (a) helping clinicians to work in virtual teams to delivery patient care across settings, (b) assisting providers in delivering evidenced-based, population-based chronic care across settings and disease conditions, (c) generating complex information to monitor outcomes, and (d) making the patient experience seamless across the care continuum (Protti, 2009). IT is not the be-all and end-all; however, it is an essential tool in this new era of increased accountability. Health care organizations that can do these things well, and have available predictive modeling tools for forecasting what is likely to happen under various scenarios, will be far better equipped to lead effectively now and in the future.

SUMMARY

The degree of federal legislation and activity that has occurred from the late 2000s through 2010s to further the adoption and meaningful use of health information technology is unprecedented. As part of the American Recovery and Affordable Act, the HITECH Act of 2009 allocated over $30 billion to incentivize hospitals and eligible practitioners to become meaningful users of EHR technology, to create the infrastructure to support health information exchange, and to train a workforce along with regional extension centers that could serve as resources to small physician practices and rural community hospitals engaged in the EHR system selection and implementation process.

Coupled with HITECH, in March 2010, President Obama signed into law the Patient Protection and Affordable Care Act. With this Act came a far greater emphasis on evaluating new models of care delivery and payment reform that will lead to improved quality and reduced costs.

Two models of care receiving considerable attention include accountable care organizations (ACOs) and patient-centered medical homes (PCMH). Both models rely on health care providers and organizations delivering coordinated and integrated care across the continuum of care, and both have significant implications from a health IT perspective. Provider organizations considering these models of care will need to have ready access to information systems that enable them to adhere to evidence-based guidelines, ensure quality and safety, manage population health, engage patients and their families in their own care, and report on quality outcomes. With new models of care come new or different methods of payment that are better aligned with the goals they are intending to achieve. Some of the payment methods include bundled payments, pay for performance, shared savings programs, capitation, and episode-of-care payments.

Central to achieving meaningful use, the implementation of new models of care, and payment reform is the ability to electronically exchange health information among different health care entities and between providers. A Nationwide Health Information Network (NwHIN) or set of standards, services, and policies that promote secure HIE over the Internet has been established. The ONC funded fifty-six state and regional HIE cooperative programs to facilitate and support HIE within states and communities. Lessons learned from leaders in twelve fully operational HIEs include creating a shared vision, engaging stakeholders, ensuring sound data use and data integrity policies, evaluating the marketplace, evaluating the impact of HIE on clinician workflow, and managing change.

Individual health care organizations and providers will also need to ensure that they have the IT capabilities needed to effectively manage care and resources under the new models of care and payment reform. Patients will need to be accurately identified and their information linked across multiple care settings. Organizations will need to ensure that they can send and receive electronic patient data in a standardized format, such as CCD and CCR, and that the data are well integrated within their existing systems and workflow. Other important IT considerations will include establishing care coordination systems, exploring systems for engaging patients in their own care, participating in disease registries, and monitoring performance and quality. Health care leaders who are well equipped with these tools as well as predictive modeling tools will be better prepared to effectively lead their organizations during this period of great change.

KEY TERMS

Accountable care organization
  (ACO)
American Recovery and Reinvestment
  Act (ARRA) of 2009
Beacon Communities
Bundled payments
Capitation or global payment
Center for Medicare and Medicaid
  Services (CMS)
EHR certification program

Episode-of-care payment
Health information exchange
Health Information Technology for
  Economic and Clinical Health
  (HITECH) Act
Health IT workforce training
  programs
Master patient indices
Medicare and Medicaid EHR
  Incentive Programs

Meaningful use

Nationwide Health Information Network (NwHIN)

Office of the National Coordinator for Health Information Technology (ONC)

Patient Centered Medical Home (PCMH)

Patient Protection and Affordable Care Act (PPACA)

Pay for performance

Privacy and security requirements

Regional Extension Centers (RECs)

Shared savings programs

Strategic HIT Advance Research Project (SHARP)

LEARNING ACTIVITIES

1. Investigate the latest meaningful use criteria for eligible professionals or eligible hospitals. Visit either a physician practice or hospital in your community. Have they participated in the Medicare or Medicaid EHR Incentive Program? Why or why not? If the organization or provider has participated in the program, what has the experience been like? What lessons have they learned? Find out the degree to which the facility uses electronic health records and what issues or challenges they have had in achieving meaningful use.

2. Evaluate different models of care within your local community and/or state. Did you find any examples of accountable care organizations or patient-centered medical homes? Explain. Working as a team, visit or interview a leader from a site that uses an innovative model of care. Describe the model, its use, challenges, and degree of patient coordination and integration. How is health IT used to support the delivery of care and reporting of outcomes?

3. Investigate one of the Beacon Communities to find out how they are using health IT to improve quality of care and access to care within their region. Be prepared to share with the class a summary of your findings. Do you think the work that this Beacon Community has done could be replicated in your community? Why or why not?

4. Explore the extent to which health information exchange is occurring within your community, region, or state. Who are the key players? What types of models of health information exchange exist? To what extent is information being exchanged across organizations for patient care purposes? What challenges have they faced? How have they overcome them, if at all?

REFERENCES

Blumenthal, D. (2010). Launching HITECH. *New England Journal of Medicine*, *362*(5), 382–385.

Buntin, M. B., Jain, S. H., & Blumenthal, D. (2010). Health information technology: Laying the infrastructure for national health reform. *Health Affairs*, *29*(6), 1214–1219.

Carson, D. S., Garr, D. R., Goforth, G. A., & Forkner, E. (2010). *The time to hesitate has passed: The age of electronic health records is here* (pp. 2–11). Columbia: South Carolina Medical Association.

Centers for Medicare and Medicaid. (n.d.). Meaningful use. Retrieved February 2013 from http://www.cms.gov/Regulations-and-Guidance/Legislation/EHRIncentive Programs/Meaningful_Use.html

Department of Health and Human Services (HHS). (2011). Meaningful use overview. Retrieved February 2013 from http://www.healthit.gov/buzz-blog /meaningful-use/resources-onc-becoming-meaningful-user-ehr

Dixon, B. E., Zafar, A., & Overhage, J. M. (2010). A framework for evaluating the costs, effort, and value of nationwide health information exchange. *Journal of the American Medical Informatics Association*, *17*, 295–301.

eHealth Initiative. (2011). Report on HIE market and vendors. Retrieved February 2013 from http://www.ehealthinitiative.org/resources/viewdownload/54-annual -surveys/221–2011-report-on-health-information-exchange-market-report-and-hie -vendor-list.html

Glaser, J. P., & Salzberg, C. (2011). *The strategic application of information technology in health care organizations* (3rd ed). San Francisco: Jossey-Bass.

Guterman, S., & Drake, H. (2010, May). *Developing innovative payment approaches: Finding the path to high performance*. New York: The Commonwealth Fund.

Health Information Management and Systems Society. (2010). Overview of HIE in era of meaningful use. Retrieved February 2013 from http://www.himss.org /content/files/12_21_2010_HIE%20OverView%20in%20HITECH.pdf

Institute of Medicine. (2000). *To err is human: Building a safer health system*. Washington, DC: National Academies Press.

Institute of Medicine. (2001). *Crossing the quality chasm: A new health system for the 21st century*. Washington, DC: National Academies Press.

Jha, A. K. (2010). Meaningful use of electronic health records: The road ahead. *Journal of the American Medical Association*, *304*(15), 1709–1710.

Jha, A. K., DesRoches, C. M., Campbell, E. G., Donelan, K., Rao, S. R., Ferris, T. G., . . . & Blumenthal, D. (2009). Use of electronic health records in US hospitals. *New England Journal of Medicine*, *360*, 1628–1638.

Kaiser Family Foundation. (2011). Summary of new health care reform. Retrieved February 2013 from http://www.kff.org/healthreform/upload/8061.pdf

Kolkman, L., & Brown, B. (2011). *The HIE formation guide: The authoritative guide for planning an HIE in your state, region, community*. Chicago: HIMSS.

Kwo, D., & Irani, M. (2008). *Integrated care organizations: The importance of integrated information systems*. NHS Alliance. Retrieved November 2012 from http://www.nhsalliance.org/default.asp

McKethan, A., Brammer, C., Fatemi, P., Kim, M., Kirtane, J., Kunzman, J., . . . & Jain, S. H. (2011). An early status report on the beacon communities' plans for transformation via health information technology. *Health Affairs, 30*(4), 782–788.

Merlis, M. (2010, August 13). Health policy brief: Accountable care organizations. Retrieved February 2013 from www.healthaffairs.org

Miller, H. D. (2011). *Transitioning to accountable care: Incremental payment reforms to support higher quality, more affordable health care*. Pittsburgh: Center for Healthcare Quality and Payment Reform.

National Alliance for Health Information Technology. (2008, April 28). *Report to the Office of the National Coordinator for Health Information Technology on defining key health information technology terms*. Department of Health and Human Services. Retrieved February 2013 from http://www.nahit.org/docs/hitterms finalreport_051508.pdf.

National eHealth Collaborative. (2011, July). *Secrets of HIE success revealed: Lessons from the leaders*. Washington, DC: Author.

Nationwide Health Information Network. (n.d.). HealthIT.gov. Retrieved February 2013 from http://www.healthit.gov/policy-researchers-implementers/nationwide -health-information-network-nwhin

Naylor, M. D., Aiken, L. H., Kurtzman, E. T., Olds, D. M., & Hirshman, K. B. (2011). The importance of transitional care in achieving health reform. *Health Affairs, 30*(4), 746–754.

Office of the National Coordinator for Health Information Technology. (2010a). Beacon community program. Retrieved February 2013 from http:// healthit.hhs.gov/portal/server.pt?open=512&objID=1805&parentname=Community Page&parentid=2&mode=2&cached=true

Office of the National Coordinator for Health Information Technology. (2010b). Strategic Health IT Advanced Research Projects (SHARP). Retrieved February 2013 from http://healthit.hhs.gov/portal/server.pt/community /healthit_hhs_gov__sharp_program/1806

Office of the National Health Information Technology Coordinator. (2011). *Federal health information technology strategic plan: 2011–2015*. Retrieved February 2013 from http://www.healthit.gov/sites/default/files/utility/final-federal-health-it -strategic-plan-0911.pdf

Patient-Centered Primary Care Collaborative. (2007). Joint principles of the patient-centered medical home. Retrieved February 2013 from http:// www.pcpcc.net/joint-principles

Protti, D. (2009). Integrated care needs: Integrated information management and technology. *Healthcare Quarterly, 13* (special issue), 24–29.

Rossignol, P. (2011). *Integrated care organizations' integrated technology requirements.* Internal position paper (unpublished). New York: Deloitte Consulting.

Rudin, R. S., Salzberg, C. A., Szolovitis, P., Volk, L. A., Simon, S. R., & Bates, D. W. (2011). Care transitions as opportunities for clinicians to use data exchange services: How often do they occur? *Journal of the American Medical Informatics Association, 18*(6), 853–859.

Sarasohn-Kahn, J. (2011). *Primary care, everywhere: Connecting the dots across the emerging health landscape.* Oakland: California HealthCare Foundation.

Scholle, S. H., Saunders, R. C., Tirodkar, M. A., Torda, P., & Pawlson, L. G. (2011). Patient-centered medical homes in the United States. *Journal of Ambulatory Care Management, 34*(1), 20–32.

Schuster, M., McGlynn, E. A., & Brook, R. H. (2005). How good is the quality of health care in the US? *Milbank Quarterly, 83*(4), 843–895.

Shortell, S. M., Casalino, L. P., & Fisher, E. S. (2010). How the Center for Medicare and Medicaid Innovation should test accountable care organizations. *Health Affairs, 29*(7), 1293–1298.

Vest, J. R., & Gamm, L. D. (2010). Health information exchange: Persistent challenges and new strategies. *Journal of the American Medical Informatics Association, 17,* 288–294.

CHAPTER 7

System Acquisition

LEARNING OBJECTIVES

- To be able to explain the process a health care organization generally goes through in selecting a health care information system.
- To be able to describe the systems development life cycle and its four major stages.
- To be able to discuss the various options for acquiring a health care information system (for example, purchasing, leasing, contracting with an application service provider, or building a system in-house) and the pros and cons of each option.
- To be able to discuss the purpose and content of a request for information and request for proposal in the system acquisition process.
- To gain insight into the problems that may occur during the system acquisition process.
- To gain an understanding of the health care IT industry and the resources available for identifying health care IT vendors and learning about their history, products, services, and reputation.

By now you should have an understanding of the various types of health care information systems and the value they can bring to health care organizations and the patients they serve. This chapter describes the typical process a health care organization goes through in acquiring or selecting a new clinical or administrative application. Acquiring an information system (IS) application can be an enormous investment for health care organizations. Besides the initial cost, there are a host of long-term costs associated with maintaining, supporting, and enhancing the system. Health care professionals need access to reliable, complete, and accurate information in order to provide effective and efficient health care services and to achieve the strategic goals of the organization. Selecting the right application, one that meets the organization's needs, is a critical step. Too often information systems are acquired without exploring all options, without evaluating costs and benefits, and without gaining sufficient input from key constituent user groups. The results can be disastrous.

This chapter describes the people who should be involved, the activities that should occur, and the questions that should be addressed in acquiring any new information system. The suggested methods are based on the authors' years of experience and on countless case studies of system acquisition successes and failures published in the health care literature.

SYSTEM ACQUISITION: A DEFINITION

In this book *system acquisition* refers to the process that occurs from the time the decision is made to select a new system (or replace an existing system) until the time a contract has been negotiated and signed. System implementation is a separate process described in the next chapter, but both are part of the systems development life cycle. The actual system selection, or acquisition, process can take anywhere from a few days to a couple of years, depending on the organization's size, structure, complexity, and needs. Factors such as whether the system is deemed a priority and whether adequate resources (time, people, and funds) are available can also directly affect the time and methods used to acquire a new system (Jones et al., 2011).

Prior to arriving at the decision to select a new system, the health care executive team should engage in a strategic IS planning process, in which the strategic goals of the organization are formulated and the ways in which information technology (IT) will be employed to aid the organization in achieving its strategic goals and objectives are discussed. We discuss the need for aligning the IT plans with the strategic goals of the organization and for determining IT priorities in Chapter Thirteen. In this chapter, we assume that a strategic IT plan exists, IT priorities have been established, the new system has been adequately budgeted, and the organization is ready to move forward with the selection process. We also assume that the organization has conducted a readiness assessment and is well equipped to move forward with the health IT project or initiative. The AHRQ National Resource Center for Health IT has publicly available a number of tools that can be helpful to health care organizations in assessing their readiness health IT projects such as EHR implementations and for ensuring that they have in place the personnel, technical, and financial resources to embark on the initiative. These tools can be found at http://healthit.ahrq.gov/Survey_Compendium.

SYSTEMS DEVELOPMENT LIFE CYCLE

No board of directors would recommend building a new health care facility without an architect's blueprint and a comprehensive assessment of the organization's and the community's needs and resources. The architect's blueprint helps ensure that the new facility has a strong foundation, is well designed, fosters the provision of high-quality care, and has the potential for growth and expansion. Similarly, the health care organization needs a blueprint to aid in the planning, selection, implementation, and support of a new health care information system. The decision to invest in a health care information system should be well aligned with the organization's overall strategic goals and should be made after careful thought and deliberation. Information systems are an investment in the organization's infrastructure, not a one-time purchase. Health care information systems require not only up-front costs and resources but also ongoing maintenance, support, upgrades, and eventually, replacement.

The process an organization generally goes through in planning, selecting, implementing, and evaluating a health care information system is known as the *systems development life cycle (SDLC)*. Although the SDLC is most commonly described in the context of software development, the process also applies when systems are purchased from a vendor or leased through an *application service provider (ASP)*. An ASP is a company that deploys, hosts, and manages one or more clinical or administrative information systems through centrally located servers (generally via the Internet), often on a fixed, per-use basis or on a subscription basis. Regardless of how the system is acquired, most health care organizations follow a structured process for selecting and implementing a new computer-based system. The systems development process itself involves participation from individuals with different backgrounds and areas of expertise. The specific mix of individuals depends on the nature and scope of the new system.

Figure 7.1. Systems development life cycle

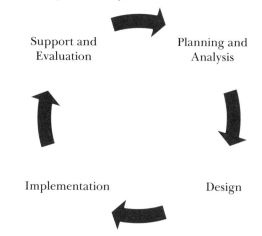

Support and
Evaluation

Planning and
Analysis

Implementation

Design

Many SDLC frameworks exist, some of which employ an incremental approach, but most have four general phases, or stages—planning and analysis, design, implementation, and support and evaluation (Wager & Lee, 2006) (see Figure 7.1). Each phase has a number of tasks that need to be performed. In this chapter we focus on the first two phases; Chapter Eight focuses on the last two.

The SDLC approach assumes that this four-phase life of an IS starts with a need and ends when the benefits of the system no longer outweigh its maintenance costs, at which point the life of a new system begins (Oz, 2012). Hence, the entire project is called a *life cycle*. After the decision has been made to explore further the need for a new information system, the feasibility of the system is assessed and the scope of the project defined (in actuality it is at times difficult to tell when this decision making ends and analysis begins). The primary focus of this *planning and analysis phase* is on the business problem, or the organization's strategy, independent of any technology that can or will be used. During this phase, it is important to examine current systems and problems in order to identify opportunities for improvement. The organization should assess the feasibility of the new system—is it technologically, financially, and operationally feasible? Furthermore, sometimes it is easy to think that implementing a new IS will solve all information management problems. Rarely, if ever, is this the case. But by critically evaluating existing systems and workflow processes, the health care team might find that current problems are rooted in ineffective procedures or lack of sufficient training. Not always is a new system needed or *the* answer to a problem.

Once it is clear that a new IS is needed, the next step is to assess the information needs of users and define the functional requirements: What functions must the system have to fulfill the need? This process can be very time consuming. However, it is vital to solicit widespread participation from end users during this early stage—to solicit and achieve buy-in. As part of the needs assessment, it is also helpful to gather, organize, and evaluate information about the environment in which the new system is to operate. Through defining system requirements, the organization specifies what the system should be able to do and the means by which it will fulfill its stated goals.

Once the team knows what the organization needs, it enters the second stage, the *design phase*, where it considers all its options. Will the new system be designed in-house? Will the organization contract with an outside developer? Or will the organization purchase a system from a health information systems vendor or contract with an ASP? A large majority of health care organizations purchase a system from a vendor or at least look first at the systems available on the market. System design is the evaluation of alternative solutions to address the business problem. It is generally in this phase that all alternatives are considered, a cost-benefit analysis is done, a system is selected, and vendor negotiations are finalized.

After the contract has been finalized or the system has been chosen, the third phase, *implementation*, begins. The implementation phase requires significant allocation of resources in completing tasks such as conducting workflow and process analyses, installing the new system, testing the system, training staff, converting data, and preparing the organization and staff for the go-live of the new system. Finally, once the system is put into operation, the *support and evaluation phase* begins. It is common to underestimate the staff and resources needed to effectively keep new and existing information systems functioning properly. No matter how much time and energy were spent on the design and build of the application, you can count on the fact that changes will need to be made, glitches fixed, and upgrades installed. Likewise, most mission-critical systems need to be functioning 99.99 percent of the time—that is, with little downtime. Sufficient resources (people, technology, infrastructure, and upgrades) need to be allocated to maintain and support the new system. Although support costs can vary widely from system to system, in most industries up to 80 percent of the IS budget is spent on maintenance (Oz, 2012). The major reason for this significant proportion is that support is the longest phase in a system's life cycle.

Moreover, maintaining and supporting the new system is not enough. Health care executives and boards want to know the value of the IT investment, thus the degree to which the new system has achieved its goals and objectives should be assessed. Eventually, the system will be replaced and the SDLC process begins again.

With this general explanation of the SDLC established, we begin by focusing on the first two phases—the planning and analysis phase and the design phase. Together they constitute what we refer to as the *system acquisition process*.

SYSTEM ACQUISITION PROCESS

To gain an understanding of and appreciation for the activities that occur during the system acquisition process, we will follow a health care facility through the selection process for a new information system—specifically, an electronic health record (EHR) system. In this case the organization, which we will call Valley Practice, is a multiphysician primary care practice.

What process should the practice use to select the EHR? Should it purchase a system from a vendor, contract with an application service provider, or seek the assistance of a system developer? Who should lead the effort? Who should be involved in the process? What EHR products are available on the market?

Exhibit 7.1. Overview of system acquisition process

- Establish project steering committee and appoint project manager.
- Define project objectives and scope of analysis.
- Screen the marketplace and review vendor profiles.
- Determine system goals.
- Determine and prioritize system requirements.
- Develop and distribute a request for proposal (RFP) or a request for information (RFI).
- Explore other options for acquiring system.
  - Contract with application service provider.
  - Contract with system developer or build in-house.
- Evaluate vendor proposals.
  - Develop evaluation criteria.
  - Hold vendor demonstrations.
  - Make site visits and check references.
  - Prepare vendor analysis.
- Conduct cost-benefit analysis.
- Prepare summary report and recommendations.
- Conduct contract negotiations.

How reputable are the vendors who develop these products? These are just a few of the many questions that should be asked in selecting a new IS.

Although the time and the resources needed to select an EHR (or any health care information system) may vary considerably from one setting to another, some fundamental issues should be addressed in any system acquisition initiative. The sections that follow the case study describe in more detail the major activities that should occur (Exhibit 7.1), relating them to the multiphysician practice scenario. We assume that the practice wishes to purchase (rather than develop) an EHR system. However, we briefly describe other options and point out how the process may differ when the EHR acquisition process occurs in a larger health care setting, such as a hospital.

CASE STUDY
Acquiring an EHR System

Valley Practice provides patient care services at three locations, all within a fifteen-mile radius, and serves nearly 100,000 patients. Valley Practice is owned and operated by seven physicians; each physician has an equal partnership. In addition to the physicians, the practice employs nine nurses, fifteen support staff, a business officer manager, an accountant, and a chief executive officer (CEO).

During a two-day strategic planning session, the physicians and management team created a mission, vision, and set of strategic goals for Valley Practice. The mission of the facility is to serve as the primary care "medical home" of individuals within the community, regardless of the patients' ability to pay. Valley Practice wishes to be recognized as a "high-tech, high-touch" practice that provides high-quality, cost-effective patient care using evidence-based standards of care. Consistent with its mission, one of the practice's strategic goals is to replace its current paper-based medical record with an EHR system. Such a system should enable providers to care for patients using up-to-date, complete, accurate information, anywhere, anytime.

Dr. John Marcus, the lead physician at Valley Practice, asked Dr. Julie Brown, the newest partner in the group, to lead the EHR project initiative. Dr. Brown joined the practice two years ago after completing an internal medicine residency at an academic medical center that had a fully integrated EHR system available in both the hospital and

(cont.)

its ambulatory care clinics. Of all the physicians at Valley Practice, Dr. Brown has had the most experience using an EHR. She has been a vocal advocate for implementing an EHR and believes it is essential to enabling the facility to achieve its strategic goals. Dr. Brown contacted the Regional Extension Center (REC) in the community for assistance with the initiative.

Dr. Brown agreed to chair the project steering committee. She invited other key individuals to serve on the committee, including Dr. Renee Ward, a senior physician in the practice; Mr. James Rowls, the CEO; Ms. Mary Matthews, RN, a nurse; and Ms. Sandy Raymond, the business officer manager. Dr. Brown suggested that the committee work with the REC to guide committee members through the system acquisition process. The physician partners approved this request, and the committee made arrangements for a representative from the REC to work with them on the selection process.

After the project steering committee was formed, Dr. Marcus met with the committee to outline its charge and deliverables. Dr. Marcus expressed his appreciation to Dr. Brown and all of the members of the committee for their willingness to participate in this important initiative. He assured them that they had his full support and the support of the entire physician team.

Dr. Marcus reviewed with the committee the mission, vision, and strategic goals of the practice as well as the committee's charge. The committee was asked to fully investigate and recommend the top three EHR products available in the vendor community. He stressed his desire that the committee members would focus on EHR vendors that have experience and a solid track record in implementing systems in physician practices similar to theirs and that have Office of the National Coordinator for Health Information Technology (ONC)–certified EHR products. He expressed concern that there is a flurry of vendors offering EHR-type products without a solid track record.

Dr. Marcus felt strongly that the EHR system needed to enable providers to access patient information from any of Valley Practice's three sites and from their homes. He also spoke of the need for the system to provide health maintenance reminders, drug interactions, and access to clinical practice guidelines or standards of care. The practice also intends to take advantage of the CMS EHR Incentive Program and achieve meaningful use. Dr. Marcus is interested in exploring what opportunities are available for health information exchange within the region. He envisions that the practice may eventually partner with specialists, hospitals, and other key stakeholders in the community to provide coordinated care across the continuum. Under the leadership of Dr. Brown, the members of the project steering committee established five project goals and the methods they would use to guide their activities. Ms. Moore, the consultant, assisted them in clearly defining these goals and discussing the various options for moving forward. They agreed to consider EHR products from only those vendors that had five or more years of experience in the industry and had a solid track record of implementations (which they defined as having done twenty-five or more). Dr. Ward, Mr. Rowls, and Ms. Matthews assumed leadership roles in verifying and prioritizing the requirements expressed by the various user groups.

The five project goals were based on Valley Practice's strategic goals. These project goals were circulated for discussion and approved by the CEO and the physician partners. Once the goals were agreed upon, the project steering committee appointed a small task group of committee members to carry out the process of defining system functionality and requirements. Because staff time was limited, the task group conducted three separate focus groups during the lunch period—one with the nurses, one with the support staff, and a third with the physicians. Ms. Moore, the consultant, conducted the focus groups, using a semistructured nominal group technique.

Concurrently with the requirements definition phase of the project, Mr. Rowls and Dr. Brown, with assistance from Ms. Moore, screened the EHR vendor marketplace. They reviewed the literature, consulted with colleagues in the state medical association, and surveyed practices in the state that they knew used an EHR system. Mr. Rowls made a few phone calls to chief information officers (CIOs) in surrounding hospitals who had experience with ambulatory care EHR to get their advice. This initial screening resulted in the identification of eight EHR vendors whose products and services seemed to meet Valley Practice's needs.

Given the fairly manageable number of vendors, Ms. Moore suggested that the project steering committee use a short-form request for proposal (RFP). This form had been developed by her consulting firm and had been used successfully by other physician practices to identify top contenders. The short-form RFPs were sent to the

(cont.)

eight vendors; six responded. Each of these six presented an initial demonstration of its EHR system on site. Following the demonstrations, the practice staff members completed evaluation forms and ranked the various vendors. After reviewing the completed RFPs and getting feedback on the vendor presentations, the committee determined that three vendors had risen to the top of the list.

Dr. Brown and Dr. Ward visited four physician practices that used EHR systems from these three finalists. Mr. Rowls checked references and prepared the final vendor analysis. A detailed cost-benefit analysis was conducted, and the three vendors were ranked. All three vendors, in rank order, were presented in the final report given to Dr. Marcus and the other physician partners.

Dr. Marcus, Dr. Brown, and Mr. Rowls spent four weeks negotiating a contract with the top contender. It was finalized and approved after legal review and after all the partners agreed to it.

Establish a Project Steering Committee

One of the first steps in any major project such as an EHR acquisition effort is to create a *project steering committee*. This committee's primary function is to plan, organize, coordinate, and manage all aspects of the acquisition process. Appointing a project manager with strong communication skills, organizational skills, and leadership abilities is critical to the project. In our Valley Practice case, the project manager was a physician partner. In larger health care organizations such as hospitals, where a CIO is employed, the CIO would likely be involved in the effort and might also be asked to lead it.

Increasingly, clinicians such as physicians and nurses with training in informatics are being called on to lead clinical system acquisition and implementation projects. Known as *chief medical informatics officers* or *nursing informatics officers*, these individuals bring to the project a clinical perspective as well as an understanding of IT and information management processes. Regardless of the discipline or background of the project manager (for example, IT, clinical, or administrative), he or she should bring to the project passion, interest, time, strong interpersonal and communication skills, and project management skills and should be someone who is well respected by the organization's leadership team and who has the political clout to lead the effort effectively.

Pulling together a strong team of individuals to serve on the project steering committee is also important. These individuals should include representatives from key constituent groups in the practice. At Valley Practice, a physician partner, a nurse, the business officer manager, and the CEO agreed to serve on the committee, along with a representative from the Regional Extension Center. Gaining project buy-in from the various user groups should begin early. This is a key reason for inviting representatives from key constituent groups to serve on the project steering committee. They should be individuals who will use the EHR system directly or whose jobs will be affected by it.

Consideration should also be given to the size of the committee; typically, having five to six members is ideal. In a large facility, however, this may not be possible. The committee for a hospital might have fifteen to twenty members, with representatives from key clinical areas such as laboratory medicine, pharmacy, and radiology in addition to representatives from the administrative, IT, nursing, and medical staffs.

It is important to have someone knowledgeable about IT serving on the project steering committee. This may be a physician, a nurse, the CEO, or an outside consultant. In a physician group practice such as Valley Practice, having an in-house IT professional is rare. The committee chair might look internally to see if someone has the requisite IT knowledge, skills, and interests and also the time to devote to the project, but also might look externally for a health care IT professional who might serve in a consultative role and help the committee direct its activities appropriately. In this case, the REC specialist may be able to provide both the technical and system selection expertise to assist Valley Practice in the acquisition process.

Define Project Objectives and Scope of Analysis

Once the project steering committee has been established, its first order of business is to clarify the charge to the committee and to define project goals. The charge describes the scope and nature of the committee's activities. The charge usually comes from senior leadership or a lead physician in the practice. Project goals should also be established and communicated in well-defined, measurable terms. What does the committee expect to achieve? What process will be used to ensure the committee's success? How will milestones be acknowledged? How will the committee communicate progress and resolve problems? What resources (such as time, personnel, and travel expenses) will the committee need to carry out its charge? What method will be used to evaluate system options? Will the committee consider contracting with a system developer to build a system or outsourcing the system to an application service provider? Or is the committee only considering systems available for purchase from a health care information systems vendor?

Once project goals are formulated, they can guide the committee's activities and also clarify the resources needed and the likely completion date for the project. Here are some examples of typical project goals:

- Assess the practice's information management needs and establish goals and objectives for the new system based on these needs.
- Conduct a review of the literature on EHR products and the market resources for these products.
- Investigate the top ten EHR system products for the ambulatory care arena.
- Visit two to four health care organizations similar to ours that have implemented an EHR system.
- Schedule vendor demonstrations for times when physicians, nurses, and others can observe and evaluate without interruptions.

As part of the goal-setting process, the committee should determine the extent to which various options will be explored. For example, the Valley Practice project steering committee decided at the onset that it was going to consider only EHR products available in the vendor community and certified by the ONC EHR. As discussed in Chapter Six, to achieve meaningful use, health care provider organizations must use certified EHR products. A listing of certified projects are available on the Office of the National Coordinator for Health Information Technology web site. Users can be assured that certified EHR products meet certain standards for content, functionality, and interoperability.

The committee further stipulated that it would consider only vendors with experience (for example, five or more years in the industry) and those with a solid track record of system installations (for example, twenty-five or more installations). The committee members felt the practice should contract with a system developer only if they were unable to find a suitable product from the vendor community—their rationale being that the practice wanted to be known as high-tech, high-touch. They also believed it was important to invest in IT personnel who could customize the application to meet practice needs and who would be able to assist the practice in achieving project and practice goals.

Screen the Marketplace and Review Vendor Profiles

Concurrently with the establishment of project goals, the project steering committee should conduct its first, cursory review of the EHR marketplace and begin investigating vendor profiles. Many resources are available to aid the committee in this effort. For example, the Valley Practice committee might obtain copies of recent market analysis reports—from research firms such as Gartner or KLAS—listing and describing the vendors that provide EHR systems for ambulatory care facilities. The committee might also attend trade shows at conferences of professional associations such as the Healthcare Information and Management Systems Society (HIMSS) and the American Medical Informatics Association (AMIA). (Appendix A provides an overview of the health care IT industry and describes a variety of resources available to health care organizations interested in learning about health care IT products, such as EHR systems, available in the vendor community.)

Determine System Goals

Besides identifying project goals, the project steering committee should define system goals. System goals can be derived by answering questions such as: What does the organization hope to accomplish by implementing an EHR system? What is it looking for in a system? If the organization intends to transform existing care processes, can the system support the new processes? Such goals often emerge during the initial strategic planning process when the decision is made to move forward with the selection of the new system. At this point, however, the committee should state its goals and needs for a new EHR system in clearly defined, specific, and measurable terms. For example, a system goal such as "select a new EHR system" is very broad and not specific. Here are some examples of specific and measurable goals for a physician practice.

Our EHR system should

- Enable the practice to provide service to patients using evidence-based standards of care.
- Aid the practice in monitoring the quality and costs of care provided to the patients served.
- Provide clinicians with access to accurate, complete, relevant patient information, on site and remotely.
- Improve staff efficiency and effectiveness.
- More fully engage patients in their own care by providing patients with ready access to their test results, immunization records, patient education materials, and other aids.
- Enable the practice to manage chronic disease patient care more effectively.

These are just a few of the types of system goals the project steering committee might establish as it investigates a new EHR for the organization. The system goals should be aligned with the strategic goals of the organization and should serve as measures of success throughout the system acquisition process.

Determine and Prioritize System Requirements

Once the goals of the new system have been established, the project steering committee should begin to determine system requirements. These requirements may address everything from what information should be available to the provider at the point of care to how the information will be secured to what type of response time is expected. The committee may use any of a variety of ways to identify system requirements. One approach is to have a subgroup of the committee conduct focus-group sessions or small-group interviews with the various user groups (physicians, nurses, billing personnel, and support staff). A second approach is to develop and administer a written or an electronic survey, customized for each user group, asking individuals to identify their information needs in light of their job role or function. A third is to assign a representative from each specific area to obtain input from users in that area. For example, the nurse on the Valley Practice project steering committee might interview the other nurses; the business office manager might interview the support staff. System requirements may also emerge as the committee examines templates provided by consultants or peer institutions, looks at vendor demonstrations and sales material, or considers new regulatory requirements the organization must meet.

The committee may also use a combination of these or other approaches. At times, however, users do not know what they want or will need. Hence, it can be extremely helpful to hold product demonstrations, meet with consultants, or visit sites already using EHR systems, so that those who will use or be affected by the EHR can see and hear what is possible. Whatever methods are chosen to seek users' information system needs, the end result should be a list of requirements and specifications that can be prioritized or ranked. This ranking should directly reflect the specific strategic goals and circumstances of the organization.

The system requirements and priorities will eventually be shared with vendors or the system developer; therefore, it is important that they be clearly defined and presented in an organized, easy-to-understand format. For example, it may be helpful to organize the requirements into categories such as *software* (system functionality, software upgrades), *technical infrastructure* (hardware requirements, network specifications, backup, disaster recovery, security), and *training and support* (initial and ongoing training, technical support). These requirements will eventually become a major component of the request for proposal (RFP) submitted to vendors or other third parties (discussed next).

Develop and Distribute the RFP or RFI

Once the organization has defined its system requirements, the next step in the acquisition process is to package these requirements into a structure that a third party can respond to, whether that third party be a development partner or a health information systems vendor. Many health care organizations package the requirements into a *request for proposal (RFP)*. The RFP provides the vendor with a comprehensive list of system requirements, features, and functions and asks the vendor to indicate whether its product or service meets each need. Vendors responding to an RFP are also generally required to submit a detailed and binding price quotation for the applications and services being sought.

RFPs tend to be highly detailed and are therefore time consuming and costly to develop and complete. However, they provide the health care organization and each vendor with a comprehensive view of the system needed. Health care IT consultants can be extremely resourceful in assisting the organization with developing and packaging the RFP. An RFP for a major health care information system acquisition generally contains the following information (sections marked with an asterisk [*] are completed by the vendor; the other sections are completed by the organization issuing the RFP):

- *Instructions for vendors:*

    Proposal deadline and contact information: where and when the RFP is due; whom to contact with questions

    Confidentiality statement and instructions: a statement that both the RFP and the responses provided by the vendor are confidential and are proprietary information

    Specific instructions for completing the RFP and any stipulations with which the vendor must comply in order to be considered

- *Organizational objectives:* type of system or application being sought; information management needs and plans.

- *Background of the organization*

    Overview of the facility: size, types of patient services, patient volume, staff composition, strategic goals of organization

    Application and technical inventory: current systems in use, hardware, software, network infrastructure

- *System goals and requirements:* goals for the system and functional requirements (may be categorized as mandatory or desirable and listed in priority order). Typically this section includes application, technical, and integration requirements. Increasingly, health care providers are interested in assessing and testing system usability. Incorporating scripted scenarios in the requirements section of the RFP that are based on existing workflow and business processes can provide meaningful information during the selection process (Corrao, Robinson, Swiernik, & Naeim, 2010; Eisenstein, Jurwishin, Kushniruk, & Nahm, 2011; IOM, 2011).

- *Vendor qualifications:* *general background of vendor, experience, number of installations, financial stability, list of current clients, standard contract, and implementation plan.

- *Proposed solutions:* *how vendor believes its product meets the goals and needs of the health care organization. Vendor may include case studies, results from system analysis projects, and other evidence of the benefits of its proposed solution.

- *Criteria for evaluating proposals:* how the health care organization will make its final decisions on product selection.

- *General contractual requirements:* *such as warranties, payment schedule, penalties for failure to meet schedules specified in contract, vendor responsibilities, and so forth.

- *Pricing and support:* *quote on cost of system, using standardized terms and forms.

The RFP may become the basis for a legally binding contract or obligation between the vendor and the solicitor, so it is important for both parties to carefully consider the wording of questions and the corresponding responses (AHIMA, 2007).

RFPs are not the only means by which to solicit information from vendors. A second approach that is often used is the *request for information (RFI)*. An RFI is less formal, considerably shorter than an RFP, and less time consuming to develop. It is often used as part of the fact-finding process to obtain basic information on the vendor's background, product descriptions, and service capabilities. Some health care organizations send out an RFI before distributing the RFP, in order to screen out vendors whose products or services are not consistent with the organization's needs or to narrow the field of vendors to a manageable number. The RFI can serve as a tool in gathering background information on vendors' products and services and in providing the project steering committee with a better sense of the health IT market place. How does one decide whether to use an RFP, an RFI, both, or neither during the system acquisition process? Several factors should be considered. Although time consuming to develop, the RFP is useful in forcing a health care organization to define its system goals and requirements and prioritize its needs. The RFP also creates a structure for objectively evaluating vendor responses and provides a record of documentation throughout the acquisition process. System acquisition can be a highly political process; by using an RFP the organization can introduce a higher degree of objectivity into that process. RFPs are also useful data collection tools when the technology being selected is established and fully developed, when there is little variability between vendor products and services, when the organization has the time to fully evaluate all options, and when the organization needs strong contract protection from the selected vendor (DeLuca & Enmark, 2002). However, not all vendors may wish to submit a response to an RFI or RFP due to costs or suitability.

There are also drawbacks to RFPs. Besides taking considerable time to develop and review, they can become cumbersome, so detail oriented that they lose their effectiveness. For instance, it is not unusual to receive three binders full of product and service information from one vendor. If ten vendors respond to an RFP (about five is ideal), the project steering committee may be overwhelmed and find it difficult to wade through and differentiate among vendor responses. Having too much information to summarize can be as crippling to a committee in its deliberations as having too little.

Therefore a scaled-back RFP or an RFI might be a desirable alternative. An RFI might be used when the health care organization is considering only a small group of vendors or products or when it is still in the exploratory stages and has not yet established its requirements. Some facilities use an even less formal process consisting primarily of site visits and system demonstrations.

Regardless of the tool(s) used, it is important for the health care organization to provide sufficient detail about its current structure, strategic IT goals, and future plans that the vendor can respond appropriately to its needs. Additionally, the RFP or RFI (or variation of either) should result in enough specific detail that the organization gets a good sense of the vendor—its services, history, vision, stability in the marketplace, and system or product functionality. The organization should be able to easily screen out vendors whose products are undeveloped or not yet fully tested (DeLuca & Enmark, 2002).

Explore Other Acquisition Options

In our Valley Practice case, the physicians and staff opted to acquire an EHR system from the vendor community. Organizations like Valley Practice often turn to the market for products that they will run on their own IT infrastructure. But there are times when they do not go to the market—they choose to leverage someone else's infrastructure (by contracting with an application service provider) or they build the application (by contracting with a system developer or using in-house staff).

Contract with an Application Service Provider

In recent years, with wider availability of high-speed or broadband Internet connections, more sophisticated vendor solutions, and a growing number of options for hosting software, the *application service provider (ASP)* approach has emerged as an alternative to buying, installing, and maintaining information systems. These services may be offered via "cloud" computing. Cloud computing is a general term that refers to both the applications delivered as services over the Internet and the hardware and software in the data centers that provide those services. An ASP is an organization with whom health care providers contract on a subscription basis to deliver an application and provide the associated services to support it. It's somewhat analogous to the option of leasing rather than purchasing a car. ASPs are also similar in concept to the shared-systems option used by many hospitals in the 1960s and 1970s, when they could not afford or did not have the IT staff available in-house to run and support software applications and hardware. In essence, another organization houses and maintains the clinical or administrative application and related hardware; the health care organization or provider simply accesses the system remotely over a network connection and pays the monthly or negotiated fees. It is worth noting that some ASPs do not physically host the application but instead contract with a third-party data center to do so (Fortin & MacDonald, 2006). Health information exchange organizations could serve as ASPs as they mature and expand their capabilities.

Why might a health care organization consider contracting with an ASP rather than purchasing an EHR system (or other application) from a vendor? There are several reasons. First, the facility may not have the IT staff needed to run or support the desired system. Hiring qualified personnel at the salaries they demand may be difficult, and retaining them may be equally challenging. Second, ASPs typically enable health care organizations to use clinical or administrative applications with fewer up-front costs and less capital. For a small physician practice, these financial arrangements can be particularly appealing. Because ASPs offer fixed monthly fees or fees based on usage, organizations are better able to predict costs. Third, by contracting with an ASP, the health care organization can focus on its core business and not get bogged down in IT support issues, although it may still have to deal with issues of system enhancements, user needs, and the selection of new systems. Other advantages to using ASPs are rapid deployment and 24/7 technical support. They also offer scalability and flexibility, so as the practice or organization grows or shrinks in size or volume, they pay only for the services used.

ASPs also have some disadvantages and limitations that the health care organization should consider in its deliberations. Although rapid deployment of the application can be a tremendous advantage to an organization, the downside is the fact that the application will likely be a standard, off-the-shelf product, with little if any customization. This means that the organization has to adapt or mold its operations to the application rather than tailoring the application to meet the operational needs of the organization. A second drawback deals with technical support. Although technical support is generally available from an ASP, it is unrealistic to think that the ASP's support personnel will have intimate knowledge of the organization and its operations. Frustrations can mount when one lacks in-house IT technical staff when and where they are needed. Third, health care providers have long been concerned about data ownership, security, and privacy—worries that increase when another organization hosts their clinical data and applications. How the ASP will secure data and maintain patient privacy should be clearly specified in the contract. Likewise, to minimize downtime, the ASP should have clear plans for backing up data, preventing disasters, and recovering data.

First Consulting prepared a report for the California HealthCare Foundation outlining developments, benefits, challenges, issues, and concerns related to the ASP model for ambulatory clinical applications (Fortin & MacDonald, 2006). It suggests health care leaders ask themselves four important questions in deciding whether an ASP approach is the right choice for their organization:

- How will the application fit into the organization's overall IT plans?
- To what extent can the organization support locally installed software?
- How willing is the organization to have another organization host a clinical application?
- What financial resources does the organization have (Fortin & MacDonald, 2006, p. 15)?

As the industry matures, we will likely see different variations and greater choices among organizations serving as ASPs. The health care executive considering whether an ASP is the right choice should thoroughly research the company and its products and consider factors such as company viability, target market, functionality, integration, implementation and training, help desk support, security, pricing, and service levels. It is important to be able to trust the ASP and to choose one wisely.

Contract with a System Developer or Build In-House

A second alternative to purchasing a system from a vendor is to contract with a developer to design a system for your organization. The developer may be employed in-house or by an outside firm. Working with a system developer can be a good option when the health care organization's needs are highly uncertain or unique and the products available on the market do not adequately meet these needs. Developing a new or innovative application can also give the organization a significant competitive advantage. The costs and time needed to develop the application can be significant, however. It is also important to consider the long-term costs. Should the developer leave, how difficult would it be to hire and retain someone to support and maintain the system? How will problems with the system be addressed? How will the application be upgraded? What long-term value will it bring the organization? These are a few of the many questions that should be addressed in considering this option. It is rare for a health care organization to develop its own major clinical information system.

Evaluate Vendor Proposals

In the Valley Practice case, the project steering committee decided to focus its efforts at first on considering only EHR products available for purchase in the vendor community. The committee came to this conclusion after its initial review of the EHR marketplace. Committee members felt there were a number of vendors whose products appeared to meet practice needs. They also felt strongly that in-house control of the EHR system was important to achieving the practice goal of becoming a high-tech, high-touch organization, because they wanted to be able to customize the application. Realizing this, the committee had budgeted for an IT director and an IT support staff member. Members felt that the long-term cost savings from implementing an EHR would justify these two new positions.

Develop Evaluation Criteria

The project steering committee at Valley Practice decided to go through the RFP process. It developed criteria by which it would review and evaluate vendor proposals. Criteria were used to grade each vendor's response to the RFP. Grading scales were established so the committee could accurately compare vendors' responses. These grading scales involved assigning more weight to required items and less weight to those deemed merely desirable. Categories of "does not meet requirement," "partially meets requirement," and

Table 7.1. Sample criteria for evaluation of RFP responses

Type of Application: *Electronic Health Record System*

Vendor Name: *The EHREHR Company*

Criteria	Meets Requirement	Partially Meets Requirement	Does Not Meet Requirement
1. Alerts user to possible drug interactions	x		
2. Provides user with list of alternate drugs	x		
3. Advises user on dosage based on patient's weight	x		
4. Allows user to enter over-the-counter medications		x (on different screen)	
5. Allows easy printout of prescriptions	x		

"meets requirement" were also used. RFP documents were compared item by item and side by side, using the grading scales established by the committee (see Table 7.1 for sample criteria). To avoid information overload, a common condition in the RFP review process, the project steering committee focused on direct responses to requirements and referred to supplemental information only as needed. Summary reports of each vendor's response to the RFP were then prepared by a small group of committee members and distributed to the committee at large.

Hold Vendor Demonstrations

During the vendor review process, it is important to host vendor system demonstrations. The purpose of these demonstrations is to give the members of the health care organization an opportunity to (1) evaluate the look and feel of the system from a user's point of view, (2) validate how much the vendor can deliver of what has been proposed, (3) conduct system usability testing, and (4) narrow the field of potential vendors. It is often a good idea to develop demonstration scripts and require all vendors to present their systems in accordance with these scripts. Scripts generally reflect the requirements outlined in the RFP and contain a moderate level of detail. For example, a script might require demonstrating the process of registering a patient or renewing a prescription. The use of scripts can ensure that all vendors are evaluated on the same basis or functionality. At the same time, it is important to allow vendors some creativity in presenting their product and services. When scripts are used, they need to be provided to vendors at least one month in advance of the demonstration, and both vendors and health care organization must adhere to them. It is also important to have end-users carry out certain functions or procedures that they would normally do in the course of the day using the vendor's system. You might ask them to complete a system usability survey after they have had a chance to use the system and practice on several records. Figure 7.2 is an example of a system usability scale questionnaire in which end-users are asked to respond to each item using a Likert scale of 1 to 5, from strongly disagree to strongly agree.

Figure 7.2. System usability scale questionnaire

Source: Brooke, 1996; Lewis & Sauro, 2009.

Criteria should be developed and used in evaluating vendor demonstrations, just as they are for reviewing vendor responses to the RFP.

Make Site Visits and Check References

After reviewing the vendors' RFPs and evaluating their product demonstrations, it is advisable to make site visits and check references. By visiting other facilities that use a vendor's products, the health care organization should gain additional insight into what the vendor would be like as a potential partner. It can be extremely beneficial to visit organizations similar to yours. For instance, in the Valley Practice case, representatives from key practice constituencies decided to visit other ambulatory care practices to see how a specific system was being used, the problems that had been encountered, and how these problems had been addressed. The Regional Extension Center specialist also provided useful information to them.

How satisfied are the staff with the system? How responsive has the vendor been to problems? How quickly have problems been resolved? To what degree has the vendor delivered on its promises? Hearing answers to such questions firsthand from a variety of users can be extremely helpful in the vendor review process.

Other Strategies for Evaluating Vendors

A host of other strategies can be used to evaluate a vendor's reputation and product and service quality. Organizational representatives might attend vendor user-group conferences, review the latest market reports, consult with colleagues in the field, seek advice from consultants, and request an extensive list of system users.

Prepare a Vendor Analysis

Throughout the vendor review process, the project steering committee members should have evaluation tools in place to document their impressions and the views of others in the organization who participate in any or all of the review activities (review of RFPs, system demonstrations, site visits, reference checks, and so forth). The committee should then prepare vendor analysis reports that summarize the major findings from each of the review activities. How do the vendors compare in reputation? In quality of their product? In quality of service? How do the systems compare in terms of their initial and ongoing costs? To what degree is the vendor's vision for product development aligned with the organization's strategic IT goals?

Figure 7.3. Cost-benefit analysis

Vendor	50 MDs	10 MDs	5 MDs	1 MD	Fin.	Tech.	Interop.	Dec. Support	Clin./ Oper. Rank	Clin./ Oper. Points
Vendor 1	$5,588	$6,178	$6,806	$13,449	3	4	4.4	3.8	2	68
Vendor 2	$6,413	$6,594	$7,413	$13,373	3	4	3.4	2.9	5	27
Vendor 3	$3,378	$4,360	$5,130	$8,842	3	4	1.9	4.2	4	28
Vendor 4	$6,899	$6,086	$7,678	$15,437	5	4	4.1	4.3	1	70
Vendor 5	$5,945	$8,494	$9,543	$34,308	4	3	3.5	3.9	6	25
Vendor 6	$4,468	$4,580	$5,654	$12,927	3	3	2.4	4.1	3	46

Note: Fin. = Financial; Tech. = Technical; Interop. = Interoperability; Dec. Support = Decision Support; Clin./Oper. Rank = Clinical and Operational Rank; Clin./Oper. Points = Clinical and Operational Points.
Source: Partners HealthCare.

Conduct a Cost-Benefit Analysis

The final analysis should include an evaluation of the cost and benefits of each proposed system. Figure 7.3 shows a comparison of six vendor products. Criteria were developed to score and rank each vendor's system. As the figure illustrates, the selection committee ranked vendor 4 the top choice.

The capital cost analysis may include software, hardware, network or infrastructure, third-party, and internal capital costs. The total cost of ownership should factor in support costs and the costs of the resources needed (including personnel) to implement and support the system. Once the initial and ongoing costs are identified, it is important to weigh them against the benefits of the systems being considered. Can the benefits be quantified? Should they be included in the final analysis?

Prepare a Summary Report and Recommendations

Assuming the capital cost analysis supports the organization in moving forward with the project, the project steering committee should compile a final report that summarizes the process and results from each major activity or event. The report may include

- System goals and criteria
- Process used

- Results of each activity and conclusions
- Cost-benefit analysis
- Final recommendation and ranking of vendors

It is generally advisable to have two or three vendors in the final ranking, in the event that problems arise with the first choice during contract negotiations, the final step in the system acquisition process.

Conduct Contract Negotiations

The final step of the system acquisition process is to negotiate a contract with the vendor. This, too, can be a time-consuming process, and therefore it is helpful to seek expert advice from business or legal advisors. The contract outlines expectations and performance requirements, who is responsible for what (for example, training, interfaces, support), when the product is to be delivered (and vendor financial liability for failing to deliver on time), how much customization can be performed by the organization purchasing the system, how confidentiality of patient information will be handled, and when payment is due. The devil is in the details, and although most technical terms are common between vendors, other language and nuances are not. Establish a schedule and a preimplementation plan that includes a timeline for implementation of the applications and an understanding of the resource requirements for all aspects of the implementation, including cultural change management, workflow redesign, application implementation, integration requirements, and infrastructure development and upgrades, all of which can consume substantial resources.

PROJECT MANAGEMENT TOOLS

Throughout the course of the system acquisition project, a lot of materials will be generated, many of which should be maintained in a project repository. A *project repository* serves as a record of the project steering committee's progress and activities. It includes such information and documents as minutes of meetings, correspondence with vendors, the request for proposal or request for information, evaluation forms, and summary reports. This repository can be extremely useful when there are changes in staff or in the composition of the committee and when the organization is planning for future projects. The project manager should assume a leadership role in ensuring that the project repository is established and maintained. Here is a sample of the typical contents of a project repository.

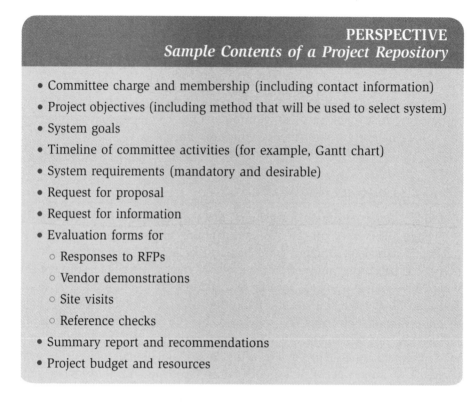

PERSPECTIVE
Sample Contents of a Project Repository

- Committee charge and membership (including contact information)
- Project objectives (including method that will be used to select system)
- System goals
- Timeline of committee activities (for example, Gantt chart)
- System requirements (mandatory and desirable)
- Request for proposal
- Request for information
- Evaluation forms for
  - Responses to RFPs
  - Vendor demonstrations
  - Site visits
  - Reference checks
- Summary report and recommendations
- Project budget and resources

Managing the various aspects of the project and coordinating activities can be a challenging task, particularly in large organizations or when a lot of people are involved and many activities are occurring simultaneously. It is important that the project manager helps those involved to establish clear roles and responsibilities for individual committee members, to set target dates, and to agree upon methods for communicating progress and problems. Many project management tools exist that can be useful here. For example, a simple Gantt chart (Figure 7.4) can document project objectives, tasks and activities, responsible parties, and target dates and milestones. A Gantt chart can also display a graphical representation of all project tasks and activities, showing which ones may occur simultaneously and which ones must be completed before another task can begin. Other tools enable one to allocate time, staff, and financial resources to each activity. (Gantt charts and other timelines can be created with software programs such as Visio or Microsoft Project. A discussion of these tools is beyond the scope of this book, but can be found in most introductory project management textbooks.)

Figure 7.4. Example of a simple Gantt chart

ID	EMR Selection Project	Start	End	Jan 2013			Feb 2013				Mar 2013				
				1/16	1/23	1/30	2/6	2/13	2/20	2/27	3/6	3/13	3/20	3/27	4/3
1	Define project objectives	1/17/2013	1/17/2013												
2	Conduct preliminary review of vendors	1/21/2013	2/8/2013		▓										
3	Determine system requirements	1/21/2013	3/15/2013		▓▓▓▓▓▓▓										
4	Conduct focus groups	2/1/2013	2/28/2013				▓▓▓								
5	Survey key user groups	2/1/2013	3/10/2013				▓▓▓▓▓								
6	Develop and administer RFP	3/15/2013	4/15/2013											▓▓	
7	Hold vendor demonstrations	4/15/2013	4/29/2013												
8	Conduct cost-benefit analysis	5/2/2013	5/13/2013												

It is important to clearly communicate progress both within the project steering committee and to individuals outside the committee. Senior management should be kept apprised of project progress, budget needs, and committee activities. Regular updates should be provided to senior management as well as other user groups involved in the process. Communication can be both formal and informal—everything from periodic update reports at executive meetings to facility newsletter briefings to informal discussions at lunch.

THINGS THAT CAN GO WRONG

Managing the system acquisition process successfully requires strong and effective leadership, planning, organizational, and communication skills. Things can and do go wrong. Upholding a high level of objectivity and fairness throughout the acquisition process is important to all parties involved. Failing to do so can hamper the overall success of the project. Following is a list of some common pitfalls in the system acquisition process, along with strategies for avoiding them.

- **Failing to manage vendor access to organizational leadership.** The vendor may schedule private time with the CEO or a board member in the hope of influencing the decision and bypassing the project steering committee entirely. It is not unusual to hear that processes or decisions have been altered after the CEO has been on a golf outing or taken a trip to the Super Bowl with a vendor. The vendor may persuade the CEO or a board member to overturn or question the decisions of the project steering committee, crippling the decision process. Hence, it should be clearly communicated to all parties (senior management, board, and vendor) that all vendor requests and communication should be channeled through the project steering committee.

- **Failing to keep the process objective (getting caught up in vendor razzle-dazzle).** Related to the need to manage vendor access to decision makers is the need to keep the process objective. The project steering committee should assume a leadership role in ensuring that there are clearly defined criteria and methods for selecting the vendor. These criteria and methods should be known to all the parties involved and should be adhered to. In addition, it is important that the committee and other organizational representatives remain unbiased and not get so impressed with the vendor's razzle-dazzle (in the form, for example, of exquisite dinners or fancy gadgets) that they fail to assess the vendor or the product objectively. Consider the politics of a situation but do not allow the vendor to drive the result—take the high road to avoid the appearance of favoritism.

- **Overdoing or underdoing the RFP.** Striking a balance between too much and too little information and detail in the RFP and also determining how much weight to give to the vendors' responses to the RFP can be challenging. The project steering committee should err on the side of being *reasonable*—that is, the committee should include enough information and detail that the vendor can appropriately respond to the organization's needs and should give the vendor responses to the RFP appropriate consideration in the final decision. Organizations should also be careful that they do not assign either too much or too little weight to the RFP process.

- **Failing to involve the leadership team and users extensively during the selection process.** A sure way to disenchant the leadership team and end-users is to fail to involve them adequately in the system acquisition process. There should be ample opportunity for people at all levels of the organization who will use or be affected by the new information system to have input into its selection. Involvement can include everything from being invited and encouraged to attend vendor presentations during uninterrupted time to being asked to join a focus group where user input is sought. It is important that the project steering committee seek input and involvement throughout the acquisition process, not simply at the end when the decision is nearly final. Far too often information system projects fail because the leadership team and end-users were not actively involved in the selection of the new system. Involving people from the very beginning helps them to be an integral part of the process and the solution.

- **Turning negotiations into a blood sport.** You want to negotiate a fair deal with the vendor and not leave the vendor's people feeling as though they have just been "beaten" in a contest. A lopsided deal results in a disenchanted partner and can create a bad climate. Understand what is required from all parties and establish performance criteria for payments and remedies for nonperformance. It is important to form a healthy, respectful long-term relationship with the vendor.

These are just a few of the many issues that can arise during the system acquisition process that the health care executive should be aware of. Failing to appropriately address these issues can interfere with the organization's ability to successfully select and implement a system that will be adopted and widely used.

SUMMARY

Acquiring or selecting a new clinical or administrative information system is a major undertaking for a health care organization. It is important that the process be managed effectively. Although the time and resources needed to select a new system will vary depending on the size, complexity, and needs of the organization, certain fundamental issues should be addressed in any system acquisition project.

This chapter discussed the various activities that occur in the system acquisition process. These activities were presented in the context of a multiphysician group practice that wishes to replace its current paper record with an EHR system by acquiring a system from a reputable vendor. Key activities in the system selection process are (1) establishing a project steering committee and appointing a strong project manager to lead the effort, (2) defining project objectives, (3) screening the vendor marketplace, (4) determining system goals, (5) establishing system requirements, (6) developing and administering a request for proposal or request for information, (7) evaluating vendor proposals, and (8) conducting a cost-benefit analysis on the various options. Other options such as contracting with an application service provider (ASP) or a system developer were also discussed. Finally, this chapter presented some of the issues that can arise during the system selection process and outlined the importance of documenting and communicating project activities and progress.

KEY TERMS

Acquisition process

Application service provider (ASP)

Contract negotiations

Cost-benefit analysis

Project repository

Project steering committee

Regional Extension Center (REC)

Request for information (RFI)

Request for proposal (RFP)

Systems development life cycle
(SDLC)
- Planning and analysis phase
- Design phase
- Implementation phase
- Support and evaluation phase

Usability testing

LEARNING ACTIVITIES

1. Interview a health care executive regarding the process last used by his or her organization to acquire a new information system. How did that process compare with the system acquisition process described in this chapter?

2. Assume you are part of a project steering committee in a rural nonprofit hospital. The hospital is interested in acquiring a new provider order entry system. You offer to screen the marketplace to see what types of computerized provider order entry systems are available. Prepare a fifteen-minute summary report of your findings to the committee at large.

3. Conduct a literature review (including an Internet search) to learn about application service provider (ASP) organizations that offer EHR systems to physician practices. Briefly summarize the EHR products available from at least three different ASPs. What criteria might you use to compare them? How do they differ in terms of service, support, and financing arrangements?

4. Find and critique a sample RFP for a health care organization. What did you like about it? What aspects of it did you feel could be improved? Explain.

5. This chapter described a typical physician practice that wishes to select an EHR system. Using the information in the Valley Practice scenario, draft a script for vendors to use in demonstrating their products and services to Valley Practice staff. Include a description of the process you used to arrive at the script.

6. Working with your classmates in small groups, assume that you are a Valley Practice committee member interested in obtaining user

feedback on the EHR vendor demonstrations. Develop a survey instrument that might be used to solicit and summarize participants' responses to each vendor demonstration. Swap the survey your group designed with another group's survey; critique each other's work.

REFERENCES

American Health Information Management Association. (2007). The RFP process for EHR systems (updated). Retrieved February 2013 from http://library.ahima.org /xpedio/groups/public/documents/ahima/bok1_047961.hcsp?dDocName=bok1 _047961.

Brooke, J. (1996). SUS: A "quick and dirty" usability scale. In P. W. Jordan, B. Thomas, I. L. McClelland, & B. A. Weerdmeester (Eds.), *Usability evaluation in industry* (pp. 189–194). London: Taylor & Francis.

Corrao, N. J., Robinson, A. G., Swiernik, M. A., & Naeim, A. (2010). Importance of testing for usability when selecting and implementing an electronic health or medical record system. *Journal of Oncology Practice, 6*(3), 120–124.

DeLuca, J., & Enmark, R. (2002). *The CEO's guide to health care information systems* (2nd ed.). San Francisco: Jossey-Bass.

Eisenstein, E. L., Jurwishin, D., Kushniruk, A.W., & Nahm, M. (2011). Defining a framework for health information technology evaluation. *Studies in Health Technology and Informatics, 164,* 94–99.

Fortin, J., & MacDonald, K. (2006). *Physician practices: Are application service providers right for you?* Oakland: California HealthCare Foundation.

Institute of Medicine. (2011). *Health IT and patient privacy: Building safer systems for better care.* Washington, DC: National Academies Press.

Jones, S. S., Koppel, R., Ridgley, M. S., Palen, T., Wu, S., & Harrison, M. I. (2011, August). *Guide to reducing unintended consequences of electronic health records.* Rockville, MD: Agency for Healthcare Research and Quality.

Lewis, J. R., & Sauro, J. (2009). The factor structure of the system usability scale. In *Proceedings of the Human Computer Interaction International Conference* (HCII 2009), San Diego, CA.

Oz, E. (2012). *Management information systems: Instructor edition* (6th ed.). Boston: Course Technology.

Wager, K. A., & Lee, F. W. (2006). Introduction to healthcare information systems. In M. Johns (Ed.), *Health information management technology: An applied approach* (2nd ed.). Chicago: American Health Information Management Association.

CHAPTER 8

System Implementation and Support

LEARNING OBJECTIVES

- To be able to discuss the process that a health care organization typically goes through in implementing a health care information system.

- To be able to appreciate the organizational and behavioral factors that can affect system acceptance and use and strategies for managing change.

- To be able to develop a sample system implementation plan for a health care information system project, including the types of individuals who should be involved.

- To gain insight into many of the things that can go wrong during system implementations and strategies that health care managers can employ to alleviate potential problems.

- To be able to discuss the importance of training, technical support, infrastructure, and ongoing maintenance and evaluation of any health care information system project.

Once a health care organization has finalized its contract with the vendor to acquire an information system, the system implementation process begins. Selecting the right system does not ensure user acceptance and success; the system must also be incorporated effectively into the day-to-day operations of the health care organization and adequately supported or maintained. Whether the system is built in-house, designed by an outside consultant, leased from an application service provider (ASP), or purchased from a vendor, it will take a substantial amount of planning and work to get the system up and running smoothly and integrated into operations.

This chapter focuses on the two final stages of the system development life cycle: implementation and then support and evaluation. It describes the planning and activities that should occur when implementing a new system. Our discussion focuses on a vendor-acquired system; however, many of the activities described also apply to systems designed in-house or by an outside developer or acquired through an ASP.

Implementing a new system (or replacing an old system) can be a massive undertaking for a health care organization. Not only are there workstations to install, databases to build, and networks to test but there are also processes to redesign, users to train, data to convert, and procedures to write. There are countless tasks and details that must be appropriately coordinated and completed if the system is to be implemented on time and within budget—and widely accepted by users. Essential to the process is ensuring that the introduction of any new health care information system or workflow change results in improved organizational performance, such as a reduction in medication errors, an improvement in care coordination, and more effective utilization of tests and procedures.

Recently concerns have been raised about the potential for EHRs to result in risk to patient safety. Health care information systems such as EHRs are enormously complex and involve not only the technology (hardware and software), but people, processes, workflow, organizational culture, politics, and the external environment (licensure, accreditation, regulatory agencies). The Institute of Medicine recently published a report that offers health care organizations and vendors suggestions on how to work collaboratively to make health IT safer (IOM, 2011). Poor user-interface designs, ineffective workflow, and lack of interoperability are all considered threats to patient safety. Several of the suggested strategies for ensuring system safety are discussed in this chapter.

Along with attending to the many activities or tasks associated with system implementation, it is equally important to address organizational and behavioral issues. Studies have shown that over half of all information system projects fail. Numerous political, cultural, behavioral, and ethical factors can affect the successful implementation and use of the new system (Ash, Anderson, & Tarczy-Hornoch, 2008; Ash et al., 2007; Sittig & Singh, 2011). We devote a section of this chapter to the organizational and behavioral issues that can arise and other things that can go wrong during the system implementation process and offer strategies for avoiding these problems. The chapter concludes by describing the importance of supporting and maintaining information systems.

SYSTEM IMPLEMENTATION PROCESS

System implementation begins once the organization has acquired the system and continues through the early stages following the *go-live* date (the date when the system is put into general use for everyone). Like the system acquisition process, the system implementation process must have a high degree of support from the senior executive team and be viewed as an organizational priority. Sufficient staff, time, and resources must be devoted to the project. Individuals involved in rolling out the new system should have sufficient resources available to them to ensure a smooth transition.

The time and resources needed to implement a new health care information system can vary considerably depending on the scope of the project, the needs and complexity of the organization, the number of applications being installed, and the number of user groups involved. There are, however, some fundamental activities that should occur during any system implementation, regardless of its size or scope:

- Organize the implementation team and identify a system champion.
- Determine project scope and expectations.
- Establish and institute a project plan.

Failing to appropriately plan for and manage these activities can lead to cost overruns, dissatisfied users, project delays, and even system sabotage. In today's environment, where capital is scarce and resources are limited, health care organizations cannot afford to mismanage implementation projects of this magnitude and importance.

Organize the Team and Identify a Champion

One of the first steps in planning for the implementation of a new system is to organize an *implementation team*. The primary role and function of the

Figure 8.1. Sample composition of implementation team

team is to plan, coordinate, budget, and manage all aspects of the new system implementation. Although the exact team composition will depend on the scope and nature of the new system, a team might include a project leader, system champion(s), key individuals from the clinical and administrative areas that are the focus of the system being acquired, vendor representatives, and information technology (IT) professionals (Figure 8.1). For large or complex projects, it is also a good idea to have someone skilled in project management principles on the team. Likewise, having a strong project leader and the right mix of people is critically important.

Implementation teams often include some of the same people involved in selecting the system; however, they may also include other individuals with knowledge and skills important to the successful deployment of the new system. For example, the implementation team will likely need at least one IT professional with technical database and network administration expertise. This person may have had some role in the selection process but is now being called on to assume a larger role in installing the software, setting up the data tables, and customizing the network infrastructure to adequately support the system and the organization's needs.

The implementation team should also include at least one *system champion*. A system champion is someone who is well respected in the organization, sees the new system as necessary to the organization's achievement of its strategic goals, and is passionate about implementing it. In many health care settings the system champion is a physician, particularly when the organization is implementing a system that will directly or indirectly affect how physicians spend their time. The physician champion serves as an advocate of the system, assumes a leadership role in gaining buy-in from other physicians and user groups, and makes sure that physicians have adequate input into the decision-making process. Other important qualities of system champions are strong communication, interpersonal, and listening skills. The system champion should be willing to assist with pilot testing, to train and coach others, and to build consensus among user groups (Miller & Sim, 2004). Numerous studies have demonstrated the importance of the system champion throughout the implementation process (Ash, Stavri, Dykstra, & Fournier, 2003; Miller, Sim, & Newman, 2003; Wager, Lee, White, Ward, & Ornstein, 2000; Yackanicz, Kerr, & Levick, 2010). When implementing clinical applications (such as computerized provider order entry [CPOE] or medication administration using bar coding) that span numerous clinical areas, such as nursing, pharmacy, and physicians, having a system champion from each division can be enormously helpful in gaining buy-in and in facilitating communication among staff. The various system champions can also assume a pivotal role in ensuring that project milestones are achieved and celebrated.

Determine Project Scope and Expectations

One of the implementation team's first items of business is to determine the scope of the project and what the organization hopes the project will achieve. To set the tone for the project, a senior health care executive should meet with the implementation team to communicate how the project relates to the organization's overall strategic goals and to assure the team of administration's commitment to the project.

The goals of the project and what the organization hopes to achieve by implementing the new system should emerge from early team discussions. The system goals defined during the system selection process (discussed in Chapter Seven) should be reviewed by the implementation team. Far too often health care organizations skip this important step and never clearly define the scope of the project or what they hope to gain as a result of the new system. At other times they define the scope of the project too broadly or scope creep occurs. The goals should be specific, measurable, attainable, relevant, and time bound (http://www.healthit.gov/providers-professionals/ehr-implementation-steps /step-1-assess-your-practice-readiness). They should also define the organization's criteria for success.

Let's look at two hypothetical examples, from two providers that we will call Mason Hospital and St. Luke's Medical Center. The implementation team at Mason Hospital defined its goal and the scope of the project and devised measures for evaluating the extent to which the hospital achieved this goal. The implementation team at St. Luke's Medical Center was responsible for completing phase 1 of a three-part project; however, the scope of the team's work was never clearly defined.

CASE STUDY

Mason Hospital

Mason Hospital decided that it wanted to implement a CPOE system. An implementation team was formed and charged with managing all aspects of the CPOE rollout. Mason Hospital's mission is to be "the premier academic community hospital in the United States." Considering how to achieve this mission, the team identified CPOE as the "building block" needed to improve quality of care, reduce errors, and create a far safer and more effective work environment for hospital medical staff. In addition to establishing this goal, the team went a step further to define what a successful CPOE implementation initiative would consist of. Team members then developed a core set of metrics—physician CPOE adoption rate, use of telephone and verbal orders in nonemergency situations, reduction in adverse drug events, reduction in duplicate orders, improved quality of documentation, and increased compliance with practice-based guidelines—that were subsequently used to track the project's success in the defined areas.

St. Luke's Medical Center

St. Luke's Medical Center set out to implement a digital medical record, planning to do so in three phases. Phase 1 would involve establishing a clinical data repository, a central database from which all ancillary clinical systems would feed. Phase 2 would consist of the implementation of CPOE and nursing documentation systems, and Phase 3 would see the elimination of all outside paper reports through the implementation of a document imaging system. St. Luke's staff felt that if they could complete all three phases, they would have, in essence, a "true" electronic or digital patient record. The implementation team did not, however, clearly define the scope of its work. Was it to complete phase 1 or all three phases? Likewise, the implementation team never defined what it hoped to accomplish or how implementation of the digital record fit into the medical center's overall mission or organizational goals. It never answered the question: How will we know if we are successful? Some project team members argued that a "digital" record was not the same as an EHR and questioned whether the team was headed down the right path. The ambiguity of the implementation team's scope of work led to disillusionment and a sense of failing to ever finish the project.

Establish and Institute a Project Plan

Once the implementation team has agreed on its goals and objectives, the next major step is to develop and implement a project plan. The project plan should have the following components:

- Major activities (also called tasks)
- Major milestones
- Estimated duration of each activity
- Any dependencies among activities (so that, for example, one task must be completed before another can begin)
- Resources and budget available (including staff whose time will be allocated to the project)
- Individuals or team members responsible for completing each activity
- Target dates
- Measures for evaluating completion and success

These are the same components one would find in most major projects. What are the major activities, or tasks, that are unique to system implementation projects? Which tasks must be completed first, second, and so forth? How should time estimates be determined and milestones defined?

System implementation projects tend to be quite large, and therefore it can be helpful to break the project into manageable components. One approach to defining components is to have the implementation team brainstorm and identify the major activities that need to be done before the go-live date. Once these tasks have been identified, they can be grouped and sequenced based on what must be done first, second, and so forth. Those tasks that can occur concurrently should also be identified. A team may find it helpful to use a consultant to guide it through the implementation process. Or the health care IT vendor may have a suggested implementation plan; the team must make sure, however, that this plan is tailored to suit the unique needs of the organization in which the new system is to be introduced.

The subsequent sections describe the major activities common to most information system implementation projects (outlined in the following list) and may serve as a guide. These activities are not necessarily in sequential order; the order used should be determined by the institution in accordance with its needs and resources.

Typical Components of an Implementation Plan

1. Workflow and process analysis

    - Analyze or evaluate current process and procedures.

    - Identify opportunities for improvement and, as appropriate, effect those changes.

    - Identify sources of data, including interfaces to other systems.

    - Determine location and number of workstations needed.

    - Redesign physical location as needed.

2. System installation

    - Determine system configuration.

    - Order and install hardware.

    - Prepare data center.

    - Upgrade or implement IT infrastructure.

    - Install software and interfaces.

    - Customize software.

    - Test, retest, and test again . . .

3. Staff training

    - Identify appropriate training method(s) to be used for each major user group.

    - Prepare training materials.

    - Train staff.

    - Test staff proficiency.

    - Update procedure manuals.

4. Conversion

    - Convert data.

    - Test system.

5. Communications

    - Establish communication mechanisms for identifying and addressing problems and concerns.

    - Communicate regularly with various constituent groups.

6. Preparation for go-live date

    - Select date when patient volume is relatively low.

    - Ensure sufficient staff are on hand.

- Set up mechanism for reporting and correcting problems and issues.
- Review and effect process reengineering.

7. System downtime procedures

  - Develop downtime procedures.
  - Train staff on downtime procedures.

Conduct Workflow and Process Analysis

One of the first activities necessary in implementing any new system is to review and evaluate the existing workflow or business processes. Members of the implementation team might also observe the current information system in use (if there is one). Does it work as described? Where are the problem areas? What are the goals and expectations of the new system? How do organizational processes need to change in order to optimize the new system's value and achieve its goals? Too often organizations never critically evaluate current business processes but plunge forward implementing the new system while still using old procedures. The result is that they simply automate their outdated and inefficient processes.

Before implementing any new system, the organization should evaluate existing procedures and processes and identify ways to improve workflow, simplify tasks, eliminate redundancy, improve quality, and improve user (customer) satisfaction. Although describing them is beyond the scope of this book, many extremely useful tools and methods are available for analyzing workflow and redesigning business processes (see, for example, *Guide to Reducing Unintended Consequences of Electronic Health Records*, by Jones et al., 2011). Observing the old system in use, listening to users' concerns, and evaluating information workflow can identify many of the changes needed. In addition, the vendor generally works with the organization to map its future workflow using flowcharts or flow diagrams. It is critical that all key areas affected by the new system participate in the workflow analysis process so that potential problems can be identified and addressed *before* the system goes live. For example, if a new CPOE application is to be implemented using a phased-in approach, where the system will go live unit by unit over a three-month process, how will the organization ensure orders are not lost or duplicated if a patient is transferred between a unit using CPOE and a unit using handwritten orders? What will downtime procedures entail? If paper orders are generated during downtime, how will these orders be stored or become part of the patient's permanent medical record?

Involving users at this early stage of the implementation process can gain initial buy-in to both the idea and the scope of the process redesign. In all likelihood, the organization will need to institute a series of process changes as a result of the new system. Workflow and processes should be evaluated critically and redesigned as needed. For example, the organization may find that it needs to do away with old forms or work steps, change job descriptions or job responsibilities, or add to or subtract from the work responsibilities of particular departments. Getting users involved in this reengineering process can lead to greater user acceptance of the new system.

Let's consider an example. Suppose a multiphysician clinic is implementing a new practice management system that includes a patient portal for appointment scheduling, prescription refills, and paying bills. The clinic might wish to begin by appointing a small team of individuals knowledgeable about analyzing workflow and processes to work with staff in studying the existing process for scheduling patient appointments, refilling prescriptions, and patient billing. This team might conduct a series of individual focus groups with schedulers, physicians and nurses, and patients, and ask questions such as these:

- Who can schedule patient appointments?
- How are patient appointments made, updated, or deleted?
- Who has access to scheduling information? From what locations?
- How well does the current system work? How efficient is the process?
- What are the major problems with the current scheduling system and process? In what ways might it be improved?

The team should tailor the focus questions so they are appropriate for each user group. The answers can then be a guide for reengineering existing processes and workflow to facilitate the new system. A similar set of questions could be asked concerning the refill of prescriptions or patient billing processes.

During the workflow analysis, the team should also examine where the new system's actual workstations will be located, how many workstations will be needed, and how information will flow between manual organizational processes (such as phone calls) and the electronic information system. Here are a few of the many questions that should be addressed in ensuring that physical layouts are conducive to the success of the new system:

- Will the workstations be portable or fixed? If users are given portable units, how will these be tracked and maintained (and protected from loss or theft)? If workstations are fixed, will they be located in safe, secure areas where patient confidentiality can be maintained?

- How will the user interact with the new system?
- Does the physical layout of each work area need to be redesigned to accommodate the new system and the new process?
- Will additional wiring be needed?
- How will the new system affect the workflow within the practice among office staff, nurses, and physicians?
- Will the e-prescribing function with local pharmacies be affected by the change?

Install System Components

The next step, which may be done concurrently with the workflow analysis, is to install the hardware, software, and network infrastructure to support the new information system and build the necessary interfaces. IT staff play a crucial role in this phase of the project. They will need to work closely with the vendor in determining system specifications and configurations and in preparing the computer center for installation. It may be, for example, that the organization's current computer network will need to be replaced or upgraded. During implementation, having adequate numbers of computer workstations placed in readily accessible locations is critical. Those involved in the planning need to determine beforehand the maximum number of individuals likely to be using the system at the same time, and accommodate this scenario. Vendors may recommend a certain number of workstations or use of hand-held devices; however, the organization must ensure the recommendations are appropriate.

Typically when a health care organization acquires a system from a vendor, quite a bit of customization is needed. IT personnel will likely work with the vendor in setting up and loading data tables, building interfaces, and running pilot tests of the hardware and software using actual patient and administrative data. It is not unlikely when purchasing a CPOE product from a vendor, for example, that the health care organization is provided a "shell" or basic framework from which to build the order sets or electronic forms. A great deal of customization and building of templates occurs. Thus, it is a good idea to pay physicians for their time involved in the project. For instance, if you need a physician's time to assist in building or reviewing order sets for the cardiology division, factor that into the resources needed for the project, perhaps by allocating two hours per week to the project for a certain period of time. Otherwise, you may be pulling physicians away from seeing patients and revenue-generating activities. It demonstrates the value placed on the physician's time and commitment to the project.

We recommend piloting the system in a unit or area before rolling out the system enterprise-wide. This test enables the implementation team to evaluate the system's effectiveness, address issues and concerns, fix bugs, and then apply the lessons learned to other units in the organization before most people even start using the system.

Consideration should be given to choosing an appropriate area (for example, a department or a location) or set of users to pilot the system. Some of the questions the implementation team should consider in identifying potential pilot sites are these:

- Which units or areas are willing and equipped to serve as a pilot site? Do they have sufficient interest, administrative support, and commitment?
- Are the staff and management teams in each of these units or areas comfortable with being system "guinea pigs"?
- Do staff have the time and resources needed to serve in this capacity?
- Is there a system champion in each unit or area who will lead the effort?

Plan, Conduct, and Evaluate Staff Training

Training is an essential component of any new system implementation. Although no one would argue with this statement, the implementation team will want to consider many issues as it develops and implements a training program. Here are a few of the questions to be answered:

- How much training is needed? Do different user groups have different training needs?
- Who should conduct the training?
- When should the training occur? What intervals of training are ideal?
- What training format is best—for example, formal, classroom-style training; one-on-one or small-group training; computer-based training; or a combination of methods?
- What is the role of the vendor in training?
- Who in the organization will manage or oversee the training? How will training be documented?
- What criteria and methods will be used to monitor training and ensure that staff are adequately trained? Will staff be tested on proficiency?

- What additional training and support are available to physicians and others after go-live?

There are various methods of training. One approach, commonly known as *train the trainer*, relies on the vendor to train selected members of the organization who will then serve as super-users and train others in their respective departments, units, or areas. These super-users should be individuals who work directly in the areas in which the system is to be used; they should know the staff in the area and have a good rapport with them. They will also serve as resources to other users once the vendor representatives have left. They may do a lot of one-on-one training, hand-holding, and other work with people in their areas until these individuals achieve a certain comfort level with the system. The main concern with this approach is that the organization may devote a great deal of time and resources to training the trainers only to have these trainers leave the institution (often because they've been lured away by career opportunities with the vendor).

Another method is to have the vendor train a pool of trainers who are knowledgeable about the entire system and who can rotate through the different areas of the organization working with staff. The trainer pool might include both IT professionals (including clinical analysts) and clinical or administrative staff such as nurses, physicians, lab managers, and business managers.

Regardless of who conducts the training, it is important to introduce fundamental or basic concepts first and allow people to master these concepts before moving on to new ones. Studies among health care organizations that have implemented clinical applications such as CPOE systems have shown that classroom training is not nearly as effective as one-on-one coaching, particularly among physicians (Holden, 2011; Metzger & Fortin, 2003). Most systems can track physician usage; physicians identified as low-volume users may be targeted for additional training.

Timing of the training is also important. Users should have ample opportunity to practice *before* the system goes live. For instance, when a nursing documentation system is being installed, nurses should have the chance to practice with it at the bedside of a typical patient. Likewise, when a CPOE system is going in, physicians should get to practice ordering a set of tests during their morning rounds. This *just-in-time training* might occur several times: for example, three months, two months, one month, and one week before the go-live date. Training might be supplemented with computer-based training modules that enable users to review concepts and functions at their own pace. Training has to be a priority and at least some of training should be in an environment free of distractions. Eventually staff will want to use the system in a "near live" or simulated environment. Additional staff should be on hand during the go-live period to assist users as needed during the transition to the new system. In general, the implementation team should work with the vendor to produce a thoughtful and creative training program.

Once the details of how the new system is to work have been determined, it is important to update procedure manuals and make the updated manuals available to the staff. Designated managers or representatives from the various areas may assume a leadership role in updating procedure manuals for their respective areas. When people must learn specific IT procedures such as how to log in, change passwords, and read common error messages, the IT department should ensure that this information appears in the procedure manuals and that the information is routinely updated and widely disseminated to the users. Procedure manuals serve as reference guides and resources for users and can be particularly useful when training new employees.

Effective training is important. Staff members need to be relatively comfortable with the application and need to know to whom they should turn if they have questions or concerns. We recommend having the users evaluate the training prior to go-live.

Convert Data and Test System

Another important task is to convert the data from the old system to the new system and then adequately test the new system. Staff involved in the data conversion must determine the sources of the data required for the new system and construct new files. It is particularly important that data be complete, accurate, and current before being converted to the new system. Data should be *cleaned* before being converted. Once converted, the data should run through a series of validation checkpoints or procedures to ensure the accuracy of the conversion.

IT staff knowledgeable in data conversion procedures should lead the effort and verify the results with key managers from the appropriate clinical and administrative areas. The specific conversion procedures used will depend on the nature of the old system and its structure as well as on the configuration of the new system.

Finally, the new system will need to be tested. The main purpose of the testing is to simulate the live environment as closely as possible and determine how well the system and accompanying procedures work. Are there programming glitches or other problems that need to be fixed? How well are the interfaces working? How does response time compare to what was expected? The system should be populated with live data and tested again. Vendors, IT staff, and user staff should all participate in the testing process. As with training, one can never test too much. A good portion of this work has to be done for the pilot testing. It may need to be repeated before going live. And the pilot lessons will guide any additional testing or conversion that needs to be done. In some cases, it may be advisable to run the old and new systems in tandem (parallel conversion) for a period of time until it is evident that the new system is operating effectively. This can reduce organizational risk. However, running parallel systems is not always feasible or appropriate. Instead, organizations may opt to implement the system using a phased approach over a period of time.

Communicate Progress or Status

Equally as important as successfully carrying out the activities discussed so far is having an effective plan for communicating the project's progress. This plan serves two primary purposes. First, it identifies how the members of the implementation team will communicate and coordinate their activities and progress. Second, it defines how progress will be communicated to key constituent groups, including but not limited to the board, the senior administrative team, the departments, and the staff at all levels of the organization affected by the new system. The communication plan may set up both formal and informal mechanisms. Formal communication may include everything from regular updates at board and administrative meetings to written briefings and articles in the facility newsletter. The purpose should be to use as many channels and mechanisms as possible to ensure that the people who need to know are fully informed and aware of the implementation plans. Informal communication is less structured but can be equally important. Implementing a new health care information system is a major undertaking, and it is important that all staff (day, evening, and night shifts) be made aware of what is happening. The methods for communication may be varied, but the message should be consistent and the information presented up-to-date and timely. For example, do not rely on e-mail communication as your primary method only to discover later that your organization's nurses do not regularly check their e-mail or have little time to read your type of message.

Prepare for Go-Live Date

A great deal of work goes into preparing for the go-live date, the day the organization transitions from the old system to the new. Assuming the implementation team has done all it can to ensure that the system is ready, the staff are well trained, and appropriate procedures are in place, the transition should be a smooth one. Additional staff should be on hand and equipped to assist users as needed. It is best to plan for the system to go live on a day when the patient census is typically low or fewer patients than usual are scheduled to be seen. Disaster recovery plans should also be in place, and staff should be well trained on what to do should the system go down or fail. Designated IT staff should monitor and assess system problems and errors.

When organizations are implementing information systems with clinical decision support, we recommend that they adhere to these "ten commandments" for effective clinical decision support.

Ten Commandments for Effective Clinical Decision Support

- Speed is everything—this is what information system users value most.

- Anticipate needs and deliver in real time—deliver information when needed.

- Fit into user's work flow—integrate suggestions with clinical practice.

- Little things can make a big difference—improve usability to "do the right thing."

- Recognize that physicians will resist stopping—offer alternatives rather than insist on stopping an action.

- Changing direction is easier than stopping—changing defaults for dose, route, or frequency of a medication can change behavior.

- Simple interventions work best—simplify guidelines by reducing to a single computer screen.

- Ask for additional information only when you really need it—the more data elements requested, the less likely a guideline will be implemented.

- Monitor impact, get feedback and respond—if certain reminders are not followed, readjust or eliminate the reminder.

- Manage and maintain your knowledge-based systems—track users' response to decision support and update to coincide with changes in medical knowledge [Bates et al., 2003].

A great deal of planning and leadership is needed in implementing a new health care information system. Despite the best-made plans, however, things can and do go wrong. The next section describes some of the unintended consequences and common organizational challenges associated with system implementation projects and offers strategies for anticipating and planning for them.

Develop and Communicate Downtime Procedures

One thing that you can count on is that systems will go down. Both scheduled and unscheduled downtime exists, and downtime procedures need to be developed and communicated well before go-live. Hopefully, the organization has invested in a stable and secure technical IT infrastructure and backup procedures and fail-safe systems are in place. But everyone needs to know what to do if the system is down, from the registration staff to the nursing staff to the medical staff and the transport team. How will orders be placed? If a paper record is kept during downtime, what is the procedure for getting the documentation in electronic form when the system is up again? How will scheduled downtime be communicated to units? And all staff members? If an organization relies heavily on computerized systems to care for patients, downtime should be minimal or near 0 percent. However, business continuity procedures must be in place to ensure patient safety and continuity of care.

MANAGING THE ORGANIZATIONAL ASPECTS

Implementing an information system in a health care facility can have a profound impact on the organization, the people who work there, and the patients they serve. Individuals may have concerns and apprehensions about the new system. They may wonder: How will the new system affect my job responsibilities or productivity? How will my workload change? Will the new system cause me more or less stress? Even individuals who welcome the new system, see the need for it, and see its potential value may worry: What will I do if the system is down? Will the system impede my relationship with my patients? Who will I turn to if I have problems or questions? Will I be expected to type my notes into the system? With the new system comes change, and change can be difficult if not managed effectively.

The human factors associated with implementing a new system should not be taken lightly. A great deal of change can occur as a result of the new system. Some of the changes may be immediately apparent; others may occur over time as the system is used more fully. Many IT implementation studies have been done in recent years, and they reveal several strategies that may lead to greater organizational acceptance and use of a new system:

- Create an appropriate environment, one where expectations are defined, met, and managed.
- Know your culture and do not underestimate user resistance.
- Allocate sufficient resources, including technical support staff and IT infrastructure.

- Provide adequate initial and ongoing training.
- Manage unintended consequences, especially those known to affect implementations such as CPOE and EHR systems.
- Establish a strong working relationship with the vendor.

More research is needed to explore the extent to which these and other strategies can lead to more widespread adoption of health care information systems, particularly clinical applications such as the CPOE and EHR systems.

Create an Appropriate Environment

If you ask a roomful of health care executives, physicians, nurses, pharmacists, or laboratory managers if they have ever experienced an IT system failure, chances are over half of the hands in the room will go up. In all likelihood the people in the room would have a much easier time describing a system failure than a system success. If you probed a little further and asked why the system was a failure, you might hear comments like these: "the system was too slow," "it was down all the time," "training was inadequate and nothing like the real thing," "there was no one to go to if you had questions or concerns," "it added to my stress and workload," and the list goes on. The fact is, the system did not meet their expectations. You might not know whether those expectations were reasonable or not.

Earlier we discussed the importance of clearly defining and communicating the goals and objectives of the new system. Related to goal definition is the management of user expectations. Different people may have different perspectives on what they expect from the new system; in addition, some will admit to having no expectations, and others will have joined the organization after the system was implemented and consequently are likely to have expectations derived from the people currently using the system.

Expectations come from what people see and hear about the system and the way they interpret what the system will do for them or for their organization. Expectations can be formed from a variety of sources—they may come from a comment made during a vendor presentation, a question that arises during training, a visit to another site that uses the same system, attendance at a professional conference, or a remark made by a colleague in the hallway.

Furthermore, the main criterion used to evaluate the system's value or success depends on the individual's expectations and point of view. For example, the chief financial officer might measure system success in terms of the financial return on investment, the chief medical director might look at impact on physicians' time and quality of care, the nursing staff might consider any change in their workload, public relations personnel might compare levels of patient satisfaction, and the IT staff might evaluate the change in the number of help desk calls made since the new system was implemented. All these approaches are measures of an information system's perceived impact on the organization or individual. However, they are not all the same, and they may not have equal importance to the organization in achieving its strategic goals.

It is therefore important for the health care executive team not only to establish and communicate clearly defined goals for the new system but also to listen to needs and expectations of the various user groups and to define, meet, and manage expectations appropriately. Ways to manage expectations include making sure users understand that the first days or weeks of system use may be rocky, that the organization may need time to adjust to a new workflow, that the technology may have bugs, and that users should not expect problem-free system operation from the start. Clear and effective communication is key in this endeavor.

In managing expectations it can be enormously helpful to conduct formative assessments of the implementation process, in which the focus is on the process as well as the outcomes. Specific metrics need to be chosen and success criteria defined to determine whether or not the system is meeting expectations (Cusack & Poon, 2011). For example, if wide-scale usage is a priority, collection of actual numbers of transactions or usage logs may be meaningful information for the leadership team. Other categories of metrics that might be helpful are clinical outcome measures, clinical process measures, provider adoption and attitude measures, patient knowledge and attitude measures, workflow impact measures, and financial impact measures. The Agency for Healthcare Research and Quality recently published the third edition of the *Health Information Exchange Evaluation Toolkit*, which can serve as a guide for project teams involved in evaluating the system implementation process or project outcomes (Cusack & Poon, 2011).

Know Your Culture and Do Not Underestimate User Resistance

Before embarking on system implementation, it is critical to know your culture. Understanding the culture is important *before* you make the investment. For example, you might ask, How engaged and ready are the physicians and other clinicians for the new system? Are they comfortable with technology? Do you have hospitalists on staff? Or are you a community hospital where the bulk of your medical staff are physicians who have admitting privileges at several hospitals and make rounds only once a day? How engaged have the physicians been in the design and build of the new system? Is there strong support? If you don't have sufficient medical staff buy-in and support or hospitalists on staff who are committed to the project, you run the risk of encountering user resistance and system failure due to inadequate use.

During the implementation process it is also important to analyze current workflow and make appropriate changes as needed. Earlier we gave an example of analyzing a patient scheduling process. Patient scheduling is a relatively straightforward process. A change in this system may not dramatically change the job responsibilities of the schedulers and may have little impact on nurses' or physicians' time. Therefore, these groups may offer little resistance to such a change. (This is not to guarantee a lack of resistance—if you mess up a practice's schedule, you can have a lot of angry people on your hands!) In contrast, changes in processes that involve the direct provision of patient care services and that do affect nurses' and physicians' time may be tougher for users to accept. The physician ordering process is a perfect example. Most physicians today are accustomed to picking up a pen and paper and handwriting an order or calling one in to the nurses' station from their phones. With CPOE, physicians may be expected to keyboard their orders directly into the system and respond to automated reminders and decision-support alerts. A process that historically took them a few seconds to do might now take several minutes, depending on the number of prompts and reminders. Moreover, physicians are now doing things that were not asked of them before—they are checking for drug interactions, responding to reminders and alerts, evaluating whether evidence-based clinical guidelines apply to the patient, and the list goes on. All these activities take time, but in the long run they will improve the quality of patient care. Therefore, it is important for physicians to be actively involved in designing the process and in seeing its value to the patient care process.

Getting physicians, nurses, and other clinicians to accept and use clinical information systems such as CPOE or EHR can be challenging even when they are involved in the implementation. At times the incentives for using the system may not be aligned with their individual needs and goals. On the one hand, for example, if the physician is expected to see a certain number of patients per day and is evaluated on patient load and if writing orders used to take thirty minutes a day with the old system and now takes sixty to ninety minutes with the new CPOE system, the physician can either see fewer patients or work more hours. One should expect to see physician resistance. On the other hand, if the physician's performance and income is related to adherence to clinical practice guidelines, using the CPOE system might improve his or her income, creating a greater chance of acceptance.

The physician's workload or productivity goals might, however, be beyond the organization's control. They might be individual goals the physician has set for himself or herself. Can or should organizations mandate the use of clinical information systems like CPOE? In effect, the organization is stating that resistance is unacceptable. Several health care facilities have instituted policies mandating physician use of CPOE, with mixed results. Physicians' acceptance of such a mandate may have a lot to do with the organizational culture, the training they received, their confidence (or lack of confidence) in the system, how the mandate was imposed, and a host of other factors. Mandating use is most common in academic medical centers where residents and fellows are expected to enter orders in a computerized system (Sklarin, Granovsky, & Hagerty-Paglia, 2011). Mandating physician use can be taxing for community hospitals or other facilities that are not the physicians' employers. Community-based physicians often see patients at more than one hospital and spend limited time at each facility. Trying to get these fairly independent physicians to buy into a facility's CPOE system and participate in the necessary training can be difficult.

To address this and related acceptance issues, the California HealthCare Foundation, in collaboration with First Consulting Group, conducted an in-depth study of ten community hospitals throughout the United States that have made significant progress in implementing CPOE (Metzger & Fortin, 2003). The study found that CPOE leaders tended to avoid the term *mandate* and instead recommended that health care executives work toward an enterprise-wide policy for universal CPOE. Key staff in participating hospitals recommended starting with a strong commitment to CPOE, delivering a consistent message that CPOE is the right thing to do, and working within the culture of the medical staff toward the goal of universal adoption. This goal might take years to achieve. Readiness for universal adoption occurred when (1) a significant number of physician CPOE adopters showed their peers what was possible, (2) sufficient progress was made toward achieving patient safety objectives, and (3) the medical staff came together with one voice to champion CPOE as the right thing to do.

It perhaps goes without saying that user acceptance occurs when users see or realize the value the health care information system brings to their work and the patients they serve. This value takes different forms. Some people may realize increased efficiency, less stress, greater organization, and improved quality of information, whereas others may find that the system enables them to provide better care, avoid medical mistakes, and make better decisions. In some cases an individual may not experience the value personally yet may come to realize the value to the organization as a whole.

Allocate Sufficient Resources

Sufficient resources are needed both during and after the new system has been implemented. User acceptance comes from confidence in the new system. Individuals want to know that the system works properly, is stable, and is secure and that someone is available to help them when they have questions, problems, or concerns. Therefore, it is important for the organization to ensure that adequate resources are devoted to implementing and supporting the system and its users. At a minimum, adequate technical staff expertise should be available as well as sufficient IT infrastructure.

We have discussed the importance of giving the implementation team sufficient support as it carries out its charge, but what forms can this support take? Some methods of supporting the team are to make available release time, additional staff, and development funds. Senior managers might allocate travel funds so team members can view the system in use in other facilities. They might decide that all implementation team members or super-users will receive 50 percent release time for the next six months to devote to the project. This release time will enable those involved to give up some of their normal job duties so they can focus on the project. Senior leaders at one health care organization in South Carolina gave sixty-four full-time staff release time for one year to devote to the implementation of a facility-wide health information system. This substantial amount of release time was indicative of the high value the executive team members placed on the project. They saw it as critical to achieving the organization's strategic goals.

Providing sufficient time and resources to the implementation phase of the project is, however, only part of the overall support needed. Studies have shown that an information system's value to the organization is typically realized over time. Value is derived as more and more people use the system, offer suggestions for enhancing it, and begin to push the system to fulfill its functionality. If users are ever to fully realize the system's value, they must have access to local technical support—someone, preferably within the organization, who is readily available, is knowledgeable about the intricacies of the system, and is able to handle both hardware and software problems. This individual should be able to work effectively with the vendor and others to find solutions to system problems. Even though it is ideal to have local technical support in-house, that may be difficult in small physician offices or community-based settings. In such cases the facility may need to consider such options as (1) devoting a significant portion of an employee's time to training so that he or she may assume a support role, (2) partnering with a neighboring organization that uses the same system to share technical support staff, or (3) contracting with a local computer firm to provide the needed assistance.

The vendor may be able to assist the organization in identifying and securing local technical support.

On busy nursing units, it can be extremely helpful to have nursing informatics analysts assigned to assist designated areas 24/7. One large academic medical center in the Southeast employs approximately eight nursing informatics specialists (in addition to the IT support) to provide additional support to nurses and other clinicians and systems users on the patient care units. The specialists wear "red" lab coats so they are easily identified and roam the halls, providing one-on-one assistance, additional training, and troubleshooting as needed.

In addition to arranging for local technical support, the organization will also need to invest resources in building and maintaining a reliable, secure IT infrastructure (servers, operating systems, and networks) to support the information system, particularly if it is a mission-critical system. Many patient information systems need to be available 24 hours a day, 7 days a week, 365 days a year. Health care professionals can come to rely on having access to timely, accurate, and complete information in caring for their patents, just as they count on having electricity, water, and other basic utilities. Failing to build the IT infrastructure that will adequately support the new clinical system can be catastrophic for the organization and its IT department.

An IT infrastructure's lifetime may be relatively short. It is reasonable to expect that within three to ten years, the hardware, software, and network will likely need to be replaced as advances are made in technology, the organization's goals and needs change, and the health care environment changes. Downtime, both scheduled and unscheduled, should be limited. For example, one hospital's goal is to have no more than nine hours of downtime a year.

Provide Adequate Training

Earlier we discussed the importance of training staff on the new system prior to the go-live date. Having a training program suited to the needs of the various user groups is very important during the implementation process. People who will use the system should be relatively comfortable with it, have had ample opportunities to use it in a safe environment, and know where to turn should they have questions or need additional assistance. It is equally important to provide ongoing training months and even years after the system has been implemented. In all likelihood the system will go through a series of upgrades, changes will be made, and users will get more comfortable with the fundamental features and will be ready to push the system to the next level. Some users will explore additional functionality on their own; others will need prodding and additional training in order to learn more advanced features.

It is also critical to provide the type of training that works best for your users' needs and learning preferences. Do not be afraid to have different training methods for different user groups (Holden, 2011). Memorial Sloan-Kettering Cancer Center is a perfect example. It is one of the world's oldest private cancer centers in the world. All of its physicians are employees of the organization. When they were first implementing their CPOE, all clinical and administrative staff underwent group training sessions (Sklarin, Granovsky, & Hagerty-Paglia, 2011). The system was not accepted by the physicians for a variety of reasons, and training was a critical issue. Once the leadership team realized this, they regrouped, changed tactics, and added three new approaches to working with the physicians: (1) they rolled out one service at a time with one hour of personalized training to each physician of that service (additional time did not seem to help); (2) support staff were stationed at the clinical areas during the implementation period for individualized assistance (similar to the "red coats" mentioned earlier); and (3) a physician champion was involved in workflow discussions and key in facilitating the placement of orders in the system and in helping ensure physician compliance (Sklarin, Granovsky, & Hagerty-Paglia, 2011). Understanding the culture and the physician training needs of the organization is vital when implementing a new system, as is a willingness to reevaluate the project. It is important to view the system as a long-term investment rather than a one-time purchase. The resources allocated or committed to the system should include not only the up-front investment in hardware and software but also the time, people, and resources needed to maintain and support it.

Manage Unintended Consequences

Management expertise and leadership are important elements to the success of any system implementation. Effective leaders help build a community of collaboration and trust. However, effective leadership also entails understanding the unintended consequences that can occur during complex system implementations and managing them. Unintended consequences can be positive, negative, or both, depending on one's perspective. Several years ago, Ash and colleagues (2007) conducted interviews with key individuals from 176 U.S. hospitals that had implemented CPOE. CPOE is one of the most complex and challenging of clinical information systems to implement. From their work, they identified eight types of unintended consequences that implementation teams should plan for and consider when implementing CPOE:

1. **More work or new work.** CPOEs can increase work due to the fact that systems may be slow, nonstandard cases may call for more steps

in ordering, training may remain an issue, some tasks may become more difficult, the computer forces the user to complete "all steps," and physicians often take on tasks that were formerly done by others.

2. **Workflow.** CPOEs can greatly alter workflow, sometimes improving workflow for some and slowing or complicating it for others.

3. **System demands.** Maintenance, training, and support efforts can be significant for an organization, not only in building the system but also in making improvements and enhancements to it.

4. **Communication.** CPOE systems affect communication within the organization; they can reduce the need to clarify orders but also lead to people failing to adequately communicate with each other in appropriate situations.

5. **Emotions.** Clinician reactions to CPOE can run the gamut from positive to negative.

6. **New kinds of errors.** Although CPOE systems are generally designed to detect and prevent errors, they can lead to new types of errors such as juxtaposition errors, in which clinicians click on the adjacent patient name or medication from a list and inadvertently enter the wrong order.

7. **Power shifts.** Shifts in power may be viewed as less of a problem than some of the other unintended consequences, but CPOE can be used to monitor physician behavior.

8. **Dependence on the system.** Clinicians become dependent on the CPOE system, so managing downtime procedures is critical. Even then, while the system is down, CPOE users view the situation as managed chaos (adapted from Ash et al., 2007).

Conflicts can also occur between paper-based and electronic systems if providers who prefer paper records annotate printouts and place them in patient charts as formal documentation, and in essence create two distinct and sometimes conflicting medical records (Jones et al., 2011).

Health care executives and implementation teams should be aware of these unintended consequences, particularly those that can adversely affect the organization, and carefully plan for and manage them.

Establish Strong Working Relationships with Vendors

Developing strong working relationships with the vendor is key. The health care executive should view the vendor as a partner, and an entity with which the organization will likely have a long-term relationship. This relationship often begins when the organization first selects a new information system and continues well after the system is live and operational. The system will have upgrades, new version releases, and ongoing maintenance contracts. It behooves both parties, the health care provider organization and the vendor, to clearly define expectations, resource needs, and timelines. It is important to have open, honest, and candid conversations when problems arise or differences in expectation occur. Equally important is for both parties to demonstrate a willingness to address needs and solve problems collaboratively.

SYSTEM SUPPORT AND EVALUATION

Information systems evolve as an organization continues to grow and change. No matter how well the system was designed and tested, errors and problems will be detected and changes will need to be made. IT staff generally assume a major role in maintaining and supporting the information systems in the health care organization. When errors or problems are detected, IT staff correct the problem or work with the vendor to see that the problem is fixed. Moreover, the vendor may detect glitches and develop upgrades or patches that will need to be installed.

Many opportunities for enhancing and improving the system's performance and functionality will arise well after the go-live date. The organization will want to ensure that the system is adequately maintained, supported, and further developed over time. Selecting and implementing a health care information system is an enormous investment. This investment must be maintained, just as one would maintain one's home.

As with other devices, information systems have a life cycle and eventually need to be replaced. Health care organizations typically go through a process whereby they plan, design, implement, and evaluate their health care information systems. Too often in the past the organization's work was viewed as done once the system went live. It has since been discovered how vital system maintenance and support resources are and how important it is to evaluate the extent to which the system goals are being achieved.

Evaluating or accessing the value of the health care information system is increasingly important. Acquiring and implementing systems requires large investments, and stakeholders, including boards of directors, are demanding to know both the actual and future value of these projects. Evaluations must be viewed as an integral component of every major health information system project and not an afterthought. In fact we believe that assessing the value of a health IT investment is enormously important and thus have devoted Chapter Seventeen entirely to the subject.

SUMMARY

Implementing a new information system in a health care organization requires a significant amount of planning and preparation. The health care organization should begin by appointing an implementation team comprising experienced individuals, including representatives from key areas in the organization, particularly areas that will be affected by or responsible for using the new system. Key users should be involved in analyzing existing processes and procedures and making recommendations for changes. A system champion should be part of the implementation team and serve as an advocate in soliciting input, representing user views, and spearheading the project. When implementing a clinical application, it is important that the system champion be a physician or clinician, someone who is able to represent the views of the care providers.

Under the direction of a highly competent implementation team, a number of important activities should occur during the system rollout. This team should assume a leadership role in ensuring that the system is effectively incorporated into the day-to-day operations of the facility. This generally requires the organization to (1) analyze workflow and processes and perform any necessary process reengineering, (2) install and configure the system, (3) train staff, (4) convert data, (5) adequately test the system, and (6) communicate project progress using appropriate forums at all levels throughout the organization. Attention should be given to the countless details associated with ensuring that downtime and backup procedures are in place, security plans have been developed, and the organization is ready for the go-live date.

During the days immediately following system implementation, the organization should have sufficient staff on hand to assist users and provide individual assistance as needed. A stable and secure IT infrastructure should be in place to ensure minimal, ideally zero, downtime and adequate response time. The IT department or other appropriate unit or representative should have a formal mechanism in place for reporting and correcting errors, bugs, and glitches in the system.

Once the system has gone live, it is critical for the organization to have in place the plans and resources needed to adequately maintain and support the new system. Technical staff and resources should be available to the users. Ongoing training should be an integral part of the organization's plans to support and further develop the new system. In addition, the leadership team should have in place a thoughtful plan for evaluating the implementation process and assessing the value of the health care information system.

Beyond taking ultimate responsibility for completion of the activities needed to implement and to support and evaluate the new system, the health care executive should assume a leadership role in managing the organizational and human aspects of the new system. Information systems can have a profound impact on health care organizations, the people who work there, and the patients they serve. Acquiring a good product and having the right technical equipment and expertise are not enough to ensure system success. Health care executives must also be attuned to the human aspects of introducing new IT into the care delivery process.

KEY TERMS

Implementation team

System champion

System implementation

Train the trainer

Unintended consequences

User resistance

Workflow and process analysis

LEARNING ACTIVITIES

1. Visit a health care organization that has recently implemented a health care information system. What process did it use to implement the system? How does that process compare with the one described in this chapter? How successful was the organization in implementing the new system? To what do staff attribute this success?

2. Search the literature for a recent article on a system implementation project. Briefly describe the process used to implement the system and the lessons learned. How might this particular facility's experiences be useful to others? Explain.

3. Physician acceptance and use of clinical information systems are often cited as challenges. What do you think the health care leadership team can or should do to foster acceptance by physicians? Assume that a handful of physicians in your organization are actively resisting a new clinical information system. How would you approach and address their resistance and concerns?

4. Assume you are working with an implementation team in installing a new nursing documentation system for a home health agency. Historically, all its nursing documentation was recorded in paper form. The home health agency has little computerization beyond basic registration information and has no IT staff. What recommendations might you offer to the implementation team as it begins the work of installing the new nursing documentation system?

5. Discuss the risks to a health care organization in failing to allocate sufficient support and resources to a newly implemented health care information system.

6. Assume you are the CEO of a large group practice (seventy-five physicians) that implemented an EHR system two years ago. The physicians are asking for an evaluation of the system and its impact on quality, costs, and patient satisfaction. Devise a plan for evaluating the EHR system's impact on the organization in these three areas.

7. Read the Executive Summary of the Institute of Medicine's (2011) report entitled *Health IT and Patient Privacy: Building Safer Systems for Better Care*. How can the introduction of health IT that is designed to enhance or improve patient quality and safety lead to patient safety concerns? Do you agree that patient safety is a partnership between the health care organization and health IT vendor when implementing health care information systems? Explain the role of each and your rationale.

REFERENCES

Ash, J. S., Anderson, N. R., & Tarczy-Hornoch, P. (2008). People and organization issues in research systems implementation. *Journal of the American Medical Informatics Association*, 15, 283–289.

Ash, J. S., Sittig, D. F., Poon, E. G., Guappone, K., Campbell, E., & Dykstra, R. (2007). The extent and importance of unintended consequences related to computerized provider order entry. *Journal of the American Medical Informatics Association*, 14(4), 415–423.

Ash, J. S., Stavri, P., Dykstra, R., & Fournier, L. (2003). Implementing computerized physician order entry: The importance of special people. *International Journal of Medical Informatics*, 69(2–3), 235–250.

Bates, D. W., Kuperman, G. J., Wang, J., Gandhi, T., Kittler, A., Volk, L., . . . & Middleton, B. (2003). Ten commandments for effective clinical decision support: Making the practice of evidence-based medicine a reality. *Journal of the American Medical Informatics Association*, 10, 523–530.

Cusack, C., & Poon, E. (2011). *Health information exchange evaluation toolkit*. Agency for Healthcare Research and Quality. Retrieved February 2013 from http://healthit.ahrq.gov/portal/server.pt/community/health_it_tools_and _resources/919/health_information_exchange_(hie)_evaluation_toolkit/27870

Holden, R. J. (2011). What stands in the way of technology-mediated patient safety improvements? A study of facilitators and barriers to physician's use of electronic health records. *Journal of Patient Safety*, 7(4), 193–203.

Institute of Medicine. (2011). *Health IT and patient privacy: Building safer systems for better care.* Washington, DC: National Academies Press.

Jones, S. S., Koppel, R., Ridgley, M. S., Palen, T., Wu, S., & Harrison, M. I. (2011, August). *Guide to reducing unintended consequences of electronic health records.* Rockville, MD: Agency for Healthcare Research and Quality.

Metzger, J., & Fortin, J. (2003). *Computerized physician order entry in community hospitals: Lessons from the field.* Oakland: California HealthCare Foundation.

Miller, R. H., & Sim, I. (2004). Physicians' use of electronic medical records: Barriers and solutions. *Health Affairs, 23*(2), 116–126.

Miller, R. H., Sim, I., & Newman, J. (2003). *Electronic medical records: Lessons from small physician practices.* Oakland: California HealthCare Foundation.

Sittig, D. F., & Singh, H. (2011). Defining health information technology-related errors: New developments since *To Err Is Human. Archives of Internal Medicine, 171*(14), 1281–1284.

Sklarin, N. T., Granovsky, S., & Hagerty-Paglia, J. (2011). Electronic health record implementation at an academic cancer center: Lessons learned and strategies for success. *American Society of Clinical Oncology,* 411–415.

Wager, K. A., Lee, F., White, A., Ward, D., & Ornstein, S. (2000). Impact of an electronic medical record system on community-based primary care practices. *Journal of the American Board of Family Practice, 13*(5), 338–348.

Yackanicz, L., Kerr, R., & Levick, D. (2010). Physician buy-in for EMRs. *Journal of Healthcare Information Management, 24*(2), 41–44.

PART THREE

Information Technology

CHAPTER 9

Technologies That Support Health Care Information Systems

LEARNING OBJECTIVES

- To gain a basic understanding of the core technologies behind health care information systems that support:
  - Data management and access
  - Networks
  - Information distribution schemes
  - Remote access technologies
  - Internet and web concepts and applications
  - Clinical and managerial decision support
  - Electronic and mobile commerce
- To be able to discuss emerging trends in information technology and the Gartner Hype Cycle.
- To be able to identify some of the major issues in the adoption of information technologies in health care organizations.
- To be able to discuss why it is important for a health care organization to adopt an overall information systems architecture.

Thus far in this book we have explored a variety of health care information systems. These systems have been presented with minimal discussion of the technology behind them. We have focused instead on how the various applications are adopted, implemented, and used. Although we do not believe that health care executives need to become information technology (IT) experts in order to make informed decisions about which health care information systems to employ in their organizations, we do believe that an exposure to some of the core technologies used to develop and implement common health care information systems is quite useful. This knowledge will help health care executives be more informed decision makers.

This chapter provides a broad overview of several core information technologies. The chapter is written with the assumption that the reader has preexisting knowledge of computer or information systems fundamentals. This chapter will not discuss basic hardware and software concepts. The focus will be on providing a working knowledge of the basic concepts, standards, and terminology associated with databases (including data warehouses), networks, and web technologies. Decision support and expert systems are introduced. The chapter begins with a discussion of the challenges faced by health care organizations adopting new technologies and concludes with a discussion of the concept and importance of the organization's overall information systems architecture. Like many other fields, IT has its own language. It is helpful for health care executives to learn IT terminology and concepts so they can communicate effectively with IT staff and vendors.

INFORMATION TECHNOLOGY ADOPTION CHALLENGES

The information technology industry in general and the health information technology industry in particular are ever-changing and evolving. New technologies are being introduced every day. How does a health care executive know when to support the adoption of the "latest and greatest" technologies? When does the organization acknowledge its current technologies are out-of-date and need upgrading? How much of the current literature about new technologies is "hype"? Which new technologies are likely to survive to become industry standards? In previous chapters we introduced specific methods for selecting health care information systems to meet the health care organizations' operations needs. The questions posed here are more general in nature and relate to the technologies upon which these systems are built. Take, for example, the use of smart phones and tablets by health care providers.

Individuals adopted those technologies for personal use with significant spill-over into the work environment. Now hospitals and other health care organizations are purchasing these devices as a part of their overall information system infrastructure and are facing the challenges associated with incorporating these devices into their overall systems. At what point should the health care executives have known that these technologies were here to stay and were something to be managed? Do the early adopters of the technologies have an advantage or a disadvantage in the market?

There are no easy answers to these questions, but Gartner, Inc., has developed a useful framework for health care executives to think about when considering adopting new technologies. The Hype Cycle (Gartner, 2012) presents a view of how a technology will evolve over time. The stated purpose is to "provide a sound source of insight to manage its deployment within the context of . . . specific business goals." The Hype Cycle (Figure 9.1) supports organizations in their decisions to adopt the technology early or wait for further maturation. There are five key phases to the cycle:

Technology Trigger. A potential technology breakthrough kicks things off. Early proof-of-concept stories and media interest trigger significant publicity. Often no usable products exist and commercial viability is unproven.

Peak of Inflated Expectations. Early publicity produces a number of success stories—often accompanied by scores of failures. Some companies take action; many do not.

Trough of Disillusionment. Interest wanes as experiments and implementations fail to deliver. Producers of the technology shake out or fail. Investments continue only if the surviving providers improve their products to the satisfaction of early adopters.

Slope of Enlightenment. More instances of how the technology can benefit the enterprise start to crystallize and become more widely understood. Second- and third-generation products appear from technology providers. More enterprises fund pilots; conservative companies remain cautious.

Plateau of Productivity. Mainstream adoption starts to take off. Criteria for assessing provider viability are more clearly defined. The technology's broad market applicability and relevance are clearly paying off (Gartner, 2012).

Figure 9.1. The hype cycle

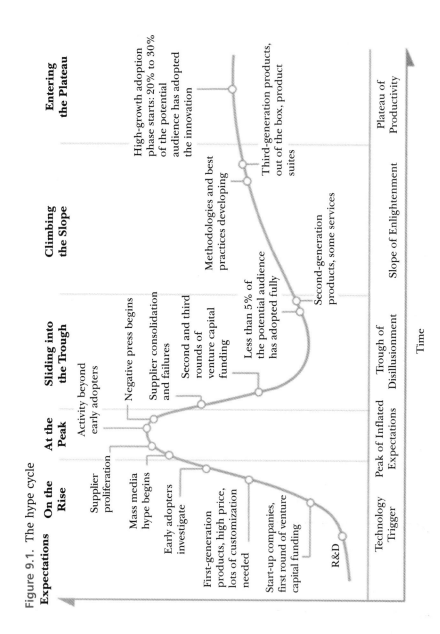

Expectations

On the Rise

Supplier proliferation

Mass media hype begins

Early adopters investigate

First-generation products, high price, lots of customization needed

Start-up companies, first round of venture capital funding

R&D

At the Peak

Activity beyond early adopters

Sliding into the Trough

Negative press begins

Supplier consolidation and failures

Second and third rounds of venture capital funding

Less than 5% of the potential audience has adopted fully

Climbing the Slope

Methodologies and best practices developing

Second-generation products, some services

Entering the Plateau

High-growth adoption phase starts: 20% to 30% of the potential audience has adopted the innovation

Third-generation products, out of the box, product suites

Technology Trigger

Peak of Inflated Expectations

Trough of Disillusionment

Slope of Enlightenment

Plateau of Productivity

Time

PERSPECTIVE
Hype Cycle for Health Care Provider Technologies and Standards, 2011

On the Rise
- 3D bioprinting
- Health care–assistive robots
- Digital pathology scanners
- Semantic web tools and health care
- Consent management

At the Peak
- IT GRCM tools
- Entity resolution and analysis
- Workflow and BPM for care coordination
- Detailed clinical models
- IHE PCD 2010

Sliding into the Trough
- GS1 health care (GDSN)
- HIPAA and HITECH
- Legacy decommissioning
- The Direct Project
- Unified communications
- HIE
- Bluetooth medical device profile
- Vendor-neutral (image) archive
- End-user experience monitoring
- ICD-10 CM (U.S.)
- Desktop virtualization
- Information life cycle management
- Mobile device management
- Semantic interoperability and health care

(cont.)

- Health care location- and condition-sensing technologies
- Interactive patient care systems

Climbing the Slope
- CCR/CCD
- SNOMED-CT
- IHE XDS
- Enterprise content management
- Strong authentication for remote access
- Server virtualization
- Service-oriented architecture
- Strong authentication for enterprise access
- Distributed antenna systems
- User provisioning
- Natural-language processing
- UMDB

Entering the Plateau
- Tablet PCs for health care
- Enterprise PKI
- Remote hosting
- Voice over Internet protocol
- CCOW
- Disaster recovery and business continuity
- HL7 CDA R2
- Single sign-on
- Speech recognition (once and done)

Off the Hype Cycle
- Basic web services
- HL7 V3 messages

Source: Gartner, 2011.

DATA MANAGEMENT AND ACCESS

All the health care applications discussed in this text require data. The electronic health record (EHR) system relies on comprehensive databases, as do other clinical applications. Data must be stored and maintained so that they can be retrieved and used within these applications. This section includes an introduction to the following topics with a focus on terminology and definitions that are most useful in the health care executive. This discussion is not meant to be all-inclusive or highly technical.

- Database models
- Database operations
- Databases on the web
- Clinical data repositories, data warehouses, and data marts
- Data mining

Database Models

Most of us are comfortable with the concept of a file. We may envision a folder with individual pieces of paper or a spreadsheet with rows that represent individual records. In whichever view, we comprehend that a file consists of records. What do records consist of? Carrying the spreadsheet example further, records consist of fields (represented on the spreadsheet as the column titles). Specific data reside within each field of each record in the spreadsheet file (see Figure 9.2).

Our spreadsheet is an example of a *traditional or flat file structure*. It is a common way to store data that works very well for simple data storage.

Figure 9.2. Traditional file structure for simplified patient registration

MRN	Patient Name	Date of Birth	Physician	Clinic	Admission Date	Next of Kin
00 01 01	Emma J. Watkins	9/23/1951	Ethel Mays	Medicine	2/2/2000	Jennifer Watson
00 01 02	Henry H. McHardy	6/22/1960	Ethel Mays	Medicine	2/3/2000	Carloline Wicher
00 01 03	Lillian V. Mitchell	10/14/1993	Olivia Carson	Medicine	12/18/2010	Harold Mitchell
00 01 05	Michael C. Collins	11/27/1997	Gerald Johnson	Pediatrics	3/25/2010	Maria Collins
00 01 11	Trevor W. Clayton	11/21/1953	Olivia Carson	Medicine	5/1/2010	Francine Clayton
01 02 04	Eloise M. Murton	5/30/1979	Hillary Puentes	OB/Gyn	9/26/2011	Geoff Black
01 02 12	William B. Anders	12/19/1931	Majorie Taylor	Cardiac	10/23/2011	William Anderson
02 01 05	Sarah L. Fitzgerald	4/23/1925	Ethel Mays	Medicine	1/5/2012	Christine Jones
02 01 06	Lois I. Griffin	2/14/1927	Majorie Taylor	Cardiac	1/6/2012	Louis Griffin
02 01 09	Ingrid N. Norris	8/12/2010	Gerald Johnson	Pediatrics	4/29/2012	Nora Norris

FIELD

RECORD

However, as data storage becomes more complex, flat file structures become very cumbersome with many data redundancies. A better approach to data management is a *database structure*.

The most common type of database in use today is a *relational database*. Two older types of databases, hierarchical and network (not to be confused with a computer network), may still exist in health care organizations as components of older, legacy applications, but because they no longer have a significant presence in the database market, they are not discussed here. A fourth type of database, the *object-oriented database*, received a lot of attention in the literature a few years ago, but suffered from lack of standardization.

The relational database is a logical structure for storing, retrieving, and manipulating data. The relational database consists of *tables* that are connected through the use of *keys*, which are common data elements. The relational database structure eliminates data redundancy. It supports both one-to-many and many-to-many relationships between the records within different tables (see Figure 9.3). A relational database is implemented through a *relational database management system (RDBMS)*. Microsoft Access is an example of an RDBMS for desktop computing; Oracle, IBM DB2, and Microsoft SQL Server are examples of the more robust proprietary RDBMSs that are used to develop larger applications. MySQL is a popular open source RDBMS.

Database Operations

The programming language most widely used in relational databases is *structured query language (SQL)*. In fact, SQL is recognized as a de facto standard for relational database functioning. The common RDBMS products support some type of SQL, but many of them also employ extensions to the basic language. The following example of a simple SQL statement would return a list of Dr. Ethel Mays's patients from the simplified patient registration database in Figure 9.3:

SELECT PATIENT, PHYSICIAN FROM PATIENTS

WHERE PHYSICIAN = "Ethel Mays"

Other basic concepts related to the relational database are *schema, data dictionary*, and *metadata*. The schema describes the actual structure of the database as it is designed. For example, the names and types of fields and relationships among records must be created. This information becomes a part of the repository of information about the database, known as the data dictionary or metadata (Oz, 2009). Creating a data dictionary is an important step in developing a health care application. It gives the developer and user a

Figure 9.3. Possible database structure for simplified patient registration

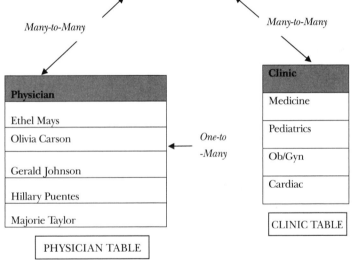

MRN	Patient Name	Date of Birth	Next of Kin	Admission Date
00 01 01	Emma J. Watkins	9/23/1951	Jennifer Watson	2/2/2000
00 01 02	Henry H. McHardy	6/22/1960	Carloline Wicher	2/3/2000
00 01 03	Lillian V. Mitchell	10/14/1993	Harold Mitchell	12/18/2010
00 01 05	Michael C. Collins	11/27/1997	Maria Collins	3/25/2010
00 01 11	Trevor W. Clayton	11/21/1953	Francine Clayton	5/1/2010
01 02 04	Eloise M. Murton	5/30/1979	Geoff Black	9/26/2011
01 02 12	William B. Anders	12/19/1931	William Anderson	10/23/2011
02 01 05	Sarah L. Fitzgerald	4/23/1925	Christine Jones	1/5/2012
02 01 06	Lois I. Griffin	2/14/1927	Louis Griffin	1/6/2012
02 01 09	Ingrid N. Norris	8/12/2010	Nora Norris	4/29/2012

clear understanding of the data elements contained in the database. Confusion about data definitions can lead to poor-quality data and even to poor decisions based on data misconceptions. A typical data dictionary allows for the documentation of

- Table names
- All attribute or field names
- A description or definition of each data element
- The data type of the field (text, number, date, and so forth)

- The format of each data element (such as DD-MM-YYYY for the date)
- The size of each field (such as eleven characters for a Social Security number, including the dashes)
- An appropriate range of values for the field (such as integers 000000 to 999999 for a medical record number)
- Whether or not the field is required (is it a primary key or a linking key?)
- Relationships among fields

The importance of a well-thought-out data dictionary cannot be overstated. When an organization is trying to link or combine databases, the data dictionary is a vital tool. Think, for example, how difficult it might be to combine information from databases with different definitions for fields with the same name.

Databases on the Web

Without online access to databases, the web would be rendered practically useless. Much of information found on the Internet is stored in a database. Technically, these online databases are essentially the same as other databases. The difference is that a special interface must be developed to work specifically in the web environment. There are several common programming languages for building these interfaces. Some of the most common are Java servlets, active server pages (ASP), and PHP. You may actually see these included in URLs that appear after web searches (Oz, 2009).

Clinical Data Repositories, Data Warehouses, and Data Marts

Many health care organizations, particularly those moving toward electronic health records, develop *clinical data repositories*. Although these databases can take different forms, in general the clinical data repository is a large database that gets data from various data stores within application systems across the organization. There is generally a process by which data are *cleaned* before they are moved from the source systems into the repository. Once the clean data are in the repository, they can be used to produce reports that integrate data from two or more data stores. In function, the clinical data repository is generally a large relational database.

A *data warehouse*, however, is functionally different from a relational database. It is a type of large database designed to support decision making in an organization. Traditionally, health care organizations have collected data in a variety of *online transactional processing (OLTP)* systems, such as the traditional relational database and clinical data repository. OLTP systems are well suited for supporting the daily operations of a health care organization but less well suited for decision support. Data stored in a typical OLTP system are always changing, making it difficult to track trends over time, for example. The data warehouse, in contrast, is specifically designed for decision support. It differs from the traditional OLTP database in several key areas, summarized in Table 9.1.

Table 9.1. Differences between OLTP databases and data warehouses

Characteristic	OLTP Database	Data Warehouse
Purpose	Support transaction processing	Support decision support
Source of data	Business transactions	Multiple files, databases—data internal and external to the firm
Data access allowed to users	Read and write	Read only
Primary data access mode	Simple database update and query	Simple and complex database queries with increasing use of data mining to recognize patterns in the data
Primary database model employed	Relational	Relational
Level of detail	Detailed transactions	Often summarized data
Availability of historical data	Very limited—typically a few weeks or months	Multiple years
Update process	Online, ongoing process as transactions are captured	Periodic process, once per week or once per month
Ease of update	Routine and easy	Complex; must combine data from many sources; data must go through a data cleanup process
Data integrity issues	Each individual transaction must be closely edited	Major effort to clean and integrate data from multiple sources

Source: Principles of Information Systems, 10th Edition, by STAIR/REYNOLDS.
© 2012. Reprinted with permission of Course Technology, a division of Thomson Learning: www.thomsonrights.com. Fax 800–730–2215.

Like a clinical data repository, a data warehouse stores data from other database sources. Creating a data warehouse involves extracting and cleaning data from a variety of organizational databases. However, the underlying structure of a data warehouse is different from the table structure of a relational database. This different structure allows data to be extracted along such dimensions as time (by week, month, or year), location, or diagnosis. Data in a data warehouse can often be accessed via *drill-down* menus that allow you to see smaller and smaller units within the same dimension. For example, you could view the number of patients with a particular diagnosis for a year, then a month in that year, then a day in that month. Or you could see how many times a procedure was performed at all locations in the health system, then see the total by region, then by facility. Even though the same data might be available in a relational database, its normalized structure makes the queries you would have to use to get at the information quite complex and difficult to execute. Data warehouses help organizations transform large quantities of data from separate transactional files into a single decision-support database. *Data marts* are structurally similar to data warehouses but generally not as large. The typical data mart is developed for a particular purpose or unit within an organization (Stair & Reynolds, 2012).

Data Mining

Data mining is another concept closely associated with large databases such as clinical data repositories and data warehouses. However, data mining (like several other IT concepts) means different things to different people. Health care application vendors may use the term *data mining* when referring to the user interface of the data warehouse or data repository. They may refer to the ability to drill down into data as data mining, for example. However, more precisely used, data mining refers to a sophisticated analysis tool that automatically discovers patterns among data in a data store. Data mining is an advanced form of decision support. Unlike passive query tools, the data mining analysis tool does not require the user to pose individual specific questions to the database. Instead, this tool is programmed to look for and extract patterns, trends, and rules. True data mining is currently used in the business community for marketing and predictive analysis (Stair & Reynolds, 2012). This analytical data mining is, however, not currently widespread in the health care community.

NETWORKS AND DATA COMMUNICATIONS

The term *data communications* refers to the transmission of electronic data within or among computers and other related devices. In this section we will take a cursory look at many of the components that go into building computer networks for the purpose of data communications. (Although the Internet is certainly a part of the overall data communications system that health care organizations use, we believe it is significant enough to warrant its own section, which follows this one.)

Devices that make up computer networks must be compatible; they must be able to communicate with one another. Much of what we introduce in this section takes the form of definitions and examples of different types of network components whose compatibility and interoperability might be an issue. Specifically, we cover the following topics as they relate to data communications, particularly in health care settings:

- Types of networks
- Network components and performance
- Network protocols and standards

Types of Networks

White (2011, p. 3) defines a computer network as "an interconnection of computers and computing equipment using either wires or radio waves and can share data and computing resources." The first distinction that is often made when describing a network is to identify it as either a *local area network (LAN)* or a *wide area network (WAN)*. LANs typically operate within a building or sometimes across several buildings belonging to a single organization and located in the same general vicinity. The actual distance a LAN covers can vary greatly. One common way to distinguish a LAN from a WAN is that the LAN will have its network hardware and software under the control of a single organization. As the Internet and its related technologies are used more by organizations, the line between LANs and WANs is becoming somewhat blurred. For our purposes, we will think of the LAN as being confined to a single geographical area and controlled by a single organization. A WAN is any network that extends beyond the LAN. WANs may be public (like the Internet) or private. They may be connected by dedicated lines, a satellite, or other media.

Each device and computer within a LAN has a *network interface card (NIC)*. These cards are generally specific to the type of LAN transmission technology being employed, such as Ethernet or Wi-Fi. (This is why you may hear the term *Ethernet card* or *Wi-Fi card* used to refer to your computer's NIC.) Clearly, most health care organizations today operate one or more LANs and use WANs as well (see Figure 9.4).

Figure 9.4. Simplified health care organization network

A few other network types or designations are commonly used in health care organizations: *virtual private networks (VPNs)* and *wireless LANs*. Virtual private networks are private networks (for example, a network for a particular health care organization) that use the Internet's public networks. VPNs utilize specific technologies to ensure secure connections over the Internet allowing remote access to the private network for authorized personnel. Wireless LANs fall under the same general definition as a LAN, but wireless technologies are employed for the connectivity.

Network Components and Performance

Networks can be set up in a variety of connectivity configurations, depending on the needs of the organization. Some of the more common connectivity configurations used by health care organizations include: workstation to LAN, workstation to Internet, LAN to LAN, LAN to WAN, and WAN to WAN. These configurations may employ technologies ranging from cellular phones to satellites and microwave towers. Truly, there are endless combinations of connectivity configurations that can be employed. In this section we will take a very high-level look at network components and performance. We will list basic network components and discuss factors that influence network performance.

In a bird's-eye view of networks, whether wired or wireless, LANs generally consist of the following components:

- *Workstations*, such as personal computers, tablets, and smart phones.
- *Servers*, which are the computers that store network software and/or shared files.
- *Switches*, which serve as a collection point for the wires and wireless signals that interconnect workstations on the network.
- *Routers*, which connect the LAN to a WAN or the Internet.
- *Connection media*, which are generally wires or wireless signals or a combination. Wireless signals require *access points* at interim locations throughout the network.

Similarly, WANs consist of the following components:

- *Nodes*, which are the devices that allow workstations to connect to the WAN; nodes also make "decisions" about where data are routed
- *High-speed transmission media*, which connects one node to another
- *Subnet*, which represents a cohesive unit of nodes and transmission media (White, 2011)

These components allow coded data signals to travel across networks. Very simply, the strength and speed of these data signals determines the quality of transmission. What factors influence the strength and speed of the signals? The technical details are beyond the scope of this chapter, but there are two components that we will discuss: media and bandwidth.

Media

Data may be transmitted on a network through several types of media. Common types of conducted media for LANs include *twisted pair wire, coaxial cable*, and *fiber-optic cable*. Common wireless media include *terrestrial* and *satellite microwave transmissions* as well as *spread spectrum radio transmissions*. Mobile phone technology and infrared technology are also being used for wireless computer data transmission (White, 2011).

- **Twisted pair.** Twisted pair wire comes in categories, ranging from the "slowest," Category 1, to the "fastest," Category 7. Traditional telephone wire is Category 1 twisted pair. Typical LAN wire is Category 5 or 6.

- **Coaxial cable.** Coaxial cable is the cable used to transmit cable television signals and connection to the Internet.

- **Fiber-optic cable.** Fiber-optic cable is made of thin glass fibers only a little bigger in diameter than a human hair. These glass "wires" are encased in insulation and plastic. The big advantage of fiber-optic cable is its ability to transmit data over longer distances than traditional twisted pair can. However, fiber-optic cable is more expensive to use.

- **Microwaves.** Microwaves are a type of radio wave with very short wavelengths. Terrestrial microwave transmission occurs between two microwave antennas. In order to receive and send microwave signals, the sending and receiving antennas must be in sight of one another. Satellite microwave transmission sends microwave signals from an antenna on the ground to an orbiting satellite and then back to another antenna on the ground.

- **Spread spectrum.** Spread spectrum wireless transmission uses another type of radio wave. Unlike conventional radio broadcasting, which uses a specific, consistent wave frequency, spread spectrum technology employs a deliberately varied signal, resulting in greater bandwidth. The popular Wi-Fi (802.11) standard for wireless computing is based on spread spectrum technology.

Bandwidth

Bandwidth is another name for the capacity of a transmission medium. Generally, the greater the capacity, or bandwidth, of the medium, the greater the speed of transmission. *Baseband* is the term used to describe communication media that carry only one transmission at a time. Ethernet twisted pair cables are examples of baseband media. *Broadband* is the term used to describe media that is capable of carrying multiple transmissions simultaneously. Fiber-optic cables and wireless connections are broadband. Multiple factors influence transmission speed, and bandwidth is only one of them, but a low bandwidth can impede transmission rates across the network. Transmission rates are expressed as *bits per second (bps)*. In other words, a medium's capacity is determined by the maximum number of bps it can carry.

Network Protocols and Standards

Data communication across computer networks is possible today because of *communication protocols and standards*. Without the common *language* of protocols, networked computers and other devices would not be able to connect with and talk to one another. The distinction between protocols and standards is often misunderstood. On the one hand, the English language is a protocol for communication. It is also a standard. People taught English by different instructors in different parts of the globe will learn (more or less) the same thing and be able to communicate with each other because there is a standard vocabulary and standards for such things as verb tense. On the other hand, the plugs for appliances are protocols—there is a specification for the two flat prongs that form the plug. But the plug is not a standard. Appliances in Switzerland use two round prongs and an American appliance cannot be plugged into a Swiss outlet.

The need for standard network protocols has been evident since the first computer networks were built. To this end the International Organization for Standardization developed the *Open Standards Interconnection (OSI)* seven-layer model. (Of historical interest, the HL7 standard name is derived from the seventh, Application, OSI layer.) Work on OSI was begun in the 1980s. Although this model was well accepted for many years as a conceptual, or reference, model for network protocols, it has not evolved into detailed specifications, as was once anticipated.

TCP/IP

The network model most commonly adopted for creating software for network communications is the Internet model, which employs *Transmission Control Protocol/Internet Protocol (TCP/IP)*. TCP/IP was first introduced in the 1970s by the U.S. government to support defense activities (Stair & Reynolds, 2012). However, it was not until the boom of the World Wide Web that this set of protocols began to dominate the computer network industry. Like the OSI model, the Internet model is a layered model. However, the Internet model has fewer layers, and unlike the OSI reference model, it represents actual protocol specifications at each layer (White, 2011). Table 9.2 lists the layers of the TCP/IP with corresponding protocols (Microsoft, 2012). This is not a complete model, but rather a simplified illustration.

Each layer of a network requires specific protocols, which must then work together to make sure that data flow from the sender to the receiver. Data flow from the Application layer down to the Network Interface layer and back again.

Table 9.2. TCP/IP layer illustration

Application	Protocols used for the exchange of user information: • The Hypertext Transfer Protocol (HTTP) is used to transfer files that make up the web pages of the World Wide Web. • The File Transfer Protocol (FTP) is used for interactive file transfer. • The Simple Mail Transfer Protocol (SMTP) is used for the transfer of mail messages and attachments. • Telnet, a terminal emulation protocol, is used for logging on remotely to network hosts. Protocols used to facilitate the use and management of TCP/IP networks: • The Domain Name System (DNS) is used to resolve a host name to an IP address. • The Routing Information Protocol (RIP) is a routing protocol. • The Simple Network Management Protocol (SNMP) is used between a network management console and network devices.
Transport (aka Host-to-Host Transport)	Core protocols are: • Transmission Control Protocol (TCP) provides the Application layer with session communication services. • User Datagram Protocol (UDP) provides the Application layer with datagram communication services.
Internet	Main Protocol is the Internet Protocol (IP) responsible for IP addressing, routing, and the fragmentation and reassembly of packets.
Network Interface	This layer is responsible for placing TCP/IP packets on the network medium and receiving TCP/IP packets off the network medium. It is independent of any specific network technology and is designed to work with a variety of standard technologies, such as Ethernet.

Table 9.3. Ethernet standards, cables, and transmission capabilities

Ethernet Standard	Cable Type	Max Transmission Speed	Max Segment Length
10BaseT	Twisted pair	10 Mbps	100 meters
100Base TX	2-pair Category 5 or higher unshielded twisted pair	100 Mbps	100 meters
100BaseFX	Fiber optic	100 Mbps	1,000 meters
1000BaseSX	Fiber optic	1000 Mbps	300 meters
1000BaseLX	Fiber optic	1000 Mbps	100 meters
1000BaseCX	Specialized balanced copper	1000 Mbps	25 meters
1000BaseT	Twisted pair (four pairs)	1000 Mbps	100 meters
10GBase-fiber	Fiber optic	10 Gbps	Various lengths
10GBase-T	Category 6 twisted pair	10 Gbps	55–100 meters
10GBae-CX4	Twin axial	10 Gbps	~30 meters

A few other network protocols are also worth mentioning, although the following list is by no means all-inclusive.

Wired Ethernet

Wired Ethernet is the most popular LAN system in use today, both in health care and in business. Ethernet is specified as an IEEE standard (802.3). It was originally developed as a joint effort by several prominent vendors: Xerox, Digital Equipment Corporation, and Intel. Ethernet systems are offered by many different network vendors and come in a variety of *speeds* and maximum *segment length*. Specific Ethernet standards require specific types of cables. The general types of cables include copper twisted pair, coaxial, and fiber-optic. Table 9.3 summarizes the Ethernet standards, transmission speed, maximum segment length, and cable type. New standards are always being developed for faster speeds and longer segments (White, 2011).

Wireless Protocols

Wireless technologies have been incorporated into health care networks. These technologies are supported by several different sets of protocols:

- **Wireless Ethernet** has gained wide acceptance for LANs. The IEEE 802.11 set of protocols, known as Wi-Fi, supports the many types of wireless LANs. 802.11a was introduced in the late 1990s and supported a bandwidth of 20MHz. The most recent 802.11 standard is 802.11ac (draft), which will support bandwidths of 80 to 160MHz.

- **Bluetooth** is a proprietary technology first introduced in 1994. It is designed to support communications over short distances, such as among cellular phones, handheld computers, and other wireless devices. Bluetooth is widely employed by health care and other industries to support wireless keyboards, mice, headsets, smart phones, and tablets.

Mobile Communications Standard and Protocols

It is an understatement to say that cellular phones have changed the way individuals and organizations operate. Mobile technologies create a tremendous opportunity for health care organizations, in spite of some significant security hurdles. (See Chapter Eleven.) In this section we will discuss 3G wireless communication, 4G wireless communication, and WiMAX.

- **3G wireless communications** standards and protocols support wireless voice and data communications in a mobile environment. The term 3G stands for third generation and introduced mobile capabilities for video, e-commerce, location-based services, gaming, and downloading music. 3G, originally called IMT-2000, was established in 1999 to be the single standard for cellular networks. However, the original standard has since split into several different standards (Stair & Reynolds, 2012).

- **4G wireless communications** is the fourth-generation mobile communications standard for cellular phones and other devices. These standards are currently evolving, but are expected to deliver the most advanced versions of multimedia and video, along with increased data transmission rates (Stair & Reynolds, 2012).

- **WiMAX** (Worldwide Interoperability for Microwave Access) is a newer wireless digital communications standard, IEEE 802.16. WiMAX, an IP-based wireless broadband access technology, can transmit signals for twenty to thirty miles in the range of millions of bits per second. The WiMAX web site describes the technology as providing "performance similar to 802.11/Wi-Fi networks with the coverage and QOS (quality of service) of cellular networks" (WiMAX, 2012).

INFORMATION DISTRIBUTION SCHEMES

Networks and databases are often described in terms of the method through which the organization distributes their information processing. Two common server-based distribution methods are *file server* and *client/server*. A third distribution method that has emerged within the past few years relies on the Internet and is referred to as *cloud computing*. All three types are found in health care information networks. A single health care organization may in fact employ one, two, or all three methods of processing distribution, depending on its computing needs and its strategic decisions regarding architecture.

Server-Based Distribution Schemes

File server systems have the application and database on a single computer. However, the end-user's workstation runs the database management system. When the user needs the data that reside on the file server, the file server will send the entire file to the computer requesting it.

Client/server systems differ from traditional file server systems in that they have multiple servers, each of which is dedicated to one or more specialized functions. For example, servers may be dedicated to database management, printing, or other program execution. The servers are accessible from other computers in the network, either all computers in the network or a designated subset. The client side of the network usually runs the applications and sends requests from the applications to the server side, which returns the requested data.

Cloud Computing

Historically, information distribution has been accomplished through the organization's LAN, but with the latest advancements and permeation of the Internet, web technologies, and handheld devices, information distribution has begun a shift toward *cloud computing*. The term comes from the common practice of showing the Internet as a cloud on network diagrams. Cloud computing refers to "a computing environment in which software and storage are provided an Internet service and accesses through a Web browser" (Stair & Reynolds, 2012, p. 281). Cloud computing can be deployed publicly or privately. Publicly provided cloud computing is offered to the general Internet public and is accessible via their computers, tablets, or smart phones. Examples of public cloud computing services include Drop Box file storage; Apple's iCloud for PC, tablet, and phone backup; as well as music and video remote sharing. More well-known sites such as Facebook, HotMail, Yahoo Mail, and YouTube are all cloud-based services that are publicly available. Privately available cloud computing services are organizationally run and offered for specific users and user groups. Some experts predict that most computing of the future will take place in the "world of cloud computing," with users accessing Internet servers through web browsers (Stair & Reynolds, 2012, p. 281).

The potential for cloud computing solutions is great. However, there are challenges, particularly in health care. Security concerns must be addressed, as well as consideration of backup, business continuity, and disaster recovery plans. Cloud computing services have been known to lose data or fail altogether (Stair & Reynolds, 2012). As with other information technology solutions, careful planning and implementation are essential.

REMOTE ACCESS TECHNOLOGIES

Health care organizations, like other businesses, have a lot of computers and software to support and maintain. They are continuously looking for efficiencies in desktop management and software distribution. *Remote access technologies* provide a mechanism for improving this efficiency across the organization. These technologies provide remote access to full desktop systems or to individual applications through a terminal or a client application. The software is accessed remotely over the Internet or LAN and operates as if it were loaded locally on the computer hard drive. This method provides easier distribution of new software, updates to existing software, and changes to software. Three commonly used remote access technologies are *Remote Desktop, Terminal Services*, and *Citrix*.

Remote Desktop is available for many different operating systems, including Windows and OS X. The technology utilized is the Remote Desktop Protocol, which provides remote access to users to another system, providing them complete control of the computer. This is a client solution and the user must load the client before remotely accessing the available computer. *Terminal Services* is often used in clinical environments where there are many remote sites. This service provides fully functional Windows-based computing on terminals where there is no true local hard drive. All applications and software are hosted on a terminal service server. *Citrix* is a direct competitor to Windows' Terminal Service and provides remote access to applications through a locally installed client. It can run on different computing devices such as desktops, tablets, and phones.

INTERNET AND WEB CONCEPTS AND APPLICATIONS

Think of how health care organizations use the Internet today. They maintain informational web pages for patients, providers, and insurers. They use Internet technologies to facilitate communications and transactions internally and with suppliers and customers. Some health care organizations have developed health information web applications or have contracted with third parties to maintain patient records electronically. Telemedicine and *electronic data interchange (EDI)* functions may be web based. The list of examples goes on. This is truly an amazing phenomenon when you consider that the vast majority of this Internet and web application development has occurred in the last two decades. Although the Internet has its early roots in an effort that began in the late 1960s, it was not until the development of the *World Wide Web (WWW)* that businesses, including health care organizations, began to see the benefit of online communications and online business transactions (e-commerce). The image that most of today's users have of the Internet is this multimedia world of the WWW; however, this is only one part of the vast network of networks known as the Internet. The WWW is the means by which the majority of users interact with the Internet, but the WWW and the Internet are not the same.

Internet use is one of the most rapidly growing aspects of health information technology. In this section we will examine the technologies that make web-based e-commerce possible for health care organizations. In this chapter we will describe the fundamentals of Internet and WWW technologies and explore a few of the more recent developments, including Web 2.0.

The Internet

What, exactly, is the Internet? The Internet is the world's largest computer network. It consists of thousands of interconnected computers (or *hosts*) that communicate using a common set of protocols, TCP/IP. The Internet is not owned or controlled by any single organization. It is not controlled by the government. In fact, there are very few specific regulations governing the Internet. One of the hallmarks of the Internet is that it allows information to be exchanged in a "free," relatively unregulated environment.

The Internet began in 1969 as a government project to improve defense communications. This precursor to today's Internet was known as the Advanced Research Projects Agency Network (ARPANET). The goal of the Advanced Research Projects Agency was to establish a network that could survive a nuclear strike; therefore, it was intentionally developed without a central point of control. This is a characteristic of the Internet that still exists today. Believe it or not, ARPANET began as a network of four computers. In the beginning ARPANET was open only to academic institutions and portions of the national defense infrastructure. As it grew, the network divided into a civilian branch and a government branch. The civilian branch became known as the Internet. In 1991, the government decided to allow businesses to link to the Internet, but not many businesses were interested in this until the WWW was introduced a couple of years later.

The use of the Internet changed dramatically when a British scientist invented the software protocol *Hypertext Transfer Protocol (HTTP)*, making way for the formation of the World Wide Web (WWW). HTTP allows full-color graphics, tables, forms, video, and animation to be shared over the Internet. This protocol is the basis for the web as we know it today. The codes used for displaying files on the WWW are called *markup languages*. (The most common markup languages are discussed in more detail later in this chapter.) The WWW is what brought multimedia and ease of use to the Internet and its applications. Since the introduction of the WWW, Internet use has exploded. There were an estimated 1,500,000 host computers on the Internet when the first web browser, Mosaic, was introduced in 1993. In 2009, this number was over 681,000,000. The emergence of user-friendly but powerful search engines such as Google, Web 2.0 (discussed later in this chapter), and the release of Internet-capable cell phones have all contributed to this tremendous growth (Stair & Reynolds, 2012).

How the Internet Works

Every computer and device that operates within the Internet has a unique identifier known as an *Internet protocol (IP)* number, or address. Specific Internet protocols (discussed earlier in this chapter) allow each computer or device on the Internet to use these IP addresses to locate other computers or devices. The IP address is a four-part number, with each part separated by a period. IP addresses may be static or dynamic. Static addresses are permanently assigned to a computer or device. A dynamic address is assigned "as needed" by a special server that recognizes when a computer or device needs an address. Dynamic IP addressing gives the organization flexibility in using its allotted IP addresses (Oz, 2009; Stair & Reynolds, 2012).

How the Web Works

The web resides on the Internet. It was designed to organize information and make it easy to find. The building blocks of the WWW are web pages.

These pages are stored and distributed through client/server software. The servers supporting the web are identified on the Internet through IP addresses, just as any other computer would be. However, these IP addresses are often associated with a

Figure 9.5. URL components

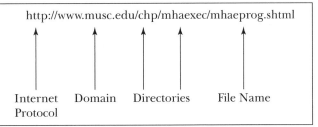

character-based address, which is easier for people to remember. The process of associating the numerical IP address with the character-based name is accomplished by a *Domain Name System (DNS)*. Individual web pages are linked to one another by means of *hyperlinks*. A group of web pages that is created for a common purpose under a single domain is called a *web site*. Web pages do not have to reside on the same server to be linked; any web page can be linked to any other. Web pages are viewed using a *web browser* such as Internet Explorer, Safari, or Firefox (Stair & Reynolds, 2012).

Think about using the WWW. How do you get to the web page you want? Typically, you type the URL (uniform resource locator) for the page (for example, http://www.musc.edu/chp/facstaff.htm) into the browser. Browser software not only allows web users to search for and retrieve specific web sites, but also allows the user to use additional software components, known as *plug-ins*, to perform functions such as viewing videos or listening to audio. Figure 9.5 shows the various components of a URL. The HTTP part of the address indicates that Hypertext Transfer Protocol is being used. HTTP is one of the protocols that make up TCP/IP. (Another TCP/IP protocol, HTTPS, is a secure variation of HTTP that employs encryption to protect the site.) The next component, www.musc.edu, is the domain name (a domain name may or may not include www). The *edu* section of the address in Figure 9.5 is the *top-level domain (TLD)*, which often indicates the type of organization that registered the domain name. Some TLDs, such as *edu, mil,* and *gov,* are restricted to use by qualified organizations. However, some, such as *com, org,* and *net,* are less restricted and can be used by any individual or organization in the appropriate generic category. The next section of the URL indicates the specific directory, or folder, where the web page resides. In our example there are two directories, but there can be several or only one. The final component of the URL is the actual name of the file to be located. In this example the file ends with the extension *shtml,* which shows that it was created, or coded, using a specific version of HTML.

Figure 9.6. HTML and XML code

HTML

```
<p>MRN: 12345<br>
Name: John Doe<br>
Date of Birth: November 21, 1953</p>
```

Tags define how the text will look and not the data the text represents.

XML

```
<patient>
<patient.id>12345</patient.id>
<patient.name>John Doe</patient.name.
<patient.date.of.birth>November 21, 1953</patient.date.of.birth>
</patient>
```

Tags define the actual data elements.

Web Languages

The code used for displaying files on the WWW is called a *markup language*. The most common markup language today is *hypertext markup language (HTML)*. HTML defines how pages look on the web by using *tags*, special codes that inform a web browser how text or other content should look. A newer markup language that many think will change the way data are captured and stored is *extensible markup language (XML)*. Unlike HTML, which defines only how pages look, XML also defines what the data enclosed in the tags are. XML has emerged as a predominant messaging standard in health care and other applications. Figure 9.6 presents examples of HTML and XML code.

Intranets and Extranets

Health care organizations and other businesses not only use the public Internet, but also use Internet protocols and services to create private networks with limited access. These Internet-based private networks are often referred to as *intranets* and *extranets*. *Intranets* can be used for virtually any type of internal network application. The network designers develop web applications that are accessible via web browsers. The user interface appears very similar to any other web application. An intranet generally uses both "public" Internet routes and internal network lines; however, it is generally a secure network that is protected from unauthorized users. For example, a hospital may set up an intranet site with employee benefits and forms that can be accessed only from authorized computers within the organization or by employees entering the organization's network through a secure mechanism. The secure path established between the Internet and an intranet, using a combination of software and hardware protections, is sometimes referred to as a *tunnel*. An *extranet* is similar to an intranet except that the network of users includes business partners of the health care organization, such as suppliers, customers, or other health care providers. Again, extranets are generally secure, limiting access to their sites (Oz, 2009).

Web Applications in Health Care

You would be hard pressed to find a health care organization today that did not have a web presence. A well-designed web site is an important component of any health care organization's public relations and customer service efforts. There a two basic ways that an organization can establish a web site: by owning and maintaining their own server or by using a hosting service. Owning and maintaining a server provides a high level of flexibility and control for the organization, but it is generally a costly option. Larger health care organizations are more likely to maintain their own web sites. Smaller organizations may opt to use a web hosting service. Regardless of who hosts their web sites, health care organizations are using them to, among other things, promote their services, provide health care information, for internal and external communications, and to provide e-commerce services. A full discussion of all health care web applications is beyond the scope of this chapter. However, in the following sections we will discuss the use of Web 2.0 applications, web portals, and web-based conferencing.

Web 2.0

The term Web 2.0 is widely accepted as a general term that describes a collection of changes to the web over the last few years. The "2.0" part of Web 2.0 reflects the view that this collection represents the second generation of web technologies and capabilities. These changes are based on the web's advancement to web-based applications that include real-time collaboration, data sharing, and social media rather than the viewing of static information. Web 2.0 applications are alive, have dynamic information, provide user and group interactivity, are rich with media content such as video and animation, as well as providing backend storage for information retention and sharing. Included within the umbrella term Web 2.0 are

- Social networking web sites
- Rich Internet applications
- Blogs
- Podcasts
- Wikis

Social Networking Web Sites

Social networking sites provide for group accessibility where the primary goal is group interactivity. These include social media sites such as Facebook and Google+ where individuals network with friends and share information. Also included are online gaming sites and online educational sites. Health care organizations and other businesses have recognized the public relations potential in creating and maintaining social networking sites.

Rich Internet Applications

Rich Internet applications are the successors of desktop applications delivered via a browser or browser plug-in. They have many, if not all, of the same qualities and abilities as a local desktop application; however, all are accessed remotely from the internet. Google, for example, has full versions of Word and Excel-like web applications that are free to use.

Blogs

Blogs are a type of social web site that allows a user or "blogger" to write about information they find interesting. Blog readers can post their reactions to and comments on the material entered by the blog author and by other readers. Health care organizations may host one or more blogs that provide pertinent health care information or commentary to the public. There are many examples of health care blogs on the web today. Some are disease-specific; others are related to the politics of health care or a health care organization.

Podcasts

Podcasts are audio or video recordings of subject matter distributed using social media tools. Most podcasts are downloaded or streamed online to a computer or mobile device. As with blogs, the use of podcasts by health care organizations is widespread. Hospital web sites include podcasts of everything from the latest surgical technique to a CEO's welcome statement.

Wikis

Wikis are used for collaborative sharing and editing of information. Wikis are accessed through the web using browsers and use a specialized markup language that is much easier to use than HTML. The most well-known wiki in use today is Wikipedia, the online collection of user-contributed knowledge on a wide range of topics. Wikis can be used by health care organizations for both internal and external collaboration.

Web Portals

Web portal is the term used to describe a web page that serves as the entry point to the web or a specific segment of the web. Portals generally include a search engine, a subject directory, daily or recent "news" headlines, and other items of specific interest. There are publicly "horizontal" portals that cover a wide range of topics. Two common public portals are iGoogle and My Yahoo!, which allow users to customize their entry to the web. Health care organizations may set up web portals (or *dashboards*) for their employees or potential clients. A client portal might include a calendar of upcoming health seminars, links to health care articles of interest, a provider directory, and a search engine for searching the greater organization web site. An employee portal might provide access to work-related resources and organizational news. The employee portal might serve as the entry point for the organization's intranet.

PERSPECTIVE
Medical University of South Carolina's Patient Portal

Like many large academic medical centers, the Medical University of South Carolina's (MUSC) web site can be accessed through several different portals. Figure 9.7 shows the entry page for the MUSCHealth.com patient portal. Existing and potential patients can find a physician by browsing by name, specialty, or condition. They can also request an appointment and view online patient education materials. The MUSCHealth.com patient portal is an important aspect of MUSC's patient service strategy.

(cont.)

Figure 9.7. MUSC patient portal example

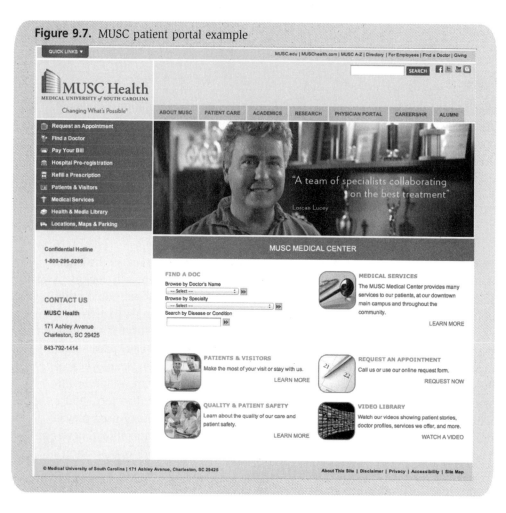

Web Conferencing

Web conferencing technologies provide health care organizations with the ability to engage in real-time online conferencing. These technologies incorporate voice, either by phone or PC microphone, and computer sharing. Some allow web cameras to broadcast video of the conference participants. Two of the most common web conferencing services are WebEx and GoToMeeting. However, there are many others, some offering high-resolution video and audio.

E-COMMERCE IN HEALTH CARE

Electronic commerce, or e-commerce, has changed the way health care organizations conduct business. E-commerce has introduced efficiencies by replacing time-consuming, paper-based business processes. Broadly defined, *e-commerce* includes business activities, such as billing, distribution, buying, selling, marketing, and providing services that are conducted electronically over computer networks. Clearly, the vast majority of health care organizations (if not all) conduct a portion of their daily business transactions over computer networks. Some of the e-commerce is directed at consumers of the organization's services and some is directed at other businesses, such as suppliers or insurance companies. In fact, the federal government now requires the electronic submission of claims for most health providers. On the consumer side of e-commerce, the widespread use of mobile devices has led to an expansion that includes mobile access to online transactions and services. This component of e-commerce is sometimes referred to as *m-commerce* (Stair & Reynolds, 2012).

As with other information technologies, the health care organization must choose e-commerce technologies that align with its overall mission and with its IT strategic plan. There are four basic components to any e-commerce system (Stair & Reynolds, 2012):

- Web server hardware. As discussed earlier, this hardware may be owned and maintained by the health care organization or by a web hosting site.
- Web server software.
- E-commerce software. This software should support several key aspects of e-commerce, including transaction processing and an electronic payment system.
- High-speed connection to the LAN and Internet.

E-commerce web sites must be well designed and maintained to build traffic and support online transactions. Just as the health care organization is concerned about the appearance of its buildings and the quality of its clients' experiences while at its "brick-and-mortar" facilities, it must be concerned with the appearance of its e-commerce site(s) and the quality of the online experience.

CLINICAL AND MANAGERIAL DECISION SUPPORT

Health care executives and providers are faced with decisions every day, multiple times per day. The success of any health care organization depends on these large and small decisions. In this section we will describe technologies that support decision making in health care today, for both clinical and managerial decisions. The types of systems that we examine are

- Decision-support systems (DSS)
- Artificial intelligence systems, including expert systems, natural language processing, fuzzy logic, and neural networks

Nobel Prize–winning economist Herbert Simon described decision making as a three-step process (Oz, 2009; Stair & Reynolds, 2012). The steps involve

1. Intelligence: collecting facts, beliefs, and ideas. In health care these facts may be stored as data elements in a variety of data stores.
2. Design: designing the methods with which to consider the data collected during intelligence. These methods may be models, formulas, algorithms, or other analytical tools. Methods are selected that will reduce the number of viable alternatives.
3. Choice: making the most promising choice from the limited set of alternatives.

Problems that face health care executives and clinicians may be *structured, unstructured*, or *semistructured*. Structured problems are also referred to as *programmable* problems, because a computer program can be written with relative ease to solve this kind of problem. Transaction-based applications can be used to solve structured, or programmable, problems. For example, a payroll system is based on known facts about each employee's salary, deductions, and so on. The "decision" of how much to write the monthly paycheck for is fairly straightforward. The unstructured and semistructured problems present much more of a challenge for computer application developers.

Decision-Support Systems

How do we harness the power of a computer to solve a problem or make a decision about a solution when the situation is not easily structured with a simple algorithm (sequence of logical steps)? The computer systems developed to tackle the unstructured or semistructured problem are called *decision-support systems (DSS)*. Decision-support system is another term that can mean slightly different things to different vendors or users. In this section we are referring primarily to the traditional, stand-alone DSS: in other words, an application that is designed for the purpose of supporting decisions. This is not the only form of decision support available to health care executives and providers today. For example, patient care or administrative applications may have components, such as data mining, that aid in decision making, but these applications might not be classified as full-blown DSS. An electronic spreadsheet, such as Excel, can also be used as a decision-support tool. Spreadsheets have built-in functions as well as the ability to use what-if statements.

The stand-alone DSS generally has three distinct components:

1. The data management module, which is an existing or built-in transactional database or data warehouse. In a clinical DSS, the data module could be a clinical data repository.

2. The model management module, which allows the user to select a model to be applied to the problem at hand. Models can be mathematical, statistical, or based on expert knowledge. The model management module of a DSS is its most complex component and may seem like a "black box" to the health care executive.

3. The dialog module, which is the user interface. This module allows the user to pose the problem to the system by selecting the data and the decision model to use on the data. The dialog module also displays results, generally in text and graphical formats.

Executive information systems (EIS) are decision-support systems specifically designed for the higher-level manager. Most of these systems have drill-down capability to allow the executive to examine a problem at different levels of granularity, and many are tied to data warehouses (Oz, 2009).

Artificial Intelligence

Artificial intelligence (AI) is a branch of computer science devoted to emulating the human mind. One very common use of AI today is incorporated into the Google search engine. When the user types a misspelled word in a string of keywords, Google will suggest alternative keywords based on the context of the query (Oz, 2009). Another form of AI was introduced as "Siri" for the iPhone. AI is a broad field with many different types of technology. Most AI is quite complex, and describing the underlying technology is beyond the scope of this text. However, we will introduce a few types of AI that may be found in health care settings, including *expert systems, natural language processing*, and *neural networks*.

Expert Systems

The hallmark of expert systems is that they use *heuristics*, or "rules of thumb," collected from experts in the particular field for which the system was built. Expert systems comprise

- A *knowledge base*, which stores all the relevant information, data, rules, and cases that will be used by the system. It is similar to a database, but the relationships are designed to match those dictated by the human experts. One of the challenges of building the knowledge base is getting the expert knowledge. Experts, being people, do not always agree on the way to approach a problem.
- An *inference engine*, which provides the expert advice from the knowledge base.
- An *explanation facility*, which allows the user to understand how the inference engine arrived at the advice it is presenting.
- A *knowledge acquisition facility*, which allows the user to update the knowledge base with new or additional expert information (Stair & Reynolds, 2012).

Natural Language Processing

Natural language processing (NLP) programs take human language (typed as text or input as voice) and translate it into a standard computer instruction, such as SQL. Suppose you typed this text into an application:

> List the names of all drugs that will treat shingles for less than $60 per month.

Or:

> What are the names of the drugs that will treat shingles for less than $60 per month?

An NLP program might recognize either form of this sentence in context and convert it to an SQL statement similar to this:

SELECT NAME FROM DRUGS

WHERE DISEASE = "SHINGLES"

AND COST ¡ 60

So far NLP programs have met with limited success. The difficulty is in identifying all of the possible meanings of words or combinations of words based on context. This problem is magnified in the health care community by medical terminology that is both complex and seems to be ever changing.

Neural Networks

Neural networks, or *neural nets*, may be used by sophisticated expert systems. They are software programs that involve "machine learning" in an attempt to mimic the way the human brain operates. This is in contrast to the traditional, step-by-step process used in other computer programming languages. Neural networks involve a very sophisticated level of programming, but they are employed in both business and health care applications today.

INFORMATION SYSTEMS ARCHITECTURE

In the preceding sections we introduced many specific technologies that can be used in health care organizations. However, a huge question remains: How does the organization choose among these technologies and ultimately bring them together into a cohesive set of health care information systems? This section answers these questions by examining health care information system architecture.

An organization's information systems require that a series of core technologies *come together*, or work together as whole, to meet the IT goals of the organization. Up to this point we have discussed the core technologies but have not discussed how they work together as a cohesive information system. The way that core technologies, along with the application software, come together should be the result of decisions about what information systems are implemented and used within the organization and how they are implemented and used. For example, the electronic health record system or the patient accounting system with which users ultimately interact involves not just the application software but also the network, servers, security systems, and so forth that all come together to make the system work effectively. This coming together should never be a haphazard process. It should be engineered.

In discussing health care information system architecture, we will cover several topics:

- A definition of architecture
- Architecture perspectives
- Architecture examples
- Observations about architecture

A Definition of Architecture

A design and a blueprint guide the coming together of a house. The coming together of information systems is guided by information systems *architecture*. For the house, the development of the blueprint and the design is influenced by the builder's objectives for the house (is it to be a single-family house or an apartment building, for example), and the desired properties of the house (energy efficient or handicap accessible, for example). For an organization's information systems, the development of an architecture is influenced by the organization's objectives (electronic health records that span multiple hospitals, for example) and the systems' desired properties (efficient to support and having a high degree of application integration, for example).

Following the design and the blueprints, the general contractor, plumbers, carpenters, and electricians use building materials to create the house. Following the architecture for the organization's information systems, the IT staff and the organization's vendors implement the core technologies and application software and integrate them to create the information systems.

Information systems architecture consists of concepts, strategies, and principles that guide an organization's technology choices and the manner in which the organization integrates and manages these choices. For example, an organization's architecture discussion concludes that the organization should use industry standard technology. This decision reflects an organizational belief that standard technology will have a lower risk of obsolescence, be easier to support, and be available from a large number of information technology vendors that use standard technology. Guided by its architecture decision, the organization chooses to implement networks that conform to a specific standard network protocol and decides to use the Windows operating system for its workstations.

Two additional terms are sometimes used either as synonyms for or in describing architecture: *platform* and *infrastructure*. In this text, however, we adhere to accepted distinctions among these three terms. For example, you might hear IT personnel say that "our systems run on a Microsoft, HP, and Cisco platform." *Platforms* are the specific vendors and technologies that an organization chooses for its information systems. You might hear of a Windows platform or web-based platform. Platform choices should be guided by architecture discussions. You might also hear IT personnel talk about the infrastructure of the health care information system. *Infrastructure* as we use it refers primarily to the organization's computer networks and, perhaps, to the applications running on those networks. Although *infrastructure* is not vendor or technology specific, it is not quite as broad a term as *architecture*, which encompasses much more than specific technologies and networks.

In creating an *infrastructure*, an organization will implement *platforms* and be guided by its IT architecture.

Architecture Perspectives

Organizations adopt various frames of reference as they approach the topic of architecture. This section will illustrate two approaches, one based on the characteristics and capabilities of the desired architecture and the other based on application integration.

Characteristics and Capabilities

Glaser (2002, p. 62) defines architecture as "the set of organizational, management, and technical strategies and tactics used to ensure that the organization's information systems have critical, organizationally defined characteristics and capabilities." For example, an organization can decide that it wants an information system that has characteristics such as being agile, efficient to support, and highly reliable.

In addition, the organization can decide that its information systems should have capabilities such as being accessible by patients from their homes or being able to incorporate clinical decision support. If it wants high reliability, it will need to make decisions about fault-tolerant computers and network redundancy. If it wants users to be able to customize their clinical information screens, this will influence its choice of a clinical information system vendor. If it wants providers to be able to structure clinical documentation, it will need to make choices about natural language processing, voice recognition, and templates in its electronic medical record.

Architecture choices are guided by organizational decisions about the capabilities and characteristics that are desired of its information systems.

Application Integration

Another way of looking at information systems architecture is to look at how applications are integrated across the organization. One often hears vendors talk about architectures such as best of breed, monolithic, and visual integration. *Best of breed* describes an architecture that allows each department to pick the best application it can find and that then attempts to integrate these applications by means of an interface engine that manages the transfer of data between these applications—for example, it can send a transaction with registration information on a new patient from the admitting system to the laboratory system.

Monolithic describes the architecture of a set of applications that all come from one vendor and that all use a common database management system and common user interface.

Visual integration architecture wraps a common browser user interface around a set of diverse applications. This interface enables the user, for example, a physician, to use one set of screens to access clinical data even though those data may come from several different applications.

This view of architecture is focused on the various approaches to the integration of applications: integration by sharing data between applications, integration by having all applications use one database, and integration by having an integrated access to data. This view does not address other aspects of architecture; for example, the means by which the organization might get information to mobile workers.

Architecture Examples

A few examples will help illustrate how architecture can guide information technology choices. Each example begins with an architecture statement and then shows some choices about core technologies and applications and the approach to implementing them that might result from this statement.

Statement. We would like to deliver an electronic health record to our small physician practices that is inexpensive, reliable, and easy to support. To do this we will

- Run the application from our computer room, reducing the need for practice staff to manage their own servers and do tasks such as backups and applying application enhancements.
- Run several practices on one server to reduce the cost.
- Obtain a high-speed network connection, and a backup connection, from our local telephone company to provide good application performance and improve reliability.

Statement. We would like to have decision-support capabilities in our clinical information systems. To do this we will

- Purchase our applications from a vendor whose product includes a very robust rules engine.
- Make sure that the rules engine has the tools necessary to author new decision support and maintain existing clinical logic.
- Ensure that the clinical information systems use a single database with codified clinical data.

Statement. We want all of our systems to be easy and efficient to support. To do this we will

- Adopt industry standard technology, making it easier to hire support staff.

- Implement proven technology—technology that has had most of the bugs worked out.

- Purchase our application systems from one vendor, reducing the support problems and the finger-pointing that can occur between vendors when problems arise.

Observations about Architecture

Organizations will often bypass the architecture discussion in their haste to "get the IT show on the road and begin implementing stuff." Haste makes waste, as people say. It is terribly important to have thoughtful architecture discussions. There are many organizations, for example, that never took the time to develop thoughtful plans for integrating applications and that then discovered, after millions of dollars of IT investments, that this oversight meant that they could not integrate these applications or that the integration would be both expensive and limited.

As we will see in Chapter Fourteen, the organizations that have been very effective in their applications of IT over many years have had a significant focus on architecture. They have realized that thoughtful approaches to agility, cost efficiency, and reliability have a significant impact on their ability to continue to apply technology to improve organizational performance. For example, information systems that are not agile can be difficult (or impossible) to change as the organization's needs evolve. This ossification can strangle an organization's progress. In addition, information systems that have reliability problems can lead an organization to be hesitant to implement new, strategically important applications—how can they be sure that this new application will not go down too often and impair their operations? In Chapter Thirteen, we will discuss planning the system architecture as a component of strategic IT planning.

Organizational leadership must take time to engage in the architecture discussion. The health care executive does not need to be involved in deciding which vendor to choose to provide network switches. But he or she does need a basic understanding of the core technologies in order to help guide the formation of the principles and strategies that will direct that decision. In the boxed example here, the application integration perspective on architecture (choosing among best of breed, monolithic, and visual integration) illustrates a typical architecture challenge that a hospital might face.

PERSPECTIVE
Choosing the System Architecture

A hospital has adopted a best-of-breed approach and, over the course of several years, has implemented separate applications that support the registration, laboratory, pharmacy, and radiology departments and the transcription of operative notes and discharge summaries. An interface engine has been implemented that enables registration transactions to flow from the registration system to the other systems.

However, the physicians and nurses have started to complain. To retrieve a patient's laboratory, pharmacy, and radiology records and transcribed materials, they have to sign into each of these systems, using a separate user name and password. To obtain an overall view of a patient's condition, they have to print out the results from each of these systems and assemble the different printouts. All of this takes too much time, and there are too many passwords to remember.

Moreover, the hospital would like to analyze its care, in an effort to improve care quality, but the current architecture does not include an integrated database of patient results.

The hospital has two emerging architectural objectives that the current architecture cannot meet:

1. Provide an integrated view of a patient's results for caregivers.
2. Efficiently support the analysis of care patterns.

To address these objectives, the hospital decides to implement a browser-based application that

- Gathers clinical data from each application and presents it in a unified view for the caregivers
- Supports the entry of one user ID and password that is synchronized with the user ID and password for each application

In addition, the hospital decides to implement a database that receives clinical results from each of the applications and stores these data for access by query tools and analysis software.

To achieve its emerging objectives, the hospital has migrated from best-of-breed architecture to visual integration architecture. The hospital has also extended to visual integration architecture by adding an integrated database for analysis purposes.

In analyzing what would be the best architecture to meet its new objectives, the hospital considered monolithic architecture. It could meet its objectives by replacing all applications with one integrated suite of applications from one vendor. However, the hospital decided that this approach would be too expensive and time consuming. Besides, the current applications (laboratory, pharmacy, and radiology) worked well; they just weren't integrated. The monolithic architecture approach to integration was examined and discarded.

SUMMARY

The value of this chapter to the health care executive is that it provides a broad overview of health care information architecture and several categories of specific information technologies. Although these technologies are not unique to health care, health care organizations use them for their information systems. We discussed various technologies used for data management and access; networks and data communications; remote access technologies; information processing distribution schemes; the Internet, intranets, and extranets; e-commerce; and clinical and managerial decision support. The Gartner Hype Cycle was introduced as a framework for examining emerging technologies.

We ended our discussion with the concept of system architecture, the way in which all the technologies in an organization fit together to support health care applications. Like many fields, IT has its own language. It is helpful for health care executives to learn IT terminology so they can communicate effectively with IT staff and vendors. The overall goal of this chapter was to provide information to support an understanding of the many components that go into health care information systems.

KEY TERMS

Access point

Artificial intelligence

Bandwidth

Baseband

Bits per second (bps)

Blog

Bluetooth

Broadband

Client/server

Clinical data repository

Clinical decision support systems

Cloud computing

Coaxial cable

Data communication

Data dictionary
Data management
Data mart
Data mining
Data warehouse
Decision support systems
Domain Name System (DNS) server
E-commerce
Electronic data interchange
Ethernet
Executive information systems
Expert systems
Extensible markup language (XML)
Extranet
Fiber-optic cable
File server
Flat file structure
4G wireless communications
Gartner Hype Cycle
Hyperlink
Hypertext markup language (HTML)
Hypertext Transfer Protocol (HTTP)
IEEE 802.11 standards
IP address
Information processing distribution schemes
Information systems architecture
Infrastructure
Infrastructure network
Internet
Internet protocol (IP) address
Intranet
Local area network (LAN)
M-commerce
Markup language
Metadata
Microwaves
Natural language processing
Network
Network interface card (NIC)
Network media
Network operating system

Neural networks
Node
Object-oriented database
Online transactional processing (OLTP)
Open Standards Interconnection (OSI) model
Platform
Podcasts
Protocol
Relational database
Relational database management system
Remote access technologies
Rich Internet applications
Router
Schema
Single sign-on system
Social networking web sites
Spread spectrum radio transmissions
Structured query language (SQL)
Subnet
Switch
3G wireless communications
Transmission Control Protocol/ Internet Protocol (TCP/IP)
Tunnel
Twisted pair wire
Uniform resource locator (URL)
Virtual private network
Web browser
Web conferencing
Web portal
Web site
Web 2.0
Workstation
Wide area network (WAN)
Wiki
WiMAX
Wireless LAN
World Wide Web

LEARNING ACTIVITIES

1. Technology is changing and evolving. Conduct a search of the Internet or print literature to identify several new or emerging technologies. Describe each technology and discuss its potential use in the management of health care information or the development of health care information systems.

2. Visit a small health care facility or physician's office. Describe the computer network that is used. Does this location use both a LAN and a WAN? What functions are limited to the LAN? Which functions use a WAN? Ask for a copy of the LAN diagram for the office (if one exists) or create one from your visit.

3. Do an Internet search and find at least one site that offers a decision-support product to health care executives. Describe the product. Can you tell from the site whether or not the product employs artificial intelligence? Can you tell which type? How useful would the product be to you as a health care executive?

4. Meet with the chief information officer or director or the IT manager in a health care organization. Ask him or her to describe the architecture used for the clinical component of the organization's health care information system. Based on this conversation, describe how this IT professional views the architecture. What process did this organization use to determine its architecture design? Does it have plans to move to a different architecture?

5. Do an Internet search of health care organizations. Which ones are using Web 2.0 technologies to establish connections with patients or other consumers? How many are engaged in e-commerce directed at consumers?

REFERENCES

Gartner. (2011, August 2). *Gartner's hype cycle special report for 2011*. Retrieved April 2012 from http://my.gartner.com/portal/server.pt?open=512&objID=260&mode=2&PageID=3460702&resId=1758314&ref=QuickSearch&sthkw=Hype+Cycle+Mobile+Technologies

Gartner. (2012). *Research methodologies*. Retrieved May 2012 from http://www.gartner.com/technology/research/methodologies/hype-cycle.jsp

Glaser, J. (2002). *The strategic application of information technology in health care organizations* (2nd ed.). San Francisco: Jossey-Bass.

Microsoft. (2012). TCP/IP protocol architecture. *TechNet*. Retrieved April 2012 from http://technet.microsoft.com/en-us/library/cc958821.aspx

Oz, E. (2009). *Management information systems: Instructor edition* (6th ed.). Boston: Course Technology.

Stair, R., & Reynolds, G. (2012). *Principles of information systems* (10th ed.). Boston: Course Technology.

White, C. (2011). *Data communications and computer networks: A business user's approach* (6th ed.). Boston: Course Technology.

WiMAX. (2012). What is WiMAX? *WiMAX Forum*. Retrieved April 2012 from http://www.wimax.com/general/what-is-wimax

CHAPTER 10

Health Care Information System Standards

LEARNING OBJECTIVES

- To be able to give examples of the four major methods by which standards are developed—ad hoc, de facto, government mandate, and consensus.

- To be able to identify the major types of health care information standards and the organizations that develop or approve them:

  - Classification standards
  - Vocabulary and terminology standards
  - Standards for electronic data interchange
  - Health record content and functional standards

- To be able to identify and discuss the role of organizations that currently have a significant impact on the adoption of health care information standards in the United States.

- To be able to identify and discuss the role of federal initiatives and legislation that have a significant impact on the adoption of health care information standards in the United States.

- To be able to discuss the Nationwide Health Information Network.

In order to achieve interoperability, portability, and data exchange, health care information systems must employ standards. Systems that conform to different standards cannot communicate with one another. For a simple analogy, think about traveling to a country where you do not speak the language. You would not be able to communicate with that country's citizens without a common language or translator. Think of the common language as the standard to which all parties agree to adhere. Once you and others agree on a common language, you and they can communicate. You may still have some problems, but generally these can be overcome.

A plethora of information technology (IT) standards, including standards for messaging, content and coding, networks, electronic data interchange, and electronic health records, are important to health care information systems. Some of these standards compete with one another. In 2004, Bazzoli had identified 450 voluntary and mandated standards from 150 organizations, and this number has certainly increased over time. It is important to recognize that, although they will not be discussed in this chapter, many IT standards that do not specifically address health care also have a tremendous impact on health care information systems, such as basic communication protocols and extensible markup language (XML), which has emerged as a messaging standard not only in business-related Internet transactions but also in health care transactions and communications.

In the sections that follow we provide an overview of the standards development process and introduce several key initiatives, some formal and some less so, that have led to the development of standards to facilitate interoperability among health care information systems. These standards will be reviewed in four main categories:

- Classification standards
- Vocabulary and terminology standards
- Data interchange standards
- Health record content and functional standards

We will conclude this chapter with a discussion of the impact of federal regulations and the efforts of the Office of the National Coordinator for Health Information Technology on the adoption of health care information standards to facilitate interoperability.

STANDARDS DEVELOPMENT PROCESS

When seeking to understand why so many different IT and health care information standards exist, it is helpful to look first at the basic standards development process that exists in the United States (and internationally) and the changes that have occurred in this process over the past decade. In general the methods used to establish health care IT standards can be divided into four categories (Hammond & Cimino, 2006):

- **Ad hoc.** A standard is established by the *ad hoc* method when a group of interested people or organizations agrees on a certain specification without any formal adoption process. The Digital Imaging and Communications in Medicine (DICOM) standard for health care imaging came about in this way.

- **De facto.** A *de facto* standard arises when a vendor or other commercial enterprise controls such a large segment of the market that its product becomes the recognized norm. The SQL database language and the Windows operating system are examples of de facto standards. XML is becoming a de facto standard for health care and other types of industry messaging.

- **Government mandate.** Standards are also established when the government mandates that the health care industry adopt them. Examples are the transaction and code sets mandated by the Health Insurance Portability and Accountability Act (HIPAA) regulations.

- **Consensus.** *Consensus*-based standards come about when representatives from various interested groups come together to reach a formal agreement on specifications. The process is generally open and involves considering comment and feedback from the industry. This method is employed by the *standards development organizations (SDOs)* accredited by the *American National Standards Institute (ANSI)*. Most health care information standards are developed by this method, including Health Level Seven (HL7) standards and Accredited Standards Committee (ASC) X12N standards.

Libicki, Schneider, Frelinger, and Slomovic (2000) outline a two-by-two matrix topology for IT standard-setting organizations. They classify the organizations that set IT standards by membership type (open to all or members only) and by process (democratic or dependent on "a strong leader"). The organizations with the most formal standard-setting processes, such as the International Organization for Standardization (ISO), ANSI, and the ANSI-accredited SDOs, fall into the member-only, democratic classification. The relationships among the various standard-setting organizations can be confusing. Not only do many of the acronyms sound similar, but the organizations themselves, as voluntary, member-based organizations, can set their own missions and goals. Therefore, although there is a formally recognized relationship among

Table 10.1. Organizations responsible for formal standards development

Organizations	Facts
International Organization for Standardization (ISO), www.iso.org	Members are national standards bodies from many different countries around the world ANSI is the U.S. national body member Oversees the flow of documentation and international approval of standards developed under the auspices of its member bodies
American National Standards Institute (ANSI), www.ansi.org	U.S. member of ISO Accredits standards development organizations (SDOs) from a wide range of industries, including health care Oversees the work of the SDOs, technical committees, subcommittees, and working groups Does *not* develop standards itself, but accredits the organizations that develop standards Publishes the 10,000+ American National Standards developed by accredited SDOs
Standards development organizations (SDOs)	Must be accredited by ANSI Develop standards in accordance with ANSI criteria
SDOs that develop health care–related standards discussed in this chapter	Can use the label "Approved American National Standard"
ASTM International (formerly American Society for Testing and Materials), www.astm.org	Currently, there are 270+ ANSI-accredited SDOs representing many industries, including health care
Health Level Seven (HL7), www.hl7.org ANSI Accredited Standards Committee (ASC) X12, www.x12.org	

ISO, ANSI, and the SDOs, there is also some overlap in activities. Table 10.1 outlines the relationships among these formal standard-setting organizations and for each one gives a brief overview of important facts and a current web site.

All the ANSI-accredited SDOs must adhere to the guidelines established for accreditation; therefore, they have similar standard-setting processes. According to ANSI, this process includes

- Consensus on a proposed standard by a group or "consensus body" that includes representatives from materially affected or interested parties
- Broad-based public review and comment on draft standards
- Consideration of and response to comments submitted by voting members of the relevant consensus body and by public review commenters
- Incorporation of approved changes into a draft standard
- Right to appeal by any participant that believes that due process principles were not sufficiently respected during the standards development in accordance with the ANSI-accredited procedures of the standards developer [ANSI, 2012]

In the last decade the IT industry in general has experienced a movement away from the process of establishing standards via the SDOs. The Internet and World Wide Web standards, for example, were developed by groups with much less formal structures. However, the SDOs continue to have a significant impact on the IT standards for the health care industry.

The HIPAA rules identify a subset of SDOs and other organizations as Designated Standards Maintenance Organizations (DSMOs), whose responsibility it is to maintain the transaction standards that fall under the HIPAA rules. The current HIPAA DSMOs are

- Accredited Standards Committee X12
- Dental Content Committee of the American Dental Association
- Health Level Seven
- National Council for Prescription Drug Programs
- National Uniform Billing Committee
- National Uniform Claim Committee

PERSPECTIVE
European Committee for Standardization (CEN)

Although the focus of this chapter is standards developed within the United States, it is important to recognize there are other standards organizations worldwide. For example, the *European Committee for Standardization (CEN)* was created in Brussels in 1975. Its current membership

(cont.)

includes National Standards Bodies from thirty-two European countries (CEN, 2012a). The CEN develops standards not only for health care, but also for other industries. CEN has a close working relationship with the major international standards organizations. In general, standards developed by ISO independently of CEN will be accepted as de facto CEN standards, provided CEN feels the standards are needed.

The Technical Committee within CEN that oversees health care informatics standards is CEN TC 251, which consists of four working groups:

- WG1: information models
- WG2: terminology and knowledge representation
- WG3: security, safety, and quality
- WG4: technology for interoperability (CEN, 2012b)

CLASSIFICATION STANDARDS

The most widely recognized coding and classification systems—ICD, Current Procedural Terminology (CPT), and diagnosis related groups (DRGs)—were discussed in Chapter One. Although these systems and the other systems discussed in this section do not meet the criteria for full clinical vocabularies, they are used to classify diagnoses and procedures and are the basis for information retrieval in health care information systems. Most were originally developed to facilitate disease and procedure information retrieval, but have been adopted to code for billing services as well. Several of the most commonly used classification systems are actually incorporated across more robust standard vocabularies such as SNOMED-CT and UMLS®.

The HIPAA rules specify specific code sets for diagnoses and procedures that are to be used in any transactions by a covered entity. The code sets required by HIPAA are

- HCPCS (ancillary services or procedures) (see Chapter One)
- CPT-4 (physicians procedures) (see Chapter One)
- CDT (dental terminology)
- ICD-9 (ICD-10 as of October 2014 for diagnoses and hospital inpatient procedures) (see Chapter One)
- NDC (national drug codes) (CMS, 2012a)

The HITECH "meaningful use" final rule (discussed in Chapter Four) also includes ICD-9, with the transition to ICD-10, as its classification standard.

Code on Dental Procedures and Nomenclature

The American Dental Association (ADA) publishes the CDT, *Code on Dental Procedures and Nomenclature*. This set of codes is designed to support accurate recording and reporting of dental treatments. The ADA (2012) strives to maintain an up-to-date set of codes that reflect actual practice. The code set is divided into twelve sections as follows (Washington Dental Service, 2012):

I.   Diagnostic (D0000–D0999)

II. Preventative (D1000–D1999)

III. Restorative (D2000–D2999)

IV. Endodontics (D3000–D3999)

V.   Periodontics (D4000–D4999)

VI. Prosthodontics (D5000–D5899)

VII. Maxillofacial prosthetics (D5900–D5999)

VIII. Implant services (D6000–D6199)

IX. Prosthodontics (D6200–D6999)

X.   Oral and maxillofacial surgery (D7000–7999)

XI. Orthodontics (D8000–8999)

XII. Adjunctive General Services (D9000–D9999)

National Drug Codes

The *National Drug Code (NDC)* is the universal product identifier for all human drugs. The Drug Listing Act of 1972 requires registered drug companies to provide the Food and Drug Administration (FDA) a current listing of all drugs "manufactured, prepared, propagated, compounded, or processed by it for commercial distribution" (FDA, 2012). The FDA, in turn, assigns the unique, three-segment NDC (listed as package code in the following example) and maintains the information in the National Drug Code Directory. The NDC Directory is updated twice each month. Data maintained for each drug include up to sixteen fields. The information for the common over-the-counter drug Tylenol PM (Extra Strength), for example, is as follows:

Product NDC: 50580–176

Product Type Name: Human OTC Drug

Proprietary Name: Tylenol PM (Extra Strength)

Non-proprietary Name: Acetaminophen and Diphenhydramine Hydrochloride

Dosage Formulation: Tablet, Coated

Route Name: Oral

Start Marketing Date: 12–01–1991

End Marketing Date: <blank field>

Marketing Category Name: OTC Monograph Final

Application Number: part338

Labeler Name: McNeil Consumer Healthcare Div. McNeil-PPC, Inc

Substance Name: Acetaminophen; Diphenhydramine Hydrochloride

Strength Number/Unit: 500 mg/1, 25 mg/1

Pharm Class: Histamine H1 Receptor Antagonists [MoA], Histamine-1 Receptor Antagonist [EPC]

Package Code: 50580–176–10

Package Description: 1 Bottle, Plastic in 1 Carton (50580–176–10) > 100 tablet, coated in 1 Bottle, Plastic

DEA classification: <blank> (FDA, 2012)

VOCABULARY AND TERMINOLOGY STANDARDS

One of the most difficult problems in exchanging health care information and building longitudinal electronic health records (EHRs) is coordinating the vast amount of health information that is generated in diverse locations for patients and populations. The vocabulary and terminology standards discussed in this section serve similar purposes—to create a common language that allows different information systems or vendor products to communicate unambiguously with one another. In a very simplified example, a standard vocabulary would ensure that the medical term "myocardial infarction," for example, is "mapped" to the term "heart attack" and that both terms share exactly the same attributes. An effective standard vocabulary must also standardize the very complex hierarchy and syntax of the language used in the health industry. This is a complicated and detailed endeavor to say the least. So it is not surprising that to date, no single vocabulary has emerged to meet all the information exchange needs of the health care sector.

The *National Committee on Vital and Health Statistics (NCVHS)* has the responsibility, under a HIPAA mandate, to recommend uniform data standards for patient medical record information (PMRI). Although no single vocabulary has been recognized by NCVHS as *the* standard, they have recommended the following as a core set of PMRI terminology standards:

- Systematized Nomenclature of Medicine—Clinical Terms (SNOMED CT)
- Logical Observation Identifiers Names and Codes (LOINC) laboratory subset
- Several federal drug terminologies, including RxNorm (NCVHS, 2003)

The HITECH "meaningful use" final rule (discussed in Chapter Four) also includes vocabulary standards—LOINC, SNOMED-CT, RxNorm, and CVX (clinical vaccines administered).

In this section we will describe SNOMED CT, LOINC, CVX, and RxNorm, along with the National Library of Medicine's Unified Medical Language® (UMLS®) (of which RxNorm is one component), which has become the standard for bibliographical searches in health care and has the potential for other uses as well.

Systematized Nomenclature of Medicine—Clinical Terms

Systematized Nomenclature of Medicine—Clinical Terms (SNOMED CT) is a comprehensive clinical terminology developed specifically to facilitate the electronic storage and retrieval of detailed clinical information. It is the result of collaboration between the College of American Pathologists (CAP) and the United Kingdom's National Health Service (NHS). SNOMED CT merges CAP's SNOMED Reference Terminology, an older classification system used to group diseases, and the NHS's Clinical Terms Version 3 (better known as Read Codes), an established clinical terminology used in Great Britain and elsewhere. As a result, SNOMED CT is based on decades of research. As of April 2007 SNOMED is owned, maintained, and distributed by the *International Health Terminology Standards Development Organisation (IHTSDO)*, a nonprofit association based in Denmark. The National Library of Medicine is the U.S. member of the IHTSDO and distributes SNOMED at no cost within the United States (NLM, 2012a).

Logical Observation Identifiers Names and Codes

The *Logical Observation Identifiers Names and Codes (LOINC)* system was developed to facilitate the electronic transmission of laboratory results to hospitals, physicians, third-party payers, and other users of laboratory data. Initiated in 1994 by the Regenstrief Institute at Indiana University, LOINC provides a standard set of universal names and codes for identifying individual laboratory and clinical results. These standard codes allow users to merge clinical results from disparate sources (LOINC, 2012).

LOINC codes have a fixed length field of seven characters. Current codes range from three to seven characters long. There are six parts in the LOINC name structure: component/analyte, property, time aspect, system, scale type, and method. The syntax for a name follows this pattern (Case, 2011):

LOINC Code: Component: Property Measured: Timing: System: Scale: Method

Example

5193–8:Hepatitis B virus surface Ab: ACnc:Pt:Ser:Qn:EIA

Clinical Vaccines Administered

The Centers for Disease Control and Prevention (CDC) National Center of Immunization and Respiratory Diseases (NCIRD) developed the Clinical Vaccines Administered (CVX) as a table for use with HL7 messaging standard (see the HL7 section later in this chapter for more explanation.) Table 10.2 is an excerpt from the full CVX table (CDC, 2012).

RxNorm

The *National Library of Medicine (NLM)* produces *RxNorm*, which serves two purposes, as "a normalized naming system for generic and brand name drugs and as a tool for supporting semantic interoperation between drug terminologies and pharmacy knowledge based systems" (NLM, 2012b). The goal of RxNorm is to allow disparate health information systems to communicate with one another in an unambiguous manner.

There are twelve separate RxNorm data files that are released on a monthly basis. The files show

- Drug names and unique identifiers
- Relationships
- Attributes
- Semantic types

Table 10.2. Excerpts from CVX (clinical vaccines administered) table

Short Description	Full Vaccine Name	CVX Code	Status	Last Date Updated	Notes
adenovirus types 4 and 7	Adenovirus, type 4 and type 7, live, oral	143	Active	3/20/2011	This vaccine is administered as two tablets.
anthrax	anthrax vaccine	24	Active	5/28/2010	
BCG	Bacillus Calmette-Guerin vaccine	19	Active	5/28/2010	
DTaP, IPV, Hib, HepB	Diphtheria and Tetanus Toxoids and Acellular Pertussis Absorbed, Inactivated Poliovirus, Haemophilus b Conjugate (Meningococcal Outer Membrane Protein Complex), and Hepatitis B (Recombinant) Vaccine	146	Active	Pending	Note that this vaccine is different from CVX 132.
influenza, seasonal, injectable	influenza, seasonal, injectable	141	Active	9/30/2010	This is one of two codes replacing CVX 15, which is being retired.
influenza, live, intranasal	influenza virus vaccine, live, attenuated, for intranasal use	111	Active	5/28/2010	Seasonal influenza

- Data history (three files)
- Obsolete data (three files)
- Metadata (two files)

The following example from the first RxNorm data file represents the "concept," Azithromycin 250 MG Oral Capsule, with the unique identifier 141962 (NLM, 2012b):

141962|ENG||||||944489|944489|141962||RXNORM|SCD|141962|Azithro mycin 250 MG Oral Capsule||N||

Unified Medical Language System

The National Library of Medicine (NLM), an agency of the National Institutes of Health, began the *Unified Medical Language System (UMLS)* project in 1986, and it is ongoing today. The purpose of the UMLS project is to "to facilitate the development of computer systems that behave as if they 'understand' the meaning of the language of biomedicine and health. The UMLS provides data for system developers as well as search and report functions for less technical users" (NLM, 2008, p. 1).

The UMLS has three basic components, called *knowledge sources:*

- **UMLS Metathesaurus®**, which contains over one million biomedical concepts from over one hundred source vocabularies. All the common health information vocabularies, including SNOMED CT, ICD, and CPT, along with approximately one hundred other vocabularies, including RxNorm, are incorporated into the metathesaurus. The metathesaurus project's goal is to incorporate and map existing vocabularies into a single system.

- **UMLS Semantic Network**, which defines 133 broad categories and fifty-four relationships between categories for labeling the biomedical domain. The semantic network contains information about the categories (such as "Disease or Syndrome" and "Virus") to which metathesaurus concepts are assigned. The semantic network also outlines the relationships among the categories (for example, "Virus" causes "Disease or Syndrome").

- **SPECIALIST Lexicon and Lexical Tools.** The lexicon contains information for many terms, component words, and English language words that do not appear in the metathesaurus.

The UMLS products are widely used in NLM's own applications, such as PubMed. They are available to other organizations free of charge, provided the users submit a license agreement (NLM, 2008).

Data Interchange Standards

The ability to exchange and integrate data among health care applications is critical to the success of any overall health care information system, whether an organizational, regional, or national level of integration is desired. Although there is some overlap, these standards differ from the vocabulary standards because their major purpose is to standardize the actual "messaging" between health care information systems. Much of the health care information standards development activity has been in the area of standards for data interchange or integration. In this section we will look at a few of the standards that have been developed for this purpose. There are others, and new needs are continually being identified. However, the following groups of standards are recognized as important to the health care sector, and together they provide examples of both broad standards addressing all types of applications and specific standards addressing one type of application.

- Health Level Seven standards
- Digital Imaging and Communications in Medicine (DICOM)
- National Council for Prescription Drug Programs (NCPDP)
- ANSI ASC X12N standards

It is important to note that the HIPAA rules include specified standards for electronic transactions, which fall into this category of data exchange standards. HIPAA specifically required covered entities to comply with specific ANSI X12N and NCPCP standards.

PERSPECTIVE
President's Council of Advisors on Science and Technology Report on Health Information Technology

In December 2011 the President's Council of Advisors on Science and Technology (PCAST) released a report calling for the adoption of a "universal exchange language" that would allow for the transfer of relevant health data while maximizing privacy. They argue that EHR's usefulness is limited primarily to the owner organization. The report supports the development of an "information technology ecosystem" to facilitate real-time exchange of patient information. PCAST specifically recommends that the Office of the National Coordinator for Health Information Technology (ONC) and CMS develop guidelines for the adoption of a universal exchange language, similar to the existing extensible markup languages, to move the industry forward from a system of traditional electronic health records to a "more medically useful and secure system in which individual bits of healthcare data are tagged with privacy and security

(cont.)

specifications." Each individual unit of pertinent health care data would be accompanied by a mandatory "metadata tag" that describes the data's attributes, provenance, and required security and privacy protections. PCAST's recommendations would not require the replacement of electronic health record systems, but would create a system of compatibility through the use of "apps" or "middleware." The report further recommends that the new guidelines be developed as a part of the meaningful use standards under HITECH, which must be achieved in stages by 2015.

Not surprisingly, the PCAST report has generated a good bit of discussion in the health care information community. It is too early to tell what the actual impact of the report will be in the establishment of interoperability standards. However, the ONC has established a work group to review and respond to the recommendations (Office of Science and Technology Policy, 2010).

Health Level Seven Standards

Health Level Seven International (HL7) is an ANSI-accredited standards development organization that was founded as an ad hoc group in 1987. HL7 was founded with a purpose of developing a *messaging standard* to support the "exchange, management, and integration of data that support clinical patient care" (Marotta, 2000). This purpose has expanded over time to include standards defining

- System integration and interoperability
- Tools and "building blocks" used to build the standards
- Messaging and document standards
- EHR functional models and profiles

Since its inception, HL7 has grown from a small group of fourteen individuals to a large organization with over 2,300 health care provider, vendor, and consultant members. HL7's five hundred corporate members represent more than 90 percent of health care information systems vendors (HL7, 2012).

HL7 v3 messaging standards incorporate the root elements of XML and, as such, are a significant change from early versions. See the HL7 Perspective for an example of HL7 v3.

PERSPECTIVE
HL7 Laboratory Results Use Case

The following object identifiers (OIDs) are used within the Good Health Hospital (GHH):

- GHH Placer Order IDs: 2.16.840.1.113883.19.1122.14
- GHH Lab Filler Order IDs: 2.16.840.1.113883.19.1122.4
- The code system for the observation within the GHH is LOINC: 2.16.840.1.113883.6.1
- The HL7 Confidentiality Code system: 2.16.840.1.113883.5.25

The HL7 v3 Message: Domain Content Excerpt

The "Domain Content" starts with its own root element: observationEvent. The elements within specify the type of observation, the ID, the time of the observation, statusCode, and the results. The value for the actual result is shown in the value element. The interpretationCode element shows that the value has been interpreted as high (H), while referenceRange provides the normal values for this particular observation.

<observationEvent>
<id root="2.16.840.1.113883.19.1122.4" extension="1045813"
assigningAuthorityName="GHH LAB Filler Orders"/>
<code code="1554-5" codeSystemName="LN"
codeSystem="2.16.840.1.113883.6.1"
displayName="GLUCOSE∧POST 12H CFST:MCNC:PT:SER/PLAS:QN"/>
<statusCode code="completed"/>
<effectiveTime value="200202150730"/>
<priorityCode code="R"/>
<confidentialityCode code="N"
codeSystem="2.16.840.1.113883.5.25"/>
<value xsi:type="PQ" value="182" unit="mg/dL"/>
<interpretationCode code="H"/>
<referenceRange>

(cont.)

```
<interpretationRange>
<value xsi:type="IVL_PQ">
<low value="70" unit="mg/dL"/>
<high value="105" unit="mg/dL"/>
</value>
<interpretationCode code="N"/>
</interpretationRange>
</referenceRange>
</assignedEntity>
</author>
```

Source: Ringholm, 2012.

Digital Imaging and Communications in Medicine

The growth of digital diagnostic imaging (such as CT scans and MRIs) gave rise to the need for a standard for the electronic transfer of these images between devices manufactured by different vendors. The American College of Radiology (ACR) and the National Electrical Manufacturers Association (NEMA) published the first standard, a precursor to the current *Digital Imaging and Communications in Medicine (DICOM)* standard, in 1985. The goals of DICOM are to "achieve compatibility and to improve workflow efficiency between imaging systems and other information systems in healthcare environments worldwide." It is used by all of the major diagnostic medical imaging vendors, which translates to its use in nearly every medical profession that uses images (DICOM, 2012).

National Council for Prescription Drug Programs

The mission of the *National Council for Prescription Drug Programs (NCPDP)* states that "NCPDP provides a forum wherein our diverse membership can develop business solutions, including ANSI-accredited standards, and guidance for promoting information exchanges related to medications, supplies, and services within the healthcare system. Through a consensus building process in collaboration with other industry organizations, our members develop these solutions to improve safety, privacy and healthcare outcomes for patients and healthcare consumers, while reducing costs in the system." To this end the NCPDP, an ANSI-accredited SDO with over 1,600 members representing the pharmacy services industry, has developed a set of standards for the electronic submission of third-party drug claims (NCPDP, 2012).

These standards not only include the Telecommunication Standards and Batch Standards required by HIPAA, but also Uniform Healthcare Payer Data Standard, Retiree Drug Subsidy Standard, the SCRIPT standard for e-prescribing (required by CMS for Medicare and Medicaid e-prescribing), and the Manufacturers Rebate Standard, among others. Of note, the SCRIPT standard currently incorporates the RxNorm, discussed earlier in this chapter, as a standardized medication nomenclature. The NCPDP Provider Identification Number is a unique identifier of over 75,000 pharmacies. As of January 2012, HIPAA requires covered entities to comply with the NCPDP Telecommunications Standard Version D.0 and Batch Standards Version 1.2 for pharmacy claims transactions (Emdeon, 2012). Table 10.3 presents excerpts from the NCPDP Data Dictionary, which outlines a few of the Transmission Header Segment requirements. The entire Data Dictionary table is over seventy pages long (CMS, 2012c).

ANSI ASC X12N Standards

The ANSI *Accredited Standards Committee (ASC)* X12 develops standards, in both X12 and XML formats, for the electronic exchange of business information. One ASC X12 subcommittee, *X12N*, has been specifically designated to deal with electronic data interchange (EDI) standards in the insurance industry, and this subcommittee has a special health care task group, known as TG2. According to the X12 TG2 web site, "the purpose of the Health Care Task group shall be the development and maintenance of data standards (both national and international) which shall support the exchange of business information for health care administration. Health care data includes, but is not limited to, such business functions as eligibility, referrals and authorizations, claims, claim status, payment and remittance advice, and provider directories." To this end ASC X12N has developed a set of standards that are monitored and updated through ASC X12N work groups. Table 10.4 lists the current X12 work group areas.

All HIPAA-covered entities were required to be compliant with the ASC X12 version 5010 by January 1, 2012. A portion of the X12 5010 Professional Claim standard is shown in Exhibit 10.1. The standard for Professional Claim alone is over ninety pages in length.

Table 10.3. Excerpts from NCPDP data dictionary

NCPDP Data Dictionary Name	Field Number	NCPDP Definition of Field	Version D.0 Format	Valid Values per the Standard
Service Provider ID Qualifier	202-B2	Code qualifying the Service Provider ID	X(02)	Blank=Not Specified 01=National Provider Identifier (NPI) 02=Blue Cross 03=Blue Shield 04=Medicare 05=Medicaid 06=UPIN 07=NCPDP Provider ID 08=State License 09=Champus 10=Health Industry Number (HIN) 11=Federal Tax ID 12=Drug Enforcement Administration (DEA) 13=State Issued 14=Plan Specific 15=HCID (HC IDea) 99=Other
Service Provider ID	201-B1	ID assigned to pharmacy or provider	X(15)	N/A
Date of Service	401-D1	Identifies date the prescription was filled or professional service rendered or subsequent payer began coverage following Part A expiration in a long-term care setting only	9(08)	Format=CCYYMMDD

Table 10.4. X12 TG2 work groups

Work Group Number	Work Group Name
WG1	Health Care Eligibility
WG2	Health Care Claims
WG3	Claim Payments
WG4	Enrollments
WG5	Claims Status
WG9	Patient Information
WG10	Health Care Services Review
WG15	Provider Information
WG20	Insurance—824 Implementation Guide
WG21	Health Care Regulation Advisory/Collaboration

Source: Accredited Standards Committee X12, 2012.

Exhibit 10.1. X12 5010 professional claim standard

5010							
Element Identifier	**Description**	**ID**	**Min. Max.**	**Usage Reg.**	**Loop**	**Loop Repeat**	**Values**
837-P 5010							
ISA	**INTERCHANGE CONTROL HEADER**		**1**	**R**	___	**1**	
ISA01	Authorization Information Qualifier	ID	2-2	R			00, 03
ISA02	Authorization Information	AN	10-10	R			
ISA03	Security Information Qualifier	ID	2-2	R			00, 01
ISA04	Security Information	AN	10-10	R			
ISA05	Interchange ID Qualifier	ID	2-2	R			01, 14, 20, 27, 28, 29, 30, 33, ZZ
ISA06	Interchange Sender ID	AN	15-15	R			

(cont.)

Exhibit 10.1. (*Continued*)

							5010
Element Identifier	**Description**	**ID**	**Min. Max.**	**Usage Reg.**	**Loop**	**Loop Repeat**	**Values**
ISA07	Interchange ID Qualifier	ID	2-2	R			01, 14, 20, 27, 28, 29, 30, 33, ZZ
ISA08	Interchange Receiver ID	AN	15-15	R			
ISA09	Interchange Date	DT	6-6	R			YYMMDD
ISA10	Interchange Time	TM	4-4	R			HHMM
ISA11	Interchange Control Standards ID		1-1	R			
ISA12	Interchange Control Version Number	ID	5-5	R			00501
ISA13	Interchange Control Number	N0	9-9	R			
ISA14	Acknowledgement Requested	ID	1-1	R			0, 1
ISA15	Usage Indicator	ID	1-1	R			P, T
ISA16	Component Element Separator	AN	1-1	R			
GS	**FUNCTIONAL GROUP HEADER**		**1**	**R**	**—**	**1**	
GS01	Functional Identifier Code	ID	2-2	R			
GS02	Application Sender Code	AN	2-15	R			
GS03	Application Receiver Code	AN	2-15	R			
GS04	Date	DT	8-8	R			CCYYMMDD
GS05	Time	TM	4-8	R			HHMM
GS06	Group Control Number	N0	1-9	R			
GS07	Responsible Agency Code	ID	1-2	R			X
GS08	Version Identifier Code	AN	1-12	R			005010X222

HEALTH RECORD CONTENT AND FUNCTIONAL STANDARDS

In this section we will look at four sets of health record content and functional standards.

- HL7 EHR-S (Electronic Health Record-System) Functional Model
- ASTM Health Record Content Standards
- Continuity of Care Document
- HITECH EHR Certification Criteria

HL7 EHR-S Functional Model

The *HL7 Health Record-System (EHR-S) Functional Model*, Release 1, is the result of a 2009 revision to the original HL7 Functional Model. The purpose of this functional model is to outline important features and functions that should be contained in an EHR. Targeted users of the functional model include vendors and care providers and it has been recognized by the ISO as an international standard (ISO 10781). The stated benefits (HL7, 2012) to the functional model are to

- Facilitate describing end-user defined benefits such as patient safety, quality outcomes, and cost efficiencies in terms of standard EHR-S functions
- Promote a common understanding of EHR functions from which developers, vendors, users, and other interested parties can plan and evaluate EHR-S functions
- Provide the necessary framework to drive the requirements and applications of next level standards, such as EHR content, coding, information models, constructs, and interoperability for information portability between subsystems of and across EHR-Ss
- Establish a standards-based method by which each realm (country) can apply these EHR functions to care settings, uses, and priorities
- Inform those concerned with secondary use of EHR data and national infrastructure what functions can be expected in an EHR system

The EHR-S Functional Model includes a functional outline, functional profiles, and assigned priorities for the functions in the profile. The functional outline is divided into three sections: Direct Care, Supportive, and

Exhibit 10.2. EHR-S overall functional model			

Direct Care	DC.1	Care Management
	DC.2	Clinical Decision Support
	DC.3	Operations Management and Communication
Supportive	S.1	Clinical Support
	S.2	Measurement, Analysis, Research and Reports
	S.3	Administrative and Financial
Information Infrastructure	IN.1	Security
	IN.2	Health Record Information and Management
	IN.3	Registry and Directory Services
	IN.4	Standard Terminologies & Terminology Services
	IN.5	Standards-based Interoperability
	IN.6	Business Rules and Management
	IN.7	Workflow Management

Source: HL7, 2007.

Information Infrastructure functions. Within these three main sections there are thirteen subsections and over 140 individual functions. Exhibit 10.2 depicts the overall functional model, and Exhibit 10.3 provides an example of two functions contained within the Information Infrastructure section.

ASTM Health Record Content Standards

ASTM International Committee E31 on Health Informatics has been working on consensus standards related to the maintenance and transfer of patient information since 1970. Since that time, several standards have been developed by E31 (ASTM, 2012):

- E2369, Specification for Continuity of Care Record (CCR), which defines a core set of information to be sent to a health care provider when a patient is referred or transferred.

Exhibit 10.3. Two functions contained within the information infrastructure section

ID#	Type	Name	Statement/Description	See Also	Conformance Criteria	Row #
IN.1	H	Security	**Statement:** Secure the access to an EHR-S and EHR information. Manage the sets of access control permissions granted within an EHR-S. Prevent unauthorized use of data, data loss, tampering and destruction. **Description:** To enforce security, all EHR-S applications must adhere to the rules established to control access and protect the privacy of EHR information. Security measures assist in preventing unauthorized use of data and protect against loss, tampering and destruction. An EHR-S must be capable of including or interfacing with standards-conformant security services to ensure that any Principal (user, organization, device, application, component, or object) accessing the system or its data is appropriately authenticated, authorized and audited in conformance with local and/or jurisdictional policies. An EHR-S should support Chains of Trust in respect of authentication, authorization, and privilege management, either intrinsically or by interfacing with relevant external services.			1
IN.1.1	F	Entity Authentication	**Statement:** Authenticate EHR-S users and/or entities before allowing access to an EHR-S. **Description:** Both users and applications are subject to authentication. The EHR-S must provide mechanisms for users and applications to be authenticated. Users will have to be authenticated when they attempt to use the application, the applications must authenticate.		1. The system **SHALL** authenticate principals prior to accessing an EHR-S application or EHR-S data.	2
					2. The system **SHALL** prevent access to EHR-S applications or EHR-S data to all non-authenticated principals.	3

Source: HL7, 2007.

- E1384, Practice for Content and Structure of the Electronic Health Record (EHR), which provides a structure for data collected in patient care records.

- E1633, Specification for Coded Values Used in the Electronic Health Record, which provides detailed value sets for use with E1384.

Continuity of Care Document

The *Continuity of Care Document (CCD)* is a standard for the electronic exchange of patient summary information, so-called "transportable" patient care information. The current CCD standard is actually a merger of two other standards, the HL7 Clinical Document Architecture (CDA) standard and the ASTM *Continuity of Care Record (CCR)*. There has been some discussion among experts about the CCR and CCD being competing standards, but HL7 has taken the position that CCD is an implementation of CCR and simply an evolution of the CCR (Rouse, 2010). Although discussed in this section, the CCD standard is not solely a content standard, but includes elements of a data exchange standard; it has an XML-based specification for patient summary data, but also includes a standard outline of its content. The current content outline for the CCD is as follows (Corepoint Health, 2012):

1. Header
2. Purpose
3. Problems
4. Procedures
5. Family history
6. Social history
7. Payers
8. Advance directives
9. Alerts
10. Medications
11. Immunizations
12. Medical equipment
13. Vital signs
14. Functional stats
15. Results
16. Encounters
17. Plan of care

HITECH EHR Certification Criteria

The details of the *Health Information Technology for Economic and Clinical Health (HITECH)* Act are discussed at length in Chapter Six. One of the significant components of this Act is the incentive program for electronic health records. To qualify for the incentive program, providers not only must ensure "meaningful use" of the EHR, but must also demonstrate that the EHR in use meets certification criteria. The certification criteria for the EHR under HITECH is divided into criteria for the Ambulatory Setting and for the Inpatient Setting. Table 10.5 outlines the EHR criteria to meet the Stage 1 Meaningful Use Objectives, along with relevant standards. For a full list of all EHR criteria, go to http://healthit.hhs.gov (HHS, 2012d). Eligible participants must meet all of the listed "Core Set" and five out of ten "Menu Set."

Federal Initiatives Affecting Health Care IT Standards

The federal government has several important initiatives related to health care information standards, several of which have been mentioned in previous sections of this chapter and in other chapters in this book. However, in this section we will take a summary view of these initiatives and their specific impact on health care IT standards. We will look at federal initiatives for health care IT standards as a part of HIPAA, CMS e-prescribing, and the Office of the National Coordinator for Health Information Technology. As discussed throughout this chapter, the HITECH Act also affects health care IT standards. However, it will not be discussed in this section. Refer to Chapter Six for a full discussion of this important, wide-sweeping legislation.

HIPAA

In August 2000, the U.S. Department of Health and Human Services published the final rule outlining the standards to be adopted by health care organizations for electronic transactions, and announced the *designated standard maintenance organizations* (DSMOs). Several modifications to this final rule have been subsequently published. In publishing this rule the federal government mandated that health care organizations adopt certain standards for electronic transactions and standard code sets for these transactions, and identified the standards organizations that would oversee the adoption of standards for HIPAA compliance. *HIPAA transaction standards* apply to all covered entities' *electronic data interchange (EDI)* related to claims and encounter information, payment and remittance advice, claims status, eligibility, enrollment and disenrollment, referrals and authorizations, coordination of benefits and premium

Table 10.5. Excerpt from HITECH EHR certification criteria core set

CERTIFICATION CRITERIA 45 CFR 170.302 & 170.304	CERTIFICATION CRITERIA 45 CFR 170.302 & 170.306
Ambulatory Setting	**Inpatient Setting**
<u>Computerized provider order entry.</u> Enable a user to electronically record, store, retrieve, and modify, at a minimum, the following order types: (1) Medications; (2) Laboratory; and (3) Radiology/imaging.	<u>Computerized provider order entry.</u> Enable a user to electronically record, store, retrieve, and modify, at a minimum, the following order types: (1) Medications; (2) Laboratory; and (3) Radiology/imaging.

<u>Drug-drug, drug-allergy interaction checks.</u>
(1) <u>Notifications.</u> Automatically and electronically generate and indicate in real-time, notifications at the point of care for drug-drug and drug-allergy contraindications based on medication list, medication allergy list, and computerized provider order entry (CPOE).
(2) <u>Adjustments.</u> Provide certain users with the ability to adjust notifications provided for drug-drug and drug-allergy interaction checks.

<u>Maintain up-to-date problem list.</u> Enable a user to electronically record, modify, and retrieve a patient's problem list for longitudinal care in accordance with:
(1) The standard specified in §170.207(a)(1); or
(2) At a minimum, the version of the standard specified in §170.207(a)(2).

<u>Electronic prescribing.</u> Enable a user to electronically generate and transmit prescriptions and prescription-related information in accordance with:
(1) The standard specified in §170.205(b)(1) or §170.205(b)(2); and
(2) The standard specified in §170.207(d).

<u>Maintain active medication list</u>. Enable a user to electronically record, modify, and retrieve a patient's active medication list as well as medication history for longitudinal care.

<u>Maintain active medication allergy list</u>. Enable a user to electronically record, modify, and retrieve a patient's active medication allergy list as well as medication allergy history for longitudinal care.

payment. The current HIPAA transaction standards are ASC X12N version 5010 (which accommodates ICD-10) along with NCPDP D.0 for certain pharmacy transactions. In addition to these transaction standards, several standard code sets, as listed earlier in the chapter, have been established for use in electronic transactions. The DSMOs, also listed earlier in this chapter, have the responsibility for the development, maintenance, and modification of relevant electronic data interchange standards (CMS, 2012a).

Centers for Medicare and Medicaid E-Prescribing

The Medicare Prescription Drug, Improvement, and Modernization Act of 2003 (MMA) established a Voluntary Prescription Drug Benefit program. There is no requirement in this Act that providers write prescriptions electronically, but those who choose to do so must comply with specific electronic prescribing (*e-prescribing*) standards. The current published CMS e-prescribing standards consist of three sets of existing health care IT standards as "foundation" standards, which include NCPDP's SCRIPT Standard for e-Prescribing, ASC X12N standard for Health Care Eligibility Benefit and Response, and NCPDP's telecommunications standard. In addition, the final rule identifies three additional electronic "tools" to be used in implementing e-prescribing: NCPDP Formulary and Benefit Standard Implementation Guide, which provides information about drugs covered under the beneficiary's benefit plan; NCPDP SCRIPT Medication History Transactions, which provides information about medications a beneficiary has been taking; and Fill Status Notification (RxFill), which allows prescribers to receive an electronic notice from the pharmacy regarding the beneficiary's prescription status (CMS, 2012b).

Office of the National Coordinator for Health Information Technology

In April 2004, President Bush established the *Office of the National Coordinator for Health Information Technology (ONC)* and charged the office with providing "leadership for the development and nationwide implementation of an interoperable health information technology infrastructure to improve the quality and efficiency of health care" (HHS, 2008). In 2009, the role of ONC was strengthened when the HITECH Act legislatively mandated ONC to provide this leadership and oversight (HHS, 2012a). Today, ONC is the "principal Federal entity charged with coordination of nationwide efforts to implement and use the most advanced health information technology and the electronic exchange of health information," which is clearly reflected in their published mission statement (HHS, 2012a).

ONC's mission:

- Promoting development of a nationwide health IT infrastructure that allows for electronic use and exchange of information that
  - Ensures secure and protected patient health information
  - Improves health care quality
  - Reduces health care costs
  - Informs medical decisions at the time and place of care
  - Includes meaningful public input in infrastructure development
  - Improves coordination of care and information among hospitals, labs, physicians, and so on
  - Improves public health activities and facilitates early identification of and rapid response to public health emergencies
  - Facilitates health and clinical research
  - Promotes early detection, prevention, and management of chronic diseases
  - Promotes a more effective marketplace
  - Improves efforts to reduce health disparities
- Providing leadership in the development, recognition, and implementation of standards and the certification of health IT products
- Health IT policy coordination
- Strategic planning for health IT adoption and health information exchange
- Establishing governance for the Nationwide Health Information Network

Current ONC initiatives, in addition to implementing HITECH, include several that influence the development and implementation of health care IT standards (HHS, 2012b): cybersecurity (discussed more fully in Chapter Eleven), Nationwide Health Information Network, and state-level initiatives for *health information exchange (HIE)*.

Nationwide Health Information Network

The *Nationwide Health Information Network (NwHIN)* is defined by ONC as a set of standards, services, and policies that enable the secure exchange of health information over the Internet (HHS, 2012c). It is not a physical network, and it does not store any health care information. The NwHIN has evolved from its earliest model of a network of networks to an operational set of standards, services, and policies. The latest evolution of the NwHIN supports "public-private healthcare interoperability and partnerships," the NwHIN Exchange. The participating organizations of the NwHIN share information using a common set of specifications, including those developed for NwHIN and other industry standards. There are currently twenty-five participating NwHIN organizations, including four federal agencies—CMS, DoD, SSA, and VA—and twenty-one private health care organizations (Sullivan, 2012).

HIEs and the NwHIN are still in the early stages of development. These efforts face daunting challenges of developing sustainable business models, managing patient privacy, ensuring effective governance, implementing data standards, and creating scalable technologies. Although establishing health IT interoperability across the country is a logical and necessary goal, achieving that goal will be a multiyear and complex undertaking.

SUMMARY

In this chapter we reviewed the processes by which health care information standards are developed and looked at some of the common standards that exist today, including standards in three main categories: classification, vocabulary, and terminology standards; data interchange standards; and health record content standards.

Multiple standard-setting organizations and health care professional organizations play a role in standards development. Standards can be developed through a formal process or by less formal mechanisms, including de facto designation.

The standards discussed in this chapter and other general IT standards enable health care information systems to be interoperable and portable and to exchange data. Without such standards, the EMR system and other health care information systems would have limited functionality.

The future of health care information systems is unknown; however, it is clear that the goal of having functional EHRs will not be realized until national standards are adopted. The government, as well as the private sector, plays a role in the development of national standards. HIPAA and HITECH, for example, have had a significant impact on the development of health care information standards. In addition, the creation of the Office of the National Coordinator for Health Information Technology has contributed to the movement toward true health care IT interoperability.

KEY TERMS

Accredited Standards Committee (ASC)
Ad hoc standard development
American National Standards Institute (ANSI)
ASTM International
Clinical Vaccines Administered (CVX)
Code on Dental Procedures and Nomenclature
Consensus standards
Content and functional standards
Continuity of Care Document (CCR)
Continuity of Care Record (CCR)
De facto standard development
Dental Content Committee of the American Dental Association (ADA DCC)
Designated standard maintenance organizations (DSMOs)
Digital Imaging and Communications in Medicine (DICOM)
Electronic data interchange standards
Electronic health record standards
E-prescribing
European Committee for Standardization (CEN)
Government mandated standards
Health information exchange (HIE)
Health Level Seven International (HL7)
HIPAA transaction standards
HL7 EHR-S Functional Model
HITECH

HITECH EHR Certification Criteria
International Health Terminology Standards Development Organisation (IHTSDO)
Logical Observation Identifiers Names and Codes (LOINC)
Messaging standards
National Committee on Vital and Health Statistics (NCVHS)
National Council for Prescription Drug Programs (NCPDP)
National Drug Codes
National Library of Medicine (NLM)
National Uniform Billing Committee (NUBC)
National Uniform Claim Committee (NUCC)
Nationwide Health Information Network (NwHIN)
Network standards
Office of the National Coordinator for Health Information Technology (ONC)
RxNorm
Standards development organizations (SDOs)
Systematized Nomenclature of Medicine—Clinical Terms (SNOMED CT)
Unified Medical Language System (UMLS)
X12N standards

LEARNING ACTIVITIES

1. Standards development is a dynamic process. Select one or more of the standards listed in this chapter and conduct an Internet search for information on that standard. Has the standard changed? What are the current issues surrounding the standard?

2. Visit a hospital IT department and speak with a clinical analyst or other person who works with clinical applications. Investigate the standards that the hospital's applications use. Discuss any issues surrounding these standards.

3. Interview the chief information officer (CIO) of a health care organization. Find out his or her views on the current state of health care IT standards or on the need for standards as the United States moves toward broader adoption of EMR systems.

4. Visit the ONC web site at http://www.dhhs.gov/healthit/onc/mission. Discuss the efforts of the ONC as they relate to the adoption of health care IT standards.

5. As you reflect on the information in this chapter and your own research, compare and contrast the intent of "classification," "functional," "content," "messaging." and "transaction" health care IT standards.

REFERENCES

Accredited Standards Committee X12. (2012). X12N/TG2: Health care purpose and scope. Retrieved March 2012 from http://www.disa.org/x12org/subcommittees /sc_home.cfm?sendTo=PurposeAndScope.cfm&doSet=TRUE&CFID=5823233&CF TOKEN=37309527

American Dental Association. (2012). *Code on Dental Procedures and Nomenclature (CDT)*. Retrieved March 2012 from http://www.ada.org/3827.aspx

American National Standards Institute. (2012). Domestic programs (American National Standards) overview. *ANSI Standards Activities*. Retrieved March 2012 from http://ansi.org/standards_activities/domestic_programs/overview.aspx ?menuid=3

ASTM. (2012). *ASTM international standards for healthcare services, products and technology*. Retrieved March 2012 from http://www.astm.org/ABOUT/images /Medical_sector.pdf

Bazzoli, F. (2004, May). NAHIT IT standards directory aims to provide common ground. *Healthcare IT News*, p. 5.

Case, J. (2011). *Using RELMA or . . . in search of the missing LOINC*. PowerPoint presentation. Retrieved March 2012 from http://loinc.org/slideshows/lab -loinc-tutorial

Centers for Disease Control and Prevention. (2012). IIS: HL7 standard code set CVX—Vaccines administered. *Vaccines and Immunizations*. Retrieved March 2012 from http://www2a.cdc.gov/nip/IIS/IISStandards/vaccines.asp?rpt=cvx

Centers for Medicare and Medicaid. (2012a). Overview. *Transaction and code sets standards*. Retrieved March 2012 from http://www.cms.gov/Transaction CodeSetsStands/

Centers for Medicare and Medicaid. (2012b). Overview. *E-prescribing*. Retrieved March 2012 from https://www.cms.gov/EPrescribing/02_Adopted%20 Standard%20and%20Transactions.asp#TopOfPage

Centers for Medicare and Medicaid. (2012c). NCPDP flat file format. *NCPDP reference manual*. Retrieved March 2012 from http://www.cms.gov/Medicare/Billing /ElectronicBillingEDITrans/downloads/NCPDPflatfile.pdf

Corepoint Health. (2012). CCD: Continuity of care document. Retrieved March 2012 from http://www.corepointhealth.com/resource-center/hl7-resources/ccd

Department of Health and Human Services (HHS). (2008). *The ONC-coordinated federal health information technology strategic plan: 2008–2012*. Retrieved August 2008 from http://www.hhs.gov/healthit/resources/HITStrategicPlanSummary.pdf

Department of Health and Human Services (HHS). (2012a). About ONC. The Office of the National Coordinator for Health Information Technology. Retrieved March 2012 from http://healthit.hhs.gov/portal/server.pt/community/healthit_hhs _gov__onc/1200

Department of Health and Human Services (HHS). (2012b). ONC initiatives. The Office of the National Coordinator for Health Information Technology. Retrieved March 2012 from http://healthit.hhs.gov/portal/server.pt/community/healthit _hhs_gov__onc_initiatives/1497

Department of Health and Human Services (HHS). (2012c). Nationwide Health Information Network: Overview. The Office of the National Coordinator for Health Information Technology. Retrieved March 2012 from http://healthit.hhs .gov/portal/server.pt/community/healthit_hhs_gov__nationwide_health _information_network/1142

Department of Health and Human Services (HHS). (2012d). Standards and certification criteria final rule. The Office of the National Coordinator for Health Information Technology. Retrieved March 2012 from http://healthit.hhs.gov /portal/server.pt?open=512&objID=1195&parentname=CommunityPage&parentid =97&mode=2&in_hi_userid=11673&cached=true

DICOM. (2012). DICOM: *Digital Imaging and Communications in Medicine*. Retrieved March 2012 from http://medical.nema.org

Emdeon. (2012). *NCPCP D.0 HIPAA 5010: Frequently asked questions*. Retrieved March 2012 from http://www.emdeon.com/5010/pdfs/HIPAA_Simplified_FAQ -NCPDP_D%200_and_5010_Version_1-0.pdf

European Committee for Standardization (CEN). (2012a). What is CEN? CEN. Retrieved April 2012 from http://www.cen.eu/cen/AboutUs/WhatisCEN/Pages /default.aspx

European Committee for Standardization (CEN). (2012b). Technical committees. CEN. Retrieved April 2012 from http://www.cen.eu/cen/Sectors/Technical CommitteesWorkshops/TCs/Pages/default.aspx

Food and Drug Administration. (2012). *National Drug Code directory*. Retrieved March 2012 from http://www.fda.gov/Drugs/InformationOnDrugs/ucm142438 .htm

Hammond, W., & Cimino, J. (2006). Biomedical informatics. In E. Shortliffe & J. Cimino (Eds.), *Standards in biomedical informatics* (pp. 265–311). New York: Springer-Verlag.

HL7. (2007). HL7 EHR system functional model release 1. Retrieved March 2012 from https://www.hl7.org/implement/standards/product_brief.cfm?product_id=18

HL7. (2012). *About HL7*. Retrieved March 2012 from http://www.hl7.org/about /index.cfm

Libicki, M., Schneider, J., Frelinger, D., & Slomovic, A. (2000). *Scaffolding the new web: Standards and standards policy for the digital economy*. Santa Monica, CA: Rand.

Logical Observation Identifiers Names and Codes. (2012). *LOINC background*. Retrieved March 2012 from http://loinc.org/background

Marotta, D. (2000). *Healthcare informatics: HL7 in the 21st century*. Retrieved March 2004 from http://www.healthcare-informatics.com/issues/2000/04_00/h17.htm

National Committee on Vital and Health Statistics. (2003, November 5). *Letter to the secretary: Recommendations for PMRI terminology standards*. Retrieved March 2012 from http://www.ncvhs.hhs.gov/031105lt3.pdf

National Council for Prescription Drug Programs. (2012). About. Retrieved March 2012 from http://www.ncpdp.org/about.aspx

National Library of Medicine. (2008). *Unified Medical Language System® basics*. Retrieved March 2012 from http://www.nlm.nih.gov/research/umls/new_users /online_learning/OVR_001.htm

National Library of Medicine. (2012a). *Unified Medical Language System: SNOMED clinical terms (SNOMED CT)*. Retrieved March 2012 from http://www.nlm.nih .gov/research/umls/Snomed/snomed_main.html

National Library of Medicine. (2012b). An overview to RxNorm. *Unified Medical Language System® UMLS®*. Retrieved March 2012 from http://www.nlm.nih.gov /research/umls/rxnorm/overview.html

Office of Science and Technology Policy. (2010, December 8). President's Council of Advisors on Science and Technology releases report on health information technology (press release). Retrieved April 2012 from http://www.whitehouse .gov/sites/default/files/microsites/ostp/pcast-health-it-release.pdf

Ringholm. (2012). *HL7 message examples version 2 and version 3*. Retrieved March 2012 from http://www.ringholm.de/docs/04300_en.htm

Rouse, M. (2010, May). Continuity of care document. SearchHealthIT. Retrieved March 2012 from http://searchhealthit.techtarget.com/definition/Continuity -of-Care-Document-CCD

Sullivan, T. (2012, March 15). ONC to stand up NwHIN Exchange in October. *Government Health IT*. Retrieved April 2012 from http://www.govhealthit.com /news/onc-stand-nwhin-exchange-october.

Washington Dental Service. (2012). *CDT procedure code information*. Retrieved March 2012 from http://www.deltadentalwa.com/Dentist/Public/ResourceCenter/CDT %20Procedure%20Codes.aspx

Security of Health Care Information Systems

By now it should be clear that much of the information in today's health care organizations is transmitted, maintained, and stored electronically. Electronic health record (EHR) systems are becoming more common, and as we have seen, even primarily paper-based health care information systems contain a large quantity of data and information that have been created and transmitted electronically. Movement toward health information exchanges (HIEs) and a Nationwide Health Information Network (NwHIN), along with the general increase in the use of Internet-based solutions for transmitting data within and among health care organizations, has led to more confidential health care information than ever before being transmitted electronically. Securing this information and the systems that support it is a crucial function in the operation of health care organizations.

In this chapter we define security, examine the need for establishing an organization-wide security program, and discuss a variety of security-related topics. We look at the various existing threats to health care information. In addition, we outline the components of the Health Insurance Portability and Accountability Act (HIPAA) security regulations, including the recent updates to the regulations under the HITECH legislation. Although security concerns certainly predate the implementation of the HIPAA Security Rule, the standards in this rule provide an excellent and comprehensive outline of the components necessary for securing health information and, to some extent, provide a framework for establishing a viable health care information security program. The chapter then continues with a look at the following topics, including examples of actual practices and procedures:

- Administrative safeguards
- Physical safeguards
- Technical safeguards

A specific discussion of business continuity and disaster recovery planning for maintaining and restoring health care information is included in the Administrative Safeguards section. The chapter concludes with a discussion of the special security issues associated with increased use of wireless networks and related devices in health care organizations, along with a discussion of the security issues raised when employees have remote access to health care organizations' computer networks.

THE HEALTH CARE ORGANIZATION'S SECURITY PROGRAM

Health care organizations must protect their information systems from a range of potential threats. Among these threats are viruses, fire in the data center, untested software, and employee theft of clinical and administrative data. Threats may involve intentional or unintentional damage to hardware, software, or data or the misuse of the organization's hardware, software, or data. The realization of any of these threats can cause significant damage to the organization. Resorting to manual operations if the computers are down for days can lead to organizational chaos. Theft of organizational data can lead to litigation by the individuals harmed by the disclosure of the data. Viruses can corrupt databases, corruption from which there may be no recovery. Health care organizations must have programs in place to combat security breaches.

The function of the health care organization's security program is to identify potential threats and implement processes to remove these threats or mitigate their ability to cause damage. For example, the use of antivirus software is designed to reduce the threat from viruses; the installation of fire protection systems in data centers is intended to reduce the damage that might be caused by a fire.

It is important to understand how patient privacy is related to security. The intentional or unintentional release of patient-identifiable information constitutes a misuse of the organization's information systems. Security in a health care organization should be designed, however, to protect not only patient-specific information but also the organization's IT assets—such as the networks, hardware, software, and applications that make up the organization's health care information systems—from potential threats, both threats that come from human beings and those that come from natural and environmental causes.

The primary challenge of developing an effective security program in a health care organization is balancing the need for security with the cost of security. An organization does not know how to calculate the likelihood that a hacker will cause serious damage or a backhoe will cut through network cables under the street. The organization may not fully understand the consequences of being without its network for four hours or four days. Hence, it may not be sure how much to spend to remove or reduce the risk. This dilemma is similar to the one posed when individuals consider obtaining long-term care insurance. None of us know whether we will or will not need this insurance, how long we might live in a long-term care facility, or the acuity of the care we may need. How much insurance should we buy?

One aspect of this challenge is maintaining a satisfactory balance between health care information system security and health care data and information availability. As we saw in Chapter One, the major purpose of maintaining health information and health records is to facilitate high-quality care for patients. On the one hand, if an organization's security measures are so stringent that they prevent appropriate access to the health information needed to care for patients, this important purpose is undermined. On the other hand, if the organization allows unrestricted access to all patient-identifiable information to all its employees, the patients' rights to privacy and confidentiality would certainly be violated and the organization's IT assets would be at considerable risk.

As health care organizations develop their security programs, they should be sure to seek input from a wide range of health care providers and other system users as well as legal counsel and technical experts. The balance between access and security should be reasonable—protecting patients' rights while allowing appropriate access.

THREATS TO HEALTH CARE INFORMATION

What are the threats to health care information systems? In general, threats to health care information systems fall into one of these three categories:

- Human threats, which can result from intentional or unintentional human tampering

- Natural and environmental threats, such as floods, fires, and power outages

- Technology malfunctions, such as a drive that fails and has no backup

Within these categories are multiple potential threats. Threats to health care information systems from human beings can be intentional or unintentional. They can be *internal*, caused by employees, or *external*, caused by individuals outside the organization. Intentional threats include theft, intentional alteration of data, and intentional destruction of data. The culprit could be a disgruntled employee, a computer hacker, or a prankster. In a Florida case several years ago, for example, the daughter of a hospital employee accessed confidential information through an unattended computer workstation in the facility's emergency room. She wrote down names and addresses of recent patients and then called to tell them that they had tested positive for HIV. Several of the recipients of these prank calls became extremely distraught (Associated Press, 1995).

Computer viruses are among the most common and virulent forms of intentional computer tampering. They pose a serious threat to computerized patient data and health care applications. (See the section on virus checking later in this chapter for more information on viruses.) Some of the causes of unintentional damage to health care information systems are lack of training in proper use of the system or human error. When users share passwords or download information from a nonsecure Internet site, for example, they create the potential for a breach in security.

Internal breaches of security are far more common than external breaches. Some of the more common forms of internal breaches of security across all industries are the installation or use of unauthorized software, use of the organization's computing resources for illegal or illicit communications or activities (porn surfing, e-mail harassment, and so forth), and the use of the organization's computing resources for personal profit.

Computer hardware used in health care information systems must also be protected from loss. In recent years there have been multiple instances of computer thefts from health care organizations, resulting in exposure of confidential patient information. Data reported by HHS Office of Civil Rights show that nearly seven million patients were affected by data breaches from September 2008 to December 2010. The majority of these breaches were caused by theft. The most common location for the breached information was a laptop computer (Keckley, Coughlin, & Gupta, 2011).

Electronic health care information is vulnerable to internal and external threats. Whether intentional or unintentional, these threats pose serious security risks. To minimize the risk and protect patients' sensitive health care information, well-established and well-implemented administrative, physical, and technical security safeguards are essential for any health care organization, regardless of size.

The security standards established by the Department of Health and Human Services under the terms of the Health Insurance Portability and Accountability Act (HIPAA) provide an excellent framework for developing an overall security plan and program for a health care institution. The regulations are designed to be flexible and scalable and are not reliant on specific technologies for implementation, making it possible for health care organizations of all sizes to be compliant.

OVERVIEW OF THE HIPAA SECURITY RULE

The final rule on the HIPAA security standards, known generally as the Security Rule, was published in the Federal Register on February 20, 2003 (68 Fed. Reg. 34, 8333–8381). It was subsequently updated by the HITECH legislation. (In Chapter Three we looked at the various components of the far-reaching HIPAA legislation. In this section we discuss the security component in greater detail. You may wish to refer back to Chapter Three for a description of how the Security Rule fits into the overall Act.) The HIPAA Security Rule is closely connected to the HIPAA Privacy Rule (also discussed in Chapter Three). However, whereas the Privacy Rule governs all protected health information

(PHI), the Security Rule governs only ePHI. *EPHI* is defined as protected health information maintained or transmitted in electronic form. The Security Rule does not distinguish between electronic forms of information or between transmission mechanisms. EPHI may be stored in any type of electronic media, such as magnetic tapes and disks, optical disks, servers, and personal computers. Transmission may take place over the Internet, on local area networks (LANs), or by disks, for example.

The *HIPAA Security Rule* was first published, in draft form, in August 1998. At that time one of the complaints was that the standards were too prescriptive and not flexible enough. As a result the standards in the final rule were defined in general terms, focusing on what should be done rather than on how it should be done. According to the Centers for Medicare and Medicaid Services (CMS, 2004), the final rule specifies "a series of administrative, technical, and physical security procedures for covered entities to use to assure the confidentiality of electronic protected health information. The standards are delineated into either required or addressable implementation specifications."

There are a few key terms to be defined before we examine the content of the HIPAA Security Rule. What is a covered entity? What is the difference between a required implementation specification and an addressable one?

The HIPAA standards govern *covered entities* (CEs), which are defined as

- A health plan.
- A health care clearinghouse.
- A health care provider who transmits protected health information in electronic form. This includes practically every type of health care organization imaginable, including hospitals, clinics, physicians' offices, nursing homes, and so forth.

The specifications contained in the Security Rule are designated as either *required* or *addressable*. A required specification must be implemented by a CE for that organization to be in compliance. However, the CE is in compliance with an addressable specification if it does any one of the following:

- Implements the specification as stated.
- Implements an alternative security measure to accomplish the purposes of the standard or specification.
- Chooses not to implement anything, provided it can demonstrate that the standard or specification is not reasonable and appropriate and that the purpose of the standard can still be met. Because the Security Rule is designed to be technology neutral, this flexibility was granted

for organizations that employ nonstandard technologies or have legitimate reasons not to need the stated specification (AHIMA, 2003).

The standards contained in the HIPAA Security Rule are divided into sections, or categories, the specifics of which we outline here. You will notice overlap among the sections. For example, contingency plans are covered under both administrative and physical safeguards, and access controls are addressed in several standards and specifications. In subsequent sections of this chapter we will look at some actual practices that might be employed by health care organizations in each of the first four categories. As you read through this outline, consider how it would work as a framework or model for a health care organization's security program.

OUTLINE OF THE HIPAA SECURITY RULE

The Administrative Safeguards section of the Final Rule contains nine standards:

1. **Security management functions.** This standard requires the CE to implement policies and procedures to prevent, detect, contain, and correct security violations. There are four implementation specifications for this standard:
   - *Risk analysis* (required). The CE must conduct an accurate and thorough assessment of the potential risks to and vulnerabilities of the confidentiality, integrity, and availability of ePHI.
   - *Risk management* (required). The CE must implement security measures that reduce risks and vulnerabilities to a reasonable and appropriate level.
   - *Sanction policy* (required). The CE must apply appropriate sanctions against workforce members who fail to comply with the CE's security policies and procedures.
   - *Information system activity review* (required). The CE must implement procedures to regularly review records of information system activity, such as audit logs, access reports, and security incident tracking reports.
2. **Assigned security responsibility.** This standard does not have any implementation specifications. It requires the CE to identify the individual responsible for overseeing development of the organization's security policies and procedures.

3. **Workforce security.** This standard requires the CE to implement policies and procedures to ensure that all members of its workforce have appropriate access to ePHI and to prevent those workforce members who do not have access from obtaining access. There are three implementation specifications for this standard:

   - *Authorization and/or supervision* (addressable). The CE must have a process for ensuring that the workforce working with ePHI has adequate authorization and supervision.

   - *Workforce clearance procedure* (addressable). There must be a process to determine what access is appropriate for each workforce member.

   - *Termination procedures* (addressable). There must be a process for terminating access to ePHI when a workforce member is no longer employed or his or her responsibilities change.

4. **Information access management.** This standard requires the CE to implement policies and procedures for authorizing access to ePHI. There are three implementation specifications within this standard. The first (not shown here) applies to health care clearinghouses, and the other two apply to health care organizations:

   - *Access authorization* (addressable). The CE must have a process for granting access to ePHI through a workstation, transaction, program, or other process.

   - *Access establishment and modification* (addressable). The CE must have a process (based on the access authorization) to establish, document, review, and modify a user's right to access a workstation, transaction, program, or process.

5. **Security awareness and training.** This standard requires the CE to implement awareness and training programs for all members of its workforce. This training should include periodic security reminders and address protection from malicious software, log-in monitoring, and password management. (These items to be addressed in training are all listed as addressable implementation specifications.)

6. **Security incident reporting.** This standard requires the CE to implement policies and procedures to address security incidents.

7. **Contingency plan.** This standard has five implementation specifications:

   - *Data backup plan* (required).

   - *Disaster recovery plan* (required).

- *Emergency mode operation plan* (required).

- *Testing and revision procedures* (addressable). The CE should periodically test and modify all contingency plans.

- *Applications and data criticality analysis* (addressable). The CE should assess the relative criticality of specific applications and data in support of its contingency plan.

8. **Evaluation.** This standard requires the CE to periodically perform technical and nontechnical evaluations in response to changes that may affect the security of ePHI.

9. **Business associate contracts and other arrangements.** This standard outlines the conditions under which a CE must have a formal agreement with business associates in order to exchange ePHI.

The Physical Safeguards section contains four standards:

1. **Facility access controls.** This standard requires the CE to implement policies and procedures to limit physical access to its electronic information systems and the facilities in which they are housed to authorized users. There are four implementation specifications with this standard:

   - *Contingency operations* (addressable). The CE should have a process for allowing facility access to support the restoration of lost data under the disaster recovery plan and emergency mode operation plan.

   - *Facility security plan* (addressable). The CE must have a process to safeguard the facility and its equipment from unauthorized access, tampering, and theft.

   - *Access control and validation* (addressable). The CE should have a process to control and validate access to facilities based on users' roles or functions.

   - *Maintenance records* (addressable). The CE should have a process to document repairs and modifications to the physical components of a facility as they relate to security.

2. **Workstation use.** This standard requires the CE to implement policies and procedures that specify the proper functions to be performed and the manner in which those functions are to be performed on a specific workstation or class of workstation that can be used to access ePHI, and that also specify the physical attributes of the surroundings of such workstations.

3. **Workstation security.** This standard requires the CE to implement physical safeguards for all workstations that are used to access ePHI and to restrict access to authorized users.

4. **Device and media controls.** This standard requires the CE to implement policies and procedures for the movement of hardware and electronic media that contain ePHI into and out of a facility and within a facility. There are four implementation specifications with this standard:

- *Disposal* (required). The CE must have a process for the final disposition of ePHI and of the hardware and electronic media on which it is stored.

- *Media reuse* (required). The CE must have a process for removal of ePHI from electronic media before the media can be reused.

- *Accountability* (addressable). The CE must maintain a record of movements of hardware and electronic media and any person responsible for these items.

- *Data backup and storage* (addressable). The CE must create a retrievable, exact copy of ePHI, when needed, before movement of equipment.

The Technical Safeguards section has five standards:

1. **Access control.** This standard requires the CE to implement technical policies and procedures for electronic information systems that maintain ePHI in order to allow access only to those persons or software programs that have been granted access rights as specified in the administrative safeguards. There are four implementation specifications within this standard:

- *Unique user identification* (required). The CE must assign a unique name or number for identifying and tracking each user's identity.

- *Emergency access procedure* (required). The CE must establish procedures for obtaining necessary ePHI in an emergency.

- *Automatic log-off* (addressable). The CE must implement electronic processes that terminate an electronic session after a predetermined time of inactivity.

- *Encryption and decryption* (addressable). The CE should implement a mechanism to encrypt and decrypt ePHI as needed.

2. **Audit controls.** This standard requires the CE to implement hardware, software, and procedures that record and examine activity in the information systems that contain ePHI.

3. **Integrity.** This standard requires the CE to implement policies and procedures to protect ePHI from improper alteration or destruction.

4. **Person or entity authentication.** This standard requires the CE to implement procedures to verify that a person or entity seeking access to ePHI is in fact the person or entity claimed.

5. **Transmission security.** This standard requires the CE to implement technical measures to guard against unauthorized access to ePHI being transmitted across a network. There are two implementation specifications with this standard:

   - *Integrity controls* (addressable). The CE must implement security measures to ensure that electronically transmitted ePHI is not improperly modified without detection.

   - *Encryption* (addressable). The CE should encrypt ePHI whenever it is deemed appropriate.

The Policies, Procedures, and Documentation section has two standards:

1. **Policies and procedures.** This standard requires the CE to establish and implement policies and procedures to comply with the standards, implementation specifications, and other requirements.

2. **Documentation.** This standard requires the CE to maintain the policies and procedures implemented to comply with the Security Rule in written form. There are three implementation specifications:

   - *Time limit* (required). The CE must retain the documentation for six years from the date of its creation or the date when it was last in effect, whichever is later.

   - *Availability* (required). The CE must make the documentation available to those persons responsible for implementing the policies and procedures.

   - *Updates* (required). The CE must review the documentation periodically and update it as needed.

HITECH EXPANSION OF THE HIPAA SECURITY RULE

In 2009, the Health Information Technology for Economic and Clinical Health (HITECH) Act was signed by President Obama. Among other things, this Act expanded the HIPAA Privacy and Security Rules. The expansion to the Security Rule includes

- Applying the requirements directly to business associates
- Establishing mandatory federal security breach reporting requirements
- Establishing new criminal and civil penalties and enforcement responsibilities for noncompliance

Under HITECH, any HIPAA-covered entity or business associate (including HIEs) that "accesses, maintains, retains, modifies, records, stores, destroys or otherwise holds, uses or discloses *unsecured protected health information*" must notify each individual affected by a breach of health information (68 Fed. Reg. 34, 8333–8381, Feb. 20, 2003). This notification must be made by first-class mail within sixty days of discovery. If more than ten individuals are involved, the entity must post the facts of the breach to a conspicuous web site or by means of major print or broadcast media. If more than five hundred individuals are involved, the entity must report the breach to "prominent media outlets." It is important to note that HITECH defines *unsecured protected health information* as PHI not secured through the use of technology or methodology specified by HHS guidance (Coppersmith, Gordon, Schermer, & Brockelman, PLC, 2012). By implementing adequate security programs that adhere to HHS guidance, health care organizations can avoid the necessity of potentially harmful and expensive public notification if a theft or loss of PHI occurs.

HITECH gave the responsibility for enforcing the HIPAA Privacy and Security Rules to the Office of Civil Rights (OCR) beginning in July 2009. Since that time they have received over five hundred complaints specific to the Security Rule. The results of these OCR enforcement activities and those for the Privacy Rule, including specific case examples, are available to the public at http://www.hhs.gov/ocr/privacy/hipaa/enforcement/index.html.

This section has provided an outline of the key components of the HIPAA security standards published in 2003 (68 Fed. Reg. 34, 8333–8381, Feb. 20, 2003) and the HITECH expansion. In the next sections we will examine some of the practices that can be employed to address the regulations and ensure that an organization has an effective security program.

ADMINISTRATIVE SAFEGUARDS

As you have seen from the HIPAA security standards outline, *administrative safeguards* cover a wide range of organizational activities. We do not attempt in this section to give a comprehensive, detailed view of all possible administrative safeguards but rather to present a few practices that can be used as part of a total administrative effort to improve the health care organization's information security program. We will discuss the following topics:

- Risk analysis and management
- Chief security officer
- System security evaluation
- Contingency, business continuity, and disaster recovery planning

Risk Analysis and Management

One of the key components of applying administrative safeguards to protect the organization's health care information is *risk analysis*. It is impossible to establish an effective risk management program if the organization is not aware of the risks or threats that exist. Risk analysis is relatively new to health care. Few organizations had implemented formal security risk assessment prior to the publication of the HIPAA rules. This in no way minimizes its importance. However, health care has had to look to other industries for examples of risk assessment processes (Reynolds, 2009; Walsh, 2003).

Steve Weil (2004) defines risk as the "likelihood that a specific threat will exploit a certain vulnerability, and the resulting impact of that event." He introduces a risk analysis process with eight parts, or steps:

1. **Boundary definition.** During the boundary definition step, the organization should develop a detailed inventory of all health information and information systems. This review can be conducted using interviews, inspections, questionnaires, or other means. The important thing in this step is to identify all the patient-specific health information, health care information systems (both internal and external), and users of the information and systems.

2. **Threat identification.** Identifying threats will result in a list of all potential threats to the organization's health care information systems. The three general types of threats that should be considered are

   a. Natural, such as floods and fires

   b. Human, which can be intentional or unintentional

   c. Environmental, such as power outages

3. **Vulnerability identification.** In this step the organization identifies all the specific vulnerabilities that exist in its own health care information systems. Generally, vulnerabilities take the form of flaws or weaknesses in system procedures or design. Software packages are available to assist with identifying vulnerabilities, but the organization may also need to conduct interviews, surveys, and the like. Some organizations may employ external consultants to help them identify the vulnerabilities in their systems.

4. **Security control analysis.** The organization also needs to conduct a thorough analysis of the security controls that are currently in place. These include both preventive controls, such as access controls and authentication procedures, and controls designed to detect actual or potential breaches, such as audit trails and alarms.

5. **Risk likelihood determination.** This step in the process involves assigning a risk rating to each area of the health care information system. There is a variety of rating systems that may be employed. Weil recommends using a fairly straightforward high-risk, medium-risk, and low-risk system of rating.

6. **Impact analysis.** This is the step in which the organization determines what the actual impact of specific security breaches would be. A breach may affect confidentiality, integrity, or availability. Impact, too, can be rated as high, medium, or low.

Table 11.1 lists the three security objectives—confidentiality, integrity, and availability, the definitions of each, and examples of potential impacts should the objective be lost or compromised (Scholl et al., 2008).

Table 11.1. Security objectives

Security Objective	Definition	Examples of Impact if Compromised
Confidentiality	Protection of information from unauthorized disclosure	Loss of public confidence, embarrassment, financial loss due to legal action
Integrity	Protection of information from improper modification	Data inaccuracy, fraud, or erroneous decisions; could lead to loss of confidentiality or system availability
Availability	Availability of functioning mission-critical IT systems	Loss of productive time, decreased end users' performance, compromised organizational mission

7. **Risk determination.** The information gathered up to this point in the risk analysis process is now brought together in order to determine the actual level of risk to specific information and specific information systems. The risk determination is based on

   a. The likelihood that a certain threat will attempt to exploit a specific vulnerability (high, medium, or low)

   b. The level of impact should the threat successfully exploit the vulnerability (high, medium, or low)

   c. The adequacy of planned or existing security controls (high, medium, or low)

   Each specific system or type of information can be assessed for each of these three factors, and then these assessments can be combined to produce an overall risk rating of high (needing immediate attention), medium (needing attention soon), or low (existing controls are acceptable).

8. **Security control recommendations.** The final step of the process is to compile a summary report on the findings of the analysis and recommendations for improving security controls.

The risk analysis should lead to the development of policies and procedures outlining risk management procedures and sanctions or consequences for employees and other individuals who do not follow the established procedures. All health care organizations should have a formal security risk management program in place. In general, this program is administered by the organization's security officer.

Chief Security Officer

Each health care organization must have a single individual who is responsible for overseeing the information security program. Generally, this individual is identified as the organization's *chief security officer*. The chief security officer may report to the chief information officer (CIO) or to another administrator in the health care organization. The role of security officer may be 100 percent of an individual's job responsibilities or only a fraction, depending on the size of the organization and the scope of its health care information systems. Regardless of the actual reporting structure, it is essential that the chief security officer be given the authority to effectively manage the security program, apply sanctions, and influence employees. As Tom Walsh (2003, p. 15) stated in identifying the importance of the security officer, "Influence can leverage the right people to get the job done."

System Security Evaluation

Chief security officers must periodically evaluate their organization's health care information systems and networks for proper technical controls and processes. There are several useful resources available to facilitate the technical security evaluation. The U.S. Department of Commerce National Institute of Standards and Technology (NIST) Computer Security Division publishes over three hundred information security documents, including the Federal Information Processing Standards (FIPS), the Special Publication (SP) 800 series and others. NIST Special Publication 800–66 provides an introductory resource for implementing the HIPAA Security Rule that references existing federal information security guidance. Although HIPAA-covered entities and business associates are not required to follow this guidance, it provides them with a description of technologies and methodologies to secure their PHI. Entities that effectively secure PHI can avoid the extensive HITECH notification requirements in the event of a breach in security (AMA, 2010).

There are also general standards for security technologies that span all types of organizations developed by the International Organization for Standardization (ISO) as ISO Standard 15408 (titled Information Technology—Security Techniques—Evaluation Criteria for IT Security). These standards, updated in 2009, allow any organization to use a common set of requirements and thus to compare the results of independent security evaluations (ISO, 2009).

Contingency, Business Continuity, and Disaster Recovery Planning

The National Institute for Standards and Technology (NIST) identifies three types of contingency-related plans: the *continuity of operations plan* (also known as business continuity plan), *contingency plan*, and *disaster recovery plan*. Table 11.2 defines and compares the typical scope of each type of plan (Scholl et al., 2008).

In reality, a health care organization is likely to have a set of plans. According to the NIST, this suite of plans is necessary "to properly prepare response, recovery, and continuity activities for disruptions affecting the organization's IT systems, business processes, and the facility" (Scholl et al., 2008). These plans must be coordinated to prevent duplication or contradiction of guidance. Ideally, all contingency plans would be coordinated to create a comprehensive, robust, enterprise-wide business continuity plan.

Table 11.2. Types of contingency-related plans

Type of Plan	Description	Scope
Continuity of operations plan (aka business continuity plan)	A predetermined set of instructions or procedures that describe how an organization's essential functions will be sustained for up to thirty days as a result of a disaster event before returning to normal operations	Addresses the organization's critical missions; not specifically IT-focused
Contingency plan	Management policy and procedures designed to maintain or restore business operations, including computer operations, possibly at an alternate location, in the event of emergencies, system failures, or disasters	Addresses the organization's IT disruptions
Disaster recovery plan	A written plan for processing critical applications in the event of a major hardware or software failure or destruction of facilities	Limited to major disruptions with long-term effects; typically IT-focused

Contingency Plan

The HIPAA Security Rule specifically addresses contingency plans for ePHI under the Administrative Safeguards section. In addition, contingency and disaster recovery planning and related activities for ePHI are mentioned in several other sections of the regulations. As outlined earlier in the chapter, there are specific components of the contingency plan that covered entities must address. The NIST offers detailed guidance in its publication 800–66, *An Introductory Resource Guide for Implementing the Health Insurance Portability and Accountability Act (HIPAA) Security Rule*, Appendix F. NIST (Scholl et al., 2008) defines contingency planning as generally including one or more of three approaches to restoring disrupted IT services:

- Restoring IT operations at an alternate location.
- Recovering IT operations using alternative equipment.
- Performing some or all of the affected business processes using non-IT (manual) means. This approach is typically only acceptable as a solution for short-term disruptions.

The NIST also offers a specific approach to developing contingency plans. The entire approach is beyond the scope of this chapter, but the following provides a brief outline of each step (Scholl et al., 2008):

1. Develop the contingency planning policy statement
2. Conduct the business impact analysis (BIA)
   a. Identify critical IT resources
   b. Identify disruption impacts
   c. Identify allowable outage times
   d. Develop recovery priorities
3. Identify preventative controls (see the Perspective for a list of potential preventative controls)
4. Develop recovery strategies
5. Develop an IT contingency plan with the following components:
   a. Supporting information (introduction, background, and so forth)
   b. Notification and activation
   c. Recovery phase
   d. Reconstitution phase
   e. Appendixes listing personnel and vendor contact lists
6. Conduct plan testing, training, and exercises
7. Maintain the plan

PERSPECTIVE
Common Preventative Controls

- Appropriately sized uninterruptible power supplies (UPSs) to provide short-term backup power to all system components
- Gasoline- or diesel-powered generators to provide long-term backup power
- Air-conditioning system with adequate excess capacity to permit failure of certain components, such as a compressor
- Fire suppression systems
- Fire and smoke detectors
- Water sensors in the computer room ceiling and floor

- Plastic tarps that may be unrolled over IT equipment to protect from water damage
- Heat-resistant and waterproof containers for backup media and vital nonelectronic records
- Emergency master system shutdown switch
- Offsite storage of backup media, nonelectronic records, and system documentation
- Technical security controls, such as cryptographic key management and least-privilege access controls
- Frequent scheduled backups

Source: Scholl et al., 2008.

Challenges to the Health Care Organization Business Continuity Plan

Rozek and Groth (2008) discuss the challenges faced by health care organizations in developing and managing a "robust" *business continuity plan (BCP)*. One challenge is the increased use of digital technology in the provision of care. This trend is likely to continue. However, the health care organization's BCP should not be driven solely by its IT needs. Another challenge in creating a robust BCP is the nature of the business structures within health care. Many are decentralized, with nearly autonomous departments. This may lead to multiple BCPs that must be coordinated into an effective enterprise-wide overall plan. A third challenge is the number and disparate nature of the business partnerships in health care. Often critical business functions are outsourced to other organizations and vendors. Departments or services may in fact be fully staffed and managed by employees of an outside partner. Health care organizations must view the development of a well-coordinated, robust, enterprise-wide BCP as an ongoing activity.

PHYSICAL SAFEGUARDS

A security program must address physical as well as technical and administrative safeguards. *Physical safeguards* involve protecting the actual computer hardware, software, data, and information from physical damage or loss due to natural, human, or environmental threats. Several specific issues related to physical security are addressed in this section:

- Assigned security responsibility
- Media controls
- Physical access controls
- Workstation security

Assigned Security Responsibility

Each component of the health care information system should be secure, and one easily identifiable employee should be responsible for that security. These individuals are in turn accountable to the chief security officer. For example, in a nursing department the department manager might be responsible for ensuring that all employees have been trained to understand and use security measures and that they know the importance of maintaining the security of patient information. The network administrator, however, might be the person responsible for assigning initial passwords and removing access from terminated employees or employees who transfer to other departments (Reynolds, 2009).

Media Controls

The physical media on which health information is stored must be physically protected. *Media controls* are the policies and procedures that govern the receipt and removal of hardware, software, and computer media such as disks and tapes into and out of the organization and also their movements inside the organization.

Media controls also encompass data storage. Backup tapes, for example, must be stored in a secure area with limited access. The final disposition of electronic media is another aspect of media controls. Policies for the destruction of patient information must address the electronic media and hardware (workstations and servers) that contain patient information. As organizations gather old computers, all patient data must be removed before this equipment goes to surplus or is otherwise disposed of (Reynolds, 2009).

Physical Access Controls

Physical access controls are designed to limit physical access to health information to persons authorized to see that information. Locks and keys are examples of physical access controls. However, it is obvious that not all workstations can be kept under lock and key. This might create a secure system, but it would not be readily available to the health care providers who need patient information. Some of the physical access control components that can be employed are equipment control; a facility security plan; procedures that verify user identity before allowing physical access to an area; a procedure for maintaining records of repairs and modifications to hardware, software, and physical facilities; and a visitor sign-in procedure. Organizations should have a system, such as an inventory control system, that tells them exactly what equipment is currently in use in their health care information system. An inventory control system generally involves marking or tagging each piece of equipment with a unique number and assigning each piece to a location and a responsible person. When equipment is moved, retired, or destroyed, that action must be documented in the inventory control system. Another form of equipment control is to install antitheft devices, such as chains that attach computers to desks, alarms, and other tools that deter thieves.

A facility security plan is one that ensures that the individuals in a certain area are authorized to have access to that area. The main computer operations of a health care organization will generally be under tight security, including video surveillance and personal security checks. Badges with photographs are common in health care facilities to help identify personnel who are authorized to access certain buildings and facilities. Some secure areas require individuals to punch a code into a keypad or swipe an identification card over a card reader before entry is allowed. The facility security plan should also have procedures for admitting visitors. Each visitor might sign in and be issued a temporary identification badge, for example. There may be areas of the organization that are not open to visitors at all (Reynolds, 2009).

Workstation Security

Workstations that allow access to patient information should be placed in areas that are secure or monitored at all times. The workstations in the reception area or other public areas should be situated so that visitors or others cannot read the screens. Devices can be placed over workstation monitors that prevent people from reading a screen unless they are directly in front of it. Another aspect of workstation security is developing clear policies for workstation use. These policies should delineate, among other things, the appropriate functions to perform on the workstation and rules for sharing workstations.

Organizations that allow personnel to work from home have additional workstation security issues. Employees working from home must be given clear guidance on appropriate use of the organization's computer resources, whether these resources involve hardware, software, or web access. Employees should access any patient-identifiable information through a secure connection, with adequate monitoring to ensure that the user is in fact the authorized employee. (Specific remote access guidelines are discussed later in this chapter.)

All the aspects of physical security require adequate training of all personnel with potential access to the health care information systems. Employees, agents, and contractors with access to locations that house patient information must all participate in security and confidentiality awareness education (Reynolds, 2009).

TECHNICAL SAFEGUARDS

Many different *technical safeguards* can be used to help secure health care information systems and the networks on which they reside. Again, we will not provide a comprehensive list of all available safeguards but will present a few representative examples. We will discuss technical safeguards related to the following topics:

- Access control
- Entity authentication
- Audit trails
- Data encryption
- Firewall protection
- Virus checking

Access Control

Only individuals with a *need to know* should have access to patient-identifiable health information. Modern computer systems, including databases and networks, allow users to access a variety of resources such as individual files, database files, and tapes and to use printers and other peripheral devices. This sharing of resources is an important component of effective health care information systems, but it requires that network administrators and database administrators set appropriate access rights for each resource. Often users of a health care information system have to be assigned network access rights and separate application access rights before they can use the system.

Control over access to health data may involve any of the following methods:

- User-based access
- Role-based access
- Context-based access

Before we discuss each of these options, a brief explanation of access rights is necessary. Traditional user-based and role-based access rights have two parameters—who and how. The *who* is a list of the users with rights to access the information or computer resource in question. This list, called an *access control list*, may be organized by individual users or by groups of users. These groups are generally defined by role or job function. For example, all coders in the health information management department would be granted the same access rights, all registered nurses in a particular job classification would be granted the same access, and so forth.

The *how* parameter of the access control scheme specifies how a user may access the resource. Typical actions users might be allowed to take are read, write, edit, execute, append, and print. Only so-called owners and administrators will be granted full rights so that they can modify or delete or create new components for the resource. Clearly, owner and administrative privileges for the use of health care information systems should be carefully monitored.

User-based access control is defined as "a security mechanism used to grant users of a system access based upon the identity of the user." With *role-based access* control (RBAC), access decisions are based on the roles individual users have within the organization. "With RBAC, rather than attempting to map an organization's security policy to a relatively low-level set of technical controls (typically, access control lists), each user is assigned to one or more predefined roles, each of which has been assigned the various privileges needed to perform the role" (63 Fed. Reg. 155, August 12, 1998). One of the benefits of role-based over user-based access is that as new applications are added, privileges are more easily assigned. Discretionary assignment of access by an administrator is limited with RBAC. Users must be assigned to a specific role in order to be assigned access to a specific application.

Context-based access control is the most stringent of the three options. Harry Smith (2001) describes it this way: "A context-based access control scheme begins with the protection afforded by either a user-based or role-based access control design and takes it one step further . . . Context-based access control takes into account the person attempting to access the data, the type of data being accessed and the *context* of the transaction in which the access attempt is made." In other words, the context-based access has three parameters to consider: the who, the how, and the context in which the data are to be accessed. The Case Study here illustrates the differences among the three types of access control (Reynolds, 2009).

CASE STUDY
Three Types of Access Control

Mary Smith is the director of the Health Information Management Department in a hospital. Under a user-based access control scheme, Mary would be allowed read-only access to the hospital's laboratory information system because of her personal identity—that is, because she is Mary Smith and uses the proper log-in and password(s) to get into the system. Under a role-based control scheme, Mary would be allowed read-only access to the hospital's lab system because she is part of the Health Information Management Department and all department employees have been granted read-only privileges for this system. If the hospital were to adopt a context-based control scheme, Mary might be allowed access to the lab system only from her own workstation or another workstation in the Health Information Services Department, provided she used her proper log-in and password. If she attempted to log in from the Emergency Department or another administrative office, she might be denied access. The context control could also involve time of day. Because Mary is a daytime employee, she might be denied access if she attempted to log in at night.

Entity Authentication

Access control mechanisms are effective means of controlling who gains entry to a health care information system only when there is a system for ensuring the identity of the individual attempting to gain access. *Entity authentication* is defined in the HIPAA Security Rule as "the corroboration that a person is the one claimed." Entity authentication associated with health care information systems should include at least (1) automatic log-off and (2) a unique user identifier (Reynolds, 2009).

Automatic log-off is a security procedure that causes a computer session to end after a predetermined period of inactivity, such as ten minutes. Multiple software products are available that allow network administrators to set automatic log-off parameters. Once installed, these log-off systems act like any other screensaver on a typical workstation, coming on after a set period of inactivity. Users are then required to enter a network password to deactivate the log-off system screen. Generally, a device driver is also installed that prevents rebooting to deactivate the log-off system. Other security measures that may be included in automatic log-off products are features that prevent users from changing the screensaver and that allow an authorized person to set local password options in case the user is not connected to the network. Failed log-in attempts may be recorded and reported on, along with statistics on user log-ins, elapsed time, and user identification.

Each user of a health care information system must be assigned a unique identifier. This identifier is a combination of characters and numbers assigned and maintained by the security system. It is used to track individual user activity. This identifier is commonly called the *user ID* or *log-on ID*. It is the *public*, or known, portion of most user log-on procedures. For example, many organizations will assign a log-on identifier that is the same as the user's e-mail address or a combination of the user's last and first name. It is generally fairly easy to identify a user by his or her log-on. John Doe's log-on identifier might be "doej," for example. Because of the public nature of the log-in, additional safeguards beyond the log-on ID are needed.

Entity authentication can be implemented in a number of different ways in a health care information system. The most common entity authentication method is a *password system*. Other mechanisms include *personal identification numbers (PINs)*, *biometric identification systems, telephone callback procedures*, and *tokens*. These implementation methods can be used alone or in combination with other systems. Security experts often encourage *layered* security systems that use more than one security mechanism. As one security expert has stated, "A series of overlapping solutions works much more effectively, even when you know the solutions are individually fallible. If you line up three security controls that are each 60 percent effective, together they're something like 90 percent effective against a given attack" (Briney, 2000).

Walsh (2003) recommends a system that uses a *two-factor* authentication. He identifies these three methods for authentication, and any two of them used together would constitute a two-factor system:

- Something you know, such as a password or personal identification number (PIN)
- Something you have, such as an ATM card, token, or swipe card
- Something you are, such as a biometric fingerprint, voice scan, or iris or retinal scan [Walsh, 2003].

Password Systems

The most common way to control access to a health care information system (or any other computer system, for that matter) is through a combination of the user ID and a password or PIN. User IDs and passwords for a system are maintained either as a part of the access control list for the network or local operating system or in a special database. The list or database is then searched for a match before the user is allowed to access the system requested. Although the user ID is not secret, the password or PIN is. Passwords are generally stored in an encrypted form for which no decryption is available (Oz, 2009; White, 2011).

Although password and PIN systems are the most common forms of entity authentication, they also provide the weakest form of security. A *password* is defined by TechTarget (2012) as an "unspaced sequence of characters used to determine that a computer user requesting access to a computer system is really that particular user." Typically, a password is made up of four to sixteen characters. One of the biggest problems with passwords is that users may share them or publicly display them. Users will often write down passwords they cannot remember. They may even tape or post the password on the computer workstation. Health care organizations must take steps to prevent this type of password misuse. Clear policies on the use and maintenance of passwords, education for employees, and meaningful sanctions for policy violators are essential.

Another common problem with passwords is that when they are simple enough to remember, they may be simple enough for someone else to guess. Passwords are encrypted, but there are software programs available, called *password crackers,* that can be used to identify an unknown or forgotten password. Unfortunately, unauthorized persons seeking to gain access to computer systems can also use these applications (TechTarget, 2012; White, 2011). Health care organizations should establish enforceable, clear guidelines for choosing passwords. The following Perspective offers some suggestions (Reynolds, 2009; TechTarget, 2012; White, 2011).

PERSPECTIVE
Password Do's and Don't's

Don't

- Pick a password that someone who knows you can easily guess (for example, do not use your Social Security number, birthday, maiden name, pet's name, child's name, or car name).
- Pick a word that can be found in the dictionary (because cracker programs can rapidly try every word in the dictionary!).

- Pick a word that is currently newsworthy.
- Pick a password that is similar to your previous password.
- Share your password with others.

Do

- Pick a combination of letters and at least one number. Pick a password with at least eight characters, mixing uppercase and lowercase if your password system is case-sensitive.
- Pick a word that you can easily remember.
- Change your password often. (Some networks require that you change your password periodically.)

Biometric Identification Systems

Because of the inherent weaknesses of password systems, other identification systems have been developed. *Biometric identification systems* employ users' biological data, in the form, for example, of a voiceprint, fingerprint, handprint, retinal scan, faceprint, or full body scan. Biometrics is beginning to play a role in health care information system security. Biometric devices consist of a reader or scanning device, software that converts the scanned information into digital form, and a database that stores the biometric data for comparison.

Telephone Callback Procedures

Telephone callback procedures are another form of entity authentication in use today. Callback is used primarily when employees have access to a health care information system from home. When a modem dials into the system, a special callback application asks for the telephone number from which the call has been placed. If this number is not an authorized number, the callback application will not allow access.

Tokens

Tokens are devices, such as key cards, that are inserted into doors or computers. With token authentication systems, identification is based on the user's possession of the token (Eng, 2001). The disadvantage of tokens is that they can be lost, misplaced, or stolen. When tokens are used in combination with a password or PIN, it is essential that the password or PIN not be written on the token or in a location near where the token is stored.

Audit Trails

Webopedia (2012) defines an *audit trail* as "a record showing who has accessed a computer system and what operations he or she has performed during a given period of time." In addition, there are separate audit trail software products that enable network administrators to monitor use of network resources. Audit trails are generated by specialized software, and they have multiple uses in securing information systems. These uses may be categorized as follows (Gopalakrishna, 2000):

- **Individual accountability.** When employees' or other individuals' actions are tracked with an audit trail, these individuals become accountable for their actions, which can be a strong deterrent to violating acceptable policies and procedures.
- **Reconstructing electronic events.** Audit trails can also be used to reconstruct how and when a computer or application was used. This can be quite useful when there is a suspected security breach, whether internal or external.
- **Problem monitoring.** Some types of auditing software can detect problems such as disk failures, overutilization of system resources, and network outages as they occur.
- **Intrusion detection.** When there are attempts to gain unauthorized access to a system, an audit system can detect them.

Data Encryption

Data encryption is used to ensure that data transferred from one location on a network to another are secure from anyone eavesdropping or seeking to intercept them. This becomes particularly important when sensitive data, such as health information, are transmitted over public networks such as the Internet or across wireless networks. Secure data are data that cannot be intercepted, copied, modified, or deleted either while in transit or stored, such as on a disk or tape.

Cryptography is the study of encryption and decryption techniques. It is a complicated science with a vast number of associated techniques. Only the basic concepts and some current authentication technologies will be discussed in this chapter. Public Key Infrastructure, wired equivalent privacy (WEP), and

Figure 11.1. Encryption procedure

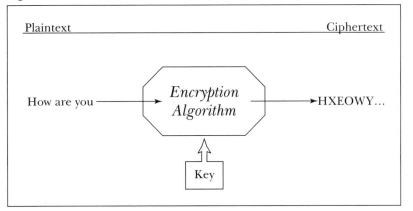

WiFi protected access (WPA) are forms of encryption being used in health care organizations today. (WEP and WPA apply specifically to wireless networks and will be discussed later in this chapter.) These protocols are used to authenticate the senders and receivers of messages transmitted over public networks, such as the Internet or wireless networks.

Some basic terms associated with encryption are plaintext, encryption algorithm, ciphertext, and key. *Plaintext* refers to data before any encryption has taken place. In other words, the original datum or message is recorded in the computer system as plaintext. An *encryption algorithm* is a computer program that converts plaintext into an enciphered form. The *ciphertext* is the data after the encryption algorithm has been applied. The *key* in an encryption and decryption procedure is unique data that are needed both to create the ciphertext and to decrypt the ciphertext back to the original message. Figure 11.1 is a simple diagram of the components of an encryption and decryption system (White, 2011).

Consider one of the simplest and earliest known forms of encryption—letter shift or Caesar cipher. The Caesar cipher replaces each plaintext letter with the letter found a fixed number of places down the alphabet. The fixed number of places in the alphabet is the "key" to unlocking the resulting ciphertext. Exhibit 11.1 illustrates the basic concepts in encryption using the Caesar cipher. In this example, the fixed number of "shift letters" is three (Felder, 1999).

This simple example and other early encryption systems used a single, private key. In other words, the same key (or code) was used to generate the ciphertext and to decrypt it. The problems with the single, private (secret) key systems were that both the sender and receiver had to have the key and that this key had to be protected from interception or tampering as well.

Exhibit 11.1. Caesar cipher encryption components

Plaintext: THE CAT IS IN THE HOUSE

Encryption Algorithm: Shift the letters in the alphabet over three places to the right.

Key:

A	B	C	D	E	F	G	H	I	J	K	L	M	N	O	P	Q	R	S	T	U	V	W	X	Y	Z
D	E	F	G	H	I	J	K	L	M	N	O	P	Q	R	S	T	U	V	W	X	Y	Z	A	B	C

Ciphertext: WKH FDW LV LQ WKH KRXVH

Public key cryptography addresses the basic problems of single, private key systems. In a public key system, there are two keys (distinct but corresponding computer codes), a *private key* and a *public key*. Basically, in this two-key system, data encrypted with the public key can be decrypted only by the private key, and data encrypted by the private key can be decrypted only by the public key. With public key cryptography, encrypted data become very difficult to break (White, 2011). Public key cryptography today is a component of *public key infrastructure (PKI)*, an entire system designed to make the use of public key cryptography practical. PKI is a combination of encryption techniques, software, and services.

The following is a simplified illustration of how public key cryptography works. A health care clinic in a major city needs to send patient information to the main hospital across town. First, encryption software ensures that the hospital sends the needed public key to the clinic, but "keeps" the corresponding private key in a secure location. The clinic software uses the public key to encrypt the data before sending it to the hospital. Now, only the hospital's system can decode the data, because it has sole possession of the corresponding private key.

Another form of public key cryptography is used to create digital signatures. Digital signatures, like other signatures, are used to authenticate electronic documents or messages. If Sam wants to send a "signed" e-mail to Sarah, he uses his digital signature, which contains his private key. When Sarah receives the e-mail, the message is authenticated with Sam's public key.

The most common encryption algorithm in use today is RSA. However, the AMA (2010) recommends advanced encryption standard (AES) as a better choice for encrypting ePHI. Encrypting ePHI is an important component of any health care organization security plan. The AMA recommends that physician practices encrypt any systems and individual files containing ePHI. They recommend that the following "most pressing problems" be addressed first, followed by all other ePHI systems:

- Backup media that must leave the facility
- E-mails containing ePHI
- Laptops containing ePHI
- Internet sessions involving ePHI
- Any other remote access sessions involving ePHI

There are several approaches to encrypting sensitive health care data (and a discussion of the specific technology is beyond the scope of this chapter), but the ultimate result should lead to a system in which the process of encrypting and decrypting involves minimal effort on the part of end users.

Firewall Protection

A *firewall* is "a system or combination of systems that supports an access control policy between two networks" (White, 2011, p. 369). The term *firewall* may be used to describe software that protects computing resources or to describe a combination of software, hardware, and policies that protects these resources. The most common place to find a firewall is between the health care organization's internal network and the Internet. This firewall prevents users who are accessing the health care network via the Internet from using certain portions of that network and also prevents internal users from accessing various portions of the Internet (Oz, 2009).

The basic types of firewalls are (1) packet filter, or network level, and (2) proxy servers, or application level. The packet filter firewall is essentially a router that has been programmed to filter out some types of data and to allow other types to pass through. The early versions of these firewalls were fairly easy to fool. As routers have become more sophisticated, the protection offered by this type of firewall has increased. The proxy server is a more complex firewall device. The proxy server firewall is software that runs on a computer that acts as the gatekeeper to an organization's network. All external transactions enter the organization's network through the proxy server. The request for information is actually "stopped" at the proxy server, where a proxy application is created. This proxy is what goes into the organization's network to retrieve the requested information (White, 2011).

As important as firewalls are to the overall security of health care information systems, they cannot protect a system from all types of attacks. Many viruses, for example, can hide inside documents that will not be stopped by a firewall.

Virus Checking

There are various methods used to maliciously attack computers and networks. One of the most common is a computer virus infection. A computer virus is defined as "a small program that alters the way a computer operates without the knowledge of the computer's users" (White, 2011, p. 389). Viruses are generally designed to cripple the computer operation by deleting, altering, or corrupting data, files, or operating system components. Following are some common types of viruses:

- A *Trojan horse* is released when the user opens an infected e-mail attachment. The malicious code is hidden within seemingly harmless code.
- A *botnet* takes over operations of the infected computer.
- A *macro virus* is programmed into an attached macro file found in spreadsheet, database, and word processing documents.
- A *boot sector virus* resides in a removable media device such as a flash drive.
- A *polymorphic virus* mutates with every infection, making it very difficult to identify.
- A *file infector virus* infects a piece of executable code. When the infected program is executed, the virus spreads to the computer.
- A *worm* copies itself from one system to another over a network without human assistance (White, 2011).

Checking for malicious software and other system attacks is an important component of a health information security program. As discussed earlier, malicious attacks are very common and can cause extensive damage and loss of productivity. Antivirus software is effective as long as the virus catalogue is updated frequently. Most antivirus software packages can be set to automatically scan the user's computer system periodically to detect and clean any viruses or other malicious software that is found.

SECURITY IN A WIRELESS ENVIRONMENT

As discussed in earlier chapters, wireless technologies are changing the way health care information systems operate. These technologies cover a wide range of capabilities. *Wireless LAN (WLAN)* devices allow users to move laptops easily from place to place within the health care organization. Bluetooth technologies allow data synchronization and application sharing across a variety of devices, such as keyboards, printers, and other peripheral devices. Handheld devices and tablets allow remote users to synchronize personal data and to access health care organizations' network services, such as calendars, e-mail, and Internet access. These technologies offer flexibility and new capabilities to health care providers and the individuals who support them (Karygiannis & Owens, 2002). However, the adoption of wireless technologies has been relatively rapid, creating concerns about the level of security they offer in an environment like the health care organization. According to a white paper written by Fluke Networks, the issues with wireless security are "exactly the same as with wired security. The problem with wireless is that it's difficult to limit the transmission media to just the areas that we control, or just the hosts we want on our network" (2003, p. 1).

WLANs consist of client devices (laptops, smart phones, and tablets) and access points (APs). The APs are designed to connect the client devices to the organization's overall (wired) network infrastructure. (The components of the WLAN are discussed in more detail in Chapter Nine.) In 2012, the National Institute of Standards and Technology recommended that organizations implement the following guidelines to improve security of WLANs (Souppaya & Scarfone, 2012). These guidelines address two main components of wireless network security—system configuration and system monitoring:

- Create standardized security configurations for common WLAN components. Standardization reduces the time and effort needed to secure the WLAN and verify its security.

- Consider the security not only of the WLAN itself, but also how it may affect the security of other networks. Care should be taken in allowing client devices access to the wired network or other wireless networks. For example, an organization should have a logically separated WLAN for external (guest) use and another for internal use.

- Establish clear policies regarding "dual connections," when a client device is connected to both a wired and wireless network at the same time.

- Ensure the organization's WLAN client devices and APs are configured and compliant with the organization WLAN policies. Organizations should standardize, automate, and centralize as much of the WLAN security configuration as possible.

- Perform attack monitoring and vulnerability monitoring to support WLAN security. Security monitoring is more important in the wireless environment because of the increased risk of unauthorized access. It is generally easier to intercept wireless network transmissions than wired transmissions.

- Conduct regular periodic technical security assessments for the organization's WLANs.

The specific capability recommendations (Souppaya & Scarfone, 2012) for continuous monitoring of WLANs include detection of

- Unauthorized WLAN devices
- WLAN devices that are misconfigured or using weak protocols
- Unusual WLAN patterns, such as high numbers of client devices using a particular AP or many failed attempts to join the WLAN
- Use of active WLAN scanners
- Denial of service attacks and other network interference
- Impersonation, such as when a device is attempting to "spoof" the identity of another device

Health care organizations that use wireless technologies should pay close attention to risk analysis for these technologies and make safeguards a part of ongoing risk management. As with other networks and information systems, the organization must know where the threats and vulnerabilities are. Securing the handheld devices, tablets, and laptop computers commonly associated with a wireless network also poses challenges for the health care organization. Clear policies, and appropriate sanctions for those violating the policies, should be established to govern the downloading of patient-specific information onto personal devices such as these.

REMOTE ACCESS SECURITY

Health care organizations, like many other modern organizations, allow personnel to work from home. This *remote access* creates additional security issues. In fact there have been a number of security incidents related to the remote use of laptops and other portable devices that store ePHI. In response to these incidents and the potential risk of HIPAA violations due to remote access, CMS issued a HIPAA security guidance document. Tables 11.3, 11.4,

Table 11.3. CMS recommendations for accessing ePHI remotely

Risks	Possible Risk Management Strategies
Log-on or password information is lost or stolen, resulting in potential unauthorized or improper access to or inappropriate viewing or modification of ePHI	Implement two-factor authentication for granting remote access to systems that contain ePHI. This process requires factors beyond general usernames and passwords to gain access to systems (such as requiring users to answer a security question such as "favorite pet's name"). Implement a technical process for creating unique usernames and performing authentication when granting remote access to a workforce member. This may be done using Remote Authentication Dial-In User Service (RADIUS) or other similar tools.
Employees access ePHI when not authorized to do so while working offsite	Develop and employ proper clearance procedures and verify training of workforce members prior to granting remote access. Establish remote access roles specific to applications and business requirements. Different remote users may require different levels of access based on job function. Ensure that the issue of unauthorized access to ePHI is appropriately addressed in the required sanction policy.
Home or other offsite workstations left unattended, risking improper access to ePHI	Establish appropriate procedures for session termination (time-out) on inactive portable or remote devices; covered entities can work with vendors to deliver systems or applications with appropriate defaults.
Contamination of systems by a virus introduced from an infected external device used to gain remote access to systems that contain ePHI	Install personal firewall software on all laptops that store or access ePHI or connect to networks on which ePHI is accessible. Install, use, and regularly update virus-protection software on all portable or remote devices that access ePHI.

Source: CMS, 2006.

Table 11.4. CMS recommendations for storing ePHI on portable devices

Risks	Possible Risk Management Strategies
Laptop or other portable device is lost or stolen, resulting in potential unauthorized or improper access to or modification of ePHI housed or accessible through the device	Identify the types of hardware and electronic media that must be tracked, such as hard drives, magnetic tapes or disks, optical disks or digital memory cards, and security equipment, and develop inventory control systems Implement process for maintaining a record of the movements of and person(s) responsible for or permitted to use hardware and electronic media containing ePHI Require use of lock-down or other locking mechanisms for unattended laptops Password-protect files Password-protect all portable or remote devices that store ePHI Require that all portable or remote devices that store ePHI employ encryption technologies of the appropriate strength Develop processes to ensure appropriate security updates are deployed to portable devices such as smart phones and PDAs Consider the use of biometrics, such as fingerprint readers, on portable devices
Use of external device to access corporate data, resulting in the loss of operationally critical ePHI on the remote device	Develop processes to ensure backup of all ePHI entered into remote systems Deploy policy to encrypt backup and archival media; ensure that policies direct the use of encryption technologies of the appropriate strength
Loss or theft of ePHI left on devices after inappropriate disposal by the organization	Establish ePHI deletion policies and media disposal procedures: at a minimum this involves complete deletion, via specialized deletion tools, of all disks and backup media prior to disposal; for systems at the end of their operational lifecycle, physical destruction may be appropriate
Data is left on an external device (accidentally or intentionally), such as in a library or hotel business center	Prohibit or prevent download of ePHI onto remote systems or devices without an operational justification Ensure workforce is appropriately trained on policies that require users to search for and delete any files intentionally or unintentionally saved to an external device Minimize use of browser-cached data in web-based applications that manage ePHI, particularly those accessed remotely
Contamination of systems by a virus introduced from a portable storage device	Install virus-protection software on all portable or remote devices that store ePHI

Source: CMS, 2006.

Table 11.5. CMS recommendations for transmitting ePHI from remote locations

Risks	Possible Risk Management Strategies
Data intercepted or modified during transmission	Prohibit transmission of ePHI via open networks, such as the Internet, where appropriate Prohibit the use of offsite devices or wireless access points (such as hotel workstations) for nonsecure access to e-mail Use more secure connections for e-mail via SSL and message-level standards such as S/MIME, SET, PEM, or PGP Implement and mandate appropriately strong encryption solutions for transmission of ePHI such as SSL or HTTPS SSL should be a minimum requirement for all Internet-facing systems that manage ePHI in any form, including corporate web-mail systems
Contamination of systems by a virus introduced from an external device used to transmit ePHI	Install virus-protection software on portable devices that can be used to transmit ePHI

Source: CMS, 2006.

and 11.5, taken from this HIPAA security guidance document, list potential risks in accessing, storing, and transmitting ePHI when using portable devices in remote locations and describe the management strategies recommended to mitigate these risks.

SUMMARY

Health information is created, maintained, and stored using computer technology. The use of this technology creates new issues in protecting patients' rights to privacy and confidentiality, and demands that health care organizations develop comprehensive information security programs. The publication of the final HIPAA Security Rule in 2003 underscores the importance of securing health information and the need for comprehensive security programs. The standards and specifications of the HIPAA rule can serve as a framework for health care organizations as they design their individual security programs.

Information security programs need to be designed to address internal and external threats to health care information systems, whether those threats are intentional or unintentional. Health information security programs should address administrative, physical, and technical safeguards. This chapter not only outlined the HIPAA security requirements but also provided a discussion of many of the common security measures that can be employed to minimize potential risks to health information.

KEY TERMS

Access control

Administrative safeguards

Assigned security responsibility

Audit trail

Automatic log-off

Biometric identification system

Business continuity plan

Chief security officer

Ciphertext

Continuity of operations plan

Contingency plan

Covered entity (CE)

Data encryption

Disaster recovery plan

Encryption algorithm

Entity authentication

Firewall

HIPAA Security Rule

Key

Media controls

Password

Personal identification number (PIN)

Physical access controls

Physical safeguards

Plaintext

Public key infrastructure (PKI)

Remote access

Risk analysis

System security evaluation

Technical safeguards

Telephone callback systems

Tokens

Virus checking

Wireless LAN (WLAN)

LEARNING ACTIVITIES

1. Do an Internet or library search for recent articles discussing the HIPAA Security Rule. From your research, write a short paper discussing the impact of these security regulations on health care organizations. How have these regulations changed the way organizations view security? Do you think the regulations are too stringent? Not stringent enough? Just right? Explain your rationale.

2. Interview a chief security officer at a hospital or other health care facility. What are the major job responsibilities of this individual? To whom does he or she report within the organization? What are the biggest challenges of the job?

3. Contact a physician's office or clinic and ask if the organization has a security plan. Discuss the process that staff undertook to complete the plan, or develop an outline of a plan for them.

4. Visit a local hospital or other health care organization's IT department. Ask to view their IT contingency plan. Determine whether or not the plan meets all of the HIPAA security requirements. Investigate whether the contingency plan is part of a broader business continuity plan.

5. Visit the Office of Civil Rights Enforcement Activities and Results web site. Read at least five case examples involving HIPAA security violations. What do these cases have in common? What are their differences? Do all of the Security Rule violations you read also involve Privacy Rule violations? What were your impressions of the types of cases you read and their resolutions?

REFERENCES

American Health Information Management Association. (2003). *Final rule for HIPAA security standards*. Chicago: Author.

American Medical Association. (2010). *HIPAA Security Rule: Frequently asked questions regarding encryption of personal health information*. Practice Management Center, American Medical Association. Retrieved April 2012 from http://www.ama-assn.org/ama1/pub/upload/mm/368/hipaa-phi-encryption.pdf

Associated Press. (1995, February 28). *7 Get fake HIV-positive calls*. Retrieved December 2004 from http://www.aegis.com/news/ap/1995/AP950248.html

Briney, A. (2000). *2000 information security industry survey*. Retrieved November 2004 from http://www.infosecuritymag.com

Centers for Medicare and Medicaid Services. (2004). *HIPAA administrative simplification: Security—Final rule*. Retrieved November 2004 from http://www .cms.hhs.gov/hipaa/hipaa2/regulations/security

Centers for Medicare and Medicaid Services. (2006, December 28). *HIPAA security guidance*. Retrieved April 2012 from http://www.hhs.gov/ocr/privacy/hipaa /administrative/securityrule/remoteuse.pdf

Coppersmith, Gordon, Schermer, & Brockelman, PLC. (2012). HITECH Act expands HIPAA Privacy and Security Rules. Retrieved March 2012 from http://www .azhha.org/member_and_media_resources/documents/HITECHAct.pdf

Eng, J. (2001). Computer network security for the radiology enterprise. *Radiology*, *220*(2), 304–309.

Felder, R. (1999, November 1). Caesar's shift. (How a Caesar cipher works). *Cobblestone*. Retrieved October 2012 from http://www.highbeam.com/doc/1G1 -62495672.html

Fluke Networks. (2003). *Wireless security notes: A brief analysis of risks*. Retrieved December 2004 from http://wp.bitpipe.com/resource/org_1014144860_961 /fnet_wireless_security_bpx.pdf

Gopalakrishna, R. (2000). *Audit trails*. Retrieved July 2004 from http://www.cerias .purdue.edu/homes/rgk/at.html

International Organization for Standardization (ISO). (2009). ISO/IEC 15408-1, 3rd ed.: Information technology—Security techniques—Evaluation criteria for IT security, Part 1, Introduction and general model. Retrieved April 2012 from http://standards.iso.org/ittf/PubliclyAvailableStandards/index.html

Karygiannis, T., & Owens, L. (2002). *Wireless network security: 802.11, Bluetooth and handheld devices (Special Publication 800–48)*. Gaithersburg, MD: National Institute of Standards and Technology.

Keckley, P. H., Coughlin S., & Gupta, S. (2011). *Issue brief: Privacy and security in health care—A fresh look*. Deloitte Center for Health Solutions. Retrieved April 2012 from http://www.deloitte.com/us/privacyandsecurityinhealthcare

Oz, E. (2009). *Management information systems: Instructor edition* (6th ed.). Boston: Course Technology.

Reynolds, R. B. (2009). The HIPAA Security Rule. In M. S. Brodnick, M. C. McCain, L. A. Rinehart-Thompson, & R. Reynolds (Eds.), *Fundamentals of law for health informatics and information management* (pp. 195–236). Chicago: American Health Information Management Association.

Rozek, P., & Groth, D. (2008). Business continuity planning. It's a critical element of disaster preparedness. Can you afford to keep it off your radar? *Health Management Technology, 29*(3), 10–12.

Scholl, M., Stine, K., Hash, J., Bowen, P., Johnson, A., Smith, C. D., & Steinberg, D. I. (2008). *An introductory resource guide for implementing the Health Insurance Portability and Accountability Act (HIPAA) Security Rule*. Gaithersburg, MD: Computer Security Division, Information Technology Laboratory, National Institute of Standards and Technology. Retrieved April 2012 from http://csrc.nist .gov/publications/nistpubs/800-66-Rev1/SP-800-66-Revision1.pdf

Smith, H. (2001). *A context-based access control model for HIPAA privacy and security compliance*. SANS Institute, Information Security Reading Room. Retrieved December 2004 from http://www.sans.org/rr/whitepapers/legal/44.php

Souppaya, M., & Scarfone, K. (2012). Guidelines for securing wireless local area networks (WLANs). *Recommendations of the National Institute of Standards and Technology* (NIST Special Publication 800–153). Retrieved April 2012 from http:// csrc.nist.gov/publications/nistpubs/800-153/sp800-153.pdf

TechTarget. (2012). Password definition. *SearchSecurity*. Retrieved April 2012 from http://searchsecurity.techtarget.com/definition/password

Walsh, T. (2003). Best practices for compliance with the final Security Rule. *Journal of Healthcare Information Management, 17*(3), 14–18.

Webopedia. (2012). Audit trail definition. Retrieved April 2012 from http://www
.webopedia.com/TERM/A/audit_trail.html

Weil, S. (2004). *The final HIPAA Security Rule: Conducting effective risk analysis.*
Retrieved April 2004 from http://www.hipaadvisory.com/action/Security
/riskanalysis.htm

White, C. (2011). *Data communications and computer networks: A business user's
approach. Instructor edition* (6th ed.). Boston: Course Technology.

PART FOUR

Senior Management IT Challenges

CHAPTER 12

Organizing Information Technology Services

LEARNING OBJECTIVES

- Describe the roles, responsibilities, and major functions of the IT department or organization.
- Discuss the role and responsibility of the chief information officer (CIO), chief medical informatics officer (CMIO), chief security officer (CSO), chief technology officer (CTO), and other key IT staff.
- Describe the different ways IT services might be organized and governed within a health care organization.
- Identify key attributes of highly effective IT organizations.
- Develop a plan for evaluating the effectiveness of the IT function within an organization.

By now you should have an understanding of health care data, the various clinical and administrative applications that are used to manage those data, and the processes of selecting, acquiring, and implementing health care information systems. You should also have a basic understanding of the core technologies that are common to many health care applications, and you can appreciate some of what it takes to ensure that information systems are reliable and secure.

In many health care organizations, an information technology (IT) function employs staff who are involved in these and other IT-related activities—everything from customizing a software application to setting up and maintaining a wireless network to performing system backups. In a solo physician practice, this responsibility may lie with the office manager or lead physician. In a large hospital setting, this responsibility may lie with the IT department in conjunction with the medical staff, the administration, and the major departmental units—for example, admissions, finance, radiology, and nursing.

Some health care organizations outsource a portion or all of their IT services; however, they are still responsible for ensuring that those services are of high quality and support the IT needs of the organization. This responsibility cannot be delegated entirely to an outside vendor or IT firm. Health care executives must manage IT resources just as they do human, financial, and other facility resources.

This chapter provides an overview of the various functions and responsibilities that one would typically find in the IT department of a large health care organization. We describe the different groups or units that are typically seen in an IT department. We review a typical organizational structure for IT and discuss the variations that are often seen in that structure and the reasons for them. This chapter also presents an overview of the senior IT management roles and the roles with which health care executives will often work in the course of projects and IT initiatives. IT outsourcing, in which the health care organization asks an outside vendor to run IT, is reviewed. Finally, we examine approaches to evaluating the efficiency and effectiveness of the IT department.

INFORMATION TECHNOLOGY FUNCTIONS

The IT department has been an integral part of most hospitals or health care systems since the early days of mainframe computing. If the health care facility was relatively large and complex and used a fair amount of information technology, one would find IT staff "behind the scenes" developing or enhancing applications, building system interfaces, maintaining databases, managing networks, performing system backups, and carrying out a host of other IT support activities. Today the IT department is becoming increasingly important, not only in hospitals but in all health care organizations that use IT to manage clinical and administrative data and processes.

Throughout this chapter we refer to the IT department usually found in a large community hospital or health care system. We chose this setting because it is typically the most complex and IT intensive. Moreover, many of the principles that apply to managing IT resources in a hospital setting also apply in other types of health care facilities, such as an ambulatory care clinic or rural community health center. The breadth and scope of the services provided may differ considerably, however, depending on the extent to which IT is used in the organization.

IT Department Responsibilities

The IT department has several responsibilities:

- Ensuring that an IT plan and strategy have been developed for the organization and that the plan and strategy are kept current as the organization evolves; these activities are discussed in Chapter Thirteen.
- Working with the organization to acquire or develop and implement needed new applications; these processes were discussed in Chapters Seven and Eight.
- Providing day-to-day support for users: for example, fixing broken personal computers, responding to questions about application use, training new users, and applying vendor-supplied upgrades to existing applications.
- Managing the IT infrastructure: for example, performing backups of databases, installing network connections for new organizational locations, monitoring system performance, and securing the infrastructure from virus attacks.
- Examining the role and relevance of emerging information technologies.

Core Functions

To fulfill their responsibilities, all IT departments have four core functions. Depending on the size of the IT group and the diversity of applications and responsibilities, a function may require several subsidiary departments or subgroups.

Operations and Technical Support

The *operations and technical support function* manages the IT infrastructure—
for example, the servers, networks, operating systems, database management
systems, and workstations. This function installs new technology, applies
upgrades, troubleshoots and repairs the infrastructure, performs "housekeeping" tasks such as backups, and responds to user problems, such as a printer
that is not working.

This function may have several IT subgroups:

- Data center management: manages the equipment in the
  organization's computer center.
- Network engineers: manage the organization's network technologies.
- Server engineers: oversee the installation of new servers and perform
  such tasks as managing server space utilization.
- Database managers: add new databases, support database query tools,
  and respond to database problems such as file corruptions.
- Security: ensure that virus protection software is current, physical access
  to the computer room is constrained, disaster recovery plans are current,
  and processes are in place to manage application and system passwords.
- Help desk: provide support to users who call in with problems such
  as broken office equipment, trouble operating an application, a
  forgotten password, or uncertainty about how to perform a specific
  task on the computer.
- Deployments: install new workstations and printers, move
  workstations when groups move to new buildings, and the like.
- Training: train organization staff on new applications and office
  software, such as presentation development applications.

Applications Management

The *applications management* group manages the processes of acquiring new
application systems, developing new application systems, implementing these
new systems, providing ongoing enhancement of applications, troubleshooting
application problems, and working with application suppliers to resolve these
problems.

This function may have several IT groups:

- Groups that focus on major classes of applications: for example, a
  financial systems group and a clinical systems group.

- Groups dedicated to specific applications (this is most likely in large organizations): for example, a group to support the applications in the clinical laboratory or in radiology.

- An applications development group (this is found in organizations that perform a significant amount of internal development).

- Groups that focus on specific types of internal development: for example, a web development group.

Specialized Groups

Health care organizations may develop groups that have very *specialized functions*, depending on the type of organization or the organization's approach to IT. For example:

- Groups that support the needs of the research community in academic medical centers

- Process redesign groups in organizations that engage in a significant degree of process reengineering during application implementation

- Decision-support groups that help users and management perform analyses and create reports from corporate databases: for example, quality-of-care reports or financial performance reports

In addition, the chief information officer (CIO), who is the most senior IT executive, is often responsible for managing the organization's telecommunications function—the staff who manage the phone system, overhead paging system, and nurse call systems. Depending on the organization's structure and the skill and interests of the CIO, one occasionally finds these other organizational functions reporting to the CIO:

- The health information management or medical records department

- The function that handles the organization's overall strategic plan development

- The marketing department

IT Administration

Depending on the size of the IT department, one may find groups that focus on supporting *IT administrative* activities. These groups may perform such tasks as

- Overseeing the development of the IT strategic plan
- Managing contracts with vendors
- Developing and monitoring the IT budget
- Providing human resource support for the IT staff
- Providing support for the management of IT projects: for example, developing project status reports or providing project management training
- Managing the space occupied by an IT department or group

A typical organizational structure for an IT department in a large academic medical center is shown in Figure 12.1.

IT Senior Leadership Roles

Within the overall IT group, several positions and roles are typically present. These roles range from senior leadership—for example, the chief information officer—to staff who do the day-in, day-out work of implementing application systems—for example, systems analysts. In the following sections we will describe several senior-level IT positions:

- Chief information officer (CIO)
- Chief technology officer (CTO)
- Chief security officer (CSO)
- Chief medical information officer (CMIO)

This is not an exhaustive list of all possible senior-level positions, but the discussion provides an overview of typical roles and functions.

The Chief Information Officer

Many midsize and large health care organizations employ a *chief information officer (CIO)*. The CIO not only manages the IT department but is also seen as the executive who can successfully lead the organization in its efforts to apply IT to advance its strategies.

The role of the CIO in health care and other industries has been the subject of research and debate over the years (Glaser & Williams, 2007). Studies conducted by College of Healthcare Information Management Executives (CHIME) (1998, 2008) have chronicled the evolution of the health care CIO. This evolution has involved debates on CIO reporting relationships, salaries, and titles

Figure 12.1. Typical IT organizational chart

Source: Courtesy of the Medical University of South Carolina.

and the role of the CIO in an organization's strategic planning. Through extensive research, CHIME has identified seven key attributes, or competencies, exhibited by high-performing CIOs (CHIME, 2008). CHIME provides intensive "boot camp" training sessions for its CIO members, to aid in their professional development of these competencies.

PERSPECTIVE
Seven Key Attributes of a High-Performing CIO

1. *Sets vision and strategy.* Collaborates well with senior leaders to set organization vision and strategy and to determine how technology can best serve the organization.

2. *Integrates information technology for business success.* Applies knowledge of the organization's systems, structures, and functions to determine how best to advance the performance of the business with technology.

3. *Makes change happen.* Is able to lead the organization in making the process changes necessary to fully capitalize on IT investments.

4. *Builds technological confidence.* Helps the business assess the value of IT investments and the steps needed to achieve that value.

5. *Partners with customers.* Interacts with internal and external customers to ensure continuous customer satisfaction.

6. *Ensures information technology talent.* Creates a work environment and community that draws, develops, and retains top IT talent.

7. *Builds networks and community* Develops and maintains professional networks with internal and external sources and effectively leverages those networks to further the effective use of IT.

Source: CHIME, 2008.

Earlier work by Earl and Feeney (1995) found that CIOs from a wide range of industries who "added value" to their respective organizations had many of these same characteristics. Earl and Feeney found that the value-added CIOs

- Obsessively and continuously focus on business imperatives so that they focus the IT direction correctly.
- Have a track record of delivery that causes IT performance problems to drop off management's agenda.

- Interpret for the rest of the leadership the meaning and nature of the IT success stories of other organizations.

- Establish and maintain good working relationships with the members of the organization's leadership.

- Establish and communicate the IT performance record.

- Concentrate the IT development efforts on those areas of the organization where the most leverage is to be gained.

- Work with the organization's leadership to develop a shared vision of the roles and contributions of IT.

- Make important general contributions to business thinking and operations.

Earl and Feeney (1995) also found that the value-added CIO, as a person, has integrity, is goal directed, is experienced with IT, and is a good consultant and communicator. Those organizations that have such a CIO tend to describe IT as critical to the organization, find that IT thinking is embedded in business thinking, note that IT initiatives are well focused, and speak highly of IT performance.

Organizational excellence in IT doesn't just happen. It is managed and led. If the health care organization decides that the effective application of IT is a major element of its strategies and plans, it will need a very good CIO. Failure to hire and retain such talent will severely hinder the organization's aspirations.

Whom the CIO should report to has been a topic of industry debate and an issue inside organizations as well. CIOs will often argue that they should report to the chief executive officer (CEO). This argument is not wrong nor is it necessarily right. The CIO does need access to the CEO and clearly should be a member of the executive committee and actively involved in strategy discussions. However, the CIO needs a boss who is a good mentor, provides appropriate political support, and is genuinely interested in the application of IT. Chief financial officers (CFOs) and chief operating officers (COOs) can be terrific in these regards. In general about one-third of all health care provider CIOs report to the CEO, one-third report to the CFO, and one-third report to the COO.

The Chief Technology Officer

The *chief technology officer (CTO)* has several responsibilities. The CTO must guide the definition and implementation of the organization's technical architecture. This role includes defining technology standards (for example, defining the operating systems and network technologies the organization will support), ensuring that the technical infrastructure is current (for example, that major vendor releases and upgrades have been applied), and ensuring that all the technologies fit. The CTO's role in ensuring fit is similar to an architect's role in ensuring that the materials used to construct a house come together in a way that results in the desired house.

The CTO is also responsible for tracking emerging technologies, identifying the ones that might provide value to the organization, assessing them, and when appropriate, working with the rest of the IT department and the organization to implement these technologies. For example, the CTO may be asked to investigate the possible usefulness of the new biometric security technologies. The CTO role is not often found in smaller organizations but is increasingly common in larger ones. In smaller organizations, the CIO also wears the CTO hat.

The Chief Security Officer

As discussed in Chapter Ten, the *chief security officer (CSO)* is a relatively new position that has emerged as a result of the growing threats to information security and the health care organization's need to comply with federal and state security regulations. The primary role and functions of the CSO are to ensure that the health care organization has an effective information security plan, that appropriate technical and administrative procedures are in place to ensure that information systems are secure and safe from tampering or misuse, and that appropriate disaster recovery procedures exist.

The Chief Medical Information Officer

Like the CSO, the *chief medical information officer (CMIO)* is a relatively new position. The CMIO position emerged as a result of the growing interest in adopting clinical information systems and the need for physician leadership in this area. The CMIO is usually a physician, and this role may be filled through a part-time commitment by a member of the organization's medical staff.

Examples of the types of responsibilities a CMIO might assume include

- Leading clinical information system initiatives such as electronic health record implementations
- Serving as physician advocate for computerized provider order entry (CPOE)
- Engaging physicians and other health care professionals in the development and use of the EHR system
- Leading the clinical informatics steering committee or other designated group that serves as the central governance forum for establishing the organization's clinical IT priorities

- Keeping a pulse on national efforts to develop EHR systems, and assuming a leadership role in areas where the national effort and the organization's agenda are synergistic
- Being highly responsive to user needs, such as training, to ensure widespread use and acceptance of clinical systems

Like the CIO and CTO, the role of the CMIO is emerging. Leviss, Kremsdorf, and Mohaideen (2006) conducted structured interviews with five CMIOs at health systems that used health information technology widely. The aim of the study was to identify individual skills and organizational structures that helped the CMIO to be effective. The Perspective here lists the recommendations that Leviss and his colleagues offer to hospital and health system leaders.

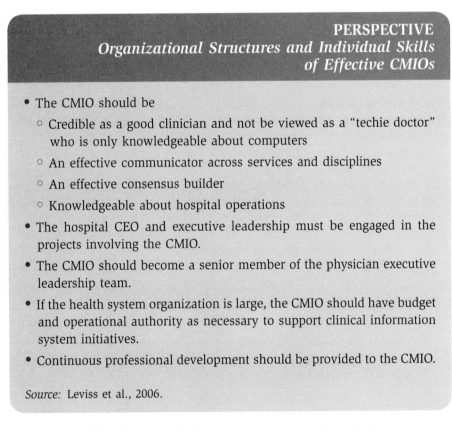

PERSPECTIVE
Organizational Structures and Individual Skills of Effective CMIOs

- The CMIO should be
  - Credible as a good clinician and not be viewed as a "techie doctor" who is only knowledgeable about computers
  - An effective communicator across services and disciplines
  - An effective consensus builder
  - Knowledgeable about hospital operations
- The hospital CEO and executive leadership must be engaged in the projects involving the CMIO.
- The CMIO should become a senior member of the physician executive leadership team.
- If the health system organization is large, the CMIO should have budget and operational authority as necessary to support clinical information system initiatives.
- Continuous professional development should be provided to the CMIO.

Source: Leviss et al., 2006.

The CIO, CTO, CSO, and CMIO all play important roles in helping to ensure that information systems acquired and implemented are consistent with the strategic goals of the health care organization, are well accepted and effectively used, and are adequately maintained and secured. Sample job descriptions for the CIO and the CMIO positions are displayed in Exhibits 12.1 and 12.2.

Exhibit 12.1. Sample CIO job description

«XX» Health Care System, Inc.
JOB DESCRIPTION

POSITION TITLE: Chief Information Officer (CIO)

DEPARTMENT: Information Systems & Telecommunications

POSITION REPORTS TO: Chief Financial Officer (CFO)

POSITION SUPERVISES: Information Systems Department, Telecommunications Department

POSITION REQUIREMENTS:

Master of Science Degree in Information Systems or other related field. Five to ten years' progressive management experience in Information Systems required. Experience with a multi-uni/integrated health care system preferred. Demonstrated successful leadership in planning, developing, and implementing management information processes, mechanisms, and systems is required. Excellent communication skills, leadership skills, negotiation skills, and motivational abilities are a must.

POSITION SUMMARY:

Responsible for «XX» Health Care System's Information Systems Division. This division includes Information Management, Health Information Management and Telecommunications for our multilocation/integrated health care system operating 24 hours a day, 365 days a year. This job description is congruent with the human and community development philosophy of the «XX». The philosophy emphasizes responsibility for human life and the dignity and worth of every person. It also promotes the creation of caring communities in which the needs of those serving and being served are met. It is expected employees will perform their jobs in accordance with the philosophy.

ESSENTIAL FUNCTIONS:

1. Knows, understands, incorporates, and demonstrates the «XX» Health Care System Mission, Visions, Values, and Management Philosophy in leadership behaviors, practices, and decisions.

2. Montiors the health care delivery environment in order to anticipate any impact on information systems and communications networks to ensure appropriate utilization of information technology.

3. Examines new systems and develops strategies directed toward increased productivity by improving the work environment through systems and people consistent with the Mission, Vision, Values, and Management Philosophy of the «XX» system.

4. Establishes systemwide information managemen/technology standards and strategies for achieving integration and interoperability of information systems, technology architecture, and selection of software applications.

Exhibit 12.1. (*Continued*)

5. Maintains responsibility for the information system operations including the development and management of operating and capital budgets, policies, human resource utilization, mission effectiveness, and the overall performance of information technology within «XX» Health Care System.

6. Develops long-range plans and associated capital and expense budgets and monitors the achievement of these plans in order to ensure the successful performance of the organization.

7. Develops information system plans and programs to improve organization effectiveness and efficiency, ensuring that the information needs of «XX» Health Care System information technology staff are met.

8. Creates a seamless process to gather information regarding operational, human resources, financial, and clinical outcomes.

9. Maintains internal and external relationships with all system users and vendors.

10. Is responsible for the installation of all new information systems and telecommunication systems for «XX» Health Care System.

11. Is a member of the Executive Team providing leadership to «XX» Health Care System.

12. Maintains the integrity and security of «XX» Health Care System's information systems, complying wtih all regulatory agencies and statutes.

13. Provides for professional growth and career opportunities for the Information System division staff.

OTHER FUNCTIONS:
All other duties as assigned.

APPROVED BY:

DEPARTMENT HEAD	**DATE**
PRESIDENT'S COUNCIL MEMBER	**DATE**
HUMAN RESOURCES DEPARTMENT	**DATE**

REVISION DATES: _____

FOR HUMAN RESOURCES DEPT. USE ONLY: ___EXEMPT ___NONEXEMPT

Exhibit 12.2. Sample CMIO job description

JOB DESCRIPTION FOR CHIEF MEDICAL INFORMATION OFFICER

BACKGROUND

The position of Chief Medical Information Officer is a newly created position and reports to the Senior Vice President Information Services, CIO. This individual will lead the development and implementation of automated support for clinicians and clinical analysts through researching, recommending, and facilitating major and advanced clinical information system initiatives for the health care system.

In this role, the incumbent will provide reviews of medical informatics experiences and approaches, develop technical and application implementation strategies, manage implementation of advanced clinical information systems, assist in the development of strategic plans for clinical information systems, and provide project management for codevelopment relationships with the vendor community.

Information technology at THE HOSPITAL is becoming highly user driven. Governed by the Quality Council, a Clinical Informatics Steering Committee and subcommittees reporting to the Clinical Informatics Steering Committee will be formed to provide a user forum for input, coordination, and integration of information technology with THE HOSPITAL. The Director of Medical Informatics will chair, lead, and support the Clinical Informatics Steering Committee.

The following are ongoing responsibilities of the CHIEF MEDICAL INFORMATION OFFICER:

Lead the implementation of a computerized patient record (CPR) system for the health care system (hospitals, clinics, physicians offices, ancillary, and therapy units). This system should embody an information model focused on the diagnosis, treatment, and process data that will be required in future treatment and preventive care.

Engage providers with varying roles including independent and employed physicians and clinicians, medical records professionals, and clinical analysts to contribute to the development and use of the CPR and analysis tools.

Lead and support the Clinical Informatics Steering Committee which serves as the principal user governance forum to determine organizational priorities in this area.

Stay attuned to the national effort to develop comprehensive, functional, and uniform medical records, and take an active role in areas where the national effort and health care system can mutually benefit.

Be highly responsive to users' needs, including training, to ensure widespread acceptance and provider use of the clinical systems.

Exhibit 12.2. (*Continued*)

The following are expected accomplishments of the Chief Medical Information Officer for the first 12 to 24 months.

Gain a thorough understanding of the personality and culture of the organization and community; evaluate and refine the strategic information plan as it relates to clinical informatics.

Develop empathy and understanding of physician needs; build relationships with physicians to gain the support of physician leadership.

Together with a team leader, evaluate the skills of the current clinical informatics team, identify needs and build a strong team by enhancing team members' skill base, motivating them and fostering a collaborative approach that values their contribution.

Design a model of the clinical database(s) to support the enterprise-wide CPR. The database(s) should support individual patient care and clinical studies across the full continuum of care.

Guided by the Quality Council, determine an approach and plan for the development and implementation of clinical systems that are components of a computerized patient record. The CPR will be designed to support clinicians in the care of patients throughout the network.

Select the products and vendors for the components of the initial phase of CPR implementation. Be on schedule, according to plan, with the implementations.

Implement physician network services, the transfer of clinical information between network sites, and the presentation of that information on a physician workstation.

The following are the desired credentials, skills, and personality characteristics of the ideal candidate (not listed in priority order):

The successful candidate will have the following profile:

A licensed physician with recent medical practice experience, graduate degree in medical informatics, and one year of work experience in medical informatics. In lieu of graduate training in medical informatics, a minimum of three years' work experience in medical informatics systems will be required.

A personable individual with excellent interpersonal and communication skills who can handle a diversity of personalities and interact effectively with people at all levels of the organization.

A strong leader with a mature sense of priorities and solid practical experience to implement the vision for the organization.

(cont.)

Exhibit 12.2. (*Continued*)

An individual who is politically savvy, has a high tolerance for ambiguity, and can work successfully in a matrix management model.

A systems thinker with strong organizational skills who can pull all the pieces together and understand how to deliver ideals.

A strong manager who is adaptable and has a strong collaborative management style.

A creative thinker with high energy and enthusiasm.

A team player and consensus builder who promotes the concept of people working together versus individual performance.

A contemporary clinician who understands major trends in health care and managed care and has extensive knowledge of currently available point-of-care products and medical informatics development.

An individual with strong self-confidence who is assertive without being arrogant or ostentatious and who possesses confidence in heavy physician interaction.

IT Staff Roles

The IT leadership team cannot carry out the organization's IT agenda unilaterally. The department's work relies heavily on highly trained, qualified professional and technical staff to perform a host of IT-related functions. In this section are brief descriptions of some key professionals who work in IT:

- The project leader
- The systems analyst
- The programmer
- The database administrator
- The network administrator
- The telecommunications specialist

The Project Leader

The *project leader* manages IT projects such as the implementation of a departmental system, deployment of infrastructure in a new medical office building, or determination of the need for a new system. At times project leaders are staff from user departments, though in general they are members of the IT department. This role will be discussed in more depth in Chapter Sixteen.

The Systems Analyst

The role of the *systems analyst* will vary considerably depending on the analyst's background and the needs of the organization. Some analysts have a strong computer programming background, whereas others have a business orientation or come from clinical disciplines, such as nursing, pharmacy, or laboratory sciences. In fact, due to the increased interest in the adoption of clinical information systems, systems analysts with clinical backgrounds in nursing, pharmacy, laboratory science, and the like (often referred to as *clinical systems analysts*) are in high demand. Most systems analysts work closely with managers and end users in identifying information system needs and problems, evaluating workflow, and determining strategies for optimizing the use and effectiveness of particular systems.

When an organization decides to develop a new information system, systems analysts are often called upon to determine what computer hardware and software will be needed. They prepare specifications, flowcharts, and process diagrams for computer programmers to follow.

They work with programmers and vendor staff to *debug*, or eliminate, errors in the system. Systems analysts may also conduct extensive testing of systems, diagnose problems, recommend solutions, and determine whether program requirements have been met. They may also prepare cost-benefit and return-on-investment analyses to help management decide whether implementing a proposed system will deliver the desired value.

The Programmer

Programmers write, test, and maintain the programs that computers must follow to perform their functions. They also conceive, design, and test logical structures for solving problems with computers. Many technical innovations in programming—advanced computing technologies and sophisticated new languages and programming tools—have redefined the role of programmers and elevated much of the programming work done today (Department of Labor, Bureau of Labor Statistics, 2008).

Programmers are often grouped into two broad types—applications programmers and systems programmers. *Applications programmers* write programs to handle specific user tasks, such as a program to track inventory within an organization. They may also revise existing packaged software or customize generic applications such as integration technologies. *Systems programmers* write programs to maintain and control infrastructure software, such as operating systems, networked systems, and database systems. They are able to change the sets of instructions that determine how the network, workstations, and central processing units within a system handle the various jobs they have been given and how they communicate with peripheral equipment such as other workstations, printers, and disk drives.

The Database Administrator

Database administrators work with database management systems software and determine ways to organize and store data. They identify user requirements, set up computer databases, and test and coordinate modifications to these systems. An organization's database administrator ensures the performance of the database systems, understands the platform on which the databases run, and adds new users to the systems. Because they may also design and implement system security, database administrators often plan and coordinate security measures. With the volume of sensitive data growing rapidly, data integrity, backup systems, and database security have become increasingly important aspects of the job for database administrators (Department of Labor, Bureau of Labor Statistics, 2008).

The Network Administrator

As discussed earlier in this book, it is essential that the organization has an adequate network or network infrastructure to support all its clinical and administrative applications and also its general applications (such as e-mail, intranets, and the like). Networks come in many variations, so *network administrators* are needed to design, test, and evaluate systems such as local area networks (LANs), wireless networks, the Internet, intranets, and other data communications systems. Networks can range from a connection between two offices in the same building to globally distributed connectivity to voice-mail and e-mail systems across a host of different health care organizations. Network administrators perform network modeling, analysis, and planning; they may also research related products and make hardware and software recommendations.

The Telecommunications Specialist

Working closely with the network administrator is the *telecommunications specialist*. These specialists manage the organization's telephone systems: for example, the central phone system, cellular telephone infrastructure, and nurse call systems. They often manage the communication network to be used by the organization in the event of a disaster. Because of the progressive convergence of voice networks and data networks, they may design voice and data communication systems, supervise the installation of those systems, and provide maintenance and other services to staff throughout the organization after the system is installed.

Comments

The distinctions between the roles and functions of IT staff may seem a bit murky in practice. In one organization, the systems analyst might do computer programming, advise on network specifications, and assist in database development. In another organization, the systems analyst might have a clinical focus and work primarily with the end users in a particular unit, such as a laboratory, identifying needs, addressing problems, working with the application vendor, and providing ongoing training and support.

The specific qualifications, roles, and functions of the various IT staff members are generally determined by the pattern of IT development and use within the organization. For example, in a large academic medical center, the IT staff may be actively involved in designing in-house applications, and therefore the organization may employ teams of IT staff to work with faculty and clinicians in developing customized IT tools. This same level of IT expertise would be rare in an organization that relies primarily on IT applications purchased from the health care IT vendor community.

Furthermore, an organization might have an in-house IT services department, yet outsource a number of IT functions, having them performed by staff outside the organization.

Staff Attributes

In addition to ensuring that it has the appropriate IT functions and IT roles (and that the individuals filling these roles are competent), the health care organization must ensure that the IT staff have certain attributes. These attributes are unlikely to arise spontaneously; they must often be managed into existence. An assessment of the IT function (as discussed later in this chapter) can highlight problems in this area and then lead to management steps designed to improve staff attributes.

High-performing IT staff have several general characteristics:

- *They execute well.* They deliver applications, infrastructure, and services that reflect a sound understanding of organizational needs. These deliverables occur on time and on budget, so that those involved in a project give the project team high marks for professional comportment.

- *They are good consultants.* They advise organizational members on the best approach to the application of IT given the problem or opportunity. They advise when IT may be inappropriate or the least important component of the solution. This advice ranges from help desk support to systems analyses to new technology recommendations to advice on the suitability of IT for furthering an aspect of organizational strategy.

- *They provide world-class support.* Information systems require daily care and feeding and problem identification and correction. This support needs to be exceptionally efficient and effective.

- *They stay current in their field of expertise.* They keep up to date on new techniques and technologies that may improve the ability of the organization to apply IT effectively.

Recruitment and Retention of IT Staff

In addition to ensuring that IT staff possess desired attributes, senior leadership may become involved in discussions centered on the attraction and retention of IT staff. Although the IT job market ebbs and flows, the market for talented and experienced IT staff is likely to be competitive for some time (Committee on Workforce Needs in Information Technology, 2001).

The changes in the health care system discussed in Chapter Six have resulted in a significant increase in the demand for health care IT professionals, in particular those with experience with electronic health record implementations. A 2010 Modern Healthcare (Conn, 2010) survey of health care executives found that

- Fifty-eight percent of respondents planned to increase IT staff in the next twelve months

- Forty percent expected to increase their IT workforce by 10 percent or more and 9 percent planned to increase between 30 percent and 50 percent

The same survey found that 49 percent reported difficulty recruiting.

Estimates of the additional IT staff needed to support payment reform changes range from a 2008 Bureau of Labor Statistics estimate of 35,000 to an Office of the National Coordinator for Health Information Technology estimate of 50,000 (Conn, 2010). An increase of 50,000 staff would represent a 50 percent increase in the current health care IT workforce.

Recruitment and retention strategies involve making choices about what work factors and management practices will be changed and how they will be changed in order to improve the organization's ability to recruit and retain. Management may need to determine whether the focus will be on salaries or career development or physical surroundings or some combination of these factors.

For example, the IT managers at Partners HealthCare were asked to identify the factors that make an organization a great place to work and then to rate the Partners IT group on those factors using letter grades. The factors identified by the managers were

- Salary and benefits
- Physical quality of the work setting; for example, well-maintained surroundings
- Caliber of IT management
- Amount of interesting work
- Importance of the organization's mission
- Opportunities for career growth
- Adequacy of communication about topics ranging from strategy to project status

The managers' grades for Partners IT on these factors are presented in Table 12.1.

Table 12.1. Managers' grades for work factors

	A	B	C	D	F
Compensation and benefits	1	14	12	3	
Work environment	4	17	4	3	2
Good management	6	13	8	3	
Interesting work	12	2			
Mission	17	12	1		
Career growth	4	19	5	2	
Communication		8	15	2	5
Status of organization	17	10	3		
TOTAL	61	95	48	13	7

Using these scores, Partners IT leadership decided to focus on

- Establishing more thorough and better-defined career paths and development programs for all staff
- Improving training opportunities, ranging from brown bag lunches with invited speakers to technical training to supervisory training to leadership training
- Reviewing work environment factors such as parking, free amenities (such as soda), and office furniture
- Improving communication through mechanisms such as sending a monthly e-mail from the CIO, webcasting staff meetings so they could be attended remotely, and having regular dinners and lunches hosted by the CIO and deputy CIO

Taking steps such as these is important. Fundamentally, people work at organizations where the work is challenging and meaningful. They work at places where they like their coworkers and respect their leadership. They work at places where they are proud of the organization, its mission, and its successes.

ORGANIZING IT STAFF AND SERVICES

Now that we have introduced the various roles and functions found in the health care IT arena, we will examine how these roles and functions can be organized. Essentially, four factors influence the structure of the IT department:

- Definition and formation of major IT units
- Degree of IT centralization or decentralization
- Core IT competencies
- Departmental attributes

Definition and Formation of Major IT Units

There is no single right way to organize IT, and a department may iterate various organizational approaches in an effort to find the one that works best for it. (No approach is free of limitations.) There are several overall approaches to structuring formal departments, and an organization may employ several approaches simultaneously.

First, many IT departments organize their staff according to major job function or service areas. For example, a department might have a communications unit that sets up and manages local area networks and access to wide area networks, a research and development unit that keeps abreast of technology advances and experiments with new products, and a data administration unit that designs and maintains the organization's databases, data warehouses, and data management applications. Under this structure, staff members working in these various areas typically have both specialized and common skills, which they then apply to a wide range of systems or applications throughout the organization.

Second, the IT staff and services may be organized along product lines. That is, IT staff might work as project teams to develop, implement, maintain, and support a particular application or suite of applications. For example, there might be an applications unit comprising five to six major project teams. One team might support the administrative and billing systems, a second might support human and facility resources, and a third might cover clinical areas such as the laboratory, pharmacy, radiology, or nursing. Each team might combine IT staff and end users from the respective area. For example, a CPOE project team might include a systems analyst, a network administrator, a database manager, and key representatives from the clinical areas of medicine, nursing, laboratory, and pharmacy. This approach enables team members to work together closely, gain extensive knowledge about a particular application or suite of applications, and engage in holistic problem solving. In fact, the IT staff on the team may be physically located near the user department.

Third, the IT staff may be organized according to critical organizational processes. For example, there may be an IT team that manages and provides IT services to support the patient revenue cycle or patient access or medical services. This arrangement would enable the IT staff to understand all the information systems issues associated with a cross-organization process and develop a comprehensive understanding of critical organizational processes. This approach recognizes that patient care is based not on processes defined by organizational silos—for example, the laboratory or admitting—but rather on processes that cut across silos. Despite the conceptual appeal of this approach, it is not common. Its rarity is due largely to the fact that most organizations are organized by departments and not cross-organization processes: for example, it is rare to see a vice president of patient access. In general it is not intelligent to have IT organized in a way that is radically different from the approach used by the organization overall.

Fourth, the IT department may support a health care organization that is an integrated delivery system (IDS); it has multiple subsidiaries and divisions and may span a wide geography. The form of the IT department in an

Figure 12.2. IT department organized by function and geography

Figure 12.3. IT department organized by function and process

IDS is invariably matrixed. Kilbridge, Classen, Bates, and Denham (2006), in a study of IT organization in integrated delivery systems, found three dimensions that defined this matrix. The *functional* dimension was devoted to IDS-wide infrastructure, such as a communications network and enterprise master person index, and the support of IDS-wide consolidated functions, such as finance. The *geographical* dimension was devoted to supporting distinct geographical sites or logically separate provider sites, such as one of the IDS's community hospitals. The *cross-continuum, process-oriented* dimension might support acute care in general or a *carve-out,* such as oncology services. Figure 12.2 depicts a two-dimensional structure based on function and geography. Figure 12.3 shows a two-dimensional structure based on function and process.

These four approaches are by no means the only ways that one might approach organizing IT staff. The CIO, in conjunction with the organization's executive team, should consider a wide range of options for organizing IT staff and resources. As part of this process, the executive team should seek input from key constituents, examine the culture of the organization and the IT department, assess the long-term goals of the organization, and ultimately employ a structure that facilitates IT staff efficiency and effectiveness. In determining the structure of the IT organization, the team may ask these strategic questions: Which approaches will be used? Do the IT groupings represent well-circumscribed clusters of like expertise or common goals? Is the resulting set of departments comprehensive in scope?

Degree of IT Centralization or Decentralization

A critical factor in determining the structure for the IT department is the degree of centralization of organizational decision making. A health care organization might be a highly structured, vertical hierarchy where decisions are made by a few senior leaders. Conversely, an organization might delegate authority to the departmental level, or to the hospital level in an integrated delivery system, resulting in decentralized decision making.

There is no right level of centralization. Centralized organizations can be as effective as decentralized organizations. There are trade-offs, however. For example, centralized organizations are more likely to be able to effect uniformity of operations and to be more rational in their allocation of capital dollars, whereas decentralized organizations are more likely to be innovative. Moreover, an organization can be centralized in some areas, such as the process for developing the budget, and decentralized in other areas, such as developing marketing plans.

Ideally, the management and structure of IT will parallel that of the executive team's management philosophy; centralized management tends to want centralized control over IT, whereas decentralized management is more likely to be comfortable with IT that can be locally responsive.

One approach is not necessarily better than the other; they both have advantages and trade-offs. Some of the advantages to centralizing IT services (Oz, 2004) are

- *Enforcement of hardware and software standards.* In a centralized structure, the organization typically develops software and hardware standards, which can lead to cost savings, facilitate the exchange of data among systems, make installations easier, and promote sharing of applications.
- *Efficient administration of resources.* Centralizing the administration of contracts and licenses and inventories of hardware and software can lead to greater efficiency.
- *Better staffing.* Because it results in a pool of IT staff from which to choose, the centralized approach may be able to identify and assign the most appropriate individuals to a particular project.

- *Easier training.* In a centralized department, staff can specialize in certain areas (hardware, software, networks) and do not need to be jacks of all trades.

- *Effective planning of shared systems.* A centralized IT services unit typically sees the big picture and can facilitate the deployment of systems that are to be used by all units of a health care system or across organizational boundaries.

- *Easier strategic IT planning.* A strategic IT plan should be well aligned with the overall strategic plan of the organization. This alignment may be easier when IT management is centralized.

- *Tighter control by senior management.* A centralized approach to managing IT services permits senior management to maintain tighter control of the IT budget and resources.

Despite the advantages of a more centralized approach to managing IT services, many health care organizations have moved in recent years to a relatively decentralized structure. Some of the advantages to a decentralized structure (Oz, 2006) are

- *Better fit of IT to business needs.* The individual IT units are familiar with their business unit's or department's needs and can develop or select systems that fit those needs more closely.

- *Quick response time.* The individual IT units are typically better equipped to respond promptly to requests or can arrange IT projects to fit the priorities of their business unit or department.

- *Encouragement of end-user development of applications.* In a decentralized IT services structure, end users are often encouraged to develop their own small applications to increase productivity.

- *Innovative use of information systems.* Given that IT staff are closer in proximity to users and know their needs, the decentralized structure may have a better chance of implementing innovative systems.

Most IT services in a health care organization are not fully centralized or decentralized but a combination of the two. For example, training and support for applications may be decentralized, with other IT functions such as application development, network support, and database management being managed centrally. The size, complexity, and culture of the health care organization might also determine the degree to which IT services should be managed centrally. For example, in an ambulatory care clinic with three sites that are fairly autonomous, it may be appropriate to divide IT services into three functional units, each dedicated to a specific clinic. In a larger, more complex organization, such as an integrated delivery network (with multiple hospitals, outpatient clinics, and physician practices), it may be appropriate to form a centralized IT services unit that is responsible for specific IT areas such as systems planning and integration, network administration, and telecommunications, with all other functions being managed at the individual facility level.

Core IT Competencies

Organizations should identify a small number of areas that constitute core IT capabilities and competencies. These are areas where getting an A+ from the "customers" matters. For example, an organization focused on transforming its care processes would want to ensure A+ competency in this area and would perhaps settle for B– competency in its supply chain operations. An organization dedicated to being very efficient would want A+ competency in areas such as supplier management and productivity improvement and would perhaps settle for a B– in delivering superb customer service.

This definition of core competencies has a bearing on the form of the IT organization. If A+ competency is desired in care transformation, the IT department should be organized into functions that specialize in supporting care transformation: for example, a clinical information systems implementation group and a care reengineering group.

Partners HealthCare, for example, defined three areas of core capabilities: base support and services, care improvement, and technical infrastructure.

Base Support and Services

The category of core capabilities at Partners HealthCare included two subcategories:

- Frontline support: for example, mobile device problem resolution
- Project management skills

The choice of these areas of emphasis resulted in many management actions and steps: for example, the selection of criteria to be used during annual performance reviews. The emphasis on frontline support also led to the creation of an IT function responsible for all frontline support activities, including the help desk, workstation deployments, training, and user account management. The emphasis on project management led to the creation of a project management office to assist in monitoring the status of all projects and a *project center of excellence* to offer training on project management and established project management standards.

Care Improvement

Central to the Partners agenda was the application of IT to improve the process of care. One consequence was to establish, as a core IT capability, the set of skills and people necessary to innovatively apply IT to medical care improvement. An applied medical informatics function was established to oversee a research and development agenda. Staff skilled in clinical information systems application development were hired. A group of experienced clinical information system implementers was established. An IT unit of health services researchers was formed to analyze deficiencies in care processes, identify IT solutions that would reduce or eliminate these deficiencies, and assess the impact of clinical information systems on care improvement. Organizational units possessing unique technical and clinical knowledge in radiology imaging systems and telemedicine were also created.

Technical Infrastructure

Because Partners HealthCare recognized the critical role of a well-conceived, well-executed, and well-supported technical architecture, infrastructure architecture and design continued to serve as a core competency. A technology strategy function was created, and the role of chief technology officer was created. Significant attention was paid to ensuring that extremely talented architectural and engineering staff were hired along with staff with terrific support skills.

Departmental Attributes

IT departments, like people, have characteristics or attributes. They may be agile or ossified. They may be risk tolerant or risk averse. These characteristics can be stated, and strategies to achieve desired characteristics can be defined and implemented. To illustrate, this section will briefly discuss two characteristics—agility and innovativeness—and discuss how they might affect the organization of IT functions. These two characteristics are representative and are generally viewed as desirable.

There are many steps that an organization can take to increase its overall agility and also that of the IT department (Glaser, 2008a). For example, it is likely to try to *chunk* its initiatives so that there are multiple points at which a project can be reasonably stopped and yet still deliver value. Thus, the rollout of an electronic health record might call for implementation at ten clinics per year but could be stopped temporarily at four clinics and still deliver value to those four. Chunking allows an organization and its departments to quickly shift emphasis from one project to another.

An agile IT department will have the ability to form and disband teams quickly (perhaps every three months) as staff move from project to project. This requires that organizational structures and reporting relationships be flexible so staff can move rapidly between projects. It also means that during a project, the project manager is (temporarily anyway) the boss of the project team members. The team members might report to someone else according to the organizational chart, but their real boss at this time is the project manager. Because team members might move rapidly from project to project, they might have several bosses during the course of a year. And a person might be the boss on one project and the subordinate on another project. Agile organizations and departments are organized less around functions and more around projects. The IT structure must accommodate continuous project team formation, and project managers must have significant authority.

An organization or department that wants to be innovative might take steps such as implementing reward systems that encourage new ideas and successful implementation of innovative applications, and also punishment systems that are loath to discipline those involved in experiments that failed (Glaser, 2008b). The innovative IT department might create dedicated research and development groups. It might form teams composed of IT staff and vendor staff in an effort to cross-fertilize each group of staff with the ideas of the other. It might also permit staff to take sabbaticals or accept internships with other departments in the organization in an effort to expand IT members' awareness of organizational operations, cultures, and issues.

IN-HOUSE VERSUS OUTSOURCED IT

For the past two decades, health care organizations have generally provided IT services in-house. By *in-house* we mean that the organization hired its own IT staff and formed its own IT department. In recent years, however, health care organizations have shown a growing interest in outsourcing part or all of their IT services. *Outsourcing IT* means that an organization asks a third party to provide the IT staff and be responsible for the management of IT.

The reasons for outsourcing IT functions are varied. Some health care organizations may simply not have staff with the skills, time, or resources needed to take on new IT projects or provide sufficient IT service. Others may choose to outsource certain IT functions, such as help desk services or web site development, so that internal IT staff can focus their time on implementing or supporting applications central to the organization's strategic goals. Still other organizations contract with a cloud computing vendor to run system applications, manage the data, and provide technical support. Outsourcing IT may enable organizations to better control costs. Because a contract is typically established for a defined scope of work to be done over a specific period of time, the IT function becomes a line item that can be more effectively budgeted over time. This does not mean, however, that outsourcing IT services is necessarily more cost-effective than providing IT services in-house. At times, new organizational leadership finds an IT function that is in disastrous condition. After years of mismanagement, applications may function poorly, the infrastructure may be unstable, and the IT staff may be demoralized. An outsourcing company may be brought in as a form of rescue mission.

A number of factors come into play and should be considered when evaluating whether outsourcing part or all of IT services is in the best interest of the organization. The following questions should be asked:

- Does our organization have IT staff with the knowledge and skills needed to provide necessary services? Effectively manage projects? Adequately support current applications and infrastructure?

- How easy or difficult is it to recruit and retain qualified IT staff?

- What are our organization's major IT priorities? How equipped is our organization to address these priorities? Do we have the right mix of skills, time, and resources?

- What benefits might be realized from outsourcing this IT function? What are the risks? Do the benefits outweigh the risks?

- What parts, if any, of the IT department does it make the most sense to outsource?

- If we opt to outsource IT services, with whom do we want to do business? How will we monitor and evaluate IT performance and service? What provisions will we make in the contract with the outsourcing company to ensure timeliness and quality of service? How will the terms of the contract be monitored?

It is important to evaluate the cost and effectiveness of the IT function and services, whether they are performed by in-house staff or outsourced. There are pros and cons to each approach, and the organization must make its decision based on its strategy goals and priorities. There is no silver bullet or one solution for all.

PERSPECTIVE
Ramifications of Payment Reform on the IT Organization

Health care organizations will become more inwardly focused on execution. Strategies are always critical. However, circumstances such as the constraints on capital and the deadlines of the HITECH incentives, coupled with care transparency and accountability, will place a premium on execution of existing strategies. Poor execution of operations improvement plans or efforts to improve patient safety will have greater consequences than in years past.

These circumstances will lead to heightened scrutiny of proposed IT initiatives. Since fewer initiatives may be funded, those that are funded must be the IT projects that address the most acute needs, have the greatest likelihood of success, and promise the greatest returns. Project proposals will have to be more rigorously assessed, with project costs, potential risks, and projected payoffs being subject to greater scrutiny.

The pressure on application project performance will increase. If fewer IT projects will be funded, and those that are funded have greater consequences, the need for the project "to deliver the goods" is elevated. There will be closer monitoring of project progress. Changes or events that lead to increased project costs or prolonged timetables will be viewed as more problematic than they have been in the past. Departments and groups that fail to alter work processes, limitations in the application, or problems with the infrastructure will draw a swifter and more potent management reaction. Management interest in understanding whether the initiative actually led to the gains promised will be greater.

There will be an increased emphasis on efficiency—for everyone, including IT. Doing more with less and having measures that show that a group is doing more with less will be required.

And all of these ramifications will occur in the context of an increase in IT sophistication by the administrative and medical staff leadership. Their years of experience with IT have taught them something—they are smarter and more sophisticated about the area. This is good for IT—a sophisticated customer is a better customer. And this can be challenging for IT—a sophisticated customer is a more demanding customer.

Source: Glaser & Kirby, 2009.

EVALUATING IT EFFECTIVENESS

Whether IT services are provided by in-house staff or are outsourced, it is important to evaluate IT performance. Is the function efficient? Does it deliver good service? Is it on top of new developments in its field? Does the function have a strong management team?

At times, health care executives become worried about the performance of an IT function. Other organizations have IT functions that seem to accomplish more or spend less. Management and physicians frequently express dissatisfaction with IT; nothing is getting done, it costs too much, or it takes too long to get a new application implemented. Many factors may result in user dissatisfaction: poor expectation setting, unclear priorities, limited funding, or inadequate IT leadership. An assessment of IT services can help management understand the nature of the problems and identify opportunities for improvement.

One desirable approach to assessing IT services is to use outside consultants. Consultants can bring a level of objectivity to the assessment process that is difficult to achieve internally. They can also share their experiences, having worked with a variety of different health care organizations and having observed different ways of handling some of the same issues or problems.

Whether the assessment is done by internal staff or by consultants, several key areas should be addressed:

- Governance
- Budget development and resource allocation
- System acquisition
- System implementation
- IT service levels

Governance

How effective is the governance structure? To what degree are IT strategies well aligned with the organization's overall strategic goals? Is the CIO actively involved in strategy discussions? Does senior leadership discuss IT agenda items on a regular basis? We will discuss governance in Chapter Fifteen.

Budget Development and Resource Allocation

The IT budget is often compared to the IT budgets of comparable health care organizations. The question behind a budget benchmark is, Are we spending too much or too little on IT? Budget benchmarks are expressed in terms of the IT operating budget as a percentage of the overall organization's operating budget and the IT capital budget as a percentage of the organization's total capital budget. On average, hospitals spend 2.7 percent of their operating budget and 15 percent of their capital budget on IT (Gartner, 2008).

These budget benchmarks are useful and in some sense required because most boards of directors expect to see them. Management has to be careful in interpreting the results, however. These percentages do not necessarily reflect the quality of IT services or the extent and size of the organization's application base or infrastructure. Hence, one can find a poorly performing IT group that has implemented little having the same percentage of the organization's budgetary resources as a world-class IT group that has implemented a stunning array of applications.

Spending a high percentage of the operating budget—for example, 4.5 percent—does not per se mean that the organization is spending too much and should reduce its IT budget. The organization may have decided to ramp up its IT investments in order to achieve certain strategic objectives. A low percentage—for example, 1 percent—does not per se mean that underinvestment is occurring and the IT budget should be significantly increased. The organization may be very efficient, or it may have decided that given its strategies its investments should be made elsewhere.

We will discuss the IT budget and resource allocation in Chapter Fifteen.

System Acquisition

How effective are system acquisitions? How long did they take? What process was used to select the systems? We discussed system acquisition in Chapter Seven.

System Implementation

Are new applications delivered on time, within budget, and according to specification? Do the participants in the implementation speak fondly of the professionalism of the IT staff or do they view IT staff as forms of demonic creatures? We discussed system implementation in Chapter Eight.

IT Service Levels

IT staff deliver service every day: for example, they manage system performance, respond to help desk calls, and manage projects. The quality of these services can be measured. An assessment of the IT function invariably reviews these measures and the management processes in place to monitor and improve IT services. IT users in the organization are interested in measures such as these:

- *Infrastructure.* Are the information systems reliable, that is, do they rarely "go down"? Are response times fast?

- *Day-to-day support.* Does the help desk quickly, patiently, and effectively resolve my problems? If I ask for a new workstation, does it arrive in a reasonable period of time?

- *Consultation.* Are the IT folks good at helping me think through my IT needs? Are they realistic in helping me to understand what the technology will and will not do?

An organization faces a challenge in defining what level of IT service it would like and also how much it is willing to pay for IT services. All of us would love to have systems analysts with world-class consulting skills, but we may not be able to afford their salaries. Similarly, all of us would love to have systems that never go down and are as fast as greased lightning, but we might not be willing to pay the cost of engineering very, very high reliability and blazing speed. The IT service conversation attempts to establish formal and measurable levels of service and the cost of providing that service. The organization seeks an informed conversation about the desirability and the cost of improving the service or the possibility of degrading the service in an effort to reduce costs.

In general it can be very difficult to measure the quality and consequences of consultative services. This makes it difficult to understand whether it is worth investing to improve the service other than at the service extremes. For example, it can be clear that you need to fire a very ineffective systems analyst and that you need to treat your all-star analyst very well. But it may not be clear whether paying $10,000 extra for an IT staff member is worth it or not.

Formal, measurable service levels can be established for many infrastructure attributes and day-to-day support. Moreover, industry benchmarks exist for these measures. Common infrastructure metrics are

- *Reliability:* for example, the percentage of time that systems have unscheduled downtime

- *Response time:* for example, how quickly an application moves from one screen to the next
- *Resiliency:* for example, how quickly a system can recover after it goes down
- *Software bugs:* for example, the number of bugs detected in an application per line of program code or hour of use

Common day-to-day support metrics are

- The percentage of help desk calls that are resolved within twenty-four hours
- The percentage of help desk calls that are not resolved after five days
- The percentage of help desk calls that are repeat calls: that is, the problem was not resolved the first time
- The time that elapses between ordering a workstation and its installation

It is important that the management team define the desired level of IT service. For example, is the goal to achieve an uptime of 99.99 percent, or does the organization want to have 90 percent of help desk calls closed within twenty-four hours? If the service levels are deemed to be inadequate, a discussion can be held with IT managers to identify the costs of achieving a higher level of service. Additional staff may be needed at the help desk, or the organization may need to develop a redundant network to improve resiliency. Conversely, if the organization needs to reduce IT costs, the management team may need to examine the service consequences of reducing the number of help desk staff.

The assessment of the IT function requires examining areas that range from strategy development to service levels. And the assessment can use a variety of data collection techniques. Exhibit 12.3 is a sample survey used by an IT services department to assess user satisfaction.

Answers to these questions provide an indication, clearly rough, of how well the IT function is being run and, to a degree, of whether the aggregate IT investment is providing value. All these questions come from common sense, management beliefs about what is involved in running an organization well, and tests of IT domain knowledge.

Exhibit 12.3. Sample user satisfaction survey

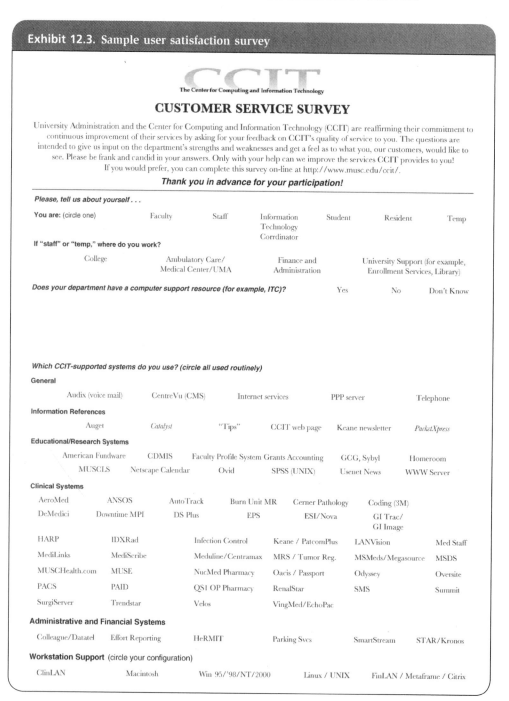

CCIT
The Center for Computing and Information Technology

CUSTOMER SERVICE SURVEY

University Administration and the Center for Computing and Information Technology (CCIT) are reaffirming their commitment to continuous improvement of their services by asking for your feedback on CCIT's quality of service to you. The questions are intended to give us input on the department's strengths and weaknesses and get a feel as to what you, our customers, would like to see. Please be frank and candid in your answers. Only with your help can we improve the services CCIT provides to you! If you would prefer, you can complete this survey on-line at http://www.musc.edu/ccit/.

Thank you in advance for your participation!

Please, tell us about yourself . . .

You are: (circle one)   Faculty   Staff   Information Technology Corrdinator   Student   Resident   Temp

If "staff" or "temp," where do you work?

College   Ambulatory Care/ Medical Center/UMA   Finance and Administration   University Support (for example, Enrollment Services, Library)

Does your department have a computer support resource (for example, ITC)?   Yes   No   Don't Know

Which CCIT-supported systems do you use? (circle all used routinely)

General

Audix (voice mail)   CentreVu (CMS)   Internet services   PPP server   Telephone

Information References

Auget   *Catalyst*   "Tips"   CCIT web page   Keane newsletter   *PacketXpress*

Educational/Research Systems

American Fundware   CDMIS   Faculty Profile System   Grants Accounting   GCG, Sybyl   Homeroom
MUSCLS   Netscape Calendar   Ovid   SPSS (UNIX)   Usenet News   WWW Server

Clinical Systems

AeroMed   ANSOS   AutoTrack   Burn Unit MR   Cerner Pathology   Coding (3M)
DeMedici   Downtime MPI   DS Plus   EPS   ESI/Nova   GI Trac/ GI Image
HARP   IDXRad   Infection Control   Keane / PatcomPlus   LANVision   Med Staff
MediLinks   MediScribe   Meduline/Centramax   MRS / Tumor Reg.   MSMeds/Megasource   MSDS
MUSCHealth.com   MUSE   NucMed Pharmacy   Oacis / Passport   Odyssey   Oversite
PACS   PAID   QS1 OP Pharmacy   RenalStar   SMS   Summit
SurgiServer   Trendstar   Velos   VingMed/EchoPac

Administrative and Financial Systems

Colleague/Datatel   Effort Reporting   HeRMIT   Parking Svcs   SmartStream   STAR/Kronos

Workstation Support (circle your configuration)

ClinLAN   Macintosh   Win 95/'98/NT/2000   Linux / UNIX   FinLAN / Metaframe / Citrix

Exhibit 12.3. (*Continued*)

Now, what do you think about us . . .

Help Desk Staff	Very satisfied	Somewhat satisfied	Neutral	Somewhat dissatisfied	Very dissatisfied
1. Requests are clearly understood	5	4	3	2	1
2. Troubleshooting skills are adequate	5	4	3	2	1
3. If not able to resolve. are able to identify right resource	5	4	3	2	1
4. Professional, friendly, diplomatic	5	4	3	2	1
5. Understands needs and priorities	5	4	3	2	1
6. Treats you with respect and consideration	5	4	3	2	1

Systems Support Staff

1. Responsive to problems/requests	5	4	3	2	1
2. Professional, friendly, diplomatic	5	4	3	2	1
3. Understands needs and priorities	5	4	3	2	1
4. Treats you with respect and consideration	5	4	3	2	1
5. Communicates well	5	4	3	2	1
6. Quality of work is high	5	4	3	2	1
7. Positive attitude	5	4	3	2	1
8. Plans/manages projects well	5	4	3	2	1

Workstation Support Staff

1. Responsive to problems/requests	5	4	3	2	1
2. Professional, friendly, diplomatic	5	4	3	2	1
3. Understands needs and priorities	5	4	3	2	1
4. Treats you with respect and consideration	5	4	3	2	1
5. Communicates well	5	4	3	2	1
6. Quality of work is high	5	4	3	2	1
7. Positive attitude	5	4	3	2	1
8. Plans/manages projects well	5	4	3	2	1

Do you have additional comments about your experiences with our staff?

Overall, how satisfied are you with CCIT? very satisfied   satisfied   neutral   not satisfied   very dissatisfied

Would you like to be interviewed? For "yes," please note your name and MUSC extension:

Thank you again for your time and assistance!

Source: © 2008 Medical University Hospital Authority. All Rights Reserved.

PERSPECTIVE
Assessing the IT Function

Glaser (2006) proposes a series of questions that can be used to assess the IT function. These questions cover the areas of infrastructure and application performance, execution, and strategic alignment.

Infrastructure and Application Performance

External and internal auditors' reports on IT controls and management. Do these reports note material problems with significant downtime, failure to perform adequate management of the data center, and adequacy of security controls?

IT infrastructure management processes. Does IT track downtime and what steps have been taken to reduce it? Are they current with vendor releases? How does IT manage virus protection? When the infrastructure has problems, what are the procedures for responding?

Execution

Achieving desired application outcomes. Picking three recent implementations, what were the objectives? To what degree were the objectives achieved? If the organization fell short in achieving objectives, why did this happen?

User engagement. Do implemented systems improve the operation of key departments? Was the training good? Were the IT group and the vendor responsive to issues and problems?

Managing the implementation. Were clear project charters developed? Are sound project management techniques used? Do most projects get done on time and on budget?

Frontline support. Does the IT organization measure its service? Has the IT organization established service goals? Was the organization's management involved in setting those goals?

Departmental IT liaisons. Who are the IT liaisons to major user departments? Do they do a good job? Do the liaisons keep the department up to date on IT plans? Are liaisons considered to be members of the department's team?

Alignment of the IT Agenda with the Organization's Agenda

IT linkage to organizational strategy. Can the major elements of the organization's strategy be mapped to the IT initiatives needed to support the strategic plan? Is there a regular senior leadership discussion of the IT agenda, and does the leadership take responsibility for making decisions about which IT initiatives to fund?

Governance. What processes and committees are used to set priorities? Is the process for setting the IT budget well understood, efficient, sufficiently rigorous, and perceived as fair? Is there a well-accepted approach for acquiring new applications?

Source: Glaser, 2006.

PERSPECTIVE
Managing Core IT Processes

Agarwal and Sambamurthy (2002) have identified eight core IT processes that must be managed well for an IT department to be effective:

1. *Human capital management* involves the development of IT staff skills and the attraction and retention of IT talent.

2. *Platform management* is a series of activities that designs the IT architecture and constructs and manages the resulting infrastructure.

3. *Relationship management* centers on developing and maintaining relationships between the IT function and the rest of the organization and on partnerships with IT vendors.

4. *Strategic planning* links the IT agenda and plans to the organization's strategy and plans.

5. *Financial management* encompasses a wide range of management processes—developing the IT budget, defining the business case for IT investments, and benchmarking IT costs.

6. *Value innovation* involves identifying new ways for IT to improve business operations and ensuring that IT investments deliver value.

7. *Solutions delivery* includes the selection, development, and implementation of applications and infrastructure.

8. *Services provisioning* centers on the day-to-day support of applications and infrastructure: for example, the help desk, workstation deployments, and user training.

Source: Agarwal & Sambamurthy, 2002.

SUMMARY

It is critical that health care organizations have access to appropriate IT staff and resources to support their health care information systems and system users. IT staff perform several common functions and have several common roles. In large organizations, the IT department often has a management team comprising the chief information officer, chief technology officer, chief security officer, and chief medical information officer, who provide leadership to ensure that the organization fulfills its IT strategies and goals. Having a CIO with strong leadership skills, vision, and experience is critical to the organization achieving its strategic IT goals. Working with the CIO and IT management team, one will often find a team of professional and technical staff including systems analysts, computer programmers, network administrators, database administrators, and web designers and support personnel. Each brings a unique set of knowledge and skills to support the IT operations of the health care organization.

The organizational structure of the IT department is influenced by several factors: definition of major units, level of centralization, core IT competencies, and desired attributes of the IT department.

IT services may be provided by in-house staff or outsourced to an outside vendor or company. Many factors come into play in deciding if and when to outsource all or part of the IT services. Availability of staff, time constraints, financial resources, and the executive management team's view of IT may determine the appropriateness of outsourcing.

Whether IT services are provided in-house or outsourced, it is important for the management team to assess the efficiency and effectiveness of IT services. The governance structure, how the IT resources are allocated, the track record of system acquisitions and system implementations, and user satisfaction with current IT service levels are some of the key elements that should be examined in any assessment. Consultants may be employed to conduct the assessment and offer the organization an outsider's objective view.

KEY TERMS

Applications management

Chief information officer (CIO)

Chief medical information officer (CMIO)

Chief security officer (CSO)

Chief technology officer (CTO)

Database administrator

Governance

IT centralization and decentralization

Network administrator

Operations and technical support

Outsourced IT

Programmer

Systems analyst

Telecommunications specialist

LEARNING ACTIVITIES

1. Visit an IT department in a health care facility in your community and interview the CIO or department director. Examine the IT department's organizational structure. What functions or services does the IT department provide? How centralized are IT services within the organization? Does the organization employ a CMIO, CSO, or CTO? If so, what are each person's job qualifications and responsibilities?

2. Find an article in the literature that outlines either the advantages or disadvantages, or both, of outsourcing IT. Discuss the findings with your classmates. What have others learned about outsourcing that may be important to your organization?

3. Plan and organize a panel discussion with CIOs from local health care facilities. Find out what some of their greatest challenges are and what a typical day is like for them. To what degree are their organizations facing workforce shortages? In what areas, if any? What strategies do they employ to recruit and retain top-notch staff?

4. Assume that your organization is concerned about employee satisfaction with IT services. How might the organization assess employee satisfaction? What methods and tools might be used? How would you use these methods and tools?

5. Investigate any one of the following roles and interview someone working in this type of position. Find out the individual's roles, responsibilities, qualifications, background, experience, and challenges.
   - Chief medical information officer
   - Chief security officer
   - Chief technology officer
   - Nursing informatics specialist
   - Clinical systems analyst
   - Biomedical informatics expert

REFERENCES

Agarwal, R., & Sambamurthy, V. (2002). *Organizing the IT function for business innovation leadership.* Chicago: Society for Information Management.

College of Healthcare Information Management Executives. (1998). *The healthcare CIO: A decade of growth.* Ann Arbor, MI: Author.

College of Healthcare Information Management Executives. (2008). *The seven CIO success factors.* Retrieved April 2008 from http://www.cio-chime.org/events /ciobootcamp/measure.asp

Committee on Workforce Needs in Information Technology. (2001). *Building a workforce for the information economy.* Washington, DC: National Academies Press.

Conn, J. (2010, May 24). Working on IT. *Modern Healthcare,* p. 28.

Department of Labor, Bureau of Labor Statistics. (2008). National employment matrix. Retrieved November 2008 from http://data.bls.gov/oep/servlet/oep .nioem.servlet.ActionServlet

Earl, M., & Feeney, D. (1995). Is your CIO adding value? *McKinsey Quarterly, 2,* 144–161.

Gartner, Inc. (2008). *Forecast: Healthcare IT spending worldwide, 2006–2011.* Stamford, CT: Author.

Glaser, J. (2006, January). Assessing the IT function in less than one day. *Healthcare Financial Management,* pp. 104–108.

Glaser, J. (2008a, April). Creating IT agility. *Healthcare Financial Management,* pp. 36–39.

Glaser, J. (2008b, February 6). The four cornerstones of innovation. *Most Wired Online.*

Glaser, J., & Kirby, J. (2009). Evolution of the healthcare CIO. *Healthcare Financial Management, 63*(11), 38–41.

Glaser, J., & Williams, R. (2007). The definitive evolution of the role of the CIO. *Journal of Healthcare Information Management, 21*(1), 9–11.

Kilbridge, P. M., Classen, D., Bates, D. W., & Denham, C. R. (2006). The National Quality Forum safe practice standard for computerized physician order entry: Updating a critical patient safety practice. *Journal of Patient Safety, 2*(4), 183–190.

Leviss, J., Kremsdorf, R., & Mohaideen, M. F. (2006). The CMIO: A new leader for health systems. *Journal of the American Medical Informatics Association, 13*(5), 573–578.

Oz, E. (2006). *Management information systems: Instructor edition* (4th ed.). Boston: Course Technology.

CHAPTER 13

IT Alignment and Strategic Planning

LEARNING OBJECTIVES

- To be able to understand the importance of an IT strategic plan.
- To review the components of the IT strategic plan.
- To be able to understand the processes for developing an information technology strategy.
- To be able to discuss the challenges of developing an IT strategy.

Information technology (IT) investments serve to advance organizational performance. These investments should enable the organization to reduce costs, improve service, enhance the quality of care, and, in general, achieve its strategic objectives. The goal of IT alignment and strategic planning is to ensure a strong and clear relationship between IT investment decisions and the health care organization's overall strategies, goals, and objectives. For example, an organization's decision to invest in a new claims adjudication system should be the clear result of a goal of improving the effectiveness of its claims processing process. An organization's decision to implement a computerized provider order entry system should reflect an organizational strategy of improving patient care.

Developing a sound alignment can be very important for one simple reason—if you define the IT agenda incorrectly or even partially correctly, you run the risk that significant organizational resources will be misdirected; the resources will not be put to furthering strategically important areas. This risk has nothing to do with how well you execute the IT direction you choose. Being on time, on budget, and on specification is of little value to the organization if it is doing the wrong thing!

IT PLANNING OBJECTIVES

The IT strategic planning process has several objectives:

- To ensure that information technology plans and activities align with the plans and activities of the organization; in other words, the IT needs of each aspect of organizational strategy are clear, and the portfolio of IT plans and activities can be mapped to organizational strategies and operational needs.

- To ensure that the alignment is comprehensive; in other words, each aspect of strategy has been addressed from an IT perspective that recognizes not all aspects of strategy have an IT component, and not all components will be funded.

- To identify non-IT organizational initiatives needed to ensure maximum leverage of the IT initiative (for example, process reengineering).

- To ensure that the organization has not missed a strategic IT opportunity, such as those that might result from new technologies.

- To develop a tactical plan that details approved project descriptions, timetables, budgets, staffing plans, and plan risk factors.

Table 13.1. IT initiatives linked to organizational goals

Goal	IT Initiatives
Research and education	Research patient data registry Genetics and genomics platform Grants management
Patient care: quality improvement	Quality measurement databases Order entry Electronic health record
Patient care: sharing data across the system	Enterprise master person index Clinical data repository Common infrastructure
Patient care: non-acute services	Nursing documentation Transition of care
Financial stability	Revenue system enhancements Payroll-personnel system Cost accounting

- To create a communication tool that can inform the organization of the IT initiatives that will and will not be undertaken.

- To establish a political process that helps ensure the plan results have sufficient organizational support.

At the end of the alignment and strategic-planning process, an organization should have an outline that at a high level resembles Table 13.1. With this outline, leadership can see the IT investments needed to advance each of the organization's strategies. For example, the goal of improving the quality of patient care may lead the organization to invest in databases to measure and report quality, computerized provider order entry (CPOE), and the EHR.

In many ways the content of Table 13.1 is deceiving. The table presents a tidy, orderly linkage between the IT agenda and the strategies of the organization. One might assume this linkage is established through a linear, rational, and straightforward series of steps. But the process of arriving at a series of connections like those in Table 13.1 is complex, iterative, and at times driven by politics and instincts.

The development of well-aligned IT strategies has been notoriously difficult for many years, and there appears to be no reason such an alignment will become significantly easier over time.

OVERVIEW OF STRATEGY

Strategy is the determination of the basic long-term goals and objectives of an organization, the adoption of the course of action, and the allocation of resources necessary to carry out those actions (Chandler, 1962). Strategy seeks to answer questions such as, Where does this organization need to go, and how will it get there? Where should the organization focus its management attention and expenditures?

The development of an organization's strategy has two major components: formulation and implementation (Henderson & Venkatraman, 1993).

Formulation

Formulation involves making decisions about the mission and goals of the organization and the activities and initiatives it will undertake to achieve them. Formulation could involve determining the following:

- Our mission is to provide high-quality medical care.
- We have a goal of reducing the cost of care while at least preserving the quality of that care.
- One of our greatest leverage points lies in reducing inappropriate and unnecessary care.
- To achieve this goal, we will emphasize reducing the number of inappropriate radiology procedures.
- We will carry out initiatives that enable us to intervene at the time of procedure ordering if we need to suggest a more cost-effective modality.

We can imagine other goals directed toward achieving this mission. For each goal, we can envision multiple leverage points, and for each leverage point, we may see multiple initiatives. The result is an inverted tree that cascades from our mission to a series of initiatives.

Formulation involves understanding competing ideas and choosing between them. In our example, we could have arrived at a different set of goals and initiatives.

We could have decided to improve quality with less emphasis on care costs. We could have decided to focus on reducing the cost per procedure. We could have decided to produce retrospective reports of radiology use by provider and used this feedback to lead to ordering behavior change rather than intervening at the time of ordering.

In IT, we also have a need for formulation. In keeping with an IT mission to use the technology to support improvement of the quality of care, we may have a goal to integrate our clinical application systems. To achieve this goal, we may decide to follow any of the following initiatives:

- Provide a common way to access all systems (single sign-on).
- Interface existing heterogeneous systems.
- Require that all applications use a common database.
- Implement a common suite of clinical applications from one vendor.

Implementation

Implementation involves making decisions about how we structure ourselves, acquire skills, establish organizational capabilities, and alter organizational processes to achieve the goals and carry out the activities we have defined during formulation of our strategy. For example, if we have decided to reduce care costs by reducing inappropriate procedure use, we may need to implement one or more of the following:

- An organizational unit of providers with health services research training to analyze care practices and identify deficiencies
- A steering committee of clinical leadership to guide these efforts and provide political support
- A provider order entry system to provide real-time feedback on order appropriateness
- Data warehouse technologies to support analyses of utilization

Using our clinical applications integration example, we may come to one of the following determinations:

- We need to acquire interface engine technology, adopt HL7 standards, and form an information systems department that manages the technology and interfaces applications.
- We need to engage external consulting assistance for selection of a clinical application suite and hire a group to implement the suite.

The implementation component of strategy development is not the development of project plans and budgets. Rather, it is the identification of the capabilities, capacities, and competencies the organization will need if it is to carry out the results of the formulation component of strategy.

VECTORS FOR ARRIVING AT IT STRATEGY

The IT strategy is developed using some combination of four vectors. These vectors are

- Organizational strategies
- Continuous improvement of core processes and information management
- Examination of the role of new information technologies
- Assessment of strategic trajectories

By a vector we mean the choice of perspectives and approaches through which an organization determines its IT investment decisions. For example, the first vector (derived from organization strategies) involves answering a question such as, "Given our strategy of improving patient safety, what IT applications will we need?" However, the third vector (determined by examining the role of new information technologies) involves answering a question such as, "There is a great deal of discussion about software as a service. Does this approach to delivering applications provide us with ways to be more effective at addressing some of our organization challenges?" Figure 13.1 illustrates the convergence of these four vectors into a series of iterative leadership discussions and debates. These debates lead to an IT agenda.

Figure 13.1. Overview of IT strategy development

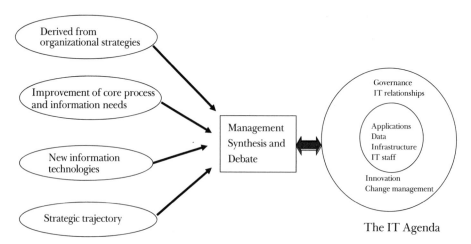

IT Strategies Derived from Organizational Strategies

The first vector involves deriving the IT agenda directly from the organization's goals and plans. For example, an organization may decide it intends to become the low-cost provider of care. It may decide to achieve this goal through implementation of disease management programs, the reengineering of inpatient care, and the reduction of unit costs for certain tests and procedures it believes are inordinately expensive.

The IT strategy development then centers on answering questions such as, "How do we apply IT to support disease management?" The answers might involve web-based publication of disease management protocols for use by providers, business intelligence technology to assess the conformance of care practice to the protocols, provider documentation systems based on disease guidelines, and CPOE systems that employ the disease guidelines to influence ordering decisions. An organization may choose all or some of these responses and develop various sequences of implementation. Nonetheless, it has developed an answer to the question of how to apply IT in support of disease management.

Most of the time the linkage between organizational strategy and IT strategy involves developing the IT ramifications of organizational initiatives, such as adding or changing services and products, growing market share, or improving service, streamlining processes, or reducing costs. At times, however, an organization may decide it needs to change or add to its core characteristics or culture. The organization may decide it needs its staff to be more care quality or service-delivery or bottom-line oriented. It may decide it needs to decentralize or recentralize decision making. It may decide to improve its ability to manage knowledge, or it may not. These characteristics (and there are many others) can point to initiatives for IT.

In cases where characteristics are to be changed, IT strategies must be developed to answer such questions as, "What is our basic IT approach to supporting a decentralized decision-making structure?" The organization might answer this question by permitting decentralized choices of applications as long as those applications meet certain standards. (For example, they may run on a common infrastructure or support common data standards.) It might answer the question of how IT supports an emphasis on knowledge management by developing an intranet service that provides access to preferred treatment guidelines.

IT Strategies to Continuously Improve Core Processes and Information Management

All organizations have a small number of core processes and information management tasks that are essential for the effective and efficient functioning of the organization. For a hospital these processes might include ensuring patient access to care, ordering tests and procedures, and managing the revenue cycle. For a restaurant these processes might include menu design, food preparation, and dining room service. For a managed care organization, information management needs might point to a requirement to understand the costs of care or the degree to which care practices vary by physician.

Using the vector of continuous improvement of core processes and information management to determine IT strategies involves defining the organization's core processes and information management needs. The organization measures the performance of core processes and uses the resulting data to develop plans to improve its performance. The organization defines core information needs, identifies the gap between the current status and its needs, and develops plans to close those gaps. These plans will often point to an IT agenda.

This vector may be a result of a strategy discussion, although this is not always the case. An organization may make ongoing efforts to improve processes regardless of the specifics of its strategic plan. For example, every year it may establish initiatives designed to reduce costs or improve services. The organization has decided that, regardless of a specific strategy, it will not thrive if core processes and information management are something other than excellent.

Table 13.2 illustrates a process orientation. It provides an organization with data on the magnitude of some problems that plague the delivery of outpatient care. These problems afflict the processes of referral, results management, and

Table 13.2. Summary of the scope of outpatient care problems

For every:	There appear to be:
1,000 patients coming in for outpatient care	14 patients with life-threatening or serious ADEs
1,000 outpatients who are taking a prescription drug	90 patients who seek medical attention because of drug complications
1,000 prescriptions written	40 prescriptions with medical errors
1,000 women with a marginally abnormal mammogram	360 who will not receive appropriate follow-up care
1,000 referrals	250 referring physicians who have not received follow-up information four weeks later
1,000 patients who qualified for secondary prevention of high cholesterol	380 will not have an LDL-C on record within three years

test ordering. The organization may decide to make IT investments in an effort to reduce or eliminate these problems. For example, e-prescribing could reduce the prevalence of adverse drug events (ADEs). Abnormal test results could be highlighted in the EHR to help ensure patient follow-up.

When this vector is used, the IT agenda is driven at least in part by a relentless year-in, year-out focus on improving core processes and information management needs.

IT Strategies That Rely on New IT Capabilities

The third vector involves considering how new IT capabilities may enable a new IT agenda or significantly alter the current agenda. For example, telemedicine capabilities may enable the organization to consider a strategy it had not previously considered, such as extending the reach of its specialists across the globe. An organization may also alter its approach to achieving an existing strategy so that, for example, it relies less on specialists visiting regional health centers and more on teleconsultation. Data mining algorithm advances might enable an organization to conduct postmarket medication surveillance and to construct a patient phenotype from EHR data to support research into the genomic basis of disease.

In this vector, the organization examines new applications and new base technologies and tries to answer the question, "Does this application or technology enable us to advance our strategies or improve our core processes in new ways?" For example, applications that support personally controlled health records might lead the organization to think of new approaches to providing feedback to the chronically ill patient. Holding new technologies up to the spotlight of organizational interest can lead to decisions to invest in a new technology.

An extreme form of this mechanism occurs when a new technology or application suggests that fundamental strategies (or even the organization's existence) may be called into question or may need to undergo significant transformation. Although IT-induced transformation is rare in health care, it is being seen in other industries. The Internet, for example, has transformed and in some cases challenged the existence of a range of companies that distribute content. Examples are companies such as bookstores, music CD stores, publishers, travel agents, and stockbrokers.

IT Strategies Based on Assessment of Strategic Trajectories

Organization and IT strategies invariably have a fixed time horizon and fixed scope. These strategies might cover a period of time two to three years into the future. They outline a bounded set of initiatives to be undertaken in that time period. Assessment of strategic trajectories asks the questions: What do we think we will be doing after that time horizon and scope? Do we think we will be doing very different kinds of things, or will we be carrying out initiatives similar to the ones we are pursuing now?

For example, we might be planning to implement an EHR. The organization believes the future will bring the broad adoption of medical homes and accountable care organizations (ACOs). These models are not widespread, but the organization believes it should strive to be well positioned to serve as an ACO. The strategic trajectory discussion asks, "What EHR capabilities are we likely to need in an ACO?"

Or we might be in the process of using IT to support joint clinical programs with other hospitals in the area. Given the federal government's emphasis on EHR interoperability, the country may see broad implementation of state-based health information exchanges. The trajectory discussion asks how these exchanges will affect our current approaches to clinical integration with affiliated providers.

The strategic trajectory discussion can be highly speculative. It might be so forward looking and speculative that the organization decides not to act today on its discussion. Yet it can also point to initiatives to be undertaken within the next year to better understand this possible future and to prepare the organization's information systems for it. For example, if we believe our information systems will eventually need to store genetic information, it would be worth understanding whether the new clinical data repository we will be selecting soon will be capable of storing these data.

THE IT ASSET

The discussion of vectors and alignment up to this point has focused generally on the development of an application agenda as the outcome. In other words, the completion of the IT strategy discussion is an inventory of systems, such as the EHR system, customer relationship management system, and clinical laboratory system, that are needed to further overall organizational strategies. However, the application inventory is a component of the larger idea of the IT asset. These areas are discussed in the following sections.

The *IT asset* is composed of those IT resources that the organization has or can obtain and that are applied to further the goals, plans, and initiatives of the organization. The IT strategy discussion identifies specific changes or enhancements to the composition of the asset—for example, the implementation of a new application—and general properties of the asset that must exist—for example, high reliability of the infrastructure. The IT asset has four components: applications, infrastructure, data, and IT staff.

Applications

Applications are the systems that users interact with: for example, scheduling, billing, and electronic health record systems. In addition to developing an inventory of applications, the organization may need to develop strategies regarding properties of the overall portfolio of applications.

For example, if the organization is an integrated delivery system, decisions will need to be made about the degree to which applications should be the same across the organization. E-mail systems ought to be the same, but is there a strategic reason to have the same clinical laboratory system across all hospitals? Should an organization buy or build its applications? Building applications is risky and often requires skills that most health care organizations do not possess. However, internally developed applications can be less expensive and can be tailored to an organization's needs.

Strategic thinking may center on the form and rigor of the justification process for new applications. Formal return on investment analyses may be emphasized so that all application decisions will emphasize cost reduction or revenue gain. Or the organization may decide to have a decision process that takes a more holistic approach to acquisition decisions, so that factors such as improving quality of care must also be considered.

In general, strategy discussions surrounding the application asset as a whole focus on, in addition to the application inventory, a few key areas:

- **Sourcing.** What are the sources for our applications? And what criteria determine the source to be used for an application? In other words, should we buy or build applications? If we buy, should we get all applications from the same vendor or will we use a small number of approved vendors?

- **Application uniformity.** For large organizations with many subsidiaries or locations, to what degree should our applications be the same at all locations? If some have to be the same but some can be different, how do we decide where we allow autonomy? This discussion often involves a trade-off between local autonomy and the central desire for efficiency and consistency.

- **Application acquisition.** What processes and steps should we use when we acquire applications? Should we subject all acquisitions to rigorous analyses? Should we use a request for proposal for all application acquisitions? This discussion is generally an assessment of the extent to which the IT acquisition process should follow the degree of rigor applied to non-IT acquisitions (of diagnostic equipment, for example).

Infrastructure

Infrastructure needs may arise from the strategic-planning process. An organization desiring to extend its IT systems to community physicians will need to ensure that it can deliver low-cost and secure network connections. Organizations placing significant emphasis on clinical information systems must ensure very high reliability of their infrastructure; computerized provider order entry systems cannot go down.

In addition to initiatives designed to add specific components to the infrastructure—for example, new software to monitor network utilization—architecture strategies will focus on the addition or enhancement of broad infrastructure capabilities and characteristics.

Capabilities are defined by completing this sentence: "We want our applications to be able to . . ." Organizations might complete that sentence with phrases such as "be accessed from home," "have logic that guides clinical decision making," or "share a pool of consistently defined data."

Characteristics refer to broad properties of the infrastructure, such as reliability, agility, supportability, integrability, and potency. An organization may be heading into the implementation of mission-critical systems and hence must ensure very high degrees of reliability in its applications and infrastructure. The organization may believe that it is in the middle of a large amount of environmental uncertainty and hence must place a premium on agility. The asset plans in these cases involve discussions and analyses that are intended to answer the questions: What steps do we need to take to significantly improve the reliability of our systems? or, If we need to change course quickly, how do we ensure an agile IT response?

Data

Data and *information* were discussed in Chapters One and Two and *data management* in Chapter Nine. Strategies surrounding data may center on the degree of data standardization across the organization, accountability for data quality and stewardship, and determination of database management and analyses technologies.

Data strategy conversations may originate with questions such as, We need to better understand the costs of our care. How do we improve the linkage between our clinical data and our financial data? or, We have to develop a much quicker response to outbreaks of epidemics. How do we link into the city's emergency rooms and quickly get data on chief complaints?

In general, strategies surrounding data focus on acquiring new types of data, defining the meaning of data, determining the organizational function responsible for maintaining that meaning, integrating existing sets of data, and obtaining technologies used to manage, analyze, and report data.

IT Staff

IT staff are the analysts, programmers, and computer operators who, day in and day out, manage and advance information systems in an organization. IT staff were discussed in Chapter Twelve. Alignment discussions may highlight the need to add IT staff with specific skills, such as web developers and clinical information system implementation staff. Organizations may decide that they need to explore outsourcing the IT function in an effort to improve IT performance or obtain difficult-to-find skills. The service orientation of the IT group may need to be improved.

In general, the IT staff strategies focus on the acquisition of new skills, the organization of the IT staff, the sourcing of the IT staff, and the characteristics of the IT department—is it, for example, innovative, service oriented, and efficient?

A NORMATIVE APPROACH TO DEVELOPING ALIGNMENT AND IT STRATEGY

You may now be asking yourself, How do I bring all of this together? In other words, is there a suggested approach an organization can take to develop its IT strategy that takes into account these various vectors? And by the way, what does an IT strategic plan look like?

Across health care organizations the approaches taken to developing, documenting, and managing an IT strategy are quite varied. Some organizations have well-developed, formal approaches that rely on the deliberations of multiple committees and leadership retreats. Other organizations have remarkably informal processes. A small number of medical staff and administrative leaders meet in informal conversations to define the organization's IT strategy. In some cases the strategy is developed during a specific time in the year, often preceding development of the annual budget. In other organizations, IT strategic planning goes on all the time and permeates a wide range of formal and informal discussions.

There is no single right way to develop an IT strategy and to ensure alignment. However, the process of developing IT strategy should be similar in approach and nature to the process used for overall strategic planning. If the organization's core approach to strategy development is informal, its approach to IT strategy development should also be informal.

Recognizing this variability, a normative approach to the development of IT strategy can be offered.

Strategy Discussion Linkage

Organizational strategy is generally discussed in senior leadership meetings. These meetings may focus specifically on strategy, or strategy may be a regular agenda item. These meetings may be supplemented with retreats centered on strategy development and with task forces and committees that are asked to develop recommendations for specific aspects of the strategy. (For example, a committee of clinical leadership might be asked to develop recommendations for improving patient safety.) These discussions will examine the organization's external environment—such as changes in reimbursement and competitive position—and internal environment—such as operational efficiency, financial health, and clinical strengths. This examination invariably results in the identification of gaps between the organization's desired position and role and its current status. This examination usually includes a review of the status and capabilities of the organization's IT capabilities and application portfolio.

Regardless of their form, the organization's CIO should be present at such meetings or kept informed of the discussion and its conclusions. If task forces and committees supplement strategy development, an IT manager should be asked to be a member. The CIO (or the IT member of a task force) should be expected to develop an assessment of the IT ramifications of strategic options and to identify areas where IT can enable new approaches to carrying out the strategy.

The CIO will not be the only member of the leadership team who will perform this role. Chief financial officers (CFOs), for example, will frequently identify the IT ramifications of plans to improve the revenue cycle. However, the CIO should be held accountable for ensuring the linkage does occur.

As strategy discussions proceed, the CIO must be able to summarize and critique the IT agenda that should be put in place to carry out the various aspects of the strategy. Exhibit 13.1 displays an IT agenda that might emerge

---

Exhibit 13.1. IT initiatives necessary to support a strategic goal for a provider

Article I. Strategic Goal
Improve service to outpatients

Article II. Problem
- Patients have to call many locations to schedule a series of appointments and services
- The quality of the response at these locations is highly variable
- Locations inconsistently capture necessary registration and insurance information
- Some locations are over capacity, whereas others are underutilized

Article III. IT Solution
- Common scheduling system for all locations
- A call center for "one-stop" access to all outpatient services
- Development of master schedules for common service groups such as preoperative testing
- Integration of scheduling system with electronic data interchange connection to payers for eligibility determination, referral authorization, and copay information
- Patient support material, such as maps and instructions, to be mailed to patients

---

from a strategy designed to improve the patient service experience in outpatient clinics. Exhibit 13.2 displays a health plan IT agenda that could result from a strategy designed to improve patient access to health information and self-service administrative tasks for a health plan.

IT Liaisons

All major departments and functions (for example, finance, nursing, and medical staff administration) should have a senior IT staff person who serves as the function's point of contact. As these functions examine ways to address their needs (for example, lower their costs and improve their services), the IT staff person can work with them to identify IT activities necessary to carry out

---

Exhibit 13.2. IT initiatives necessary to support a strategic goal for a health plan

Article IV. Strategic Goal

- Improve service to subscribers

- Reduce costs

Article V. Problem

- Subscribers have difficulty finding high-quality health information

- The costs of performing routine administrative transactions such as change of address and responding to benefits questions is increasing

- Subscriber perceptions of the quality of service in performing these transactions is low

Article VI. IT Solution

- A plan portal that provides:
  - Health content from high-quality sources
  - Access to chronic disease services and discussion groups
  - Subscriber ability to use self-service to perform routine administrative transactions
  - Subscriber access to benefit information
  - Functions that enable subscribers to ask questions
  - Plan ratings of provider quality

- A plan-sponsored provider portal that enables:
  - Subscribers to conduct routine transactions with their provider, such as requesting an appointment or renewing a prescription
  - Electronic visits for certain conditions such as back pain
  - Subscribers to ask care questions of their provider

---

their endeavors. This identification often emerges with recommendations to implement new applications that advance the performance of a function, such as a medication administration record application to improve the nursing workflow. Exhibit 13.3 provides an example of output from a nursing leadership discussion on improving patient safety through the use of a nursing documentation system.

Exhibit 13.3. System support of nursing documentation

Section 6.1. Problem Statement
- Both the admitting physician(s) and nurse document medication history in their admission note.
- Points of failure have been noted:
  - Incompleteness due to time or recall constraints, lack of knowledge, or lack of clear documentation requirements
  - Incorrectness due to errors in memory, transcription between documents, and illegibility
  - Multiple inconsistent records due to failure to resolve conflicting accounts by different caregivers
- Most of the clinical information required to support appropriate clinician decision making is obtained during the history-taking process.

Section 6.2. Technology Interventions and Goals
- A core set of clinical data should be made available to the clinician at the point of decision making:
  - Demographics
  - Principle diagnoses and other medical conditions
  - Drug allergies
  - Current and previous relevant medications
  - Laboratory and radiology reports
- Required information should be gathered only once:
  - Multidisciplinary system of structured, templated documentation
  - Clinical decision support rules, associated to specific disciplines, should guide gathering
  - Workflow should support the mobile care giver with integrated wireless access to clinical information
- Needed applications could be implemented in phases:
  - Nursing admission assessment
  - Multidisciplinary admission assessment
  - Planning and progress
  - Nursing discharge plan
  - Multidisciplinary discharge plan

Table 13.3. Potential value proposition of mobile device technology

Value				
Function	Revenue	Cost Savings	Care Quality	Patient Service
Medical information or textbooks	L	L	M	L
Lab test orders	M	L	L	L
Medication orders	H	M	H	M
Results retrieval	L	M	M	L
Patient charting	M	L	M	L
Charge capture	H	M	L	M
Supply management	L	H	L	L

Legend: H = high, M = medium, L = low.

New Technology Review

The CIO should be asked to discuss, as part of the strategy discussion or in a periodic presentation in senior leadership forums, new technologies and their possible contributions to the goals and plans of the organization. These presentations may lead to suggestions that the organization form a task force to closely examine a new technology. For example, a multidisciplinary task force could be formed to examine the role of mobile devices in nursing care, materials management, and service provision to referring physicians. Table 13.3 provides an example of a review of the potential contribution of mobile device technology; various potential uses of the technology are assessed according to their expected ability to increase revenue, reduce costs, improve care quality, and improve patient service.

Synthesis of Discussions

The CIO should be asked to synthesize or summarize the conclusions of these discussions. This synthesis will invariably be needed during development of the annual budget. And the synthesis will be a necessary component of the documentation and presentation of the organization's strategic plan. Table 13.4 presents an example of such a synthesis.

The organization should expect the process of synthesis will require debate and discussion; for example, trade-offs will need to be reviewed, priorities set, and the organization's willingness to implement embryonic technologies determined. This synthesis and prioritization process can occur in the course of leadership meetings, through the work of a committee charged to develop an

Table 13.4. Summary of IT strategic planning

Strategic Challenge	IT Agenda
Capacity and growth management	Emergency department tracking Inpatient electronic bed board Ambulatory clinic patient tracking
Quality and safety	Inpatient order entry Anticoagulation therapy unit Online discharge summaries Medication administration record
Performance improvement	Registration system overhaul Anatomic pathology Pharmacy Order communication Transfusion and donor services
Budget management and external reviews	Disaster recovery Joint Commission preparation Privacy policy review

initial set of recommendations, and during discussions internal to the IT management team.

An example of an approach to prioritizing recommendations is to give each member of the committee $100 to be distributed across the recommendations. The amount a member gives to each recommendation reflects his or her sense of its importance. For example, a member could give one recommendation $90 and another $10, or give five recommendations $20 each. In the former case, the committee member believes that only two recommendations are important and that the first recommendation is nine times more important than the second. In the latter case, the member believes that five recommendations are of equal importance. The distributed dollars are summed across the members, with a ranking of recommendations emerging.

The leadership should not feel compelled to accept the ranking as a definitive output. Rather, the process of scoring will reveal that members of the leadership team will rate recommendations differently. For example, some members will rate a project as having a high contribution to patient quality while others will view that contribution as low. The discussion that investigates these discrepancies can help the team understand the recommendation more fully and lead to a consensus that strengthens political support for the recommendation. Moreover, if the leadership team decides to approve a recommendation with a low score, it should ask itself why it views the recommendation as more important than the score would suggest.

Figure 13.2. IT initiative priorities

Column goal headings (diagonal): Enhances Patient Care · Strengthens Community Outreach · Strengthens Physician Integration · Strengthens Employee Support · Enhances Operational Efficiency · Minimizes Investment Level · Invests in Current Scalable Technology · Supports Growth with Strong ROI · Addresses Significant System Deficiency · Addresses Compliance Issues (Must Do) · Mandatory Technology Building Block

Key: Moderate | High | Must Do

	Service	People	Financial	Growth	Quality and Safety	Infra-structure	Overall Priority
Clinical Applications							
1. Physician Order Entry	✓	✓	✓		✓	✓	Start Now
2. Patient Care Documentation	✓		✓		✓	✓	Plan It
3. Clinical Data Repository		✓	✓	✓	✓		Start Now
4. Computerized Medical Record		✓	✓				Delay It
5. PACS (Phase I)	✓		✓		✓		Start Now
6. Expand Physician Practice Mgmt		✓	✓ ✓	✓			Plan It
7. Departmental Systems							Ongoing
Data Integration							
8. Integration Engine				✓	✓	✓	Plan It
Administrative and Financial Systems							
9. General Financials			✓	✓			Plan It
10. Materials Management		✓	✓	✓			Plan It
11. Scheduling Application	✓	✓	✓		✓		Plan It
12. Decision Support System			✓ ✓		✓		Start Now
Emerging Technologies							
13. Wireless LAN and WAN		✓	✓	✓ ✓			Plan It
14. Voice Recognition		✓	✓	✓			Start Now
Infrastructure							
15. Server Consolidations or Upgrades						✓	Plan It
16. Network Upgrades						✓	Ongoing
17. Security: SSO, HIPAA, Policies			✓		✓ ✓	✓	Plan It
Governance							
18. Project and Change Mgmt Office		✓	✓ ✓			✓	Start Now
19. US Governance (Steering, Bus. Liaisions, SLAs)		✓	✓ ✓				Ongoing

For an example of the scoring of proposed IT initiatives, see Figure 13.2. It lists categories of organizational goals (for example, enhance patient care), along with goals within the categories. The leadership of the organization, through a series of meetings and presentations, has scored the contribution of the IT initiative to the strategic goals of the organization. The contribution to each goal may be critical (*must do*), *high*, *moderate*, or none. These scores are based on data but nonetheless are fundamentally judgment calls. The scoring and prioritization will result in a set of initiatives deemed to be the most

Figure 13.3. IT plan timetable and budget

Hospital IT Migration Path	Priority	Funded	FY2012 Capital (in $1000) Actual	FY2013 Capital Expense (in $1000) Low	High	FY2014 Capital Expense (in $1000) Low	High	FY2015 Capital Expense (in $1000) Low	High	Annual Recurring Operate
Clinical Applications										
1. Physician Order Entry	Start Now	Funded	$ 200		$ 1,800					$ 270
2. Patient Care Documentation	Plan It			$ 333	$ 467	$ 167	$ 233			$ 70
3. Clinical Data Repository	Start Now				$ 25					$ 4
4. Computerized Medical Record	Delay It					$ 50	$ 125	$ 150	$ 375	
5. PACS (Phase I)	Start Now			$ 500	$ 500					$ 75
6. Expand of Physician Practice Mgmt	Plan It					$ 50	$ 150			
7. Departmental Systems	Ongoing			$ 167	$ 333	$ 167	$ 333	$ 167	$ 333	$ 50
Data Integration										
8. Integration Engine	Plan It			$ 100	$ 200					
Administrative and Financial Systems										
9. General Financials	Plan It					$ 300	$ 500			
10. Materials Management	Plan It					$ 200	$ 333	$ 100	$ 167	
11. Scheduling Application	Plan It					$ 75	$ 150	$ 225	$ 450	
12. Decision Support System	Start Now	$ 100		$ 50						8
Emerging Technologies										
13. Wireless LAN & WAN	Plan It					$ 167	$ 667	$ 83	$ 333	$ 75
14. Voice Recognition	Start Now	Pending		$ 100	$ 300					$ 45
Infrastructure										
15. Server Consolidations / Upgrades	Plan It			$ 250	$ 500					$ 75
16. Network Upgrades	Ongoing	Funded	$ 100	$ 33	$ 133	$ 33	$ 133	$ 33	$ 133	$ 20
17. Security - SSO, HIPAA, Policies	Plan It			$ 33	$ 67	$ 17	$ 33			$ 10
Governance										
18. Project / Change Mgmt Office	Start Now	Funded		$ 10	$ 20					$ 3
19. US Governance (Steering, Bus. Liasons, SLA's)	Ongoing	N/A		N/A	N/A	N/A	N/A	N/A	N/A	N/A

Timeline / FTE Staffing (FY11 Q4; FY2012 Q1–Q4; FY2013 Q1–Q4; FY2014 Q1–Q4):
1. Physician Order Entry: 1, 4, 4, 4
2. Patient Care Documentation: 1, 3, 3
3. Clinical Data Repository: 0.5, 1, 1, 1, 1
5. PACS (Phase I): 0.5, 1
6. Expand of Physician Practice Mgmt: 1, 1, 1, 1
7. Departmental Systems: 1, 1, 1, 1, 1, 1, 1, 1, 1, 1, 1, 1
8. Integration Engine: 1, 1
9. General Financials: 1, 2, 2
10. Materials Management: 1, 2, 2
11. Scheduling Application: 1, 2, 2, 2
13. Wireless LAN & WAN: 0.5, 0.5, 0.5
14. Voice Recognition: 0.5, 0.5, 0.5, 0.5
15. Server Consolidations / Upgrades: 0.5, 0.5, 0.8
16. Network Upgrades: 1, 1, 1, 1, 1, 1, 1, 1, 1, 1, 1, 1, 1
17. Security - SSO, HIPAA, Policies: 1, 0.5, 0.5
18. Project / Change Mgmt Office: 1, 1, 1, 1
19. US Governance: 1, 3, 3, 3, 3, 3, 3, 3, 3, 3, 3

important. The IT staff will then construct preliminary budgets, staff needs, and timelines for these projects.

Figure 13.3 provides an overview of the timeline for these initiatives and the cost of each. Management will discuss various timeline scenarios, will consider project interdependence, and ensure that the IT department and the organization are not overwhelmed by too many initiatives to complete all at once. The organization will use the budget estimates to determine how much IT it can afford. Often there is not enough money to pay for all the desired IT initiatives, and some initiatives with high and moderate scores will be deferred or eliminated as projects. The final plan, including timelines and budgets, will become the basis for assessing progress throughout the year.

Overall, a core role of the organization's chief information officer is to work with the rest of the leadership team to develop the process that leads to alignment and strategic linkage.

Once all is said and done, the alignment process should produce these results:

- An inventory of the IT initiatives that will be undertaken. (These initiatives may include new applications and projects designed to improve the IT asset.)
- A diagram or chart that illustrates the linkage between the initiatives and the organization's strategy and goals.
- An overview of the timeline and the major interdependencies between initiatives.
- A high-level analysis of the budget needed to carry out these initiatives.
- An assessment of any material risks to carrying out the IT agenda, and a review of the strategies needed to reduce those risks.

It is important to recognize the amount and level of discussion, compromise, and negotiation that go into the strategic alignment process. Producing these results without going through the preceding thoughtful process will be of little real benefit.

IT STRATEGY AND ALIGNMENT CHALLENGES

Creating IT strategy and alignment is a complicated organizational process. The following sections present a series of observations about that process.

Planning Methodologies

Formal processes and methodologies that help organizations develop IT plans, whether based on derived linkage or the examination of more fundamental characteristics of organizations, can be very helpful. If well executed, they can do all of the following:

- Lead to the identification of a portfolio of IT applications and initiatives that are well linked to the organization's strategy.
- Identify alternatives and approaches that might not have been understood without the process.
- Contribute to a more thorough analysis of the major aspects of the plan.

- Enhance and ensure necessary leadership participation and support.
- Help the organization be more decisive.
- Ensure the allocation of resources among competing alternatives is rational and politically defensible.
- Enhance communication of the developed plan.

In addition to formal IT strategic planning methodologies, organizations will often use strategy frameworks that help them frame issues and opportunities. For example, Porter's Competitive Forces Model (Porter, 1980) identifies strategic options such as competing on cost, differentiating based on quality, and attempting to raise barriers to the entry of other competitors. In using this model, the organization will make choices about its overall competitive position.

Models such as this help the leadership engage in a broader and more conceptual approach to strategy development.

Persistence of the Alignment Problem

Despite the apparent simplicity of the normative process we have described, and the many examinations of the topic by academics and consultants, achieving *IT alignment* has been a top concern of senior organizational leadership for several decades. For example, a survey of CIOs from across multiple industries found improving IT alignment with business objectives to be the number-one IT top management priority in 2007 (Alter, 2007). There are several reasons for the persistent difficulty of achieving alignment (Bensaou & Earl, 1998):

- Business strategies are often not clear or are volatile.
- IT opportunities are poorly understood.
- The organization is unable to resolve the different priorities of different parts of the organization.

Weill and Broadbent (1998) note that effective IT alignment requires organizational leadership to clearly understand and strategically and tactically integrate (1) the organization's strategic context (its strategies and market position), (2) the organization's environment, (3) the IT strategy, and (4) the IT portfolio (for example, the current applications, technologies, and staff skills). Understanding and integrating these four continuously evolving and complex areas is exceptionally difficult.

At least two more reasons can be added to this listing of factors that make alignment difficult. First, the organization may find it has not achieved the gains apparently achieved by others it has heard or read about, nor have the vendors' promises of the technologies materialized. Second, the value of IT, particularly infrastructure, is often difficult to quantify, and the value proposition is fuzzy and uncertain; for example, What is the value of improved security of applications?

In both these cases the organization is unsure whether the IT investment will lead to the desired strategic gain or value. This is not strictly an alignment problem. However, alignment does assume the organization believes it has a reasonable ability to achieve desired IT gains.

The Limitations of Alignment

Although alignment is important, it will not guarantee effective application of IT. Planning methodologies and effective use of vectors cannot, by themselves, overcome weaknesses in other factors that can significantly diminish the likelihood that IT investments will lead to improved organization performance. These weaknesses include poor relationships between IT staff and the rest of the organization, incompetent leadership, weak financial conditions, and ill-conceived IT governance mechanisms. IT strategy also cannot overcome unclear overall strategies and cannot necessarily compensate for material competitive weaknesses.

If one has mediocre painting skills, a class on painting technique will make one a better painter but will not turn one into Picasso. Similarly, superb alignment techniques will not turn an organization limited in its ability to implement IT effectively into one brilliant at IT use. Perhaps this reason, more than any other, is why the alignment issue persists as a top-ranked IT issue. Organizations are searching for IT excellence in the wrong place; it cannot be delivered purely by alignment prowess.

Alignment at Maturity

Organizations that have a history of IT excellence appear to evolve to a state where their alignment process is *methodology-less*. A study by Earl (1993) of organizations in the United Kingdom with a history of IT excellence found that their IT planning processes had several characteristics.

IT Planning Was Not a Separate Process

IT planning and the strategic discussion of IT occurred as an integral part of the organization's strategic planning processes and management discussions.

In these organizations, management did not think of separating out an IT discussion during the course of strategy development any more than it would run separate finance or human resource planning processes. IT planning was an unseverable, intertwined component of the normal management conversation. This would suggest not having a separate IT steering committee.

IT Planning Had Neither a Beginning nor an End

In many organizations, IT planning processes start in a particular month every year and are completed within a more or less set period. In the studied organizations, the IT planning and strategy conversation went on all the time. This does not mean that an organization doesn't have to have a temporally demarked, annual budget process. Rather, it means that IT planning is a continuous process that reflects the continuous change in the environment.

IT Planning Involved Shared Decision Making and Shared Learning

IT leadership informed organizational leadership of the potential contribution of new technologies and the constraints of current technologies. Organizational leadership ensured that IT leadership understood the business plans, strategies, and their constraints. The IT budget and annual tactical plan resulted from shared analyses of IT opportunities and a set of IT priorities.

The IT Plan Emphasized Themes

A provider organization may have themes of improving care quality, reducing costs, and improving patient service. During the course of any given year, IT will have initiatives that are intended to advance the organization along these themes. The mixture of initiatives will change from year to year, but the themes endure for many years. Because themes endure year after year, organizations develop competence around these themes. They become, for example, progressively better at managing costs and improving patient service. This growing prowess extends into IT. Organizations become more skilled at understanding which IT opportunities hold the most promise and at managing implementation of these applications. And the IT staff becomes more skilled at knowing how to apply IT to support such themes as improving care quality and at helping leadership assess the value of new technologies and applications.

IT Strategy Is Not Always Necessary

There are many times in IT activities when the goal, or the core approach to achieving the goal, is not particularly strategic, and *strategy formulation* and *implementation* are not needed. Replacing an inpatient pharmacy system, enhancing help desk support, and upgrading the network, although requiring well-executed projects, do not always require leadership to engage in conversations about organizational goals or to take a strategic look at organizational capabilities and skills.

There are many times when it is unlikely that the way an organization achieves a goal will create a distinct competitive advantage. For example, an organization may decide it needs to provide personal health records to patients, but it does not expect that that application, or its implementation, will be so superior to a competitor's personal health record that an advantage accrues to the organization.

Much of what IT does is not strategic, nor does it require strategic thinking. Many IT projects do not require thoughtful discussions of fundamental approaches to achieving organizational goals or significant changes in the IT asset.

IT Alignment and Strategy Summary

The development of IT alignment and strategic linkage is a complex undertaking. Four vectors, each complex, must converge. Organizational strategy is often volatile and uncertain and will invariably be developed in multiple forums, making it difficult to have a static, comprehensive picture of the strategy. The ability of IT to support a strategy can be unclear and the trade-offs between IT options can be difficult to assess. The complexity of this undertaking is manifest in the frequent citing of IT alignment in surveys of major organizational issues and problems. There are no simple answers to this problem. At the end of the day, good alignment requires talented leaders (including the CIO) who have effective debates and discussions regarding strategies and who have very good instincts and understandings about the organization's strategy and the potential contribution of IT.

It appears that organizations that are mature in their IT use have evolved these IT alignment processes to the point where they are no longer distinguishable as separate processes. This observation should not be construed as advice to cease using planning approaches or disband effective IT steering committees. Such an evolution, to the degree that it is normative, may occur naturally, just as kids will eventually grow up (at least most of them will).

CHARACTERISTICS OF STRATEGIC THINKING

Strategic thinking and discussion have several characteristics. Strategic thinking centers on discussions of ideas and issues that lead to the determination of goals and initiatives (formulation) and the definition of organizational capabilities and competencies needed (implementation) if we are to implement those goals and initiatives.

The consequences of being wrong are generally serious. An application software company that had a strategy that did not include the Internet revolution is generally paying dearly for that strategy (if it is still in business). Several health care provider organizations have been badly damaged by pay-for-performance strategies based on capitated payment.

A strategic decision has clear and illuminating ramifications for many other decisions. For example, an organization can decide that a critical component of an EHR is the introduction of decision support that guides a provider's decisions on ordering and referring. Such a strategy tells the organization that a provider order entry application and medical logic processors are critical aspects of its clinical systems portfolio. The organization would know it needs a group of physicians and organizational processes to develop and monitor decision rules. The organization would know it needs to code data for medications, lab tests, procedures, and problems, since these data form the basis for many rules. These decisions fall naturally from a strategy of centering on decision support.

Strategic decisions often involve changes in the core understandings that guide organizational activity. Any time the understandings that underlie an organization undergo fundamental change, the organization's activities, market position, processes, and structure can undergo significant change. For example, a move to protocol-driven care, adoption of risk arrangements, and the creation of a continuum of care all involve the adoption of new organizational concepts and will necessitate some level of fundamental change.

The implementation of strategic decisions will require significant resources and intense political activity. Extensive resource commitments and political activity are the natural consequence of and antecedent to the introduction of major organizational change.

Strategies take time, multiple iterations, and lots of analysis to develop, and they must be monitored. Organizations rarely fully understand either the consequences of their strategies or the complete set of organizational activities and investments required to implement them. Strategies can be wrong or off by fifteen degrees. The organization learns as it adjusts itself and assesses the effectiveness of its strategies.

A strategic discussion often involves frequent, sudden shifts in altitude. At one moment the leadership team is operating at thirty thousand feet while discussing principles and concepts. Seconds later it is examining ground-level issues associated with those principles. And then it returns to the stratosphere to refine those principles. Great strategic thinkers are very comfortable with high and low altitudes and frequently shift between them. Great strategies have sound high-level ideas that have been tested against the reality of the ground.

In IT, we often bypass several critical strategic decisions and prematurely move to execution questions. For example, "Should we use applications that are based on cloud computing?" is a premature question. The question needs a formulation or implementation-strategic context before it can be answered.

One might be able to arrive at the cloud question through a line of reasoning as follows:

1. Major goals in development of our technical architecture are the creation of the attribute of architectural agility and the reduction in the costs of our infrastructure (formulation).

2. We would define agility as the ability to scale our systems rapidly (formulation).

3. If we could run our applications on a cloud arrangement, that might enable quick processor and storage expansion and put in place a cost structure that is directly related to resource consumption (formulation).

4. If we pursue this technology, we will need, among other things, to partner with a vendor, move our applications to this environment, and put together a contract (implementation).

Unless one has started from some level of strategic thinking, it is hard to give a good answer to the cloud computing question.

SUMMARY

IT planning has several objectives: the alignment of IT with the strategies, plans, and initiatives of the organization; the development of support for the plan; and the preparation of tactical plans.

IT strategies are developed through four vectors. Each vector is complex, and the integration of the vectors is challenging.

IT planning is a very important organizational process. However, alignment of IT with the organization has been and remains a major challenge. This process is quite difficult. IT planning prowess cannot guarantee organizational excellence in applying IT.

KEY TERMS

Alignment challenges and limitations
IT alignment
IT asset

IT strategy vectors
Strategy formulation
Strategy implementation

LEARNING ACTIVITIES

1. Describe how an EHR system can advance the strategies of a health care provider organization.

2. Describe how a customer relationship management system can advance the strategies of a payer organization.

3. Pick an example of a new technology, such as personal health records. Discuss how this technology might leverage the strategy of a provider or a payer organization.

4. If a health care organization has a strategy of lowering its costs of care, what types of IT applications might it consider? If the organization has a strategy of improving the quality of its care, what types of IT applications might it consider? Compare the two lists of applications.

REFERENCES

Alter, A. (2007, December). Top trends for 2008. *CIO Insight*, *88*, 37–40.

Bensaou, M., & Earl, M. (1998). The right mind-set for managing information technology. *Harvard Business Review*, *76*(5), 119–128.

Chandler, A. (1962). *Strategy and structure*. Cambridge, MA: MIT Press.

Earl, M. (1993). Experiences in strategic information systems planning. *MIS Quarterly*, *17*(1), 1–24.

Henderson, J., & Venkatraman, N. (1993). Strategic alignment: Leveraging information technology for transforming organizations. *IBM Systems Journal*, *32*(1), 4–16.

Porter, M. (1980). *Competitive strategy*. New York: Free Press.

Weill, P., & Broadbent, M. (1998). *Leveraging the new infrastructure*. Boston: Harvard Business School Press.

Strategy Considerations

Chapter Thirteen discussed the alignment of the organization's overall strategy with its IT strategy. In this chapter we review lessons learned about the strategic application of IT across a range of industries and organizations. These lessons form strategy considerations and conclusions that should be understood by organization leaders as they shape their IT strategy. This chapter will discuss the following considerations:

- Complementary strategies
- Strategy evolution
- Governing concepts
- The competitive value of IT

COMPLEMENTARY STRATEGIES

Complementary strategies are organizational initiatives that do not involve the IT asset per se but are needed for the IT strategy to succeed.[1]

Complementary strategies come in two basic forms. They can (1) enable the organization to be broadly more effective in applying IT and realizing its value across a wide range of initiatives, and (2) they can be designed to improve the success of a specific initiative.

Broad Leverage

Broad leverage strategies result from an understanding that a set of IT strategies points to the need to elevate some aspects of organizational IT–related competency.

As an example, a broad leverage strategy might result from the leadership observation that for most of the health care industry, the technology and applications being implemented today are available to all industry participants, including competitors. Any provider organization can acquire and implement systems from Allscripts, Cerner, GE, Epic, or Siemens. Why would one provider believe its electronic health record (EHR) could provide an advantage if its competitor can buy the same system?

This observation might indicate that an advantage could be obtained if one or both of two things were to happen. First, one organization might do a more thoughtful and effective job than its competitors at understanding and then effecting changes in processes associated with the system to be implemented. The application does not provide an advantage, but the way it is implemented does. We see the difference execution makes every day in each of our lives. Implementation of an application is analogous to the difference between a great restaurant and a mediocre one or between a terrific movie and a terrible one. In neither case is the idea (for example, "Let's make meals and sell them") or the fact that one responds to the idea (for example, "We've hired a cook and purchased silverware") the advantage. It is the manner of execution that distinguishes. To a degree this advantage is a result of process change and innovation prowess.

Second, one organization might be consistently able to outrun the other. If an organization is able to develop the means to implement applications and change processes faster or for less cost, it may be able to outrun its competition, even if its implementations, one-for-one, are of no higher quality than its competitors'. Perhaps over a certain period of time one organization implements four applications, whereas the other implements three. Or perhaps for a given amount of capital, one organization implements five applications, whereas the other implements three.

In this example, the organization concludes it needs to strengthen its ability to manage process change and develop approaches to rapid (and inexpensive) implementation of applications.

We will discuss the two core broad leverage strategies—change management and IT governance—in Chapters Fifteen and Sixteen. While these two broad leverage areas are the most important, they are not the only examples.

Organizations that expect to engage in significant levels of IT research and development can develop strategies to improve their ability to manage industry collaborations through establishment of business development capabilities, processes for managing intellectual property, and means to avoid conflicts of interest. If an organization's strategy calls for extending its systems into other organizations, it will need to be better at protecting confidential information.

Initiative-Specific Strategies

Initiative-specific strategies result from an examination of the factors, conditions, and relationships that should or must exist if a proposed IT initiative is to succeed. For example, a strategy of improving the quality of care through disease management will lead to IT asset initiatives and other complementary strategies, such as potentially increasing the number of primary care providers. A strategy of growing market share will call for IT responses and the development of joint clinical programs with affiliates.

Two examples from Partners HealthCare should help to illustrate initiative-specific strategies.

In 2004, Partners decided to implement EHRs across its network of community-based and academic medical center physicians. This application was seen as an essential contributor to organizational strategies to reduce care costs, improve care quality, and increase the safety of care. Motivating physicians to fully use the EHR (for example, motivating physicians to use e-prescribing rather than scripts) can be challenging. In addition, the costs of an EHR can cripple community physician interest.

Partners had pay-for-performance incentive arrangements with its regional health plans. As part of its contract negotiations it obtained a financial reward for physicians who used an EHR. (The government has pursued a similar path with its *meaningful use* incentives.) This reward would not fully cover the costs of an EHR, but it did significantly drop the cost hurdle. These arrangements were accompanied by a media campaign (for example, newspaper advertorials) to signal Partners EHR intentions to its patients and providers. Eventually Partners informed its physicians they must use the EHR if they were to be included in its managed care contracts; the carrot had become a stick.

This set of approaches (advertorials, incentives, and mandates) was an essential initiative-specific complementary strategy to the organization's EHR efforts. The complementary strategy involved implementation of a diverse and evolving set of EHR adoption incentives.

In 1996, the Health Insurance Portability and Accountability Act (HIPAA) required the use of standard electronic exchange of health insurance transactions, such as eligibility determination, between providers and health plans. Partners determined this capability had no strategic value and, in fact, should be viewed as a commodity (Glaser, 2003).

In effect, electronic insurance transactions should be viewed as analogous to e-mail. Having e-mail does not distinguish one organization from another; one therefore wants the cheapest e-mail possible, assuming some standard set of defined features and functions exists.

Moreover, Partners realized the value of an exchange increased significantly as the number of participants increased and that regional health plans and other providers faced similar exchange needs and might be interested in working together to create this exchange capability. The result was a regional consortium of providers and health plans, the New England Health-Care EDI Network (NEHEN), which pooled resources and created a shared health insurance transaction infrastructure. This pooling established a critical mass of exchange participants, and was able to achieve the exchange scale necessary to cover a majority of patients seen in Partners hospitals, clinics, and physician practices. The exchange costs were amortized across several organizations.

Through collaboration, NEHEN participants were able to obtain required, noncompetitive capabilities for significantly reduced costs. The resulting infrastructure enabled HIPAA compliance and kept the insurance transaction costs well below commercial offerings.

The strategy of creating the NEHEN collaborative was an important complementary strategy to Partners' needs to obtain this exchange capability.

Summary of Complementary Strategies

The development and execution of an effective IT strategy does require that the organization identify and prioritize application initiatives and establish an IT asset direction. However, it may require that the organization examine and develop strategies for its broad and initiative-specific IT complementary strategies. Broad complementary strategies are developed through discussions about how to make the organization more effective in its IT efforts. Initiative-specific strategies arise from an assessment of initiative critical success factors and the determination of the best course of action to tackle those factors.

STRATEGY EVOLUTION

Strategies evolve. They evolve because the environment changes, the industry changes, and organizations learn as they go. This education leads to alterations in plans. As the organization's strategy evolves, so does the IT strategy.[2]

At times the evolution cannot be anticipated. Few people would have predicted the impact of the World Wide Web or the collapse of the stock and credit markets in 2008. It is difficult to factor unknown but major phenomena into strategy formulation and implementation. The organization must hope it reacts well (and doesn't overreact or underreact) to unforeseen events and that it has the patience and judgment to sort through the noise and see the emerging reality.

At times this evolution can be seen with at least some clarity. Most providers expect that accountability for care performance will increase and that chronic diseases will afflict a larger portion of the population. The foreseeable evolution is generally factored into the development of the organization's strategy and its evolution.

Sometimes strategy evolution can be anticipated because it is clear the current strategy will run its course. For example, a provider may conclude its efforts to increase market share have been successful and further increases are not necessary or prudent. Cost-reduction efforts may have gone as far as they can go for the time being.

IT strategy must react to unforeseen developments (such as reduced capital budgets during the financial crisis), and IT is usually factored into foreseeable evolutions. This "evolution" has two major ramifications:

- The organization must be prepared to adjust (and perhaps abandon) a current IT strategy due to changes in the environment including the technology.

- An organization may believe that its IT efforts will bring a form of competitive advantage. The organization must understand that that advantage is often brief; evolution requires that new advantages are constantly being examined and implemented.

One aspect of evolution (completion of the course of an IT strategy) is discussed next.

This evolution will occur once its current intense focus on EHR implementation is largely behind an organization. At some point—and this is true of all system implementations—the implementation is done. What does an organization do then?

To be fair, the organization will not really be done. There are invariably bolt-on applications that remain to be implemented and new technologies, such as new mobile devices, that may still be in the rollout phase. However, the long, expensive, and difficult task of implementing an EHR may be largely complete.

If organization members have completed an implementation, what should they do next?

It is hard to believe these providers will have arrived at the peak of health care information technology existence. They can go no further. They can lay off all of their IT staff except the data center staff. The organization need merely apply application upgrades from time to time.

However, if implementation of the EHR can be considered Phase I, then there must be a new phase, a Phase II. The discussion of the evolution of the IT strategy may note that Phase II has three major classes of activity: continuous improvement of processes, leveraging of data, and system extensions.

Continuous Improvement of Processes

The organizational imperative to relentlessly and continuously improve core processes of care, operations, and the revenue cycle never ends. Process change is not only an important component of EHR implementation, it is also an important activity after EHR implementation. With the EHR in place, the organization can now apply the technology to facilitate change.

Moreover, implementation does not mean problem lists are complete, all medications are written using order entry, or health maintenance reminders are being followed. Adoption does not mean that care has been improved.

Phase II could involve ongoing efforts, now EHR-enabled, to improve core processes. The organization must have mechanisms to identify process improvement opportunities, teams that can effect needed changes, and a means to measure the results.

Phase II would require efforts to ensure the implemented EHR is being used effectively. The organization would need to provide ongoing training, approaches to integrating EHR use into the workflow, and data to measure the effectiveness of use (for example, the percent of radiology orders that are written electronically).

Leveraging of Data

Implementation of the EHR will result in the steady accumulation of potentially large amounts of patient data. These data can be leveraged. Potential leverage opportunities include the following:

- Support of analyses needed by continuous process improvement efforts
- Development or extension of pay-for-performance contracts; for example, contracts can change from incentives that reward an appropriate number of visits by a diabetic to incentives that reward achievement of hemoglobin A1c targets
- Pharmacovigilance, that is, the early detection of medications that result in severe adverse effects
- Comparison of differences in outcomes between different, competing medical products and medications
- Support of clinical research, perhaps through integration of genomic and EHR data

Phase II could focus on leveraging EHR data for multiple purposes. This phase would require mechanisms to identify and assess data leverage opportunities, staff skilled in data analyses, staff skilled in care or operations analyses, information technology to support business intelligence activities, and workflow improvement efforts to increase the quality and completeness of data capture.

System Extensions

The EHR can be extended outside the walls of the organization. There are three major types of extension.

First, the EHR can be extended to patients. Personal health records (PHRs) and remote monitoring of the chronically ill can be implemented. Second, the organization's EHR can be integrated to varying degrees with the EHRs of other organizations to support clinical affiliations. This extension might involve the electronic exchange of clinical data or the use of one organization's EHR by the other. Third, the EHR can be extended to support very specific workflows such as e-prescribing transaction integration with pharmacies and pharmacy benefits managers.

Phase II means the organization has developed interoperability strategies, understands how to manage information technology infrastructure that is shared with other organizations, and has identified the best approaches to using the EHR to involve patients more directly in their care.

Observations about Strategy Evolution

Three observations can be made about Phase II and about strategy evolution in general.

First, planning for Phase II must start while the organization is in Phase I; aspects of Phase II need not wait for Phase I to be completed. If continuous process improvement is a key activity of Phase II, then the EHR technology being implemented in Phase I must be chosen such that it provides the rules and workflow engines needed in Phase II. The leveraging of the data and PHR implementation can begin well before every outpatient clinic and physician office has an EHR.

Second, there are parallels to these phases in other industries. The airline industry initially focused on online reservation systems. Once those systems were broadly implemented, the industry began to appreciate the ability to leverage data (frequent flier programs and yield management systems) and the value of system extension (systems to manage baggage movement between carriers and the ability to check in to a flight from home).

Third, while the organization is in Phase I, the mature forms of Phase II are not always well understood. For example, significant aspects of data leverage are not well understood. Although there may be impressive clinical research and pharmacovigilance opportunities, these opportunities are largely hypothetical. EHR data can have myriad problems that make such leverage opportunities problematic. Many of the leverage opportunities today are visions rather than proven realities.

For example, although there is much discussion of PHRs, there is not a mature understanding of their value. Similarly, the United States is struggling to find models that enable the widespread sustainability of health information exchanges (HIEs). (EHRs, PHRs, and HIEs were discussed in Chapter Nine.)

Summary of Strategy Evolution

Strategies evolve. For the evolution that cannot be anticipated, the organization must work hard to thoughtfully respond. For the evolution that can be anticipated, strategies can reflect expected evolution. A form of this anticipation is when the strategy reaches a natural closure point; in such a case, development of a new strategy after the current strategy must be discussed so the organization is well positioned for the next phase.

GOVERNING CONCEPTS ✳ Implementation ≠ Stop.

Governing concepts refer to how the organization views a particular IT challenge or opportunity. These concepts have great power since they frame management's understanding of the challenges and opportunities they confront. For example, an organization can view the EHR as a necessary expense that will cost physicians time. Or it can view the EHR as an essential contributor to efforts to transform care. The concept chosen will determine whether the EHR is viewed as a critical strategic response or not. The organization can view employee use of social networking sites as a drain on productivity or as a means for employees to engage in useful interactions with colleagues and patients. The concept chosen will determine whether use of such sites is supported or prohibited.[3]

Governing concepts also illuminate a wide range of subsequent decisions. To help illustrate the importance of these concepts and their wide-ranging impact, we will discuss applications using the concept of foundations.

A foundation provides the broad ability to perform a *never-ending* series of application-leveraged small, medium, and occasionally large advances and improvements. There are several examples of application foundations.

Provider order entry systems can be used as a foundation to improve physician decision making. Once implemented, the organization can, on an ongoing basis, introduce a series of decision-support rules and guides. These rules can address medication safety issues, improve the appropriateness of test and procedure orders, and assure that data relevant to an order are displayed to the physician. These rules and guides can be implemented over the course of many years. No single rule may turn the tide in an organization's efforts to improve care. But in aggregate they can be leveraged to effect significant improvements.

Software to support patient-provider communication can be used as a foundation to more closely engage patients in their care. The software can be used to support the management of diabetes, help patients manage their medications, provide information to address health care questions, and support development of communities of people with a chronic disease.

This view of applications as foundations has several ramifications and illuminates several subsequent decisions.

Implementation Never Stops

There may be a flurry of intense effort as the foundation is laid. The initial introduction of provider order entry and the electronic health record is difficult work that requires great skill and significant resources. However, once the foundation has been laid, implementation continues as the foundation is leveraged.

If implementation never stops, then management and clinical mechanisms must exist to manage the ongoing implementation. These mechanisms must continuously identify the next area to be leveraged, ensure that the requisite analyses are performed, install needed software modifications and enhancements, and reengineer relevant processes. In effect, these processes and mechanisms must continue the tasks that one sees prior to going live.

Architecture Becomes Very Important

The foundation must be able to support an implementation that never ends. The foundation must be able to evolve gracefully. Tools that enable rule development, the safe addition of local modifications, the incorporation of new data types and coding conventions, and efficient interoperability with other systems become essential. The foundation must be able to capitalize on new technologies in a manner that is efficient and minimally disruptive.

In many ways, the architecture, technologies, and tools that enable ongoing implementation may be more important than the current functionality of the application.

The "Feature-Centric" Request for Proposal Becomes Less Important

The request for proposal (RFP) involves the organization stating all of the application features and functions that it needs or perhaps ever will need. The RFP process implies that all functionality ever needed must be understood and defined. Although one should try to understand up front as much as one can about the functionality that is needed, there is little likelihood one can anticipate all that will be needed.

The view of a foundation leads one to try to implement functionality in a continuous series of modest-sized chunks. The organization learns during and after each implementation of a chunk, and this learning makes it smarter about the nature of the following chunks. In effect, one has an ongoing incremental learning process rather than one large "cramming for a test." Over time, this learning process and iterative implementations will result in a large amount of functionality. But that functionality is likely to be rooted in a deeper understanding of what is needed.

This learning process iteratively defines functionality requirements. The utility of the RFP that attempts to comprehensively define functionality needs before there is organizational experience with the application is diminished. The utility of the RFP that attempts to understand the ability of the architecture and technology to enable iterative learning becomes elevated.

Determining Return on Investment Is Difficult

Assessing the return on investment (ROI) of a foundation is a more difficult exercise than determining the ROI or net present value (NPV) of an application. The organization may understand the ROI of the proposed next step, but it may not know how to calculate an ROI of a to-be-determined series of an indefinite number of steps. Although the ROI analysis should never conclude the ROI cannot be assessed because "we don't know how we'll evolve," it is inherently difficult to state the outcome of a never-ending implementation. Despite the analytical challenges posed, the organization is much more likely to see a return if it views its task as the implementation of a foundation than if it views its task as the serial implementation of individual applications.

Foundation Replacement

Foundation replacement ought to be rare if the application suite is effectively evolving as the organization changes and matures in its understanding of the ways to apply the system. Foundation replacement would occur under one of four unusual circumstances:

1. The vendor goes out of business and the support disappears.
2. A new vendor arrives with products that have dramatically superior capabilities or lower costs.
3. There has been a serious failure of the foundation to incorporate new technologies.
4. The care or business model on which the foundation is based undergoes such radical change that the foundation becomes useless. For example, a foundation built for a home for a family of four would be useless if the decision were made to change the structure into an apartment building.

Summary of Governing Concepts

Governing concepts have great power (for good or for ill). An incorrect or limited core view of an information technology or its uses can blind an organization to the potential for significant gain. A view that is too infatuated with a technology can lead the organization on a path toward disappointment. A thoughtful view can provide significant guidance.

These concepts are important because they determine whether an organization will invest in information technology or not and how the organization intends to apply the technology. And they are important because they can illuminate a wide range of additional understandings and decisions. For example, the ramifications cited earlier would not necessarily have been understood if the EHR were viewed conceptually as "an application." An important strategic question that should be posed early in the IT discussion is, "Are we thinking about this the right way?"

✗THE COMPETITIVE VALUE OF IT✗

For decades organizations across many industries have attempted to use (and at times succeeded in using) IT to achieve a competitive advantage. Decades ago airlines used travel reservation systems as an advantage, listing their flights before those of a competitor. At one time banks used personal computer–based banking as an IT-based advantage, making it easier for customers to manage their assets from home and reducing the need to visit a branch bank. Amazon is a superb example of an organization that used IT to achieve an advantage over its retail rivals. Amazon was able to offer goods without incurring the expense of setting up hundreds of retail stores.[4]

Sources of Advantage

These efforts have shown that IT can enable a significant improvement in organizational performance and assist in achieving an advantage, especially when it is used to leverage core organizational processes, to support the collection of critical data, or to differentiate between organizational products and services.

Leverage of Organizational Processes

Information technology can be applied in an effort to improve organizational processes by making them faster, less error prone, less expensive, and more convenient. However, improved organizational competitive position through process gains is not an automatic result of IT implementation.

The right processes must be chosen. The leverage of processes is most effective when the processes being addressed are critical, core processes that customers use to judge the performance of the organization or to define the core business of the organization.

For example, patients are more likely to judge a provider organization on the basis of its ambulatory scheduling processes and billing processes than they are on its accounts payable and human resources processes. Making diagnostic and therapeutic decisions is a core provider organization process that is the backbone of its business.

Organizations must also examine and redesign processes. If underlying problems with processes are not remedied, the IT investment can be wasted or diluted. IT applications can result in existing processes continuing to perform poorly, only faster. Moreover, it can be harder to fix flawed processes after the application of IT since the new, IT-supported process now has an additional source of complexity, cost, and ossification to address: the new computer system.

IT can be applied to significant competitive advantage if processes are chosen wisely and are reengineered skillfully.

Rapid and Accurate Provision of Critical Data

Organizations define critical elements of their plans, operations, and environment. These elements must be monitored to ensure the plan is working, service and care quality are high, the organization's fiscal situation is sound, and the environment is behaving as anticipated. Clearly data are required to perform such monitoring.

In addition to their utility in monitoring, data can be used to guide management actions. Airlines use data on passenger use of specific routes to effect real-time adjustment of fares. Internet-based retailers use purchase data to target their advertisements.

However, obtaining and reporting critical data is not easy.

Data quality may be limited and incomplete. For example, while physicians are using an EHR, they may not be recording all of a patient's problems, and many of their entries are free text. There may be confusion about which patients belong on specific physician panels. There can be significant disagreements about the definition of "a visit."

Using IT to improve performance through the capture of critical data requires addressing process problems that hinder data capture, developing user incentives to record good data, and engaging in difficult conversations about data meaning.

Product and Service Differentiation

IT can be used to differentiate and customize products and services. For example, supermarkets send information to customers about upcoming sales. This information is often based on knowledge of prior customer purchases. Hence, a family that has purchased diapers and baby food will be seen as a household with young children. Information on sales of products directed to young parents will be sent to that household and not to households in which the purchase patterns indicate a single male. The supermarket is attempting to differentiate its service by helping the household plan its purchases around specials.

Customization and differentiation often rely upon data. Effective customization presumes that we know something about the customer. Differentiation assumes that we know something about the customer's criteria for evaluating our organization so we can differentiate our processes, products, and services in ways that are deemed to have value.

Customization and differentiation often center on organizational processes. These processes can be made distinctive, but this requires a solid understanding of the needs of patients, providers, and other customers. Using IT to send a text message to a patient telling him or her that the doctor is running late and hence their appointment is delayed recognizes that all people value convenience and good service.

Leveraging IT to differentiate products and services requires that organizations address process and data issues and have insight into customer needs and desires.

Observations on IT Use for Competitive Advantage

IT has been used competitively by hundreds of organizations across a range of industries over the course of multiple decades. These experiences have taught us several overall lessons.

Obtaining and Sustaining an Advantage

It is very difficult to obtain a competitive advantage based solely on the implementation of a particular application or technology. Competitors, noting the advantage, are quick to attempt to copy the application, lure away the original developers, or obtain a version of the application from the same or different vendor. Moreover, the advantage rarely results from the system, since most of the time advantage results from skilled process changes that thoughtfully understand how to differentiate an organization from its competitors.

The advantage does not come from the application system. In an industry where most applications can be purchased from a vendor, it is almost impossible for the application to provide an advantage. If you can buy an EHR from vendor X, so can your competitor, and any advantage is short-lived.

Moreover, the fact that an organization has implemented an EHR does not mean it has achieved a competitive advantage over a rival that has not implemented one. In fact, it may have hurt itself relative to its competitor. Its performance may be no better, yet it may have reduced its operating margin and shrunk its capital because of the costs of the EHR.

Some organizations can achieve an advantage that persists because they leverage some other assets that are quite difficult for their competitors to also garner. Such assets can include market share, access to capital, brand-name recognition, and proprietary know-how. For example, a well-known academic medical center may be able to leverage its brand name and base of foreign-born physicians who trained at the medical center to establish a telemedicine-based international consultation service.

Lacking these assets, any sustained IT-enabled advantage occurs because the organization is continuously more effective at process change and gathering critical data than its competitors and because an organization is able to effect performance improvements faster and more efficiently than its competitors.

McAfee and Brynjolfsson (2008) note a significant separation in the spread in profit margin, over time, between those companies performing in the top 25 percent of their industry versus those performing in the bottom 25 percent (see Figure 14.1). The gap between winners and losers was widening. McAfee and Brynjolfsson's explanation was that IT has become more potent in its

Figure 14.1. Profit performance differences in high IT–use industries

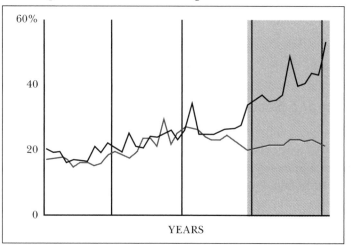

ability to leverage process improvement and information management. This potency enabled organizations that were more effective in applying technology to outdistance competitors that were less effective in IT. As an analogy, a skilled carpenter and a novice will be similarly effective in constructing a house if both use crude tools. But if you give them both sophisticated tools, the skilled carpenter will significantly outperform the novice.

Competitive Baggage

The pursuit of IT as a source of competitive advantage can result in excess baggage, which can take several forms.

Significant investment of capital for IT can cause an increase in capital costs and in IT operating budgets (depreciation and interest) and, as a result, can erode margins. If several competitors are making similar investments, they may all arrive at a position where the customer sees better service or lower prices, but none of the competitors has developed systems that truly differentiate one from the other. Despite this lack of differentiation, the competitors may very well have all reduced their margins through their costly investments. ATMs are an example (Lake, 1998). No bank distinguishes itself because of its ATM capabilities. Customers, however, are better off. The banks must now carry the cost of operating the ATMs and funding periodic upgrades in ATM technology. For the health care provider, investment in web-based consumer content may have a similar outcome.

Extensive use of IT results in dependency on IT. This dependence can affect many resources, from staff to infrastructure. Investment in technologies leaves organizations dependent on their ability to continue to attract and retain scarce and expensive talent. Failure to plan for this dependency can leave the organization exposed when staff turnover occurs. Similarly, organizations that have become reliant on an electronic health record, with a corresponding intolerance of downtime, are dependent on having a highly reliable and high-performing technical infrastructure. Pursuit of a competitive advantage needs to plan for the dependencies that will be incurred.

IT rigidity can result from poor architecture design or poor partnership selection. Many hospitals have seen, belatedly, the consequences of failure to design for application integration as they attempt to integrate systems acquired over years of a best-of-breed strategy. The pursuit of the advantage to each department of implementing the best product on the market failed to consider the infrastructure properties (the ability to integrate applications efficiently) that would be needed to continue to innovate efficiently later.

IT Arms Race

Organizations can find themselves in an IT arms race in which prudence has fled and conversation has been replaced by the innate desire to outfeature the competitors. The original thoughtfulness surrounding the use of IT to improve processes of care, expand market share, or reduce costs has been replaced by ego.

Organizations, overly sensitive to the IT market and grasping for an advantage, can pursue new technologies and ideas well before the utility of the idea, if any, is known. These organizations do not want to be left behind in pursuit of the latest technology, or they may fear ending up as also-rans. A very large number of ideas, technologies, and management techniques fail to live up to their initial hype. The desire to achieve a competitive advantage can cause organizations to lose their senses, perspective, and at times, appropriate caution.

Blinded by Governing Concepts

Governing concepts that were poorly constructed or that fail to evolve can blind organizations to new opportunities. For example, the belief that personal computers were only for hobbyists and had no major role in a large organization was true in 1978 but had become dead wrong by 1984. The belief that the Internet was a realm of interest solely to hackers, voyeurs, and academics also became wrong very quickly. Organizations often hold to beliefs and concepts long after they should be buried. This is particularly likely to happen when the initial belief led to an IT innovation that was very successful. People and organizations are loath to jettison beliefs that "got them here." Such blindness has put companies out of business (Christensen, 1997).

Technology Is a Tool

Information technology can provide a competitive advantage. However, IT has no magic properties. In particular, technology cannot overcome poor strategies, inadequate management, inept execution, or major organizational limitations. For example, a system that enables a reduction in nursing staff may not realize the salary savings desired if the average nurse's salary is very high or the staff are unionized. Information systems are tools.

In a large number of cases in which IT is used as a competitive weapon, the IT system leverages an existing capability (Freedman, 1991). If that capability is weak, IT may not be able to overcome the weakness. Organizations won't use, for example, a supply ordering system if the supplies are inferior in quality, comparatively expensive, and of limited scope. The experiences of Internet-based e-tailers have highlighted the problems created by sloppy inventory management, poor understanding of customer buying behaviors such as returning purchases, and insufficient knowledge of customer price tolerance.

Referring physicians will not find valuable, and probably will not use, a system that gives them access to hospital data if the consulting physicians at the hospital are remiss in getting their consult notes completed on time or at all.

Other factors that can limit the utility of the IT tool have been seen (Cash, McFarlan, & McKenney, 1992):

- Introducing applications too early, with the result that the organization has been unable to overcome not-ready-for-prime-time technology and an unreceptive customer environment.

- Having an inadequate understanding of buying dynamics across market segments. An academic medical center that hopes its consumer-oriented web page will lead to increased admissions may not have fully comprehended its own referral process and that 80 percent of referrals to it are made by the patient's physician.

- Being too far ahead of the customer's comfort level. For example, a large percentage of the public today is uncomfortable with the idea of transmitting individually identifiable health data over the Internet. This discomfort has not been assuaged by the incorporation of advanced security and encryption technologies into these systems.

Finally, the pace of technology evolution is rapid, and new technologies are arriving that enable new ways of supporting processes, gathering data, and differentiating and customizing products and services. In many cases where a significant advantage was obtained, organizations have been quick to assess new technologies and thoughtful in their application. The incorporation of radio frequency ID and the Internet into health care organization activities are examples of effectively leveraging new technologies. This behavior suggests that

- Organizations should have a function that scans for new industry-relevant technologies and engages in evaluating them and experimenting with them.

- To assess new technology well, organizations must develop an understanding of the characteristics of that technology that provide value: for example, what is it about Web 2.0 that might produce a significant improvement in care delivery capabilities? This assessment also involves the development of governing concepts.

- Organizations should be careful not to fall in love with their current technology; they need to be able to ruthlessly jettison technology as its ability to provide a competitive distinction wanes. = planned obsolescence.

If the objectives of a building are not well understood, its design flawed, the carpenter unskilled, and certain tools missing, the quality of the hammer and saw used to build it are irrelevant. In those cases where a significant organizational advantage has been realized, superior strategy, a deep understanding of the business, an ability to execute complex transformations of the business and its core processes, and an ability to capitalize upon IT prowess led to the gains. IT was necessary but not sufficient.

Singles and Grand Slams

When one looks back at organizations that have been effective in the strategic application of IT over a reasonably long time, one sees what looks like a series of singles punctuated by an occasional leap, a grand slam (McKenney, Copeland, & Mason, 1995). One doesn't see a progression of grand slams or, in the parlance of the industry, killer applications (Downes & Mui, 1998). In the course of improving processes, differentiating services, and gathering data, organizations carry out a series of initiatives that improve their performance. The vast majority of these initiatives do not by themselves fundamentally alter the competitive position of the organization, but in the aggregate they make a significant contribution, just as the difference between a great hotel and a mediocre hotel is not solely the presence of clean sheets or hot water but one thousand of such things.

In addition, at various points in time, the organization may have an insight that leads to a major leap in its application of IT to its performance. For example, airlines, having developed their initial travel reservation systems, continued to improve them. At some point they realized that the data gathered by a reservation system had enormous potency and frequent flyer programs resulted. American Hospital Supply, having developed its supply ordering system, continued to improve it. At some point it realized that it was in a materials management partnership with its hospital customers and not strictly in the supply ordering business. No organization has ever delivered a series of killer, or grand slam, applications in rapid succession.

Organizations must develop their IT asset in such a way that they can effect the types of continuous improvement that managers and medical staff will see as possible, day in and day out. For example, in an ideal world an organization would be able to capitalize on the improvements in ambulatory scheduling that a middle manager thinks up and also be able to capitalize on a thousand other good ideas and opportunities. The organization must also develop antennae that sense the possibility of a leap, and the ability to focus that enables it to effect the systems needed to make the leap. Ensuring that these antennae are working is one of the key functions of the chief information officer. The resulting pattern may look like the graph line in Figure 14.2—continuous improvement (singles) in performance using IT punctuated by periodic leaps or grand slams.

It is also clear that organizations have a limited ability to see more than one leap at a time. Hence, they should be cautious about visions that are too visionary or that have a very long time horizon. Organizations have great

Figure 14.2. Singles and grand slams

difficulty understanding a world that is significantly different from the one they inhabit now or that can be only vaguely understood in the context of the next leap. We might understand frequent flyer programs now, but they were not well understood, nor was their competitive value well understood, at the time they were conceived. Moreover, the organizational changes required to support and capitalize on a leap can take years—five to seven years at times (McKenney, Copeland, & Mason, 1995).

Summary of the Competitive Value of IT

Information technology itself cannot provide a competitive advantage that is sustainable for a long time. In general, competitors can acquire similar technology in one to two years or less. IT can provide an advantage if it is used to thoughtfully improve core processes, provide critical data, and support product or service differentiation. Any pursuit of an IT-based advantage should understand the risks of the IT hangover and be wary of allowing this pursuit to devolve into a pointless feature and capability race.

PERSPECTIVE
How Great Companies Use IT

In his seminal book *Good to Great*, Jim Collins (2001) identified companies that made and sustained a transition from being a good company to being a great company. His research noted that these companies had several consistent orientations to IT. They

- Avoided IT fads, but were pioneers in the application of carefully selected technologies.
- Became pioneers when the technology showed great promise in leveraging that which they were already good at doing (their core competency) and that which they were passionate about doing well.
- Used IT to accelerate their momentum toward being a great company, but did not use IT to create that momentum. In other words, IT came after the vision had been set and the organization had begun to move toward that vision. IT was not used to create the vision and start the movement.
- Responded to technology change with great thoughtfulness and creativity, driven by a burning desire to turn unrealized potential into results.

(cont.)

Mediocre companies often reacted to technology out of fear, adopting it because they were worried about being left behind.

- Achieved dramatically better results with IT than did rival companies using the exact same technology.
- Rarely mentioned IT as being critical to their success.
- "Crawled, walked and then ran" with new IT even when they were undergoing radical change.

Source: Collins, 2001, p. 162.

SUMMARY

The strategic application of information technology begins with a linkage of the organization's overall strategy to its IT strategy. That link will identify IT asset–related initiatives.

As they engage in IT strategy formulation and implementation, organizations must be knowledgeable about a series of IT strategy considerations and conclusions such as complementary strategies, strategy evolution, governing concepts, and IT use as a source of competitive advantage.

KEY TERMS

Complementary strategies
Governing concepts

The competitive value of IT
Strategy evolution

LEARNING ACTIVITIES

1. Describe the initiative-specific complementary strategies that might accompany an initiative to significantly increase the use of a provider organization–sponsored personal health record.

2. Summarize how an organization that views itself as an innovator might develop different IT strategies than an organization that views itself as a conservative adopter of new technologies and practices.

3. Pick an example of an organization outside of health care, outline its use of IT to improve a competitive position, and describe how that effort might inform competitive use in health care.

NOTES

1. This section adapted with permission of Healthcare Financial Management Association from J. Glaser, "The Importance of Companion IT Strategies," *Healthcare Financial Management*, April 2009, *63*(4), 38–42.

2. Portions of this section are reprinted, with permission, from J. Glaser, "What Happens after EHR Implementation Is Done?" *Most Wired Online*, July 11, 2007, published by Health Forum, Inc., an American Hospital Association company. Copyright © 2007. Health Forum, Inc. All rights reserved.

3. Portions of this section are reprinted, with permission, from J. Glaser, "Applications as Foundations: Laying the Groundwork for Evolution," *Most Wired Online*, September 6, 2006, published by Health Forum, Inc., an American Hospital Association company. Copyright © 2006. Health Forum, Inc. All rights reserved.

4. This section adapted with permission of Healthcare Financial Management Association from J. Glaser, "The Competitive Value of Healthcare IT," *Healthcare Financial Management*, July 2007, *61*(7), 36–40.

REFERENCES

Cash, J., McFarlan, W., & McKenney, J. (1992). *Corporate information systems management: The issues facing senior executives*. Burr Ridge, IL: Irwin.

Christensen, C. (1997). *The innovator's dilemma*. Boston: Harvard Business School Press.

Collins, J. (2001). *Good to great*. New York: HarperCollins.

Downes, L., & Mui, C. (1998). *Unleashing the killer app*. Boston: Harvard Business School Press.

Freedman, D. (1991, July). The myth of strategic I.S. *CIO*, pp. 34–41.

Glaser, J. (2003, March). Analyzing information technology value. *Healthcare Financial Management*, pp. 98–104.

Lake, K. (1998). Cashing in on your ATM network. *McKinsey Quarterly*, *1*, 173–178.

McAfee, A., & Brynjolfsson, E. (2008, July–August). Investing in the IT that makes a competitive difference. *Harvard Business Review*, *86*(7–8), 98–107.

McKenney, J., Copeland, D., & Mason, R. (1995). *Waves of change: Business evolution through information technology*. Boston: Harvard Business School Press.

CHAPTER 15

IT Governance and Management

LEARNING OBJECTIVES

- To be able to understand the scope and importance of information technology governance.
- To review the IT roles and responsibilities of users, the IT department, and senior management.
- To review the factors that enable sustained excellence in the application of IT.
- To be able to discuss the components of an IT budget and the processes for developing the budget.

In this chapter we discuss an eclectic but important set of information technology (IT) governance and management processes, structures, and issues. Developing, managing, and evolving IT governance and management mechanisms is often a central topic for organizational leadership. In this chapter we will cover the following areas:

- **IT governance.** IT governance is composed of the processes, reporting relationships, roles, and committees that an organization develops to make decisions about IT resources and activities and to manage the execution of those decisions. These decisions involve such issues as setting priorities, determining budgets, defining project management approaches, and addressing IT problems.

- **IT effectiveness.** Over the years several organizations have demonstrated exceptional effectiveness in applying IT; they include American Express, Bank of America, Schwab, and American Airlines. This chapter discusses what the management of these organizations did that led to such effectiveness. It also examines the attributes of IT-savvy senior leadership.

- **IT budget.** Developing the IT budget is a complex exercise. Organizations always have more IT proposals than can be funded. Some proposals are strategically important and others involve routine maintenance of existing infrastructure, making proposal comparison difficult. Although complex and difficult, the effective development of the IT budget is a critical management responsibility.

IT GOVERNANCE

IT governance refers to the principles, processes, and organizational structure that govern the IT resources (Drazen & Straisor, 1995). When solid governance exists, the organization is able to give a coherent answer to the following questions:

- Who sets priorities for IT, and how are those priorities set?

- What organizational structures are needed to support the linkage between IT and the rest of the organization?

- Who is responsible for implementing information system plans, and what principles will guide the implementation process?

- How are IT responsibilities distributed between IT and the rest of the organization and between centralized and decentralized (local) IT groups in an integrated delivery system?

- How are IT budgets developed?

At its core, governance involves

- Determining the distribution of the responsibility for making decisions, the scope of the decisions that can be made by different organizational functions, and the processes to be used for making decisions
- Defining the roles that various organizational members and committees fulfill for IT—for example, which committee should monitor progress in clinical information systems, and what is the role of a department head during the implementation of a new system for his or her department?
- Developing IT-centric organizational processes for making decisions in such key areas as

  IT strategy development

  IT prioritization and budgeting

  IT project management

  IT architecture and infrastructure management
- Defining policies and procedures that govern the use of IT—for example, if a user wants to buy a new network for use in his or her department, what policies and procedures govern that decision?

PERSPECTIVE
The Foundation of IT Governance

Peter Weill and Jeanne Ross have identified five major areas that form the foundation of IT governance. The organization's governance mechanisms need to create structures and processes for these areas.

- **IT principles:** high-level statements about how IT is used in the business.
- **IT architecture:** an integrated set of technical choices to guide the organization in satisfying business needs. The architecture is a set of policies, procedures, and rules for the use of IT and for evolving IT in a direction that improves IT support for the organization.
- **IT infrastructure strategies:** strategies for the existing technical infrastructure (and IT support staff) that ensure the delivery of reliable, secure, and efficient services.

(cont.)

- **Business application needs:** processes for identifying the needed applications.
- **IT investment and prioritization:** mechanisms for making decisions about project approvals and budgets.

Source: Weill & Ross, 2004, p. 27.

Developing and maintaining an effective and efficient IT governance structure is a complex exercise. Moreover, governance is never static. Continuous refinements may be needed as the organization discovers imperfections in roles, responsibilities, and processes.

Governance Characteristics

Well-developed governance mechanisms have several characteristics.

They are perceived as objective and fair. No organizational decision-making mechanisms are free from politics, and some decisions will be made as part of "side deals." It is exceptionally rare for all managers of an organization to agree with any particular decision. No matter how good an individual is at performing his or her IT governance role, there will be members of the organization who will view that individual as a lower life form. Nonetheless, organizational participants should generally view governance as fair, objective, well reasoned, and having integrity. The ability of governance to govern is highly dependent on the willingness of organizational participants to be governed.

They are efficient and timely. Governance mechanisms should arrive at decisions quickly, and governance processes should be efficient, removing as much bureaucracy as possible.

They make authority clear. Committees and individuals who have decision authority should have a clear understanding of the scope of their authority. Individuals who have IT roles should understand those roles. The organization's management must have a consistent understanding of its approach to IT governance. There will always be occasions where decision rights are murky, roles are confusing, or processes are unnecessarily complex, but these occasions should be few.

They can change as the organization, its environment, and its understanding of technology changes. For example, several organizations spun off portions of their IT groups to create e-commerce departments intended to support the organization's undertakings during the Internet frenzy from 1999 to 2001. This spinning off was an effort to, among other objectives, free e-commerce initiatives from the normal bureaucracy of these organizations' governance structures. This separation was meant to allow the e-commerce groups to operate in "Internet time." These groups have been largely dismantled as a more mature understanding of the role of the Internet developed. Likewise, the potential regional efforts to effect interoperability between clinical information systems will require new governance mechanisms that bring representatives from the partnering organizations together to deal with interorganizational IT issues.

Governance mechanisms evolve as IT technology and the organization's use of that technology evolve.

Linkage of Governance to Strategies

Governance structures and the distribution of responsibilities should be heavily influenced by basic strategic objectives. For example, the desire of several provider organizations to be integrated will have ramifications for governance design. In this section we present two examples of governance that is linked to a strategic objective.

Governance to support the *integration* of the hospitals and physician practices of an integrated delivery system (IDS) might have these characteristics:

- A central IDS IT committee develops the IT priorities, to maintain the perspective of overall integration and to ensure that initiatives that support integration of care are given a higher priority than those that do not.
- A centralized IT department or group exists, and it has authority over local IT groups.
- IT budgets developed locally are subject to central approval.
- The IT plan specifies the means by which an integrated infrastructure, including integrated applications, will be achieved and the boundaries of that plan: for example, local organizations are free to select from a set of patient care system options but, whatever the selection, the patient care system must interface with the IDS clinical data repository.

- Members of the IDS are constrained in their selection of applications to support ancillary departments, having to choose from those on an "approved" list.

- Certain pieces of data—for example, payer class or patient problems—and certain identifiers—for example, patient identifier and provider identifier—have to use a common dictionary or standard.

This approach is designed to ensure that the applications used by all the organizations within the IDS can be well integrated. The need for this high degree of application integration originates in the IDS's strategy of integrating its care. This approach (referring back to our discussion in Chapter Fourteen) represents one of the organization's governing concepts, its definition of integration.

Governance to support the ability of the IDS member organizations to be *locally responsive* might have these characteristics:

- A small, central IT group is created to assist in local IT plan development; develop technical, data, and application standards; and perform technical research and development. This group has an advisory and coordination relationship with the local IT organizations.

- Local IT steering committees develop local IT plans according to processes and criteria defined locally. A central IT steering committee with an advisory role reviews these plans to identify and advise on areas of potential redundancy or serious inconsistency.

- IT budgets are developed locally according to overall budget guidelines established centrally—for example, there are rules for capitalizing new systems and selecting the duration to use for depreciation.

- Certain pieces of data are standardized to ensure that the IDS can prepare consolidated financial statements and patient activity counts.

- Local sites are free to, for example, select any departmental system, but that system must be able to support centrally defined security requirements.

This approach reflects a strategy of ensuring that each IDS member has the latitude to respond to local market needs. This approach also reflects a governing concept in the form of a definition of integration. Each of the examples we have just given offers a different definition of integration, and both definitions are correct. As a result of these different definitions, IT governance will be different in these organizations, and both approaches to governance are correct.

IT governance structures and approaches must be designed so that they further organizational goals and strategies. They should not be brought into existence purely to perform some normative task. For example, the thinking that says "all organizations have IT steering committees with a broad representation of senior leadership and hence so should we" is misguided. If the organization has, for example, an objective of being locally responsive, that may mean that no central steering committee should exist or that its powers should be limited.

IT, User, and Senior Management Responsibilities

Effective application of IT involves the thoughtful distribution of IT responsibilities between the IT department, users of applications and IT services, and senior management. In general, these responsibilities address decision-making rights and roles. Although different organizations will arrive at different distributions of these responsibilities, and an organization's distribution may change over time, there is a fairly normative distribution (Applegate, Austin, & McFarlan, 2003).

IT Department Responsibilities

The IT department should be responsible for the following:

- Developing and managing the long-term architectural plan and ensuring that IT projects conform to that plan.
- Developing a process to establish, maintain, and evolve IT standards in several areas:
  - Telecommunications protocols and platforms
  - Client devices, such as workstations and mobile devices, and client software configurations
  - Server technologies, middleware, and database management systems
  - Programming languages
  - IT documentation procedures, formats, and revision policies
  - Data definitions (this responsibility is generally shared with the organization function, such as finance and health information management, that manages the integrity and meaning of the data)
  - IT disaster and recovery plans
  - IT security policies and incident response procedures

- Developing procedures that enable the assessment of sourcing options for new initiatives, such as building versus buying new applications or leveraging existing vendor partner offerings versus utilizing a new vendor when making an application purchase

- Maintaining an inventory of installed and planned systems and services and developing plans for the maintenance of systems or the planned obsolescence of applications and platforms

- Managing the professional growth and development of the IT staff

- Establishing communication mechanisms that help the organization understand the IT agenda, challenges, and services and new opportunities to apply IT

- Maintaining effective relationships with preferred IT suppliers of products and services [Applegate, Austin, & McFarlan, 2003, p. 56].[1]

The scope and depth of these responsibilities may vary. Some of the responsibilities of the IT group may be delegated to others. For example, some non-IT departments may be permitted to have their own IT staff and manage their own systems. This should be done only with the approval of senior management. And the IT department should be asked to provide oversight of the departmental IT group to ensure that professional standards are maintained and that no activities that compromise the organization's systems are undertaken. For example, the IT department can ensure that virus control procedures and software are effectively applied.

The organization may decide that the IT department should have almost imperial authority in carrying out its responsibilities or that its role should be closer to advisor to senior management. Organizations generally arrive at a level of authority in between imperial and advisory—a level based on experience and recent history.

In general, the IT department is responsible for making sure that both individual and organizational information systems are reliable, secure, efficient, current, and supportable. It is also usually responsible for managing the relationship with suppliers of IT products and services and ensuring that the processes that lead to new IT purchases are rigorous.

User Responsibilities

IT users (primarily middle managers and supervisors) have several IT-related responsibilities:

- Understanding the scope and quality of IT activities that are supporting their area or function

- Ensuring that the goals of IT initiatives reflect an accurate assessment of the function's needs and challenges and that the estimates of the function's resources (personnel time, funds, and management attention) needed by IT initiatives—to support the implementation of a new system, for example—are realistic

- Developing and reviewing specifications for IT projects and ensuring that ongoing feedback is provided to the IT organization on implementation issues, application enhancements and IT support, ensuring, for example, that the new application has the functionality needed by the user department

- Ensuring that the applications used by a department are functioning properly, such as by periodically testing the accuracy of system-generated reports and checking that passwords are deleted when staff leave the organization

- Participating in developing and maintaining the IT agenda and priorities [Applegate, Austin, & McFarlan, 2003, p. 62]

These responsibilities constitute a minimal set. In Chapter Eight, we discussed an additional, and more significant, set of responsibilities during the implementation of new applications.

Senior Management Responsibilities

The primary IT responsibilities of the senior leadership are as follows:

- Ensuring that the organization has a comprehensive, thoughtful, and flexible IT strategy

- Ensuring an appropriate balance between the perspectives and agendas of the IT organization and the users—for example, the IT organization may want a new application that has the most advanced technology, while the user department wants the application that has been used in the industry for a long time

- Establishing standard processes for budgeting, acquiring, implementing, and supporting IT applications and infrastructure

- Ensuring that IT purchases and supplier relationships conform to organizational policies and practices—for example, contracts with IT vendors need to use standard organizational contract language

- Developing, modifying, and enforcing the responsibilities and roles of the IT organization and users

- Ensuring that the IT applications and activities conform to all relevant regulations and required management controls and risk mitigation processes and procedures
- Encouraging the thoughtful review of new IT opportunities and appropriate IT experimentation [Applegate, Austin, & McFarlan, 2003, p. 68]

PERSPECTIVE
Principles for IT Investments and Management

Charlie Feld and Donna Stoddard have identified three principles for effective IT investments and management. They note that the responsibility for developing and implementing these principles lies with the organization's senior leadership.

1. **A long-term IT renewal plan linked to corporate strategy.** Organizations need IT plans that are focused on achieving the organization's overall strategy and goals. The organization must develop this IT renewal plan and remain focused, often over the course of many years, on its execution.

2. **A simplified, unifying corporate technology platform.** This IT platform must be well architected and be defined and developed from the perspective of the overall organization rather than the accumulation of the perspectives of multiple departments and functions.

3. **A highly functional, performance-oriented IT organization.** The IT organization must be skilled, experienced, organized, goal-directed, responsive, and continuously work on establishing great working relationships with the rest of the organization.

Source: Feld & Stoddard, 2004, p. 3.

Although organizations will vary in the ways they distribute decision-making responsibility and roles and the ways in which they implement them, problems may arise when the distribution between groups is markedly skewed (Applegate, Austin, & McFarlan, 2003).

Too much user responsibility can lead to a series of uncoordinated and undermanaged user investments in information technology. This can result in

- An inability to achieve integration between highly heterogeneous systems.
- Insufficient attention to infrastructure, resulting in application instability.
- High IT costs, due to insufficient economies of scale, significant levels of redundant activity, and the cost of supporting a high number of heterogeneous systems.
- A failure to leverage IT opportunities because of user ignorance or fear of IT—for example, users won't invest in needed applications because they are afraid to do so.
- A lack of, or uneven, rigor applied to the assessment of the value of IT initiatives—for example, insufficient homework may be done and an application selected that has serious functional limitations.

Too much IT responsibility can lead to

- Too much emphasis on technology, to the detriment of the fit of an application with the user function's need—for example, when a promising application does not completely satisfy the IT department's technical standards, IT will not allow its acquisition.
- A failure to achieve the value of an application due to user resistance to a solution imposed by IT: "We in the IT department have decided that we know what you need. We don't trust your ability to make an intelligent decision."
- Too much rigor applied to IT investment decisions; excessive bureaucracy can stifle innovation.
- A very high proportion of the IT budget devoted to infrastructure, to the detriment of application initiatives, as the IT department seeks to achieve ever greater levels (though perhaps not necessary levels) of reliability, security, and agility.
- Reduction in business innovation when IT is unwilling to experiment with new technologies that might have stability and supportability problems.

Either extreme can clearly create problems. And no compromise position will make the IT department and the IT users happy with all facets of the outcome. An outcome of "the best answer we can develop but not an answer that satisfies all" is an inevitable result of the leadership discussion of responsibility and role distribution.

Specific Governance Structures

In any organization there may be a plethora of committees and a series of complex reporting relationships and accountabilities, all of which need to operate with a fair degree of harmony in order for governance to be effective. Among them should be five core structures for governing IT:

1. Board responsibility for IT.

2. A senior leadership forum that guides the development of the IT agenda, finalizes the IT budget, develops major IT-centric policies, and addresses any significant IT issue that cannot be resolved elsewhere. This core structure includes subcommittees, designated by the forum, that have specific roles and responsibilities—for example, a privacy committee or a care improvement committee that is charged with overseeing the implementation of a clinical information system.

3. Initiative- and project-specific committees and roles (this structure will be discussed in Chapter Sixteen).

4. IT liaison relationships.

5. A chief information officer (CIO) and other IT staff (described in Chapter Twelve).

The Board

The health care organization's board holds the fundamental accountability for the performance of the organization, including the IT function. The board must decide how it will carry out its responsibility with respect to IT.

At a minimum this responsibility involves receiving a periodic update (perhaps annually), at a board meeting, from the CIO about the status of the IT agenda and the issues confronting the effective use of IT. In addition, financial information system controls and IT risk mitigation are often identified and discussed by the board's audit committee, and the IT budget is discussed by the finance committee.

Some organizations create an IT committee of the board. Realizing that the normal board agenda might not always allow sufficient time for discussion of important IT issues and that not all board members have deep experience in IT, the board can appoint a committee of board members who are seasoned IT professionals (IT academics, CIOs of regional organizations, and leaders in the IT industry). The committee, chaired by a trustee, need not be composed entirely of board members. IT professionals who are not on the board may serve as members, too. This committee informs the board of its assessments of a wide range of IT challenges and initiatives and makes recommendations about these issues.

The charter for such a committee might charge the committee to

- Review and critique IT application, technical, and organizational strategies
- Review and critique overall IT tactical plans and budgets
- Discuss and provide advice on major IT issues and challenges
- Explore opportunities to leverage vendor partnerships

Committee meeting agenda items might include

- Assessments of the value of clinical information systems
- Long-term plans for the organization's financial systems
- IT staff recruitment and retention issues
- The annual IT budget

Organizational leaders should not believe, however, that appointing an IT committee gets the board off the hook for having to deal with IT issues. Rather, this committee should be viewed as a way for all board members to continue their efforts to become more knowledgeable and comfortable with the IT conversation.

Senior Leadership Organizational Forum

Most health care organizations have a committee called something like the executive committee. Composed of the senior leadership of the organization, this committee is the forum in which strategy discussions occur and major decisions regarding operations, budgets, and initiatives are made. It is highly desirable to have the CIO as a member of this committee.

Major IT decisions should be made at the meetings of this committee. These decisions will cover a gamut of topics, such as approving the outcome of a major system selection process, defining changes in direction that may be needed during the course of significant implementations, setting IT budget targets, and ratifying the IT component of the strategic-planning efforts.

This role does not preclude the executive committee from assigning IT-related tasks or discussions to other committees. For example, a medical staff leadership committee may be asked to develop policies regarding physician use of computerized provider order entry. A committee of department heads may be asked to select a new application to support registration and scheduling. A committee of human resource staff may be charged with developing policies regarding organizational staff use of the Internet while at work.

The executive committee, major departments and functions, and several high-level committees will regularly be confronted with IT topics and issues that do not arise from the organization's IT plan and agenda. For example, a board member may ask if the organization should outsource its IT function. Several influential physicians may suggest that the organization assess a new information technology that seems to be getting a lot of hype. The CEO may ask how the organization should (or whether it should) respond to an external event: for example, a new Institute of Medicine report. The organization may need to address new regulations: for example, rules being issued by CMS.

When it is not clear which person or committee should address these issues or topics, they could be brought forth during an executive committee meeting for triage. (Alternatively, the CEO, CIO, chief financial officer [CFO], or chief operating officer [COO] may decide where an issue should be handled.) The executive committee can form a task force to examine the issue and develop recommendations, or it can request that an existing forum or function address the issue. For example, a task force of clinicians and IT staff could be asked to examine the ramifications of a new Institute of Medicine report. The organization's compliance department could be charged with developing the organization's response to new regulations.

Some organizations create an IT steering committee and charge this committee with addressing all IT issues and decisions. The use of such committees is uneven in health care organizations. Approximately half have such a committee, and most of these committees are not regarded as functioning effectively.

If an organization has an IT steering committee that works well, it should leave it alone. In general, however, such committees are not a good idea. They tend not to be composed of the most senior leadership, and hence their links to the thinking process of the CEO and the executive committee are not strong. They tend to view IT issues in isolation from the overall issues facing the organization, and few IT issues can be dealt with well in isolation. And committee members often wind up fighting each other over parochial slices of the pie during the IT budget discussion.

IT steering committees are often seen as a senior leadership effort to get "IT problems" off their plate and onto someone else's plate. This is an abdication of responsibility.

IT Liaison Relationships

All major functions and departments of the organization—for example, finance, human resources, member services, medical staff affairs, and nursing—should have an IT liaison. The IT liaison is responsible for:

- Developing effective working relationships with the leadership of each major function
- Ensuring that the IT issues and needs of these functions are understood and communicated to the IT department and the executive committee
- Working with function leadership to ensure appropriate IT representation on function task forces and committees that are addressing initiatives that will require IT support
- Ensuring that the organization's IT strategy, plans and policies, and procedures are discussed with function leadership

The IT liaison role is an invaluable one. It ensures that the IT department and the IT strategy receive needed feedback and that function leaders understand the directions and challenges of the IT agenda. It also promotes an effective collaboration between IT and the other functions and departments.

PERSPECTIVE
Improving Coordination and Working Relationships

Carol Brown and Vallabh Sambamurthy have identified five mechanisms used by IT groups to improve their coordination and working relationships with the rest of the organization.

1. **Integrators** are individuals who are responsible for linking a particular organization department or function with the IT department. An integrator might be a CIO who is a participant in senior management forums. An integrator might also be an IT person who is responsible for working with the finance department on IT initiatives that are centered on that function; such a person might have a title such as manager, financial information systems.

2. **Groups** are committees and task forces that regularly bring IT staff and organization staff together to work collectively on IT issues. These

(cont.)

groups could include, for example, the information systems steering committee or a standing joint meeting between IT and nursing to address current IT issues and review the status of ongoing IT initiatives.

3. **Processes** are organizational approaches to management activity such as developing the IT budget, selecting new applications, and implementing new systems. These processes invariably involve both IT and non-IT staff.

4. **Informal relationship building** includes a series of activities such as one-on-one meetings, IT staff presentations at department head meetings, and co-location of IT staff and user staff.

5. **Human resource practices** include training IT staff on team building, offering user feedback to IT staff during their reviews, and having IT staff spend time in a user area observing work.

Source: Brown & Sambamurthy, 1999, p. 68.

Variations

The specific governance structures just described are typical in medium-sized and large provider or payer organizations. In other types of health care settings, these structures will be different.

A medium-sized physician group might not have a separate board. The physicians and the practice manager might make up both the board and the senior leadership forum. The group might not need a CIO. Instead the practice administrator might manage contracts and relationships with companies that provide practice management systems and support workstations and printers. The practice administrator also might perform all user liaison functions.

A division within a state department of public health would not have a board, but it should have a forum where division leadership can discuss IT issues. IT decisions might be made there or at meetings of the leadership of the overall department. Similarly, the CIO for the department might not have organized IT in a way that results in a division CIO. And the staff of the department CIO might provide user liaison functions for the division.

Despite these variations, effective management of IT still requires

- A senior management forum where major IT decisions are made
- A person responsible for day-to-day management of the IT function and for ensuring that an IT strategy exists

- Mechanisms for ensuring that IT relationships have been established with major organizational functions

In addition, although the structures will vary, the guidance for the respective roles of the IT group, users, and management remains the same. The desirable attributes of the person responsible for IT are unchanged. And the properties of good governance do not change.

PERSPECTIVE
Archetypes of IT Governance Decision Making

Peter Weill and Jeanne Ross have identified six archetypes of IT governance. Each archetype describes an approach to defining how core IT decisions such as budget allocation are made.

1. **Business monarchy:** a group of business executives, often an executive committee; may include the CIO
2. **IT monarchy:** a group of IT executives or the CIO individually
3. **Feudal:** a committee of business unit leaders or key process owners
4. **Federal:** a committee of senior leadership and business unit leaders; may include IT leadership and senior managers
5. **IT duopoly:** IT executives and one other group—for example, IT leadership and finance leadership
6. **Anarchy:** each individual or business unit on its own

Any one health care organization may have several of these forms of governance but apply them in different areas. For example, a business monarchy may decide IT strategy, but an IT monarchy may be used to establish architecture standards. In addition, an IT duopoly may be asked to select and implement a new revenue management system.

Source: Weill & Ross, 2004, p. 59.

IT EFFECTIVENESS

Several studies have examined organizations that have been particularly effective in the use of IT (McKenney, Copeland, & Mason, 1995; Ross, Beath, &

Goodhue 1996; Sambamurthy & Zmud, 1996; Weill & Broadbent, 1998). Determining effectiveness is difficult, and these studies have defined organizations that show effectiveness in IT in a variety of ways. Among them are organizations that have developed information systems that defined an industry (as Amazon has altered the retail industry, for example), organizations that have a reputation for being effective over decades, and organizations that have demonstrated exceptional IT innovation.

The studies have attempted to identify those organizational factors or attributes that have led to or created the environment in which effectiveness has occurred. In other words, the studies have sought to answer the question, What are the organizational attributes that result in some organizations developing truly remarkable IT prowess?

If an organization understands these attributes and desires to be very effective in its use of IT, then it is in a position to develop strategies and approaches to create or modify its own attributes. For example, one attribute is having strong working relationships between the IT function and the rest of the organization. If an organization finds that its own relationships are weak or dysfunctional, strategies and plans can be created to improve them.

The studies suggest that organizations that aspire to high levels of effectiveness and innovation in their application of IT must take steps to ensure that the core capacity of the organization to achieve such effectiveness is developed. It is a critical IT responsibility of organizational leadership to continuously (year in and year out) identify and effect steps needed to improve overall effectiveness in IT. The development of this capacity is a challenge different from the challenge of identifying specific opportunities to use IT in the course of improving operations or enhancing management decision making. For an analogy, consider running. A runner's training, injury management, and diet are designed to ensure the core capacity to run a marathon. This capacity development is different from developing an approach to running a specific marathon, which must consider the nature of the course, the competing runners, and the weather.

Although having somewhat different conclusions (resulting in part from somewhat different study questions), the studies have much in common regarding capacity development.

Individuals and leadership matter. It is critical that the organization possess talented, skilled, and experienced individuals. These individuals will occupy a variety of roles: CEO, CIO, IT staff, and user middle managers. These individuals must be strong contributors. Although such an observation may seem trite, too often organizations, dazzled by the technology or the glorified experiences of others, embark on technology crusades and substantive investments that they have insufficient talent or leadership to effect well. The studies found that leadership is essential. It is an essential trait of the organization's senior management (or executive sponsors), the CIO, and the project team. Leaders must understand the vision, communicate the vision, be able to recruit and motivate a team, and have the staying power to see the innovation through several years of work with disappointments, setbacks, and political problems along the way.

Relationships are critical. Not only must the individual players be strong, but the team must be strong. There are critical senior executive, IT executive, and project team roles that must be filled by highly competent individuals, and great chemistry must exist between the individuals in these distinct roles. Substitutions among team members, even when involving a replacement by an equally strong individual, can diminish the team. This is as true in IT innovation as it is in sports. Political turbulence diminishes the ability to develop a healthy set of relationships among organizational players.

The technology and the technical infrastructure both enable and hinder. New technologies can provide new opportunities for organizations to embark on major transformations of their activities. This implies that the health care CIO must have not only superior business and clinical understanding but also superior understanding of the technology. This does not imply that CIOs must be able to rewrite operating systems as well as the best system programmers, but it does mean that they must have superior understanding of the maturity, capabilities, and possible evolution of various information technologies. Several innovations have occurred because an IT group was able to identify and adopt an emerging technology that could make a significant contribution to addressing a current organizational challenge. The studies also stress the importance of well-developed technical architecture. Great architecture matters. Possessing state-of-the-art technology can be far less important than having a well-architected infrastructure.

The organization must encourage innovation. The organization's (and the IT department's) culture and leadership must encourage innovation and experimentation. This encouragement needs to be practical and goal directed: a real business problem, crisis, or opportunity must exist, and the project must have budgets, political protection, and deliverables.

True innovation takes time. Creating visionary applications or industry-dominant designs or an exceptional IT asset takes time and a lot of work. In the organizations studied by McKenney, Copeland, and Mason (1995), it often took five to seven years for the innovation to fully mature and for the organization to recast itself. Applications and designs will proceed through phases that are as normative as the passage from being a child to being an adult. Innovation, like the maturation of a human being, will see some variations in timing, depth, and success in moving through phases.

Evaluation of IT opportunities must be thoughtful. Visionary and dominant-design IT innovations should be analyzed and studied thoroughly. Nonetheless, organizations engaged in these innovations should also understand that a large amount of vision, management instinct, and "feel" guides the decision to initiate investment and continue investment. The organization that has had more experiences with IT, and more successful experiences, will be more effective in the evaluation (and execution) of IT initiatives.

Processes, data, and differentiation form the basis of an IT innovation. All the innovations studied were launched from management's fundamental understanding of current organizational limitations. Innovations should focus on the core elements discussed in Chapter Fourteen as the basis for achieving an IT-based advantage: significant leveraging of processes, expanding and capitalizing on the ability to gather critical data, and achieving a high level of organizational differentiation. Often an organization can pursue all three simultaneously. At other times an organization may evolve from one core element to another as the competition responds or as it sees new leverage points.

Alignment must be mature and strong. The alignment between the IT activities and the business challenges or opportunities must be strong. It should also be mature in the sense that it depends on close working relationships rather than methodologies.

The IT asset is critical. Strong IT staff, well-crafted architecture, and a superb CIO are critical contributors to success. There is substantial overlap between the factors identified in these studies and the components of the IT asset.

Robert Dvorak, Endre Holen, David Mark, and William Meehan have identified six principles at work in a high-performance IT function:

1. IT is a business-driven line activity and not a technology-driven IT staff function. Non-IT managers are responsible for selecting, implementing, and realizing the benefits of new applications. IT managers are responsible for providing cost-effective infrastructure to enable the applications.

2. IT funding decisions are made on the basis of value. Funding decisions require thorough business cases. IT decisions are based on business judgment and not technology judgment.

3. The IT environment emphasizes simplicity and flexibility. IT standards are centrally determined and enforced. Technology choices are conservative, and packaged applications are used wherever possible.

4. IT investments have to deliver near-term business results. The 80–20 rule is followed for applications, and projects are monitored relentlessly against milestones.

5. The IT operation engages in year-to-year operation productivity improvements.

6. A business-smart IT function and an IT-smart business organization are created. Senior leadership is involved in and conversant with IT decisions. IT managers spend time developing an understanding of the business.

Source: Dvorak, Holen, Mark, & Meehan, 1997, p. 166.

Weill and Aral (2006) identify these five characteristics of "IT savvy" organizations:

1. They use IT such as social networking sites, e-mail, and Twitter extensively for internal and external communication.

(cont.)

2. They rely extensively on the web to extend processes such as airline flight management, provider-sponsored personal health records, and retail purchasing to internal and external customers.

3. They have automated a very large percentage of their transactions, internally and with customers and suppliers.

4. They have company-wide IT skills; businesspeople have a deep IT understanding, and IT people have a deep business understanding.

5. Senior and midlevel management are extensively involved in IT strategy development, project prioritization, application implementation, and IT policy development.

Source: Weill & Aral, 2006.

Earl and Feeney (2000) assessed the characteristics and behaviors of senior leaders (in this case CEOs) who were actively engaged and successful in the strategic use of IT. These leaders were convinced that IT could and would change the organization. They placed the IT discussion high on the strategic agenda. They looked to IT to identify opportunities to make significant improvements in organizational performance, rather than viewing the IT agenda as secondary to strategy development. They devoted personal time to understanding how their industry and their organization would evolve as IT evolved. And they encouraged other members of the leadership team to do the same.

Earl and Feeney (2000) observed five management behaviors in these leaders:

1. They studied, rather than avoided, IT. They devoted time to learning about new technologies and, through discussion and introspection, developed an understanding of the ways in which new technologies might alter organizational strategies and operations.

2. They incorporated IT into their vision of the future of the organization and discussed the role of IT when communicating that vision.

3. They actively engaged in IT architecture discussions and high-level decisions. They took time to evaluate major new IT proposals and their implications. They were visibly supportive of architecture standards. They established funds for the exploration of promising new technologies.

4. They made sure that IT was closely linked to core management processes:

They integrated the IT discussion tightly into the overall strategy development process. This often involved setting up teams to examine aspects of the strategy and having both IT and business leaders at the table.

They made sure IT investments were evaluated as one component of the total investment needed by a strategy. The IT investments were not relegated to a separate discussion.

They ensured strong business sponsorship for all IT investments. Business sponsors were accountable for managing the IT initiatives and ensuring the success of the undertaking.

5. They continuously pressured the IT department to improve its efficiency and effectiveness and to be visionary in its thinking.

CEOs and other members of the leadership team have an extraordinary impact on the tone, values, and direction of an organization. Hence, their beliefs and daily behaviors have a significant impact on how effectively and strategically information technology is applied within an organization.

IT BUDGET

Developing budgets is one of the most critical management undertakings; it is the process that makes strategy real since it involves the commitment of resources. The budget process forces management to make choices between initiatives and investments and requires analysis of the scope and impact of any initiative—for example, it forces answers to questions such as, Will this initiative enable us to reduce supply costs by 3 percent?

Developing the IT budget is challenging for several reasons:

- The IT projects proposed at any one time are eclectic. In addition to the IT initiatives proposed as a result of the alignment and strategic planning process, other initiatives may be put forward by clinical or administrative departments that desire to improve some aspect of their performance. Also on the table may be IT projects designed to improve infrastructure—for example, a proposal to upgrade servers. These initiatives will all be different in character and in the return they offer, making them difficult to compare.

- Dozens, if not hundreds, of IT proposals may be made, making it challenging to fully understand all the requests.

- The aggregate request for capital and operating budgets can be too expensive. It is not unusual for requests to total three to four times more money than the organization can afford. Even if it wanted to fund all of the requests, the organization doesn't have enough money to do so.

And yet the budget process requires that the organization grapple with these complexities and arrive at a budget answer.

Basic Budget Categories

To facilitate the development of the IT budget, the organization should develop some basic categories that organize the budget discussion.

Capital and Operating

The first category distinguishes between capital and operating budgets. Financial management courses are the best place to learn about these two categories. In brief, however, capital budgets are the funds associated with purchasing and deploying an asset. Common capital items in IT budgets are hardware and applications. Operating budgets are the funds associated with using and maintaining the asset. Common operating items in IT budgets are hardware maintenance contracts and the salaries of IT analysts. In an analogous fashion, the purchase of a car is a capital expense. Gasoline and tune-ups are operating expenses. Both capital and operating budgets are prepared for IT initiatives.

Support, Ongoing, and New IT

Support refers to those IT costs (staff, hardware, and software licenses) necessary to support and maintain the applications and infrastructure that are in place now. Software maintenance contracts ensure that applications receive appropriate upgrades and bug fixes. Staff are needed to run the computer rooms and perform minor enhancements. Disk drives may need to be replaced. Failure to fund support activities can make it much more difficult to ensure the reliability of systems or to evolve applications to accommodate ongoing needs—for example, adding a new test to the dictionary for a laboratory system or introducing a new plan type into the patient accounting system.

Ongoing projects are those application implementations begun in a prior year and still under way. The implementation of a patient accounting system or a computerized provider order entry system can take several years. Hence a capital and operating budget is needed for several years to continue the implementation.

New projects are just that—there is a proposal for a new application or infrastructure application. The IT strategy may call for new systems to support nursing. Concerns over network security may lead to requests for new software to deter the efforts of hackers.

Support Current Operations or Strategic Plan

Proposals may be directed to supporting current operations, perhaps by responding to new regulations or streamlining the workflow in a department. Proposals may also be explicitly linked to an aspect of the health care organization's strategic plan—they might call for applications to support a strategic emphasis on disease management, for example.

Budget Targets

During the budget process, organizations define targets for the budget overall and for its components. For example, the organization might state that it would like to keep the overall growth in its operating budget to 2 percent but is willing to allow 5 percent growth in the IT operating budget. The organization might also direct that within that overall 5 percent growth, the budget for support should not grow by more than 3 percent, but the budget for new projects and ongoing projects combined can grow by 11 percent. Table 15.1 illustrates the application of overall and selective operating budget targets.

Similarly, targets can be set for the capital budget. For example, perhaps it will be decided that the capital budget for support should remain flat but that given the decision to invest in an electronic health record system, the overall capital budget will increase to accommodate the capital required by the EHR investment.

Table 15.1. Target increases in an IT operating budget

	Support Operations	Strategic Initiatives	Overall Target
Ongoing and new	9%	15%	11%
Support	3%	3%	3%
OVERALL TARGET	4%	7%	5%

Management Development of IT Budget Categories

The management discussion of the IT budget begins with the discussion of its categories and targets. Should the organization develop categories such as support, ongoing, and new? Should it assign selective budget targets by category? What should those targets be? There are no rules for this conversation. There is no optimal outcome.

However, the categories can be used to achieve various objectives. On the one hand, support often accounts for 70 to 80 percent of the IT operating budget and 20 to 30 percent of its capital budget. The organization can decide that support must work well but is of modest strategic value. Hences, the budget orientation is to be efficient with support. The budget target should be sufficient to cover salary growth and increases in maintenance contracts, but it should also encourage ongoing efforts to be more efficient. Efficiency can be gained, for example, by asking the IT function every year to achieve a 2 percent improvement in efficiency. On the other hand, an IT agenda with several important strategic initiatives may lead the organization to conclude that it will allow a 7 percent growth in the operating budget to support strategic initiatives but a more modest 4 percent growth in initiatives to support operations.

Whatever the outcome of the management discussion, the IT budget categories should remain consistent from year to year so that annual comparisons of the budget can be made. Moreover, stability in definitions enables the management team to develop a common language and concepts during budget discussions. However, the targets may change annually, depending on the fiscal health of the organization and the strategic importance of the IT agenda.

IT Budget Development

In addition to formulating the categories already discussed, organizational leadership will need to develop the process through which the IT budget is discussed, prioritized, and approved. In other words, it must answer the question, What processes will we use to decide which projects will be approved subject to our targets? An example of a budget process is outlined in this section and illustrated in Figure 15.1.

This process example has five components, and the steps described here use some typical targets.

First, the IT department submits an operating budget to support the applications and infrastructure that will be in place as of the beginning of the fiscal year (the support budget). This budget might be targeted to a 3 percent increase over the support budget for the prior fiscal year. The 3 percent increase reflects inflation, salary increases, a recognition that new systems were implemented during the fiscal year and will require support, and an acknowledgment that

Figure 15.1. IT budget decision-making process

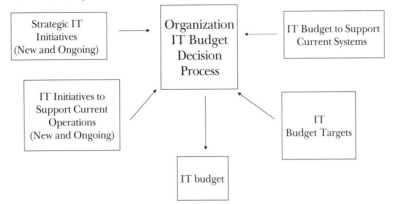

infrastructure (workstations, remote locations, and storage) consumption will increase. A figure for capital to support applications and infrastructure is also submitted, and it might be targeted to be the same as that budgeted in the prior fiscal year. If the support operating and capital budgets achieve their targets, there is minimal management discussion of those budgets.

Second, IT leadership reviews the strategic IT initiatives (new and ongoing) with the senior leadership of the organization. This review may occur in a forum such as the executive committee. This committee, mindful of its targets, determines which strategic initiatives will be funded. If the budget being sought to support strategic IT initiatives is large or a major increase over the previous year, there will be discussions about the budget with the board.

Third, the organization must decide which new and ongoing initiatives that support current operations—for example, a new clinical laboratory or contract management system—will be funded. These discussions must occur in the forum where the overall operations budget is discussed. The forums in which such discussions occur are generally organizational meetings that routinely discuss operations and that number among their members the managers of major departments and functions. Budget requests for new IT applications are reviewed in the same conversation that discusses budget requests for new clinical services or improvement of the organization's physical plant.

Fourth, both the strategy budget discussion and the operations budget discussion follow a set of ground rules:

- The IT budget is discussed in the same conversations that discuss non-IT budget requests. This will result in trade-offs between IT expenditures and other expenditures. This integration forces the organization to examine where it believes its monies are best spent, asking, for example, Should we invest in this IT proposal or should we invest in hiring staff to expand a clinical service? Following this process also means that IT requests and other budget requests are treated no differently.

- The level of analytical rigor required of the IT projects is the same as that required of any other requested budget item.

- Where appropriate, a sponsor—for example, a clinical vice president or a CFO—defends the IT requests that support his or her department in front of his or her colleagues. The IT staff or CIO should be asked to defend infrastructure investments—for example, major changes to the network—but should not be asked to defend applications.

The ground rule that sponsors should present their own IT requests deserves a bit more discussion, because the issue of who defends the request has several important ramifications, particularly for initiatives designed to improve current operations. Having this ground rule has the following results:

It forces assessment of trade-offs between IT and non-IT investments. The sponsor will determine whether to present the IT proposal or some other, perhaps non-IT, proposal. Sponsors are choosing which investments are the most important to them.

It forces accountability for investment results. The sponsor and his or her colleagues know that if the IT proposal is approved, there will be less money available for other initiatives. The defender also knows that the value being promised must be delivered or his or her credibility in next year's budget discussion will be diminished.

It improves management comfort when dealing with IT proposals. Managers can be more comfortable with the IT proposal if one of their operations colleagues is defending it. The defender also learns how to be comfortable when presenting IT proposals.

It gets IT out of the role of defending other people's operation improvement initiatives. However, the IT function must still support the budget requests of others by providing data on the costs and capabilities of the proposed applications and the time frames and resources required to implement them. If the IT function believes that the proposed initiative lacks merit or is too risky, IT staff need to ensure that this opinion is heard during the budget approval process.

In the fifth and final step of the process, the operations and strategic budget recommendations are reviewed and discussed at an executive committee meeting. The executive committee can accept the recommendations, request further refinement (perhaps cuts) of the budget, or determine that a discussion of the budget is required at an upcoming board meeting.

SUMMARY

The management and leadership of an organization play significant roles in determining the effectiveness of information technology. This chapter discussed the role of developing and maintaining IT governance mechanisms—the processes, procedures, and roles that the organization uses to make IT decisions. These decisions cover diverse terrain: budgets, roles, and responsibility distribution and the process for resolution of IT issues.

Health care executives must also take steps to improve the overall ability of the organization to apply IT. These steps may involve working on improving IT-user relationships, managing IT architecture, developing approaches to IT experimentation, ensuring IT strategic alignment, and developing the skills of the IT staff.

An annual responsibility of the leadership is determining the IT budget. Developing this budget is difficult. Comparing diverse and numerous IT proposals is challenging. However, the budget process can be made easier (although not easy) by establishing clear definitions of budget categories, category targets, and the process for IT proposal review.

KEY TERMS

IT budget

IT effectiveness

IT governance

IT steering committee

IT, user, and senior management responsibilities

LEARNING ACTIVITIES

1. Interview a member of the senior leadership team of a health care organization on the subject of IT governance. Describe the organization's approach to IT governance and assess its effectiveness.

2. Interview a health care CIO and a member of the senior leadership team of the same health care organization separately. Ask each of them to describe the process of preparing the IT budget. Compare and discuss their responses.

3. Interview a health care CIO and a member of the senior leadership team of the same health care organization separately. Ask each of

them to describe the distribution of IT and user responsibilities. Compare and discuss their responses.

4. Assume that you are a consultant who has been asked to assess the effectiveness of an organization in applying IT. Construct a questionnaire (twenty questions) to guide the interviews of organizational leaders that you would conduct to determine effectiveness.

NOTE

1. Lists quoted from Applegate, Austin, & McFarlan, 2003, McGraw-Hill © 2002, are reproduced with permission of The McGraw-Hill Companies.

REFERENCES

Applegate, L., Austin, R., & McFarlan, W. (2003). *Corporate information strategy and management* (6th ed.). Boston: McGraw-Hill.

Brown, C., & Sambamurthy, V. (1999). *Repositioning the IT organization to enable business transformation.* Chicago: Society for Information Management.

Drazen, E., & Straisor, D. (1995). *Information support in an integrated delivery system.* Paper presented at the annual Healthcare Information and Management Systems (HIMSS) conference, Chicago.

Dvorak, R., Holen, E., Mark, D., & Meehan, W., III. (1997). Six principles of high-performance IT. *McKinsey Quarterly, 3,* 164–177.

Earl, M., & Feeney, D. (2000). How to be a CEO for the information age. *MIT Sloan Management Review, 41*(2), 11–23.

Feld, C., & Stoddard, D. (2004). Getting IT right. *Harvard Business Review, 82*(2), 72–79.

McKenney, J., Copeland, D., & Mason, R. (1995). *Waves of change: Business evolution through information technology.* Boston: Harvard Business School Press.

Ross, J., Beath, C., & Goodhue, D. (1996). Develop long-term competitiveness through IT assets. *MIT Sloan Management Review, 38*(1), 31–42.

Sambamurthy, V., & Zmud, R. (1996). *Information technology and innovation: Strategies for success.* Morristown, NJ: Financial Executives Research Foundation.

Weill, P., & Aral, S., (2006). Generating premium returns on your IT investments. *MIT Sloan Management Review, 47*(2), 54–60.

Weill, P., & Broadbent, M. (1998). *Leveraging the new infrastructure.* Boston: Harvard Business School Press.

Weill, P., & Ross, J. (2004). *IT governance: How top performers manage IT decision rights for superior results.* Boston: Harvard Business School Press.

CHAPTER 16

Management's Role in Major IT Initiatives

LEARNING OBJECTIVES

- To be able to understand the different types of organizational change associated with IT initiatives.
- To be able to discuss the strategies for effecting organizational change.
- To review the structures and processes used to manage IT projects.
- To review the factors that contribute to IT project failures.

Health care organizations routinely undertake projects or initiatives designed to improve the performance of the organization or advance its strategies through the use of information technologies. Many of these projects involve the implementation of a major application system, and often these projects are labeled "IT projects." Examples of such projects include implementing computerized provider order entry, streamlining the front-end processes of registration and scheduling, and enhancing the discharge process.

This chapter discusses the role of management in these IT projects. The strategy may have been defined and the IT agenda may have been aligned; now it is time to execute the plan. What role should management play during the execution of IT initiatives? What structures, processes, and roles should be in place to make sure that the initiatives are well managed?

This chapter covers three major topics:

- Managing organizational change due to IT initiatives
- Managing IT projects
- Understanding factors that contribute to IT initiative failures

MANAGING CHANGE DUE TO IT

A majority of IT initiatives involve or require organizational change—change in processes or organizational structure or the expansion or contraction of roles or services. IT-enabled change and IT-driven change have several possible origins:

- The new IT system has capabilities different from those of the previous system and hence the workflow that surrounds the system has to change and the tasks that staff perform have to change. For example, if a new electronic health record system automatically generates letters for patients with normal test results, then the individuals who used to generate these letters will no longer have to do this task.

- The discussion surrounding the desired capabilities of a new application can lead to a reassessment of current processes, workflow, and distribution of tasks across staff and a decision to make changes in processes that extend well beyond the computer system. For example, the analysis surrounding a new patient accounting system might highlight problems that occur during registration and scheduling (such as failure to check insurance coverage during appointment check-in) that hinder the optimal performance of patient accounting.

In this way a new system becomes a catalyst for a comprehensive set of changes.

- The health care organization's strategy may call for significant changes in the way the organization operates and delivers care. For example, the organization may decide to move aggressively to protocol-driven care. This transformation has extensive ramifications for processes, roles, and workflow and for the design of applications. New IT systems will be critical contributors to the changes needed, but they are not the epicenter of the change discussion.

Change management is an essential skill for the leaders of health care organizations. Although the need for this skill is not confined to situations that involve the implementation of major applications, change management is a facet of virtually all implementations of such applications.

Types of Organizational Change

Keen (1997) identified four categories of *organizational change*:

- Incremental
- Step-shift
- Radical
- Fundamental

Incremental Change

Incremental change occurs through a series (at times continuous) of small to medium-sized changes to processes, tasks, and roles. Each change carries relatively low risk, can be completed quickly, and is often accomplished without the need for substantial analysis or leadership intervention. At times, organizations establish an overall emphasis on continuous change and create groups to help departments make changes and measure change impact. Techniques such as LEAN and Six Sigma emphasize continuous, incremental change. Continuous, incremental change can be seen as plodding and lacking bold vision. However, this perception misses the power of such change over the course of time and the occurrence of such change across many facets of the organization. One should remember that the Grand Canyon was formed from continuous, incremental erosion.

The implementation of an application can involve change that is incremental. This is particularly true when the application is an upgrade of an existing application and has new reports and features that require modest alterations to existing workflow.

One outcome of continuous change may be the recognition that current application systems are progressively becoming a poor fit with the evolving organization. After several years of dealing with a growing gap between the capabilities of an application and the direction of an evolving organization, the organization may decide to purchase a new application, one that is a better fit.

Step-Shift Change

In step-shift change the leadership is committed to making significant changes but is not changing the basic direction of the organization or how it generates value. Examples of such change include a focused effort to significantly reduce the cost of care or improve patient safety, the addition of a non-acute business line in an organization that has previously focused on acute care, and a major effort to improve the patient service experience in the outpatient clinics. Step-shift change involves an intense focus on a critical aspect of the organization and, for the areas within that focus, major changes in processes, roles, and tasks. Step-shift change is often driven by a strategic realization that the basis of competition has evolved to the point that in the absence of such change, the organization's success is in some degree of peril.

This type of change invariably leads to the implementation of major new applications. An emphasis on patient safety may lead to the implementation of computerized provider order entry, and an effort to improve the patient experience in outpatient care may result in the implementation of a new registration and scheduling application. At times the leadership responsible for implementing a new application will realize that this implementation creates the opportunity to effect step-shift change, asking, for example, Why don't we take advantage of this new outpatient system to make significant improvements in the service experience?

Radical Change

Radical change leaves the organization and its core mission intact but significantly alters the way the organization carries out its business. The creation of an integrated delivery system from a collection of previously independent organizations is an example of radical change. The movement from fee-for-service reimbursement to full capitation (that is, fixed fee per patient per year) is radical change. Radical change always requires some changes, at times extensive changes, in the IT application portfolio. Because the way work is done has changed significantly across many facets of the organization, applications that fit the way work was previously done may no longer be helpful.

In health care it is rare that IT will cause or lead to a decision to undergo radical organizational change. The Internet frenzy that occurred in the early part of this century led many health care organizations to wonder whether the Internet would cause radical change. For example, if patients could look up medical information on the Internet, would this significantly reduce their need for physicians? This radical change did not occur, although use of the Internet has led to incremental change and some step-shift change in health care.

Fundamental Change

With fundamental change the leadership is committed to creating what will in effect be a new organization that is in a different business from the one the current organization engages in. This fundamental change has occurred for some companies. For example, the now deservedly maligned Enron changed its core business from acquiring and managing natural gas pipelines to managing a complex web of businesses that included a global broadband network and the trading of paper products. A health care example would be an acute care provider that closes all its beds and becomes a diagnostic imaging center. Fundamental change is risky, and the failure rate is very high.

Clearly, in these cases the entire IT application suite may need to be jettisoned and replaced with new applications that support the new business.

Effecting Organizational Change

The management strategies required to manage change depend on the type of change. As one moves from incremental to fundamental change, the magnitude and risk of the change increase enormously, as does the uncertainty about the form and success of the outcome.

In this section we will present some normative approaches to managing a blend of step-shift and radical change. Fundamental change is rare in health care. Incremental change carries less risk and hence requires less management. Note, however, that a program of continuous incremental change is in effect a form of step-shift change.

Managing change of this magnitude (step-shift to radical) is deceptively simple and quite hard at the same time. It is the same duality encountered in raising children. At one level it is easy; all you have to do is feed, teach, protect, and love them. At another level, especially during the teenage years, it can be an exceptionally complicated, exasperating, and scary experience.

Managing change has several necessary aspects (Keen, 1997):

- Leadership
- Language and vision
- Connection and trust
- Incentives
- Planning, implementing, and iterating

Leadership

Change must be led. Leadership, often in the form of a committee of leaders, will be necessary to

- Define the nature of the change
- Communicate the rationale for and approach to the change
- Identify, procure, and deploy necessary resources
- Resolve issues and alter direction as needed
- Monitor the progress of the change initiative

This leadership committee needs to be chaired by an appropriate senior leader. If the change affects the entire organization, the CEO should chair the committee. If the change is focused on a specific area, the most senior leader who oversees that area should chair the committee.

Language and Vision

The staff who are experiencing the change must understand the nature of the change. They must know what the world will look like (to the degree that this is clear) when the change has been completed, how their roles and work life will be different, and why making this change is important. The absence of this vision or a failure to communicate the importance of the vision elevates the risk that staff will resist the change and through subtle and not-so-subtle means cause the change to grind to a halt. Change is hard for people. They must understand the nature of the change and why they should go through with what they will experience as a difficult transition.

Leaders might describe the vision, the desired outcome of efforts to improve the outpatient service experience, in this way:

- Patients should be able to get an appointment for a time that is most convenient for them.

- Patients should not have to wait longer than ten minutes in the reception area before a provider can see them.
- We should communicate clearly with patients about their disease and the treatment that we will provide.
- We should seek to eliminate administrative and insurance busywork from the professional lives of our providers.

These examples illustrate a thoughtful use of language. They first and foremost focus on patients. But the organization also wants to improve the lives of its providers. The examples use the word *should* rather than the word *must* because it is thought that staff won't believe the organization can pull off 100 percent achievement of these goals, and leaders do not want to establish goals seen as unrealistic. The examples also use the word *we* rather than the word *you*. *We* means that this vision will be achieved through a team effort, rather than implying that those hearing this message have to bear this challenge without leadership's help.

Connection and Trust

Achieving connection means that leadership takes every opportunity to present the vision throughout the organization. Leaders may use department head meetings, medical staff forums, one-on-one conversations in the hallway, internal publications, and e-mail to communicate the vision and to keep communicating the vision. Even when they start to feel ill because they have communicated the vision one thousand times, they have to communicate it another one thousand times. A lot of this communication has to be done in person, where others can see the leaders, rather than hiding behind an e-mail. The communication must invite feedback, criticism, and challenges.

The members of the organization must trust the integrity, intelligence, compassion, and skill of the leadership. Trust is earned or lost by everything that leaders do or don't do. The members must also trust that leaders have thoughtfully come to the conclusion that the difficult change has excellent reasons behind it and represents the best option for the organization. Organizational members are willing to rise to a challenge, often to heroic levels, if they trust their leaders. Trust requires that leaders act in the best interests of the staff and the organization and that leaders listen and respond to the organization's concerns.

Incentives

Organizational members must be motivated to support significant change. At times, excitement with the vision will be sufficient incentive. Alternatively, fear of what will happen if the organization fails to move toward the vision may serve as an incentive. Although important, neither fear nor rapture is necessarily sufficient.

If organizational members will lose their jobs or have their roles changed significantly, education that prepares them for new roles and/or new jobs must be offered. Bonuses may be offered to key individuals, awarded according to the success of the change and each person's contribution to the change. At times, frankly, support is obtained through old-fashioned horse-trading—if the other person will support the change, you will deliver something that is of interest to him or her (space, extra staff, a promotion). Incentives may also take the form of awards—for example, plaques and dinners for two—to staff who go above and beyond the call of duty during the change effort.

Planning, Implementing, and Iterating

Change must be planned. These plans describe the tasks and task sequences necessary to effect the change. Tasks can range from redesigning forms to managing the staged implementation of application systems to retraining staff. Tasks must be allotted resources, and staff accountable for task performance must be designated.

Implementation of the plan is obviously necessary. Because few organizational changes of any magnitude will be fully understood beforehand, problems will be encountered during implementation. New forms may fail to capture necessary data. The estimate of the time needed to register a patient may be wrong and long lines may form at the registration desk. The planners may have forgotten to identify how certain information would flow from one department to another.

These problems are in addition to the problems that occur, for example, when task timetables slip and dependent tasks fall idle or are in trouble. The implementation of the application has been delayed and will not be ready when the staff move to the new building—what do we do? Iteration and adjustment will be necessary as the organization handles problems created when tasks encounter trouble, and learns about glitches with the new processes and workflows.

MANAGING IT PROJECTS

Within the overall change agenda, projects will be formed, managed, and completed. In large change initiatives, the IT project may be one of several projects. For several step-shift changes, the change management agenda may be composed almost entirely of the implementation of an application system.

Change management places an emphasis on many of the "softer," although still critical, aspects of management and leadership: communicating vision, establishing trust, and developing incentives. *Project management* is a "harder" aspect of management. Project management centers on a set of management disciplines and practices that, when executed well, increase the likelihood that a project will deliver the desired results. Project management has several objectives:

- Clearly define the scope and goals of the project.
- Identify accountability for the successful completion of the project and associated project tasks.
- Define the processes for making project-related decisions.
- Identify the project's tasks and task sequence and interdependencies.
- Determine the resource and time requirements of the project.
- Ensure appropriate communication with relevant stakeholders about project status and issues.

Different projects require different management strategies. Projects that are pilots or experiments require less formal oversight (and are not helped by large amounts of formal oversight) than large, multiyear, multimillion-dollar undertakings. Projects carried out by two or more organizations working together will have decision-making structures different from those found in projects done by several departments in one organization.

In this chapter we discuss a normative approach to managing relatively large projects within one organization. (Much of the following discussion is adapted from Spurr, 2003.) This approach is put in place once the need for the project has been established (through the IT strategy, for example), the project objectives have been defined, the budget has been approved, and the major stakeholders have been identified.

Project Roles

Four roles are important in the management of large projects:

- Business sponsor
- Business owner
- Project manager
- IT manager

Business Sponsor

The *business sponsor* is the individual who holds overall accountability for the project. The sponsor should represent the area of the organization that is the major recipient of the performance improvement that the project intends to deliver. For example, a project that involves implementing a new claims processing system may have the chief financial officer as the business sponsor. A project to improve nursing workflow may ask the chief nursing officer to serve as business sponsor. A project that affects a large portion of the organization may have the chief executive officer as the business sponsor.

The sponsor's management or executive level should be appropriate to the magnitude of the decisions and the support that the project will require. The more significant the undertaking, the higher the organizational level of the sponsor.

The business sponsor has several duties; he or she

- Secures funding and needed business resources—for example, the commitment of people's time to work on the project.
- Has final decision-making and sign-off accountability for project scope, resources, and approaches to resolving project problems.
- Identifies and supports the business owner(s) (discussed in the next section).
- Promotes the project internally and externally, and obtains the buy-in from business constituents.
- Chairs the project steering committee and is responsible for steering committee participation during the life of the project
- Helps define deliverables, objectives, scope, and success criteria with identified business owners and the project manager.
- Helps remove business obstacles to meeting the project timeline and producing deliverables, as appropriate.

Business Owner

A *business owner* generally has day-to-day responsibility for running a function or a department: for example, a business owner might be the director of the clinical laboratories. A project may need the involvement of several business owners. For example, the success of a new patient accounting system may depend on processes that occur during registration and scheduling (and hence the director of outpatient clinics and the director of the admitting department will both be business owners) and may also depend on adequate physician documentation of the care provided (and hence the administrator of the medical group will be another business owner).

Business owners often work on the project team. Among their several responsibilities they

- Represent their department or function at steering committee and project team meetings.
- Secure and coordinate necessary business and departmental resources.
- Remove business obstacles to meeting the project timeline and producing deliverables, as appropriate.
- Work jointly with the project manager on several tasks (as described in the next section).

Project Manager

The *project manager* does just that—manages the project. He or she is the person who provides the day-to-day direction setting, conflict resolution, and communication needed by the project team. The project manager may be an IT staffer or a person in the business, or function, benefiting from the project. Among their several responsibilities, project managers:

- Identify and obtain needed resources.
- Deliver the project on time, on budget, and according to specification.
- Communicate progress to sponsors, stakeholders, and team members.
- Ensure that diligent risk monitoring is in place and appropriate risk mitigation plans have been developed.
- Identify and manage the resolution of issues and problems.
- Maintain the project plan.
- Manage project scope.

The project manager works closely with the business owners and business sponsor in performing these tasks. Together they set meeting agendas, manage the meetings, track project progress, communicate project status, escalate issues as appropriate, and resolve deviations and issues related to the project plan.

IT Manager

The *IT manager* is the senior IT person assigned to the project. He or she may be the boss of the project manager. In performing his or her responsibilities, the IT manager

- Represents the IT department.
- Has final IT decision-making authority and sign-off accountability.
- Helps remove IT obstacles to meeting project timelines and producing deliverables.
- Promotes the project internally and externally, and obtains buy-in from IT constituents.

Project Committees

These four roles may employ two or three major committees to provide project guidance and management: a project steering committee, a project team, and a project review committee.

Project Steering Committee

The *project steering committee* provides overall guidance and management oversight of the project. The steering committee has the authority to resolve changes in scope that affect the budget, milestones, and deliverables. This committee is expected to resolve issues and address risks that cannot be handled by the project team. It also manages communications with the leadership of the organization and the project team. The project steering committee may be the same committee that leads the overall change process or a subcommittee of that group.

The business sponsor should chair this committee. Its members should be representatives of the major areas of the organization that will be affected by the project and whose efforts are necessary if the project is to succeed. Returning to an earlier example, a steering committee overseeing the implementation of a new patient accounting system might include the director of outpatient clinics, the director of the admitting department, and the medical group administrator as members. The senior IT manager should also be on this committee. Depending on the size and importance of the project, this person could be the CIO. It is rare for the chair of the steering committee to be an IT person, though having an IT person as a cochair is not uncommon.

Project Team

The *project team* may not be called a committee, but it will meet regularly and it does have responsibilities. The project manager chairs the project team. This team

- Manages the performance of the project work.
- Resolves day-to-day project issues.
- Manages and allocates resources as necessary to do the work.
- Works with the steering committee and business owners, as necessary, to resolve problems; assess potential changes in scope, timeline, or budget; and communicate the status of the project.

Project team members may be business owners, business owners' staff, IT managers, or IT managers' staff.

Project Review Committee

If the organization has a relatively large number of simultaneously active IT projects (say, fifty or so), a project review committee can be helpful. The project review committee focuses on a subset of all IT projects, those deemed to be the most important to the organization or the riskiest, or both. The review committee checks the status of each project in this subset to determine if the project is proceeding well or likely to be heading into trouble. If trouble is on the horizon, the committee discusses ways to reduce the threats to the project. The committee also looks for opportunities to leverage the work from one project across other projects and checks for areas where redundant work or work at cross-purposes may be occurring. For example, two projects may need large numbers of workstations deployed during the same interval of time. If the IT group that deploys workstations could not handle this volume, the project review committee would discuss ways to resolve this problem.

The review committee serves as a second pair of eyes on critical projects and has the ability to move resources between projects. For example, if Project A is experiencing instability with its core infrastructure, the review committee can pull network engineers and database server team members from Project B to help out on Project A. The review committee is often chaired by a senior IT person and is composed largely of IT project managers.

Key Project Elements

Over the course of decades and millions of projects, a set of management disciplines and processes has been developed to help ensure that projects succeed. This collected set of practices is referred to as *project management*. One will see these disciplines and processes in action in any well-run project. Excellent project management does not ensure project success. However, without such project management the risks of failure skyrocket, particularly for large projects. The elements of project management (above and beyond the roles just described) are reviewed in the following sections. These elements are created or established after the project proposal has been approved.

Project Charter

The *project charter* is a document that describes the purpose, scope, objectives, costs, and schedule for the project. This document also discusses the roles and responsibilities of the individuals and functions that must contribute to the project. The project charter serves three basic objectives:

- It ensures that planning assumptions or potentially ambiguous objectives are discussed and resolved (this occurs during development of the charter).
- It prevents participants from developing different understandings of the project intent, timeline, or cost.
- It enables the project leadership to communicate as necessary with the organization about the project.

The project charter sets out these project elements:

- Project overview and objectives
- Application features and capabilities (vision of the solution)
- Project scope and limitations
- Metrics for determining project success
- Budget and overall timetable
- Project organization
- Project management strategies

Appendix B contains an example of a project charter.

Project Plan

The project charter provides an overview of the project. The *project plan* provides the details of the tasks, phases, and resources needed, by task and phase and timeline. The project plan is the tool used by the project team during the day-to-day management of the project. The project plan has several components:

- Project phases and tasks. A phase may have multiple tasks. For example, there may be a phase called "conduct analysis," and it may involve such tasks as "review admitting department forms," "document the admitting workflow," and "document the discharge workflow."
- The sequence of phases and tasks.
- Interdependencies between phases and tasks.
- The duration of phases and tasks.
- Staff resources needed, by phase and task.

Several software tools are available that assist project managers in developing project plans. These tools enable the project manager to develop the plan (as described earlier), prepare plan charts and resource use by phase and task, and model the impact on the plan if timelines change or resource availability alters.

Figure 16.1 is an example of a project timeline with project phases. Table 16.1 illustrates an analysis of project resources (staff) that shows project team members' time commitment by activity.

Project Plan and Charter Considerations

Developing project plans and charters requires skill and experience. Managers are often in forums (such as project steering committee meetings) where they are asked to review, critique, and approve a project plan. What should they look for in these plans?

To a large degree, the reputations of project managers precede them. If project managers have proven themselves over the course of many projects, then their plans are likely to be generally sound. If project managers are novices or have an uneven track record, their plans may require greater scrutiny. Regardless of track record, there are several cues that a project plan is as solid as one can make it at the inception of the project. (See page 538.)

Figure 16.1. Project timeline with project phases

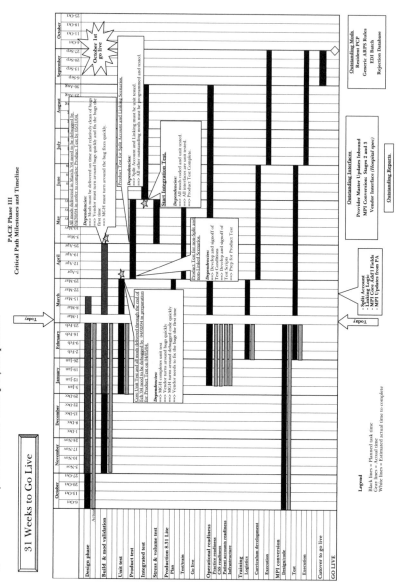

Table 16.1. Project resource analysis

Analysis Project	Activity	Start Activity	Finish Activity	% Allocated[a]
Susan Smith				
CRIS—> Cancer Registry Data Load	Application design	11/3/2012	11/10/2012	18.95%
CRIS—> Cancer Registry Data Load	Application testing	11/3/2012	12/12/2012	25.38%
CRIS—> Cancer Registry Data Load	Data mapping specification	11/3/2012	11/19/2012	17.25%
CRIS—> Cancer Registry Data Load	Functional analysis	11/3/2012	11/14/2012	35.00%
CRIS Minor Enhancements	CRIS breast minor enhancements analysis	11/3/2012	11/2/2013	4.75%
CRIS Minor Enhancements	CRIS breast minor enhancements testing	11/3/2012	11/2/2013	4.75%
CRIS/STIP GI Development and Implementation	GI CRA form design/analysis	11/3/2012	1/29/2013	5.38%
CRIS/STIP GI Development and Implementation	GI follow-up form design/analysis	11/3/2012	2/6/2013	5.75%
Renal STIP/CRIS	Renal CRIS analysis	11/3/2012	2/5/2013	
	Administration	11/3/2012	9/30/2013	12.63%
	Support work	11/3/2012	9/30/2013	55.50%
James Jones				
BICS Modernization	Background research	11/3/2012	10/28/2013	19.50%
BICS Modernization	Develop overall project plan	11/3/2012	12/13/2012	8.50%
BICS Modernization	E-mail coding	11/3/2012	1/15/2013	10.00%
Gartner TCO Analysis	Collect data and input into template—Rd 1	11/3/2012	11/11/2012	8.55%
LDRPS Implementation	Plan building pilot group	11/3/2012	12/1/2012	11.00%
Document Management	VDRNETS security testing	11/3/2012	11/11/2012	
	Administration	11/3/2012	9/30/2013	19.50%
	Support work	11/3/2012	9/30/2013	24.40%

[a]Percentage of employee's time devoted to a project during the interval bounded by the "start activity" date and the "finish activity" date.

- The project charter is clear and explicit. Fuzzy objectives and vague understandings of resource needs indicate that the plan needs further discussion and development.

- The leaders of the departments and functions that will be affected by the plan or that need to devote resources to the plan have reviewed the charter and plan, their concerns have been heard and addressed, and they have publicly committed to performing the work needed in the plan.

- The project timelines have been reviewed by multiple parties for reasonableness, and these timelines have taken into consideration factors that will affect the plan—for example, key staff going on vacation or organizational energies being diverted to develop the annual budget—and any uncertainties that might exist for particular phases or tasks—for example, if it is not fully clear how a specific task will be performed, that task timeline should have some "slack" built into it.

- The resources needed have been committed. The budget has been approved. Staff needed by the plan can be named, and their managers have taken steps to free up the staff time needed by the plan.

- The accountabilities for the plan and for each plan phase and task are explicit.

- Project risks have been comprehensively assessed, and thoughtful approaches to addressing each risk developed. Some examples of project risks are unproven information technology, a deterioration in the organization's financial condition, and turnover of project staff.

- A reasonable amount of contingency planning has addressed inevitable problems and current uncertainties. In general, projects should add 10 percent to the timeline and 10 percent to the budget to reflect the time and dollar cost of inevitable problems. For very complex projects, it is not unusual to see 20 to 25 percent of the budget and the duration of some tasks labeled "unknown" or "unclear."

Project Status Report

The *project status report* documents and communicates the current condition of the project. This report is generally prepared monthly and distributed to project participants and stakeholders. The status report often provides matter for discussion at steering committee meetings. It typically covers recent accomplishments and decisions, work in progress, upcoming milestones, and issues that require resolution (see the example in Exhibit 16.1). It may use a color

Exhibit 16.1. Sample project status report

**Electronic Medication Administration Record (E-Mar)—
Status Report**

Reporting Period: July 2012
Business Sponsor: Sally Salisbury, RN, Vice President Patient Care
Services

Business Owners: Amy Leron, RN, Director of Nursing Quality and
Practice; William Farnsworth, RPh, Director of Pharmacy

IT Managers: Cindy Mason, RNC, Corporate Director of Clinical Systems
Management; Sue Kimit, CIO-BWH

ARTICLE I. PROJECT SCHEDULE

Activity	Planned	Revised	Actual Delivery
Functional specification requirements completed	01/12	07/12	07/12
Technical Specifications completed	02/12	11/28/12	
Wireless Infrastructure in place for pilot pods	02/12	9/15/12	
Wireless Infrastructure in place for training room (Ledge Site)	02/12	07/12	07/12
Wireless Infrastructure in place for pharmacy	02/12	05/12	06/12
Wireless Infrastructure in place for all adult inpatient pods	03/12	09/26/12	
Bar Code development— Medications	6/12	08/29/12	
Bar Code development—Patient ID band Implementation	05/12	08/15/12	
Bar Code development—Clinical Staff Implementation (employee ID)	05/12	08/15/12	
Bar Code Imager Selection	02/12	04/12	04/12
Adult Pharmacy development	06/12	08/12	
Adult Pharmacy application pilot	08/12	08/12	
Code Freeze (pilot)	04/12	09/15/12	
Integrated Testing (pilot)	04/12	9/15/12–10/25/12	

(cont.)

Exhibit 16.1. (*Continued*)

Activity	Planned	Revised	Actual Delivery
Section 1.01 PILOT			
Section 1.02 Hardware Purchase (notebook, imager)	06/12	07/12	07/12
Create Image/Test Fujitsu Lifebook	06/12	07/12	07/12
Hiring/Training Support Staff	07/12	09/26/12	
Hardware Deployment	08/12	10/27/12	
Training—Planning complete	06/12	07/12	07/12
Training—Development complete	07/12	10/01/12	
Training—Conduct Classes	08/12	10/14/12–10/25/12	
Implementation	06/12	10/12	
Evaluation of pilot	07/12	12/12	
Section 1.03			
Section 1.04 ROLLOUT			
Rollout Implementation Plan	09/12	08/29/12	
Hiring Support Staff	12/12	01/13	
Training Support Staff	01/13	01/ 13	
Hardware Deployment	07/12	2/13–5/13	
Training—Planning	08/12	12/13	
Training—Development	09/12	01/ 13	
Training—Conduct Classes	09/12	02/01/13–05/12/13	
Implementation Begin	10/12	02/16/13	
Implementation End	04/13	05/21/13	

ARTICLE II. ACCOMPLISHMENTS

• The functional requirements for the pilot have been agreed upon and finalized.

ARTICLE III. DECISIONS

• The pilot date was revised to 10/27–11/21. The additional time is needed to complete the application development for upcoming changes to OE, such as the new KCL scales and PCA templates.

• The format for the Medical Record Copy of the e-mar was approved by Health Information Systems.

ARTICLE IV. WORK IN PROGRESS

• Completing the bar-coded Employee ID badge. This should be ready for testing during the second week in August.

Exhibit 16.1. (*Continued*)

- Completing the bar-coded patient ID band, which can be finalized when the font software arrives.
- Programming for recently finalized e-mar specifications—scales, tapers, various templates, downtime procedures, reports, etc.
- Programming for BICS changes necessary for e-mar.
- Jeff Smith is working with several cart vendors to secure carts for the pilot.
- Wiring/cabling for the wireless network on the inpatient pods begins 8/4 and continues through 9/26.
- Planning for integration testing.
- Unit testing.

ARTICLE V. ISSUES
- Accessing BICS from the web pod monitor is inconsistent and slow; the platform architecture specialists are investigating a solution, and it's being tested now.
- The font software for patient ID bands has been delayed; Emily Johnson is working to expedite this so that final development can occur.

ARTICLE VI. UPCOMING ACTIVITIES
- ID badge replacement scheduled for RNs and pharmacists 8/14–8/22.
- The pharmacy will conduct a pilot of its new web system beginning on 8/25.

scheme to graphically depict the status of a project—for example, green to indicate the task or phase is proceeding well, yellow to indicate the task or phase may be facing a timeline or other problem, and red to indicate the task or phase is in trouble and requires attention. When a plethora of tasks and phases are tagged with red, then the project is experiencing significant difficulty. Conversely, a sea of green indicates that the project is going well.

The preparation, distribution, and discussion of the project status report are part of the overall project communication plan. Other important communications might include quarterly project presentations at meetings of the organization's department heads, articles about the project in the organization's internal newsletter, and presentations at specific leadership forums—for example, at a medical staff forum or at a meeting of the board or of the executive committee.

UNDERSTANDING IT INITIATIVE FAILURES

The failure rate of IT initiatives is surprisingly high. Project failure occurs when a project is significantly over budget, takes much longer than the estimated timeline, or has to be terminated because so many problems have occurred that proceeding is no longer judged to be viable. Cook (2007) finds that 35 percent of IT projects were successful, whereas 19 percent failed. The remaining 46 percent delivered a useful product but suffered from budget overruns, prolonged timetables, and application feature shortfalls.

Cash, McFarlan, and McKenney (1992) note that two major categories of risk confront significant IT investments: strategy failures and implementation failures. The project failure rates suggest that management should be more worried about IT implementation than IT strategy. IT strategy is sexier and more visionary than implementation. However, a very large number of strategies and visions go nowhere or are diminished because the organization is unable to implement them.

Why is this failure rate so high? What happens? In the sections that follow, we will examine several classes of barriers that hinder large IT projects.

Lack of Clarity of Purpose

Any project or initiative is destined for trouble if its objectives and purpose are unclear. Sometimes the purpose of a project is only partially clear. For example, an organization may have decided that it should implement an electronic health record in an effort to "improve the quality and efficiency of care." However, it is not really clear to the leadership and staff how the EHR will be used to improve care. Will problems associated with finding a patient's record be solved? Will the record be used to gather data about care quality? Will the record be used to support outpatient medication ordering and reduce medication error rates?

All these questions can be answered yes, but if the organization never gets beyond the slogan of "improve the quality and efficiency of care," the scope of the project will be murky. The definition of care improvement is left up to the project participant to interpret. And the scope and timetable of the project cannot possibly be precise because project objectives are too fuzzy.

Lack of Belief in the Project

At times the objectives are very clear, but the members of the organization are not convinced that the project is worth doing at all. Because the project will change the work life of many members and require that they participate in design and implementation, they need to be sufficiently convinced that the project will improve their lives or is necessary if the organization is to thrive. They will legitimately ask, What's in it for me? Unconvinced of the need for the project, they will resist it. A resistant organization will likely doom any project. Projects that are viewed as illegitimate by a large portion of the people in an organization rarely succeed.

Insufficient Leadership Support

The organization's leaders may be committed to the undertaking yet not demonstrate that commitment. For example, leaders may not devote sufficient time to the project or may decide to send subordinates to meetings. This broadcasts a signal to the organization that the leaders have other, "more important" things to do. Tough project decisions may get made in a way that shows the leaders are not as serious as their rhetoric, because when push came to shove, they caved in.

Members of the leadership team may have voted yes to proceed with a project, but their votes may not have included their reservations about the utility of the project or the way it was put together. Once problems are encountered in the project (and all projects encounter problems), this qualified leadership support evaporates, and the silent reservations become public statements such as, "I knew that this would never work."

Organizational Inertia

Even when the organization is willing to engage in a project, inertia can hinder it. People are busy. They are stressed. They have jobs to do. Some of the changes are threatening. Staff may believe these changes leave them less skilled or less instrumental or with reduced power. Or they may not have a good understanding of their work life after the change, and they may imagine that an uncertain outcome cannot be a good outcome.

Projects add work on top of the workload of often already overburdened people. Projects add stress for often already stressed people. As a result, despite the valiant efforts of leadership and the expenditure of significant resources, a project may slowly grind to a halt because too many members find ways to avoid or not deal with the efforts and changes the initiative requires. Bringing significant change to a large portion of the organization is very hard because, if nothing else, there is so much inertia to overcome.

Organizational Baggage

Organizations have baggage. Baggage comes in many forms. Some organizations have no history of competence in making significant organizational change. They have never learned how to mobilize the organization's members. They do not know how to handle conflict. They are unsure how to assemble and leverage multidisciplinary teams. They have never mastered staying the course over years during the execution of complex agendas. These organizations are "incompetent," and this incompetence extends well beyond IT, although it clearly includes IT initiatives.

An organization may have tried initiatives "like this" before and failed. The proponents of the initiative may have failed at other initiatives. Organizations have very long memories, and their members may be thinking something like, "The same clowns who brought us that last fiasco are back with an even better idea." The odor from prior failures significantly taints the credibility of newly proposed initiatives and helps to ensure that organizational acceptance will be weak.

Lack of an Appropriate Reward System

Aspects of organizational policies, incentives, and practices can hinder a project. The organization's incentive system may not be structured to reward multidisciplinary behavior—for example, physicians may be rewarded for research prowess or clinical excellence but not for sitting on committees to design new clinical processes. An integrated delivery system may have encouraged its member hospitals to be self-sufficient. As a result, management practices that involve working across hospitals never matured, and the organization does not know how (even if it is willing) to work across hospitals.

Lack of Candor

Organizations can create environments that do not encourage healthy debate. Such environments can result when leadership is intolerant of being challenged or has an inflated sense of its worth and does not believe that it needs team effort to get things done. The lack of a climate that encourages conflict and can manage conflict means that initiative problems will not get resolved. Moreover, organizational members, not having had their voices heard, will tolerate the initiative only out of the hope that they will outlast the initiative and the leadership.

Sometimes the project team is uncomfortable delivering bad news. Project teams will screw up and make mistakes. Sometimes they really screw up and make really big mistakes. Because they may be embarrassed or worried that they will be admonished, they hide the mistakes from the leadership and attempt to fix the problems without "anyone having to know." This attempt to hide bad news is a recipe for disaster. It is unrealistic to expect problems to go unnoticed; invariably the leadership team finds out about the problem and its trust in the project team erodes. At times leadership has to look in the mirror to see if its own intolerance for bad news in effect created the problem.

Project Complexity

Project complexity is determined by many factors:

- The number of people whose work will be changed by the project and the depth of those changes
- The number of organizational processes that will be changed and the depth of those changes
- The number of processes linking the organization and other organizations that will be changed and the depth of those changes
- The interval over which all this change will occur: for example, will it occur quickly or gradually?

If the change is significant in scale, scope, and depth, then it becomes very difficult (often impossible) for the people managing the project to truly understand what the project needs to do. The design will be imperfect. The process changes will not integrate well. And many curves will be thrown the project's way as the implementation unfolds and people realize their mistakes and understand what they failed to understand initially.

Sometimes complex projects disappear in an organizational mushroom cloud. The complexity overwhelms the organization and causes the project to crash suddenly. More common is "death by ants"—no single bite (or project problem) will kill the project, but a thousand will. The organization is overwhelmed by the thousand small problems and inefficiencies and terminates the undertaking.

Managers should remember that complexity is relative. Organizations generally have developed a competency to manage projects up to a certain level and type of complexity. Projects that require competency beyond that level are inherently risky. A project that is risky for one organization may not be risky for another. For example, an organization that typically manages projects that cost $2 million, take ten person-years of effort, and affect 300 people will struggle with a project that costs $20 million and takes one hundred person-years of effort (Cash, McFarlan, & McKenney, 1992).

Failure to Respect Uncertainty

Significant organizational change brings a great deal of uncertainty with it. The leadership may be correct in its understanding of where the organization needs to go and the scope of the changes needed. However, it is highly unlikely that anyone really understands the full impact of the change and how new processes, tasks, and roles will really work. At best, leadership has a good approximation of the new organization. The belief that a particular outcome is certain can be a problem in itself.

Agility and the ability to detect when a change is not working and to alter its direction are very important. Detection requires that the organization listens to the feedback of those who are waist deep in the change, and is able to discern the difference between the organizational noise that comes with any change and the organizational noise that reflects real problems. Altering direction requires that the leadership not cling to ideas that cannot work and also be willing to admit to the organization that it was wrong about some aspects of the change.

Initiative Undernourishment

There may be a temptation, particularly as the leadership tries to accomplish as much as it can with a constrained budget, to tell a project team, "I know you asked for ten people, but we're going to push you to do it with five." The leadership may believe that such bravado will make the team work extra hard and, through heroic efforts, complete the project in a grand fashion. However, bravado may turn out to be bellicose stupidity. This approach may doom a project, despite the valiant efforts of the team to do the impossible.

Another form of undernourishment involves placing staff other than the best staff on the initiative. If the initiative is very important, then it merits using the best staff possible and freeing up their time so they can focus on the initiative. An organization's best staff are always in demand, and there can be a temptation to say that it would be too difficult to pull them away from other pressing issues. They are needed elsewhere and this decision is difficult. However, if the initiative is critical to the organization, then those other demands are less important and can be given to someone else. Critical organizational initiatives should not be staffed with the junior varsity.

Failure to Anticipate Short-Term Disruptions

Any major change will lead to short-term problems and disruptions in operations. Even though current processes can be made better, they are working and staff know how to make them work. When processes are changed, there is a shakeout period as staff adjust and learn how to make the new processes work well. At times, adjusting to the new application system is the core of the disruption. A shakeout can go on for months and degrade organizational performance. Service will deteriorate. Days in accounts receivable will climb. Balls will be dropped in many areas. The organization can misinterpret these problems as a sign that the initiative is failing.

Listening closely to the issues and suggestions of the front line is essential during this time. These staff need to know that their problems are being heard and that their ideas for fixing these problems are being acted upon. People often know exactly what needs to be done to remove system disruptions. Listening to and acting on their advice also improves their buy-in to the change.

While working hard to minimize the duration and depth of disruption, the organization also needs to be tolerant during this period and to appreciate the low-grade form of hell that staff are enduring. It is critical that this period be kept as short and as pain free as possible. If the disruption lasts too long, staff may conclude that the change is not working and abandon their support.

Invisible Progress

Sometimes initiatives are launched with great fanfare. Speeches are made outlining the rationale for the initiative. Teams are formed. Budgets are established. The organization is ready to move. Then nothing seems to be happening.

Large, complex initiatives often involve large amounts of preparatory analysis and work. These initiatives may also involve implementing a significant IT foundation of new networks and databases. And even though the project teams are busy, the rest of the organization sees no progress and comes to believe that the initiative is being held hostage. Action-oriented managers want to know what happened to the action.

Change initiatives and IT projects need to communicate their progress regularly, even when that progress is largely unseen by the organization. In a similar fashion the progress made in digging a new tunnel might be invisible to the motorist until the tunnel is open, but the tunnel diggers can report regularly on the work that is being done underground.

If possible, the project should seek to produce a series of short-term deliverables, even if they are small. For example, while the IT team is performing foundational work, the organization might go ahead and make some process changes without waiting for the implementation of the application. Deliverables demonstrate that progress is being made and help to sustain organizational commitment to the initiative. Organizational commitment is like a slowly leaking balloon; it must be constantly reinflated.

Lack of Technology Stability and Maturity

Information technology may be obviously immature. New technologies are being introduced all the time, and it takes time for them to work through their kinks and achieve an acceptable level of stability, supportability, and maturity. Some forms of social networking are current examples of information technologies that are in their youth.

Organizations can become involved in projects that require immature technology to play a critical role. This clearly elevates the risk of the project. The technology will suffer from performance problems, and the organization's IT staff and the technology supplier may have a limited ability to identify and resolve technology problems. Organizational members, tired of the instability, become tired of the project and it fails.

In general, it is not common, nor should it be often necessary, for a project to hinge on the adequate performance of new technology. A thoughtful assessment that a new technology has potentially extraordinary promise and that the organization can achieve differential value by being an early adopter should precede any such decision. Even in these cases, pilot projects that provide experience with the new technology while limiting the scope of its implementation (which minimizes potential damage) are highly recommended.

The organization should remember that technology maturity is also relative. Even if the rest of the world has used a technology, if it is new to your vendor and new to your IT staff, then it should be considered immature. Your vendor and staff will need to learn, often the hard way, how to manage and support this technology.

Projects can also get into trouble when the amount of technology change is extensive. For example, the organization may be attempting to implement, over a short period of time, applications from several different vendors that involve different operating systems, network requirements, security models, and database management systems. This broad scope can overwhelm the IT department's ability to respond to technology misbehavior.

How to Avoid These Mistakes

Major IT projects fail in many ways. However, a large number of these failures involve management action or inaction. Few management teams and senior leaders start IT projects hoping that failure is the outcome. Summarizing our discussion in this chapter produces a set of recommendations that can help organizations reduce the risk of failure:

- Ensure that the objectives of the IT initiative are clear.
- Communicate the objectives and the initiative, and test the degree to which organizational members have bought into them.
- Publicly demonstrate conviction by "being there" and showing resolve during tough decisions.
- Respect organizational inertia, and keep hammering away at it.
- Distance the project from any organizational baggage, perhaps through a thoughtful choice of project sponsors and managers.
- Change the reward system if necessary to create incentives for participants to work toward project success.
- Accept and welcome the debate that surrounds projects, invite bad news, and do not hang those who make mistakes.
- Address complexity by breaking the project into manageable pieces, and test for evidence that the project might be at risk from trying to do too much all at once.
- Realize that there is much you do not know about how to change the organization or the form of new processes; be prepared to change direction and listen and respond to those who are on the front line.
- Supply resources for the project appropriately, and assign the project to your best team.
- Try to limit the duration and depth of the short-term operational disruption, but accept that it will occur.
- Ensure and communicate regular, visible progress.
- Be wary of new technology and projects that involve a broad scope of information technology change.

These steps, along with solid project management, can dramatically reduce the risk that an IT project will fail. However, these steps are not foolproof. Major IT projects, particularly those accompanied by major organizational change, will always have a nontrivial level of risk.

There will also be times when a review of the failure factors indicates that a project is too risky. The organization may not be ready; there may be too much baggage, too much inertia to overcome; the best team may not be available; the organization may not be good at handling conflict; or the project may require too much new information technology. Projects with considerable risk should not be undertaken until progress has been made in addressing the failure factors. Management of IT project risk is a critical contributor to IT success.

PERSPECTIVE
Critical Success Factors

Jay Toole outlines several critical success factors for successful clinical information system (CIS) implementation and transformation of clinical processes.

- Set realistic and clear expectations for the outcomes that will result from implementing the CIS.
- Recognize that implementing a CIS and transforming care processes is an operational initiative and not an IT initiative.
- Operational executives must take ownership of the implementation and related transformation and must be held accountable for its success.
- Clinicians must actively participate in the CIS design and implementation.
- A liaison person knowledgeable in both IT and medical issues should be designated to keep the physicians engaged in the implementation process.
- A strong project manager with CIS implementation experience needs to be dedicated to the initiative. He or she must have dedicated staff resources with the right mix of clinical, operational and technical expertise.
- A well-defined implementation plan and the ability to monitor and track results against the plan are crucial.
- Incentives must be aligned and these incentives should reward all participants for successful implementation and achievement of predefined outcomes.

Source: Toole, 2003, p. 157.

PERSPECTIVE
IT Project Implementation Checklist

Andrew McAfee has developed a short checklist for managers who are overseeing the implementation of IT projects. This checklist covers critical project management actions necessary to avoid disaster.

- Treat the implementation as a business change effort and not as a technology installation. Project leadership should come from the business side, and the business sponsor should be given the authority to make project decisions and be held accountable for project outcomes.

- Devote the necessary resources to the project. This means putting your best people on the project and avoiding cutting corners on budgets and the use of outside expertise.

- Make sure that goals, scope, and expectations are clear from the outset. Projects get in trouble when they are overhyped, scope is allowed to expand without discipline, and goals are fuzzy.

- Track the project's progress, results, and scope. Sound project management—for example, status reports, milestones, methodical reviews of proposals to change scope, and budget tracking—must be in place.

- Test the new system every way that you can before you go live. Testing and retesting helps minimize unpleasant surprises, technology problems, and poor fit with workflow.

- Secure top management commitment. The leadership must believe in the project—its goals, scope, and the project team. Leadership must also soberly understand the magnitude and difficulty of the undertaking.

Source: Adapted from McAfee, 2003, p. 85.

SUMMARY

The leadership of health care organizations plays an essential role in managing the change that invariably accompanies the implementation of an IT application. This role is particularly important in step-shift, radical, and fundamental change. The leadership must lead, establish a vision, communicate, manage trust, plan the change, implement the change, and iterate as the organization experiences the change.

The hard science of implementation requires the creation of roles such as the business sponsor and project managers, and committees such as the project steering committee and project teams. Solid project management techniques must be in place—for example, project charters and project plans must be created, and project communication must be carried out.

There are many ways that a project failure can occur; unclear objectives, embryonic information technology, or neglecting to anticipate short-term operational disruptions may lead to failure, for example. It is the responsibility of the organization's leadership to minimize the occurrence and severity of factors that threaten to undermine the change.

KEY TERMS

Business owner

Business sponsor

IT initiative failures

IT manager

Managing IT projects

Organizational change

Project charter

Project committees

Project management

Project manager

Project plan

Project roles

Project status report

Project steering committee

Project team

LEARNING ACTIVITIES

1. Attend a project team meeting for each of two different projects. Describe the project and the challenges facing the project teams. Comment on the differences between the teams and the projects.

2. Interview the business sponsor of a major project. Describe the role of this business sponsor. Discuss the scope of the project and its objectives. Describe the change strategy for the project.

3. Interview a project manager. Describe the factors and skills that he or she associates with successful projects.

REFERENCES

Cash, J., McFarlan, W., & McKenney, J. (1992). *Corporate information systems management: The issues facing senior executives.* Burr Ridge, IL: Irwin.

Cook, R. (2007, July 20). How to spot a failing project. *CIO.* Retrieved November 2008 from http://www.cio.com/article/124309/How_to_Spot_a_Failing_Project

Keen, P. (1997). *The process edge.* Boston: Harvard Business School Press.

McAfee, A. (2003). When too much IT knowledge is a dangerous thing. *MIT Sloan Management Review, 44*(2), 83–89.

Spurr, C. (2003). Information systems project management at Partners HealthCare. Internal document, Partners HealthCare.

Toole, J. (2003). The need for transformation. In *Health care technology* (Vol. 1). San Francisco: Montgomery Research.

CHAPTER 17

Assessing and Achieving Value in Health Care Information Systems

LEARNING OBJECTIVES

- To be able to discuss the nature of IT-enabled value.
- To review the components of the IT project proposal.
- To be able to understand steps to improve IT project value realization.
- To be able to discuss why IT investments can fail to deliver returns.
- To review factors that challenge the realization of IT value.

Virtually all the discussion in this book has focused on the knowledge and management processes necessary to achieve one fundamental objective: organizational investments in IT resulting in a desired value. That value might be the furtherance of organizational strategies, improvement in the performance of core processes, or the enhancement of decision making. Achieving value requires the alignment of IT with overall strategies, thoughtful governance, solid information system selection and implementation approaches, and effective organizational change.

Failure to achieve desired value can result in significant problems for the organization. Money is wasted. Execution of strategies is hamstrung. Organizational processes can be damaged.

This chapter carries the IT value discussion further. Specifically, it covers the following topics:

- The definition of IT-enabled value
- The IT project proposal
- Steps to improve value realization
- Why IT fails to deliver returns
- Analyses of the IT value challenge

DEFINITION OF IT-ENABLED VALUE

We can make several observations about IT-enabled value:

- IT value can be both tangible and intangible.
- IT value can be significant.
- IT value can be variable across organizations.
- IT value can be diverse across IT proposals.
- A single IT investment can have a diverse value proposition.
- Different IT investments have different objectives and hence different value propositions and value assessment techniques.

These observations will be discussed in more detail in the following sections.

Both Tangible and Intangible

Tangible value can be measured whereas intangible value is very difficult, perhaps practically impossible, to measure.

Some tangible value can be measured in terms of dollars:

- Increases in revenue.
- Reductions in labor costs: for example, through staff layoffs, overtime reductions, or shifting work to less expensive staff.
- Reductions in supplies needed: for example, paper.
- Reductions in maintenance costs for computer systems.
- Reductions in use of patient care services: for example, fewer lab tests are performed or care is conducted in less expensive settings.

Some tangible value can be measured in terms of process improvements:

- Fewer errors
- Faster turnaround times for test results
- Reductions in elapsed time to get an appointment
- A quicker admissions process
- Improvement in access to data

Some tangible value can be measured in terms of strategically important operational and market outcomes:

- Growth in market share
- Reduction in turnover
- Increase in brand awareness
- Increase in patient and provider satisfaction
- Improvement in reliability of computer systems

In contrast, intangible value can be very difficult to measure. The organization is trying to measure such things as

- Improving in decision making
- Improving in communication
- Improving in compliance
- Improving in collaboration
- Increasing in agility
- Becoming more state of the art

- Improving in organizational competencies—for example, becoming better at managing chronic disease
- Becoming more customer friendly

Significant

IT can be leveraged to achieve significant organization value. Some example studies are cited next.

A study that compared the quality of diabetes care between physician practices that used electronic health records and practices that did not found that the EHR sites had composite standards for diabetes care that were 35.1 percent higher than paper-based sites and had 15 percent better care outcomes (Cebul, Love, Jain, & Herbert, 2011).

EMC (a company that makes data storage devices and other information technologies) reported a reduction of $200 million in health care costs over ten years through the use of data analytics, lifestyle coaches, and remote patient monitoring to help employees manage health risks and chronic diseases (Mosquera, 2011).

A cross-sectional study of hospitals in Texas (Amarasingham, Plantinga, Diener-West, Gaskin, & Powe, 2009) found that higher levels of the automation of notes and patient records were associated with a 15 percent decrease in the adjusted odds of a fatal hospitalization. Higher scores in the use of computerized provider order entry (CPOE) were associated with 9 percent and 55 percent decreases in the adjusted odds of death for myocardial infarction and coronary artery bypass graft procedures, respectively. For all cases of hospitalization, higher levels of clinical decision-support use were associated with a 16 percent decrease in the adjusted odds of complications. And higher levels of CPOE, results reporting, and clinical decision support were associated with lower costs for all hospital admissions.

Variable

Even when they implement the same system, not all organizations experience the same value. As discussed earlier, organizational factors such as change management prowess and governance have a significant impact on an organization's ability to be successful in implementing health information technology.

As an example of variability, two children's hospitals implemented the same electronic health record (including CPOE) in their pediatric intensive care units. One hospital experienced a significant increase in mortality (Han et al., 2005), while the other did not (Del Beccaro, Jeffries, Eisenberg, & Harry, 2006). The hospital that did experience an increase in mortality noted that several implementation factors contributed to the deterioration in quality; specific order sets for critical care were not created, changes in workflow were not well executed, and orders for patients arriving via critical care transportation could not be written before the patient arrived at the hospital, delaying life-saving treatments.

Even when organizations have comparable implementation skill levels, the value achieved can vary because different organizations decide to focus on different objectives. For example, some organizations may decide to improve diabetes care, while others may emphasize the reduction in care costs. Hence, if an outcome is of modest interest to an organization and it devotes few resources to achieving that outcome, it should not be surprised if the outcome does not materialize.

Diverse across Proposals

Consider three proposals (real ones from a large integrated delivery system) that might be in front of organizational leadership for review and approval: a disaster notification system, a document imaging system, and an e-procurement system. Each offers a different type of value to the organization.

The disaster notification system would enable the organization to page critical personnel, inform them that a disaster—for example, a train wreck or biotoxin outbreak—had taken place, and tell them the extent of the disaster and the steps they would need to take to help the organization respond to the disaster. The system would cost $520,000. The value would be "better pre-paredness for a disaster."

The document imaging system would be used to electronically store and retrieve scanned images of paper documents, such as payment reconciliations, received from insurance companies. The system would cost $2.8 million, but would save the organization $1.8 million per year ($9 million over the life of the system) due to reductions in the labor required to look for paper documents and in the insurance claim write-offs that occur because a document cannot be located.

The e-procurement system would enable users to order supplies, ensure that the ordering person had the authority to purchase supplies, transmit the order to the supplier, and track the receipt of the supplies. Data from this system could be used to support the standardization of supplies: that is, to reduce the number of different supplies used. Such standardization might save $500,000 to $3 million per year. The actual savings would depend on physician willingness to standardize. The system would cost $2.5 million.

These proposals reflect a diversity of value, ranging from "better disaster response" to a clear financial return (document imaging) to a return with such a wide potential range (e-procurement) that it could be a great investment (if you really could save $3 million a year) or a terrible investment (if you could save only $500,000 a year).

Diverse in a Single Investment

Picture archiving and communication systems (PACS) are used to store radiology (and other) images, support interpretation of images, and distribute the information to the physician providing direct patient care. These systems are an example of the diversity of value that can result from one IT investment. A PACS can

- Reduce costs for radiology film and the need for film librarians.
- Improve service to the physician delivering care, through improved access to images.
- Improve productivity for the radiologists and for the physicians delivering care (both groups reduce the time they spend looking for images).
- Generate revenue, if the organization uses the PACS to offer radiology services to physician groups in the community.

This one investment has a diverse value proposition; it has the potential to deliver cost reduction, productivity gains, service improvements, and revenue gains.

Different Analyses for Different Objectives

The Committee to Study the Impact of Information Technology on the Performance of Service Activities (1994), organized by the National Research Council, has identified six categories of IT investments in service industries, reflecting different objectives. The techniques used to assess IT investment value should vary by the type of objective that the IT investment intends to support. One technique does not fit all IT investments.

PERSPECTIVE
Four Types of IT Investment

Jeanne Ross and Cynthia Beath studied the IT investment approaches of thirty companies from a wide range of industries. They identified four classes of investment:

- **Transformation.** These IT investments had an impact that would affect the entire organization or a large number of business units. The intent of the investment was to effect a significant improvement in overall performance or change the nature of the organization.
- **Renewal.** Renewal investments were intended to upgrade core IT infrastructure and applications or reduce the costs or improve the quality of IT services. Examples of these investments include application replacements, upgrades of the network, or expansion of data storage.
- **Process improvement.** These IT investments sought to improve the operations of a specific business entity—for example, to reduce costs and improve service.
- **Experiments.** Experiments were designed to evaluate new information technologies and test new types of applications. Given the results of the experiments, the organization would decide whether broad adoption was desirable.

Different organizations will allocate their IT budgets differently across these classes. An office products company had an investment mix of experiments (15 percent), process improvement (40 percent), renewal (25 percent), and transformation (20 percent). An insurance firm had an investment mix of experiments (3 percent), process improvement (25 percent), renewal (18 percent), and transformation (53 percent).

The investment allocation is often an after-the-fact consideration—the allocation is not planned, it just "happens." However, ideally, the organization decides its desired allocation structure and does so before the budget discussions. An organization with an ambitious and perhaps radical strategy may allocate a very large portion of its IT investment to the transformation class, whereas an organization with a conservative, stay-the-course strategy may have a large process improvement portion to its IT investments.

Source: Ross & Beath, 2002, p. 54.

Infrastructure

IT investments may be for infrastructure that enables other investments or applications to be implemented and deliver desired capabilities. Examples of infrastructure are data communication networks, workstations, and clinical data repositories. A delivery system–wide network enables a large organization to implement applications to consolidate clinical laboratories, implement organization-wide collaboration tools, and share patient health data between providers.

It is difficult to quantitatively assess the impact or value of infrastructure investments because

- They enable applications. Without those applications, infrastructure has no value. Hence, infrastructure value is indirect and depends on application value.
- The allocation of infrastructure value across applications is complex. When millions of dollars are invested in a data communication network, it may be difficult or impossible to determine how much of that investment should be allocated to the ability to create delivery system–wide EHRs.
- A good IT infrastructure is often determined by its agility, its potency, and its ability to facilitate integration of applications. It is very difficult to assign return on investment numbers or any meaningful numerical value to most of these characteristics. What, for instance, is the value of being agile enough to speed up the time it takes to develop and enhance applications?

Information system infrastructure is as hard to evaluate as other organizational infrastructure, such as having talented, educated staff. As with other infrastructure,

- Evaluation is often instinctive and experientially based.
- In general, underinvesting can severely limit the organization.
- Investment decisions involve choosing between alternatives that are assessed for their ability to achieve agreed-upon goals. For example, if an organization wishes to improve security, it might ask whether it should invest in network monitoring tools or enhanced virus protection. Which of these investments would enable it to make the most progress toward its goal?

Mandated

Information system investment may be necessary because of mandated initiatives. Mandated initiatives might involve reporting quality data to accrediting organizations, making required changes in billing formats, or improving disaster notification systems. Assessing these initiatives is generally approached by identifying the least expensive and the quickest to implement alternative that will achieve the needed level of compliance.

Cost Reduction

Information system investments directed to cost reduction are generally highly amenable to return-on-investment (ROI) and other quantifiable dollar-impact analyses. The ability to conduct a quantifiable ROI analysis is rarely the question. The ability of management to effect the predicted cost reduction or cost avoidance is often a far more germane question.

Specific New Products and Services

IT can be critical to the development of new products and services. At times the information system delivers the new service, and at other times it is itself the product. Examples of information system–based new services include bank cash-management programs and programs that award airline mileage for credit card purchases. A new service offered by some health care providers is a personal health record that enables a patient to communicate with his or her physician and to access care guidelines and consumer-oriented medical textbooks.

The value of some of these new products and services can be quantifiably assessed in terms of a monetary return. These assessments include analyses of potential new revenue, either directly from the service or from service-induced use of other products and services. A return-on-investment analysis will need to be supplemented by techniques such as sensitivity analyses of consumer response. Despite these analyses, the value of this IT investment usually has a speculative component. This component involves consumer utilization, competitor response, and impact on related businesses.

Quality Improvement

Information system investments are often directed to improving the quality of service or medical care. These investments may be intended to reduce waiting times, improve the ability of physicians to locate information, improve treatment outcomes, or reduce errors in treatment. Evaluation of these initiatives, although quantifiable, is generally done in terms of service parameters that are known or believed to be important determinants of organizational success. These parameters might be measures of aspects of organizational processes that customers encounter and then use to judge the organization—for example, waiting times in the physician's office. A quantifiable dollar outcome for the service of care quality improvement can be very difficult to predict. Service quality is often necessary to protect current business, and the effect of a failure to continuously improve service or medical care can be difficult to project.

Major Strategic Initiative

Strategic initiatives in information technology are intended to significantly change the competitive position of the organization or redefine the core nature of the enterprise. In health care it is rare that information systems are the centerpiece of a redefinition of the organization. However, other industries have attempted IT-centric transformations. Amazon is an effort to transform retailing. Schwab.com is an undertaking intended to redefine the brokerage industry through the use of the web. There can be an ROI core or component to analyses of such initiatives, because they often involve major reshaping or reengineering of fundamental organizational processes. However, assessing the ROIs of these initiatives and their related information systems with a high degree of accuracy can be very difficult. Several factors contribute to this difficulty:

- These major strategic initiatives usually recast the organization's markets and its roles. The outcome of the recasting, although visionary, can be difficult to see with clarity and certainty.
- The recasting is evolutionary; the organization learns and alters itself as it progresses, over what are often lengthy periods of time. It is difficult to be prescriptive about this evolutionary process. Most accountable care organizations are confronting this phenomenon.
- Market and competitor responses can be difficult to predict.

IT value is diverse and complex. This diversity indicates the power of IT and the diversity of its use. Nonetheless, the complexity of the value proposition means that it is difficult to make choices between IT investments and also difficult to assess whether the investment ultimately chosen delivered the desired value or not.

THE IT PROJECT PROPOSAL

The *IT project proposal* is a cornerstone in examining value. Clearly, ensuring that all proposals are well crafted does not ensure value. To achieve value, alignment with organizational strategies must occur, factors for sustained IT excellence must be managed, budget processes for making choices between investments must exist, and projects must be well managed. However, the proposal (as discussed in Chapter Fifteen) does describe the intended outcome of the IT investment. The proposal requests money and an organizational commitment to devote management attention and staff effort to implementing an information system. The proposal describes why this investment of time, effort, and money is worth it—that is, the proposal describes the value that will result.

In Chapter Fifteen we also discussed budget meetings and management forums that might review IT proposals and determine whether a proposal should be accepted. In this section we discuss the value portion of the proposal and some common problems encountered with it.

Sources of Value Information

As project proponents develop their case for an IT investment, they may be unsure of the full gamut of potential value or of the degree to which a desired value can be truly realized. The organization may not have had experience with the proposed application and may have insufficient analyst resources to perform its own assessment. It may not be able to answer such questions as, What types of gains have organizations seen as a result of implementing an electronic health record (EHR) system? To what degree will IT be a major contributor to our efforts to streamline operating room throughput?

Information about potential value can be obtained from several sources (discussed in Appendix A). Conferences often feature presentations that describe the efforts of specific individuals or organizations in accomplishing initiatives of interest to many others. Industry publications may offer relevant articles and analyses. Several industry research organizations—for example, Gartner and the Advisory Board—can offer advice. Consultants can be retained who have worked with clients who are facing or have addressed similar questions. Vendors of applications can describe the outcomes experienced by their customers. And colleagues can be contacted to determine the experiences of their organizations.

Garnering an understanding of the results of others is useful but insufficient. It is worth knowing that Organization Y adopted computerized provider order entry (CPOE) and reduced unnecessary testing by X percent. However, one must also understand the CPOE features that were critical in achieving that result and the management steps taken and the process changes made in concert with the CPOE implementation.

Formal Financial Analysis

Most proposals should be subjected to formal financial analyses regardless of their value proposition. Several types of financial measures are used by organizations. An organization's finance department will work with leadership to determine which measures will be used and how these measures will be compiled.

Two common financial measures are net present value and internal rate of return:

- *Net present value* is calculated by subtracting the initial investment from the future cash flows that result from the investment. The cash can be generated by new revenue or cost savings. The future cash is discounted, or reduced, by a standard rate to reflect the fact that a dollar earned one or more years from now is worth less than a dollar one has today (the rate depends on the time period considered). If the cash generated exceeds the initial investment by a certain amount or percentage, the organization may conclude that the IT investment is a good one.

- *Internal rate of return (IRR)* is the discount rate at which the present value of an investment's future cash flow equals the cost of the investment. Another way to look at this is to ask, Given the amount of the investment and its promised cash, what rate of return am I getting on my investment? On the one hand, a return of 1 percent is not a good return (just as one would not think that a 1 percent return on one's savings was good). On the other hand, a 30 percent return is very good.

Table 17.1 shows the typical form of a financial analysis for an IT application.

Comparing Different Types of Value

Given the diversity of value, it is very challenging to compare IT proposals that have different value propositions. How does one compare a proposal that promises to increase revenue and improve collaboration to one that offers improved compliance, faster turnaround times, and reduced supply costs?

At the end of the day, judgment is used to choose one proposal over another. Health care executives review the various proposals and associated

Table 17.1. Financial analysis of a patient accounting document imaging system

	Current Year	Year 1	Year 2	Year 3	Year 4	Year 5	Year 6	Year 7
COSTS								
One-time capital expense	$1,497,466	$1,302,534						
System operations								
System maintenance	—	288,000	$288,000	$288,000	$288,000	$288,000	$288,000	$288,000
System maintenance	—	152,256	152,256	152,256	152,256	152,256	152,256	152,256
TOTAL COSTS	1,497,466	1,742,790	440,256	440,256	440,256	440,256	440,256	440,256
BENEFITS								
Revenue gains								
Rebilling of small secondary balances	—	651,000	868,000	868,000	868,000	868,000	868,000	868,000
Medicaid billing documentation	—	225,000	300,000	300,000	300,000	300,000	300,000	300,000
Disallowed Medicare bad debt audit	—	—	—	—	100,000	100,000	100,000	100,000
Staff savings								
Projected staff savings	—	36,508	136,040	156,504	169,065	169,065	169,065	171,096
Operating savings								
Projected operating savings	—	64,382	77,015	218,231	222,550	226,436	226,543	229,935
TOTAL BENEFITS	—	976,891	1,381,055	1,542,735	1,659,615	1,663,502	1,663,608	1,669,031
CASH FLOW	(1,497,466)	(765,899)	940,799	1,102,479	1,219,359	1,223,246	1,223,352	1,228,775
CUMULATIVE CASH FLOW	(1,497,466)	(2,263,365)	(1,322,566)	(220,087)	999,272	2,222,517	3,445,869	4,674,644
NPV (12% discount)	1,998,068							
IRR	33%							

value statements and make choices based on their sense of organizational priorities, available monies, and the likelihood that the proposed value will be seen. These judgments can be aided by developing a scoring approach that allows leaders to apply a common metric across proposals. For example, the organization might decide to score each proposal according to how much value it promises to deliver in each of the following areas:

- Revenue impact
- Cost reduction
- Patient or customer satisfaction
- Quality of work life
- Quality of care
- Regulatory compliance
- Potential learning value

In this approach, each of these areas in each proposal is assigned a score, ranging from 5 (significant contribution to the area) to 1 (minimal or no contribution). The scores are then totaled for each proposal, and in theory, one picks those proposals with the highest aggregate scores. In practice, IT investment decisions are rarely that purely algorithmic. However, such scoring can be very helpful in sorting through complex and diverse value propositions:

- Scoring forces the leadership team to discuss why different members of the team assigned different scores—why, for example, did one person assign a score of 2 for the revenue impact of a particular proposal and another person assign a 4? These discussions can clarify people's understandings of proposal objectives and help the team arrive at a consensus on each project.
- Scoring means that the leadership team will have to defend any decision not to fund a project with a high score or to fund one with a low score. In the latter case, team members will have to discuss why they are all in favor of a project when it has such a low score.

The organization can decide which proposal areas to score and which not to score. Some organizations give different areas different weights—for example, reducing costs might be considered twice as important as improving organizational learning. The resulting scores are not binding, but they can be helpful in arriving at a decision about which projects will be approved and what value is being sought. (A form of this scoring process was displayed earlier in Figure 13.2).

PERSPECTIVE
Prerequisites for Effective IT Project Prioritization

Jeanne Ross and Emmett Johnson (2009) identified four prerequisites to effective IT project prioritization.

Explicit Operating Vision of the Business. An operating vision is more than the sum of the operations of individual departments. Rather, it is a solid understanding of how the organization wants to operate as a whole. For example, how will the organization manage patients with a chronic disease? What processes must be in place to ensure a superior patient experience?

Operating visions lead to enterprise-wide requirements for integration and standardization. IT projects should support this vision and conform to these requirements.

Business Process Owners. Process owners are those senior leaders who are responsible for the performance of core organization processes, such as patient access. These owners must sponsor IT initiatives and be held accountable for their successful completion and value delivery. These owners are in a good position to understand the IT priorities of their processes.

Transparent IT Operating Costs. Organizational leadership must understand IT costs and the drivers of those costs. This understanding prepares them to thoughtfully assess the risks and benefits of proposed new systems and to identify alternative approaches to achieving desired process gains.

Rigorous Project Governance. Excellent IT governance must exist for the overall IT agenda (as discussed in Chapter Fifteen) and for individual projects (as discussed in Chapter Sixteen).

Source: Ross & Johnson, 2009.

Tactics for Reducing the Budget

Proposals for IT initiatives may originate from a wide variety of sources in an organization. The IT group will submit proposals, as will department directors and physicians. Many of these proposals will not be directly related to an overall strategy but may nevertheless be "good ideas" that if implemented

Table 17.2. Requests for new information system projects

Community General Hospital

Project Name	Operating Cost
TOTAL	$2,222,704
Clinical portfolio development	38,716
Enterprise monitoring	70,133
HIPAA security initiative	36,950
Accounting of disclosure—HIPAA	35,126
Ambulatory Center patient tracking	62,841
Bar-coding infrastructure	64,670
Capacity management	155,922
Chart tracking	34,876
Clinical data repository	139,902
CRP research facility	7,026
Emergency Department data warehouse	261,584
Emergency Department order entry	182,412
Medication administration system	315,323
Order communications	377,228
Transfusion services replacement system	89,772
Wireless infrastructure	44,886
Next-generation order entry	3,403
Graduate medical education duty hours	163,763

would lead to improved organizational performance. So it is common for an organization to have more proposals than it can fund. For example, during the IT budget discussion, the leadership team may decide that although it is looking at $2.2 million in requests, the organization can afford to spend only $1.7 million, so $500,000 worth of requests must be denied. Table 17.2 presents a sample list of requests.

Reducing the budget in situations like this requires a value discussion. The leadership is declaring some initiatives to have more value than others. Scoring initiatives according to criteria is one approach to addressing this challenge.

In addition to such scoring, other assessment tactics can be employed, prior to the scoring, to assist leaders in making reduction decisions.

- Some requests are mandatory. They may be mandatory because of a regulation requirement (such as a new Medicare Rule) or because a current system is so obsolete that it is in danger of crashing—permanently—and it must be replaced soon. These requests must be funded.

- Some projects can be delayed. They are worthwhile, but a decision on them can be put off until next year. The requester will get by in the meantime.

- Key groups within IT, such as the staff who manage clinical information systems, may already have so much on their plate that they cannot possibly take on another project. Although the organization wants to do the project, it would be ill advised to do so now, and so the project can be deferred to next year.

- The user department proposing the application may not have strong management or may be experiencing some upheaval; hence, implementing a new system at this time would be risky. The project could be denied or delayed until the management issues have been resolved.

- The value proposition or the resource estimates, or both, are shaky. The leadership team does not trust the proposal, so it could be denied or sent back for further analysis. Further analysis means that the proposal will be examined again next year.

- Less expensive ways of addressing the problems cited in the proposal may exist, such as a less expensive application or a non-IT approach. The proposal could be sent back for further analysis.

- The proposal is valuable, and the leadership team would like to move it forward. However, the team may reduce the budget, enabling progress to occur but at a slower pace. This delays realizing the value but ensures that resources are devoted to making progress.

These tactics are routinely employed during budget discussions aimed at trying to get as much value as possible given finite resources.

Common Proposal Problems

During the review of IT investment proposals, organizational leadership might encounter several problems related to the estimates of value and the estimates of the resources needed to obtain the value. If undetected, these problems might lead to a significant overstatement of potential return. An overstatement, obviously, may result in significant organizational unhappiness when the value that people thought they would see never materializes and never could have materialized.

Fractions of Effort

Proposal analyses might indicate that the new IT initiative will save fractions of staff time; for example, that each nurse will spend fifteen minutes less per shift on clerical tasks. To suggest a total value, the proposal might multiply as follows (this example is highly simplified): 200 nurses × 15 minutes saved per 8-hour shift × 250 shifts worked per year = 12,500 hours saved. The math might be correct, and the conclusion that 12,500 hours will become available for doing other work such as direct patient care might also be correct. But the analysis will be incorrect if it then concludes that the organization would thus "save" the salary dollars of six nurses (assuming 2,000 hours worked per year per nurse).

Saving fractions of staff effort does not always lead to salary savings, even when there are large numbers of staff, because there may be no practical way to realize the savings—to, for example, lay off six nurses. If, for example, there are six nurses working each eight-hour shift in a particular nursing unit, the fifteen minutes saved per nurse would lead to a total savings of 1.5 hours per shift. But if one were then to lay off one nurse on a shift, it would reduce the nursing capacity on that shift by eight hours, damaging the unit's ability to deliver care. Saving fractions of staff effort does not lead to salary savings when staff are geographically highly fragmented or when they work in small units or teams. It leads to possible salary savings only when staff work in very large groups and some work of the reduced staff can be redistributed to others.

Reliance on Complex Behavior

Proposals may project with great certainty that people will use systems in specific ways. For example, several organizations expect that consumers will use Internet-based quality report cards to choose their physicians and hospitals. However, few consumers actually rely on such sites. Organizations may expect that nurses will readily adopt systems that help them discharge patients faster. However, nurses often delay entering discharge transactions so that they can grab a moment of peace in an otherwise overwhelmingly busy day.

System use is often not what was anticipated. This is particularly true when the organization has no experience with the relevant class of users or with the introduction of IT into certain types of tasks. The original value projection can be thrown off by the complex behaviors of system users. People do not always behave as we expect or want them to. If user behavior is uncertain, the organization would be wise to pilot an application and learn from this demonstration.

Unwarranted Optimism

Project proponents are often guilty of optimism that reflects a departure from reality. Proponents may be guilty of any of four mistakes:

- They assume that nothing will go wrong with the project.
- They assume that they are in full control of all variables that might affect the project—even, for example, quality of vendor products and organizational politics.
- They believe that they know exactly what changes in work processes will be needed and what system features must be present, when what they really have, at best, are close approximations of what must happen.
- They believe that everyone can give full time to the project and forget that people get sick or have babies and that distracting problems unrelated to the project will occur, such as a sudden deterioration in the organization's fiscal performance, and demand attention.

Decisions based on such optimism eventually result in overruns in project budgets and timetables and compromises in system goals. Overruns and compromises change the value proposition.

Shaky Extrapolations

Projects often achieve gains in the first year of their implementation, and proponents are quick to project that such gains will continue during the remaining life of the project. For example, an organization may see 10 percent of its physicians move from using dictation when developing a progress note to using structured, computer-based templates. The organization may then erroneously extrapolate that each year will see an additional 10 percent shift. In fact the first year might be the only year in which such a gain will occur. The organization has merely convinced the more computer facile physicians to change, and the rest of the physicians have no interest in ever changing.

Underestimating the Effort

Project proposals might count the IT staff effort in the estimates of project costs but not count the time that users and managers will have to devote to the project. A patient care system proposal, for instance, may not include the time that will be spent by dozens of nurses working on system design, developing workflow changes, and attending training. These efforts are real costs. They often lead to the need to hire temporary nurses to provide coverage on the inpatient care units, or they might lead to a reduced patient census because there are fewer nursing hours available for patient care. Such miscounting of effort understates the cost of the project.

Fairy-Tale Savings

IT project proposals may note that the project can reduce the expenses of a department or function, including costs for staff, supplies, and effort devoted to correcting mistakes that occur with paper-based processes. Department managers will swear in project approval forums that such savings are real. However, when asked if they will reduce their budgets to reflect the savings that will occur, these same managers may become significantly less convinced that the savings will result. They may comment that the freed-up staff effort or supplies budgets can be redeployed to other tasks or expenses. The managers may be right that the expenses should be redeployed, and all managers are nervous when asked to reduce their budgets and still do the same amount of work. However, the savings expected have now disappeared.

Failure to Account for Postimplementation Costs

After a system goes live, the costs of the system do not go away. System maintenance contracts are necessary. Hardware upgrades will be required. Staff may be needed to provide enhancements to the application. These support costs may not be as large as the costs of implementation. But they are costs that will be incurred every year, and over the course of several years they can add up to some big numbers. Proposals often fail to adequately account for support costs.

STEPS TO IMPROVE VALUE REALIZATION

Achieving value from IT investments requires management effort. There is no computer genie that descends on the organization once the system is live and waves its wand and—shazzam!—value has occurred. Achieving value is hard work but doable work. Management can take several steps to realize value (Dragoon, 2003; Glaser, 2003a, 2003b). These steps are discussed in the sections that follow.

Make Sure the Homework Was Done

IT investment decisions are often based on proposals that are not resting on solid ground. The proposer has not done the necessary homework, and this elevates the risk of a suboptimal return.

Clearly, the track record of the investment proposer will have a significant influence on the investment decision and on leaders' thinking about whether or not the investment will deliver value. However, regardless of the proposer's track record, an IT proposal should enable the leadership team to respond with a strong yes to each of the following questions:

- Is it clear how the plan advances the organization's strategy?
- Is it clear how care will improve, costs will be reduced, or service will be improved? Are the measures of current performance and expected improvement well researched and realistic? Have the related changes in operations, workflow, and organizational processes been defined?
- Are the senior leaders whose areas are the focus of the IT plan clearly supportive? Could they give the project proposal presentation?
- Are the resource requirements well understood and convincingly presented? Have these requirements been compared to those experienced by other organizations undertaking similar initiatives?
- Have the investment risks been identified, and is there an approach to addressing these risks?
- Do we have the right people assigned to the project, have we freed up their time, and are they well organized?

Answering with a no, a maybe, or an equivocal yes to any of these questions should lead one to believe that the discussion is perhaps focusing on an expense rather than an investment.

Require Formal Project Proposals

It is a fact of organizational life that projects are approved as a result of hallway conversations or discussions on the golf course. Organizational life is a political life. While recognizing this reality, the organization should require that every IT project be written up in the format of a proposal and that each proposal should be reviewed and subjected to scrutiny before the organization will commit to supporting it. However, an organization may also decide that small projects—for example, those that involve less than $25,000 in costs and less than 120 person-hours—can be handled more informally.

Increase Accountability for Investment Results

Few meaningful organizational initiatives are accomplished without establishing appropriate accountability for results. Accountability for IT investment results can be improved by taking three major steps.

First, the business owner of the IT investment should defend the investment—for example, the director of clinical laboratories should defend the request for a new laboratory system and the director of nursing should defend the need for a new nursing system. The IT staff will need to work with the business owner to define IT costs, establish likely implementation time frames, and sort through application alternatives. The IT staff should never defend an application investment.

Second, as was discussed in Chapter Sixteen, project sponsors and business owners must be defined, and they must understand the accountability that they now have for the successful completion of the project.

Third, the presentation of these projects should occur in a forum that routinely reviews such requests. Seeing many proposals, and their results, over the course of time will enable the forum participants to develop a seasoned understanding of good versus not-so-good proposals. Forum members are also able to compare and contrast proposals as they decide which ones should be approved. A manager might wonder (and it's a good question), "If I approve this proposal, does that mean that we won't have resources for another project that I might like even better?" Examining as many proposals together as possible enables the organization to take a portfolio view of its potential investments.

Figure 17.1 displays an example of a project investment portfolio represented graphically. The size of each bubble reflects the magnitude of a

Figure 17.1. IT investment portfolio

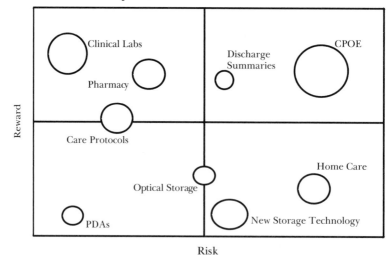

Source: Adapted from Arlotto & Oakes, 2003.

particular IT investment. The axes are labeled "reward" (the size of the expected value) and "risk" (the relative risk that the project will not deliver the value). Other axes may be used. One commonly used set of axes consists of "support of operations" and "support of strategic initiatives."

Diagrams such as the one in Figure 17.1 serve several functions:

- They summarize IT activity on one piece of paper, allowing leaders to consider a new request in the context of prior commitments.
- They help to ensure a balanced portfolio, promptly revealing imbalances such as a clustering of projects in the high-risk quadrant.
- They help to ensure that the approved projects cover an appropriate spectrum of organizational needs—for example, that projects are directed to revenue cycle improvement, to operational improvement, and to patient safety.

PERSPECTIVE
Types of Portfolio Investments

Peter Weill and Sinan Aral (2006) note that organizations should manage their IT investments as a portfolio. Specifically they describe four types of IT investments in a portfolio.

Infrastructure. Infrastructure refers to the core information technology that serves as the foundation for all applications. Examples of infrastructure include networks, servers, operating systems, and mobile devices.

Transactional. Transactional systems are those applications that support the core operations processes. Examples of transactional systems include CPOE, scheduling, clinical laboratory automation, and clinician documentation.

Informational. Informational IT assets are those that support decision making such as clinical decision support, quality measurement and analyses, market assessment, and budget performance.

Strategic. Strategic investments are IT systems that are critical to the furthering of an organization's strategy. These investments could be infrastructure, transactional, and informational, but they differ in that they are clearly directed to furthering a strategic initiative as distinct from being helpful to support ongoing operations.

(cont.)

Weill and Aral note that different industries have different allocations of IT investments across these categories. Financial services emphasize infrastructure in an effort to ensure high reliability and low costs. On the other hand, retail has emphasized informational as they seek to understand customer buying patterns.

Source: Weill & Aral, 2006.

Conduct Postimplementation Audits

Rarely do organizations revisit their IT investments to determine if the promised value was actually achieved. They tend to believe that once the implementation is over and the change settles in, value will have been automatically achieved. This is unlikely.

Postimplementation audits can be conducted to identify value achievement progress and the steps still needed to achieve maximum gain. An organization might decide to audit two to four systems each year, selecting systems that have been live for at least six months. During the course of the audit meeting, these five questions can be asked:

1. What goals were expected at the time the project investment was approved?
2. How close have we come to achieving those original goals?
3. What do we need to do to close the goal gap?
4. How much have we invested in system implementation, and how does that compare to our original budget?
5. If we had to implement this system again, what would we do differently?

Postimplementation audits assist value achievement by

- Signaling leadership interest in ensuring the delivery of results
- Identifying steps that still need to be taken to ensure value
- Supporting organizational learning about IT value realization
- Reinforcing accountability for results

Celebrate Value Achievement

Business value should be celebrated. Organizations usually hold parties shortly after applications go live. These parties are appropriate; a lot of people worked very hard to get the system up and running and used. However, up and running and used does not mean that value has been delivered. In addition to go-live parties, organizations should consider business value parties; celebrations conducted once the value has been achieved—for example, a party that celebrates the achievement of service improvement goals. Go-live parties alone risk sending the inappropriate signal that implementation is the end point of the IT initiative. Value delivery is the end point.

Leverage Organizational Governance

The creation of an IT committee of the board of directors can enhance organizational efforts to achieve value from IT investments. At times the leadership team of an organization is uncomfortable with some or all of the IT conversation. Board members may not understand why infrastructure is so expensive or why large implementations can take so long and cost so much. They may feel uncomfortable with the complexity of determining the likely value to be obtained from IT investments. The creation of a subcommittee made up of the board members most experienced with such discussions can help to ensure that hard questions are being asked and that the answers are sound.

Shorten the Deliverables Cycle

When possible, projects should have short deliverable cycles. In other words, rather than asking the organization to wait twelve or eighteen months to see the first fruits of its application implementation labors, make an effort to deliver a sequence of smaller implementations. For example, one might conduct pilots of an application in a subset of the organization, followed by a staged rollout. Or one might plan for serial implementation of the first 25 percent of the application features.

Pilots, staged rollouts, and serial implementations are not always doable. Where they are possible, however, they enable the organization to achieve some value earlier rather than later, support organizational learning about which system capabilities are really important and which were only thought to be important, facilitate the development of reengineered operational processes, and create the appearance (whose importance is not to be underestimated) of more value delivery.

Benchmark Value

Organizations should benchmark their performance in achieving value against the performance of their peers. These benchmarks might focus on process performance—for example, days in accounts receivable or average time to get an appointment. An important aspect of value benchmarking is the identification of the critical IT application capabilities and related operational changes that enabled the achievement of superior results. This understanding of how other organizations achieved superior IT-enabled performance can guide an organization's efforts to continuously achieve as much value as possible from its IT investments.

Communicate Value

Once a year the information technology department should develop a communication plan for the twelve months ahead. This plan should indicate which presentations will be made in which forums and how often IT-centric columns will appear in organizational newsletters. The plan should list three or so major themes—for example, specific regional integration strategies or efforts to improve IT service—that will be the focus of these communications. Communication plans try to remedy the fact that even when value is being delivered, most people in the organization may not be fully aware of it.

WHY IT FAILS TO DELIVER RETURNS

It is not uncommon to hear leaders of health care organizations complain about the lack of value obtained from IT investments. These leaders may see IT as a necessary expense that must be tightly controlled rather than as an investment that can be a true enabler. New health care managers often walk into organizations where the leadership mind-set features this set of conclusions:

> **The magnitude of the organization's IT operating and capital budgets is large.** IT operating costs may consume 3 percent of the total operating budget, and IT capital may claim 15 to 30 percent of all capital. Although 3 percent may appear small, it can be the difference between a negative operating margin and a positive margin. A 15 to 30 percent IT consumption of capital invariably means that funding for biomedical equipment (which can mean new revenue) and buildings (which can help the organization appear patient and staff friendly and can support the growth of clinical services) is diminished. IT can be seen as taking money away from "worthwhile initiatives."

The projected growth in IT budgets exceeds the growth in other budget categories. Provider organizations may permit overall operating budgets to increase at a rate close to the inflation rate (recently 3 to 4 percent). However, expenditures on IT often experience growth rates of 10 to 15 percent. At some point an organization will note that the IT budget growth rate may single-handedly lead to insolvency.

Regardless of the amount spent, some members of the leadership team feel that not enough is being spent. Worthwhile proposals go unfunded every year. Infrastructure replacement and upgrades seem never ending: "I thought we upgraded our network two years ago. Are you back already?"

It is difficult to evaluate IT capital requests. At times this difficulty is a reflection of a poorly written or fatuous proposal. However, it can be genuinely difficult to compare a proposal directed at improving service to one directed at improving care quality to one directed at increasing revenue to one needed to achieve some level of regulatory compliance.

When asked to "list three instances over the last five years where IT investments have resulted in clear and unarguable returns to the organization," leaders may return blank stares. However, the conversation may be difficult to stop when they are asked to "list three major IT investment disappointments that have occurred over the last five years."

If the value from information technology can be significant, why does one hear these management concerns? There are several reasons why IT investments become simply IT expenses. The organization

- Fails to clearly link IT investments and organizational strategy.
- Asks the wrong question.
- Conducts the wrong analysis.
- Does not state its investment goals.
- Does not manage outcomes.
- Leaps to an inappropriate solution.
- Mangles the project management.
- Fails to learn from studies of IT effectiveness.

Failing to Clearly Link IT Investments and Organizational Strategy

The linkage between IT investments and the organization's strategy was discussed in Chapter Thirteen. When strategies and investments are not aligned, the IT department, even if it is executing well, may be working on the wrong things or trying to support a flawed overall organizational strategy.

Linkage failures can occur because

- The organizational strategy is no more than a slogan or a buzzword with the depth of a bumper sticker, making any investment toward achieving it ill considered.

- The IT department thinks it understands the strategy but it does not, resulting in implementation of the IT version of the strategy rather than the organization's version.

- The strategists (for a variety of reasons) will not engage in the IT discussion, forcing IT leaders to be mind readers.

- The linkage is superficial: for example, "Patient care systems can reduce nursing labor costs but we haven't thought through how that will happen."

- The IT strategy conversation is separated from the organizational strategy conversation, perhaps as a result of the creation of an information systems steering committee, reducing the likelihood of alignment.

- The organizational strategy evolves faster than IT can respond.

Asking the Wrong Question

Rarely should one ask the question, What is the ROI of a computer system? This makes as much sense as asking, What is the ROI of a chain saw? If one wants to make a dress, a chain saw is a waste of money. If one wants to cut down some trees, one can begin to think about the return on a chain saw investment. One will want to compare that investment to other investments, such as an investment in an ax. One will also want to consider the user. If the chain saw is to be used by a ten-year-old child, the investment might be ill advised. If the chain saw is to be used by a skilled lumberjack, the investment might be worth it.

An organization can determine the ROI of an investment in a tool only if it knows the task to be performed and the skill level of the participants who are to perform the task. Moreover, a positive ROI is not an inherent property of an IT investment. The organization has to manage a return into existence.

Hence, instead of asking, What is the ROI of a computer system? organizational leaders should ask questions such as these:

- What are the steps and investments, including IT steps and investments, that we need to take or make in order to achieve our goals?
- Which business manager owns the achievement of these goals? Does this person have our confidence?
- Do the cost, risk, and time frame associated with implementing this set of investments, including the IT investment, seem appropriate given our goals?
- Have we assessed the trade-offs and opportunity costs?
- Are we comfortable with our ability to execute?

Conducting the Wrong Analysis

There are times when determining ROI is the appropriate investment analysis technique. If a set of investments is intended to reduce clerical staff, an ROI can be calculated. However, there are times when an ROI calculation is clearly inappropriate. What is the ROI of software that supports collaboration? One could calculate the ROI, but it is hard to imagine an organization basing its investment decision on that analysis. Would an ROI analysis have captured the strategic value of the Amazon.com system or the value of social networking sites? Few strategic IT investments have impacts that are fully captured by an ROI analysis. Moreover, strategic impact is rarely fully understood until years after implementation. Whatever ROI analysis might have been done would have invariably been wrong.

As discussed earlier, the objective of the IT investment points to the appropriate approach to the analysis of its return. Sometimes organizations apply financial techniques such as internal rate of return in a manner that is overzealous and ignores other analysis approaches. This misapplication of technique can clearly lead to highly worthwhile initiatives being deemed unworthy of funding.

Not Stating Investment Goals

Statements about the positive contributions the investment will make to organizational performance often accompany IT proposals. Statements about specific numerical goals for this improvement are less common. If the investment is intended to reduce medical errors, will it reduce errors by 50 percent or 80 percent or some other number? If it is intended to reduce claim denials, will it reduce them to 5 percent or 2 percent, and how much revenue will be realized as a result of this reduction?

Failure to be numerically explicit about goals can create three fundamental value problems:

- The organization may not know how well it performs now. If the current error rate or denial rate is not known, it is hard to believe that the leadership has studied the problem well enough to be fairly sure that an IT investment will achieve the desired gains. The IT proposal sounds more like a guess about what is needed.

- The organization may never know whether it got the desired value or not. If the proposal does not state a goal, the organization will never know whether the 20 percent reduction in errors it has achieved is as far as it can go or whether it is only halfway to its desired goal. It does not know whether it should continue to work on the error problem or whether it should move on to the next performance issue.

- It will be difficult to hold someone accountable for performance improvement when the organization is unable to track how well he or she is doing.

Not Managing Outcomes

Related to the failure to state goals is the failure to manage outcomes into existence. Once the project is approved and the system is up, management goes off to the next challenge, seemingly unaware that the work of value realization has just begun.

Figure 17.2 depicts a reduction in days in accounts receivable (AR) at a Partners HealthCare physician practice. During the interval depicted, a new practice management system was implemented. The practice did not see a precipitous decline in days in AR (a sign of improved revenue performance) in the time immediately following the implementation in the second quarter of 1997. The practice did see a progressive improvement in days in AR because someone was managing that improvement.

If the gain in revenue performance had been an "automatic" result of the information system implementation, the practice would have seen a sharp drop in days in AR. Instead it saw a gradual improvement over time. This gradual change reflects that

Figure 17.2. Days in accounts receivable before and after implementation of practice management system

- The gain occurred through day-in, day-out changes in operational processes, fine-tuning of system capabilities, and follow-ups in staff training.
- A person had to be in charge of obtaining this improvement. Someone had to identify and make operational changes, manage changes in system capabilities, and ensure that needed training occurred.

Leaping to an Inappropriate Solution

At times the IT discussion of a new application succumbs to advanced states of technical arousal. Project participants become overwhelmed by the prospect of using sexy new technology and state-of-the-art gizmos and lose their senses and understanding of why they are having this discussion in the first place. Sexiness and state-of-the-art-ness become the criteria for making system decisions.

In addition, the comparison of two alternative vendor products can turn into a features war. The discussion may focus on the number of features as a way of distinguishing products and fail to ask whether this numerical difference has any real impact on the value that is desired.

Both sexiness and features have their place in the system selection decision. However, they are secondary to the discussion that centers on the capabilities needed to effect specific performance goals. Sexiness and features may be irrelevant to the performance improvement discussion.

Mangling the Project Management

One guaranteed way to reduce value is to mangle the management of the implementation project. Implementation failures or significant budget and timetable overruns or really unhappy users—any of these can dilute value.

Among the many factors that can lead to mangled project management are these:

- The project's scope is poorly defined.
- The accountability is unclear.
- The project participants are marginally skilled.
- The magnitude of the task is underestimated.
- Users feel like victims rather than participants.
- All the world has a vote and can vote at any time.

Many of these factors were discussed in Chapters Seven and Sixteen.

Failing to Learn from Studies of IT Effectiveness

Organizations may fail to invest in the IT abilities discussed in Chapter Fifteen, such as good relationships between the IT function and the rest of the organization and a well-architected infrastructure. This investment failure increases the likelihood that the percentage of projects that fail to deliver value will be higher than it should be.

ANALYSES OF THE IT VALUE CHALLENGE

The IT investment and value challenge plagues all industries. It is not a problem peculiar to health care. The challenge has been with us for fifty years, ever since organizations began to spend money on big mainframes. This challenge is complex and persistent, and we should not believe we can fully solve it. We should believe we can be better at dealing with it. This section highlights the conclusions of several studies and articles that have examined this challenge.

Factors That Hinder Value Return

The Committee to Study the Impact of Information Technology on the Performance of Service Activities (1994) found these major contributors to failures to achieve a solid return on IT investments:

- The organization's overall strategy is wrong, or its assessment of its competitive environment is inadequate.

- The strategy is fine, but the necessary IT applications and infrastructure are not defined appropriately. The information system, if it is solving a problem, is solving the wrong problem.

- The organization fails to identify and draw together well all the investments and initiatives necessary to carry out its plans. The IT investment then falters because other changes, such as reorganization or reengineering, fail to occur.

- The organization fails to execute the IT plan well. Poor planning or less than stellar management can diminish the return from any investment.

Value may also be diluted by factors outside the organization's control. Weill and Broadbent (1998) noted that the more strategic the IT investment, the more its value can be diluted. An IT investment directed to increasing market share may have its value diluted by non-IT decisions and events—for example, pricing decisions, competitors' actions, and customers' reactions. IT investments that are less strategic but have business value—for example, improving nursing productivity—may be diluted by outside factors—for example, shortages of nursing staff. And the value of an IT investment directed toward improving infrastructure characteristics may be diluted by outside factors—for example, unanticipated technology immaturity or business difficulties confronting a vendor.

The Investment-Performance Relationship

A study by Strassmann (1990) examined the relationship between IT expenditures and organizational effectiveness. Data from an *Information Week* survey of the top one hundred users of information technology were used to correlate IT expenditures per employee with profits per employee. Strassmann concluded that there is no overall obvious direct relationship between expenditure and organizational performance. This finding has been observed in several other studies (for example, Keen, 1997). It leads to several conclusions:

- Spending more on IT is no guarantee that the organization will be better off. There has never been a direct correlation between spending and outcomes. Paying more for care does not give one correspondingly better care. Clearly, one can spend so little that nothing effective can be done. And one can spend so much that waste is guaranteed. But moving IT expenditures from 2 percent of the operating budget to

3 percent of the operating budget does not inherently lead to a 50 percent increase in desirable outcomes.

- Information technology is a tool, and its utility as a tool is largely determined by the tool user and his or her task. Spending a large amount of money on a chain saw for someone who doesn't know how to use one is a waste. Spending more money on tools for the casual saw user who trims an apple tree every now and then is also a waste. However, skilled loggers might say that if a chain saw blade were longer and the saw's engine more powerful, they would be able to cut 10 percent more trees in a given period of time. The investment needed to enhance the loggers' saws might lead to superior performance. Organizational effectiveness in applying IT has an enormous effect on the likelihood of a useful outcome from increased IT investment.

- Factors other than the appropriateness of the tool to the task also influence the relationship between IT investment and organizational performance. These factors include the nature of the work (for example, IT is likely to have a greater impact on bank performance than on consulting firm performance), the basis of competition in an industry (for example, cost per unit of manufactured output versus prowess in marketing), and an organization's relative competitive position in the market.

The Value of the Overall Investment

Many analyses and academic studies have been directed to answering this broad question: How can an organization assess the value of its overall investments in IT? Assessing the value of the aggregate IT investment is different from assessing the value of a single initiative or other specific investment. And it is also different from assessing the caliber of the IT department. Developing a definitive, accurate, and well-accepted way to answer this question has so far eluded all industries and may continue to be elusive. Nonetheless there are some basic questions that can be asked in pursuit of answering the larger question. Interpreting the answers to these basic questions is a subjective exercise, making it difficult to derive numerical scores. Bresnahan (1998) suggests five questions:

1. How does IT influence the customer experience?

2. Do patients and physicians, for example, find that organizational processes are more efficient, less error prone, and more convenient?

3. Does IT enable or retard growth? Can the IT organization support effectively the demands of a merger? Can IT support the creation of

clinical product lines—for example, cardiology—across the integrated delivery system?

4. Does IT favorably affect productivity?

5. Does IT advance organizational innovation and learning?

IT as a Commodity

Carr (2003) has equated IT with commodities—soybeans, for example. Carr's argument is that core information technologies, such as fast, inexpensive processors and storage, are readily available to all organizations and hence cannot provide a competitive advantage. Organizations can no more achieve value from IT than an automobile manufacturer can achieve value by buying better steel than a competitor does or a grocer can achieve value by stocking better sugar than a competitor does. In this view, IT, steel, and sugar are all commodities.

Responding to Carr's argument, Brown and Hagel (2003) make three observations about IT value:

1. "Extracting value from IT requires innovation in business practices." (p. 110) If an organization merely computerizes existing processes without rectifying (or at times eliminating) process problems, it may have merely made process problems occur faster. In addition, those processes are now more expensive because there is a computer system to support. Providing appointment scheduling systems may not make waiting times any shorter or enhance patients' ability to get an appointment when they need one.

   All IT initiatives should be accompanied by efforts to materially improve the processes that the system is designed to support. IT often enables the organization to think differently about a process or expand its options for improving a process. If the process thinking is narrow or unimaginative, the value that could have been achieved will have been lost, with the organization settling for an expensive way to achieve minimal gain. For example, if Amazon had thought that the Internet enabled it to simply replace the catalogue and telephone as a way of ordering something, it would have missed ideas such as presenting products to the customer based on data about prior orders or enabling customers to leave their own ratings of books and music.

2. "IT's economic impact comes from incremental innovations rather than from 'big bang' initiatives." (p. 110) Organizations will often introduce very large computer systems and process change "all at

once." Two examples of such big bangs are the replacement of all systems related to the revenue cycle and the introduction of a new patient care system over the course of a few weeks.

Big bang implementations are very tricky and highly risky. They may be haunted by series of technical problems. Moreover, these systems introduce an enormous number of process changes affecting many people. It is exceptionally difficult to understand the ramifications of such change during the analysis and design stages that precede implementation. A full understanding is impossible. As a result, the implementing organization risks material damage. This damage destroys value. It may set the organization back, and even if the organization grinds its way through the disruption, the resulting trauma may make the organization unwilling to engage in future ambitious IT initiatives.

In contrast, IT implementations (and related process changes) that are more incremental and iterative reduce the risk of organizational damage and permit the organization to learn. The organization has time to understand the value impact of phase n and then can alter its course before it embarks upon phase $n + 1$. Moreover, incremental change leads the organization's members to understand that change, and realizing value, are never-ending aspects of organizational life rather than things to be endured every couple of years.

3. "The strategic impact of IT investments comes from the cumulative effect of sustained initiatives to innovate business practices in the near term." (p. 111) If economic value is derived from a series of thoughtful, incremental steps, then the aggregate effect of those steps should be a competitive advantage. Most of the time, organizations that wind up dominating an industry do so through incremental movement over the course of several years (Collins, 2001). This observation is consistent with our view in Chapter Fourteen. Persistent innovation by a talented team, over the course of years, will result in significant strategic gains. The organization has learned how to improve itself, year in and year out. Strategic value is a marathon. It is a long race that is run and won one mile at a time.

SUMMARY

IT value is complex, multifaceted, and diverse across and within proposed initiatives. The techniques used to analyze value must vary with the nature of the value.

The project proposal is the core means for assessing the potential value of an IT initiative. IT proposals have a commonly accepted structure. And approaches exist for comparing proposals with different types of value propositions. Project proposals often present problems in the way they estimate value—for example, they may unrealistically combine fractions of effort saved, fail to appreciate the complex behavior of system users, or underestimate the full costs of the project.

Many factors can dilute the value realized from an IT investment. Poor linkage between the IT agenda and the organizational strategy, the failure to set goals, and the failure to manage the realization of value all contribute to dilution.

There are steps that can be taken to improve the achievement of IT value. Leadership can ensure that project proponents have done their homework, that accountability for results has been established, that formal proposals are used, and that postimplementation audits are conducted. Even though there are many approaches and factors that can enhance the realization of IT-enabled value, the challenges of achieving this value will remain a management issue for the foreseeable future.

Health care organization leaders often feel ill equipped to address the IT investment and value challenge. However, no new management techniques are required to evaluate IT plans, proposals, and progress. Leadership teams are often asked to make decisions that involve strategic hunches (such as a belief that developing a continuum of care would be of value) about areas where they may have limited domain knowledge (new surgical modalities) and where the value is fuzzy (improved morale). Organizational leaders should treat IT investments just as they would treat other types of investments; if they don't understand, believe, or trust the proposal, or its proponent, they shouldn't approve it.

KEY TERMS

Failure to deliver returns
IT project proposals

IT value
Value realization

LEARNING ACTIVITIES

1. Interview the CIO of a local health care provider or payer. Discuss how his or her organization assesses the value of IT investments and ensures that the value is delivered.

2. Select two articles from a health care IT trade journal that describe the value an organization received from its IT investments. Critique and compare the articles.

3. Select two examples of intangible value. Propose one or more approaches that an organization might use to measure each of those values.

4. Prepare a defense of the value of a significant investment in an electronic health record system.

REFERENCES

Amarasingham, R., Plantinga, L., Diener-West, M., Gaskin, D. J., & Powe, N. R. (2009). Clinical information technologies and inpatient outcomes. *Archives of Internal Medicine, 169*(2), 108–114.

Arlotto, P., & Oakes, J. (2003). *Return on investment: Maximizing the value of healthcare information technology.* Chicago: Healthcare Information and Management Systems Society.

Bresnahan, J. (1998, July 15). What good is technology? *CIO Enterprise,* pp. 25–26, 28, 30.

Brown, J., & Hagel, J. (2003). Does IT matter? *Harvard Business Review, 81,* 109–112.

Carr, N. (2003). IT doesn't matter. *Harvard Business Review, 81,* 41–49.

Cebul, R. D., Love, T. E., Jain, A. K., & Herbert, C. J. (2011). Electronic health records and the quality of diabetes care. *New England Journal of Medicine, 365,* 825–833.

Collins, J. (2001). *Good to great.* New York: HarperCollins.

Committee to Study the Impact of Information Technology on the Performance of Service Activities. (1994). *Information technology in the service society.* Washington, DC: National Academies Press.

Del Beccaro, M. A., Jeffries, H. E., Eisenberg, M. A., & Harry, E. D. (2006). Computerized provider order entry implementation: No association with increased mortality rates in an intensive care unit. *Pediatrics, 118*(1), 290–295.

Dragoon, A. (2003, August 15). Deciding factors. *CIO,* pp. 49–59.

Glaser, J. (2003a, March). Analyzing information technology value. *Healthcare Financial Management,* pp. 98–104.

Glaser, J. (2003b, September). When IT excellence goes the distance. *Healthcare Financial Management,* pp. 102–106.

Han, Y. Y., Carcillo, J. A., Venkataraman, S. T., Clark, R.S.B., Watson, R. S., Nguyen, T. C., Bayir, H., & Orr, R. A. (2005). Unexpected increased mortality after implementation of a commercially sold computerized physician order entry system. *Pediatrics, 116*(6), 1506–1512.

Keen, P. (1997). *The process edge*. Boston: Harvard Business School Press.

Mosquera, M. (2011). How PHRs boosted shareholder value at EMC. Government Health IT. Retrieved August 2011 from http://govhealthit.com/news/some -employers-say-phrs-cut-healthcare-costs

Ross, J., & Beath, C. (2002). Beyond the business case: New approaches to IT investment. *MIT Sloan Management Review, 43*(2), 51–59.

Ross, J. W., & Johnson, E. (2009). Prioritizing IT investments. *Research Briefing, Vol. IX*(3). Cambridge, MA: MIT Center for Information Systems Research.

Strassmann, P. (1990). *The business value of computers*. New Canaan, CT: Information Economics Press.

Weill, P., & Aral, S. (2006). Generating premium returns on your IT investments. *MIT Sloan Management Review, 47*(2), 54–60.

Weill, P., & Broadbent, M. (1998). *Leveraging the new infrastructure*. Boston: Harvard Business School Press.

CHAPTER 18

Health IT Leadership
A Compendium of Case Studies

Faculty and others who teach health administration students are often in search of case studies that can be used to help students apply theory and concepts to real-life IT management situations, encourage problem solving and critical thinking, and foster discussion and collaboration among students. This chapter provides a compendium of case studies from a variety of health care organizations and settings. It is intended to serve as a supplement to the preceding chapters and as a resource to faculty and students. Many of these case studies were originally written by working health care executives enrolled as students in the doctoral program in health administration offered at the Medical University of South Carolina. We wish to acknowledge and thank these students for allowing us to share their stories and experiences with you:

Penney Burlingame	Randall Jones
Barbara Chelton	Catrin Jones-Nazar
Stuart Fine	Ronald Kintz
David Freed	George Mikatarian
David Gehant	Michael Moran
Patricia Givens	Lorie Shoemaker
Victoria Harkins	Gary Wilde

Each case begins with background information that includes a description of the setting, the current information system (IS) challenge facing the organization, and the factors that are felt to have contributed to the current situation. (All real names and identifying information have been changed from the original cases to protect the identity of the individuals and organizations involved.) Following each case is a set of recommended discussion questions. To the extent possible, the cases are organized by major theme, such as strategic IS planning, system acquisition, and system implementation. (See Table 18.1.)

We hope you find the cases thought-provoking and useful in applying the concepts covered in this book to what is happening in health care organizations throughout our nation. We have also included at the end of the chapter a listing of other published cases that may be useful to you and your students.

Table 18.1. List of cases and major themes

Title of Case	Major Theme(s)
Case 1: Board Support for a Capital Project	Strategic planning and IT alignment; IT governance
Case 2: The Decision to Develop an IT Strategic Plan	Strategic planning and IT alignment
Case 3: Selection of a Patient Safety Strategy	Strategic planning and IT alignment

Table 18.1. (*Continued*)

Title of Case	Major Theme(s)
Case 4: Strategic IS Planning for the Hospital ED	Strategic planning and IT alignment
Case 5: Planning an EHR Implementation	IT strategy; system implementation
Case 6: Implementing a Capacity Management Information System	System acquisition
Case 7: Implementing a Telemedicine Solution	System acquisition; use of emerging technologies
Case 8: Replacing a Practice Management System	IT governance; system implementation
Case 9: Conversion to an EHR Messaging System	System implementation; project management
Case 10: Concerns and Workarounds with a Clinical Documentation System	System implementation; project management
Case 11: Strategies for Implementing CPOE	System implementation; project management
Case 12: Implementing a Syndromic Surveillance System	IT strategy; system implementation
Case 13: The Admitting System Crashes	Disaster recovery
Case 14: Breaching the Security of an Internet Patient Portal	IT security
Case 15: Assessing the Value and Impact of CPOE	Assessing the value of an HIT investment
Case 16: Selecting an EHR for Dermatology Practice	System acquisition
Case 17: Watson's Ambulatory EHR Transition	System acquisition
Case 18: Assessing the Value of Health IT Investment	Value assessment

CASE 1: BOARD SUPPORT FOR A CAPITAL PROJECT

Major themes: strategic planning and IT alignment; IT governance

Background Information

Lakeland Medical Center is a 210-bed public hospital located in the Southeast. It is governed by a politically appointed nine-member board and serves a market of approximately 100,000 people. The hospital has been financially successful, but in recent years several capital investments have not brought high returns. As a result, project investment decisions became more conservative and oriented toward financial returns. Competitive forces have continued to grow in the market, and significant internal expense items (such as the organization's pension program, paid leave bank, and health insurance program) have put strains on Lakeland's financial resources.

Revenue continues to grow at an average rate of about 10 percent each year, but controlling expenses remains a challenge. Bad debt has grown from $5 million last year to a budgeted amount of $14 million this year. The hospital continues to accomplish high patient and employee satisfaction scores, high quality scores, and an A+ credit rating. Debt is approximately $55 million, and cash reserves are approximately $95 million. Total operating revenues are approximately $130 million. The hospital employs 940 staff members. The average length of stay is 4.3 days. Annual capital expenditure is $4 million.

Information Systems Challenge

In 2008, the installation of computed radiography (CR) components to build a picture archiving and communication system (PACS) began, at an estimated total cost of $1 million. In 2009, $400,000 was spent for additional CR components. But in 2010, the board of directors (with three new members) did not approve the request of $1.9 million for completion of the PACS, saying that it represented far too large a percentage of the organization's annual capital budget. A year later Lakeland is still in need of completing the PACS program, with a board that is unlikely to approve the expenditure.

A number of factors are contributing to the board's decision not to authorize the additional $1.9 million for completion of the PACS, including

- Leadership's inability to guarantee to the board's satisfaction a financial return on the proposed investment.
- The board's perception that the radiologists are not committed to the hospital and to the community because none of the radiologists live in the community.
- The board's perception that the cardiologists are not committed to the hospital or to the community. The five cardiologists on staff are considered to be uncooperative among themselves and not supportive of the hospital's goals.
- Poor leadership within the IT department for providing the proper guidance on acquisition and implementation.
- The board's philosophy that Lakeland Medical Center should be more *high-touch* and less *high-tech*, and thus there is a philosophical difference over the need for a PACS.

- Jealousy among the medical staff that the diagnostic imaging department continues to obtain capital approvals for large items representing a major percentage of the annual capital budget. Thus, many influential members of the medical staff, such as surgeons, are not supportive of the expenditure.

- A few vocal employees speaking directly to board members expressing their concern that the PACS implementation will result in job loss for them.

- Leadership's inability to make a connection between this capital project and the strategic goals of the organization.

The chief of staff, Dr. Mary White, firmly believes that a PACS will increase patient and physician satisfaction because waiting times for results will decrease, enhance patient education, improve staff and physician productivity, improve clinical outcomes, improve patient safety, eliminate lost films, reduce medical liability, assist in reducing patient length of stay, and increase revenue potential. She believes it is management's challenge to understand the key issues of the board and to present the necessary supportive information for ultimate approval of the PACS program.

Discussion Questions

1. Conduct a role-play. Divide into four teams—the Lakeland Medical Center administrative team, the board, the medical staff, and the hospital and community at large. Assume the role of your constituent group and answer these questions: What are your views on this proposal? What are your major concerns? What questions do you have? And for whom? Do you think this is a case of someone failing to do his or her homework in putting together a sound business plan for the PACS project, or do you think there are bigger issues at play here? Explain your answers as necessary.

2. Assume that the CEO believes that the PACS project is well aligned with Lakeland's strategic goals but that this case hasn't been made clear to the board. How might Lakeland build this case? Who should lead that effort? What work needs to be done that has not occurred yet?

3. Are the board's concerns about medical staff commitment relevant in this case? Why or why not?

4. Develop a strategy for addressing the board's concerns and winning their buy-in and approval for the PACS project. Include in your description the who, what, where, when, and how.

CASE 2: THE DECISION TO DEVELOP AN IT STRATEGIC PLAN

Major themes: strategic planning and IT alignment

Background Information

Meadow Hills Hospital is a 211-bed acute care hospital with 400 members on its medical staff. Meadow serves a population of 300,000. There are three other similarly sized hospitals in the region. As an organization, Meadow Hills is very well run. It has a good reputation in the community and is considered to be technically advanced based on its investments in imaging technology. The organization is also in a strong financial position, with $238 million in reserves.

Meadow Hills has never had an information technology strategic plan.

Information Systems Challenge

The IT function reports to the Meadow Hills chief financial officer (CFO). The CEO and other members of the senior leadership team have largely left IT decisions up to the CFO. As a result, the organization's financial systems are very well developed. Computerized provider order entry (CPOE), an electronic health record (EHR) system, and a PACS have not been implemented. IT support for departments such as nursing, pharmacy, laboratory, imaging, and risk management is limited.

The Meadow Hills IT team is well regarded and the limited IT support for clinical processes has not drawn complaints from the nursing or medical staff. The organization does not currently have a chief information officer (CIO).

The CEO has never felt the need to pay attention to IT. However, he is worried that reimbursement based on care quality will arrive at Meadow Hills soon. He also believes that the Meadow Hills Clinical Laboratory and Imaging Center would be more competitive if it had stronger IT support; rival labs and imaging centers are able to offer electronic access to test results. And he suspects that the lack of IT support may eventually lead to nurses and physicians choosing to practice elsewhere.

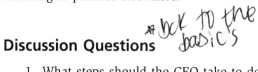

Discussion Questions

1. What steps should the CEO take to develop an IT strategy for the organization?
2. Are there unique risks to the ability of Meadow Hills Hospital to develop and implement an IT strategy?

3. Meadow Hills appears to have been successful despite years without an IT strategy. Why is this?

CASE 3: SELECTION OF A PATIENT SAFETY STRATEGY

Major themes: strategic planning and IT alignment

Background Information

Langley Mason Health (LMH) is located in North Reno County, the largest public health care district in the state of Nevada, serving an 850-square-mile area encompassing seven distinctly different communities. The health district was founded in 1937 by a registered nurse and dietician who opened a small medical facility on a former poultry farm. Today the health system comprises Langley Medical Center, a 317-bed tertiary medical center and level II trauma center; Mason Hospital, a 107-bed community hospital; and Mason Continuing Care Center and Villa Langley, two part-skilled nursing facilities (SNFs); a home care division; an ambulatory surgery center; and an outpatient behavioral medicine center.

In anticipation of expected population growth in North Reno County and to meet the state-mandated seismic requirements, LMH developed an aggressive facilities master plan (FMP) that includes plans to build a state-of-the-art 453-bed replacement hospital for its Langley Medical Center campus, double the size of its Mason Hospital, and build satellite clinics in four of its outlying communities. The cost associated with actualizing this FMP is estimated to be $1 billion. Several years ago, LMH undertook and successfully passed the largest health care bond measure in the state's history and in so doing secured $496 million in general obligation bonds to help fund its massive facilities expansion project. The remaining funds must come from revenue bonds, growth strategies, philanthropic efforts, and strong operational performance over the next ten years. Additionally, $5 million of routine capital funds will be diverted every fiscal year for the next five years to help offset the huge capital outlay that will be necessary to equip the new facilities. That leaves LMH with only $10 million per year to spend on routine maintenance, equipment, and technology for all its facilities. LMH is committed to patient safety and is building what the leadership team hopes will be one of the safest hospital-of-the-future facilities. The challenge is to provide for patient safety and safe medication practices given the minimal capital dollars available to spend today.

LMH developed an IT strategic plan in late 2010, with the following ten goals identified:

- Empower health consumers and physicians.
- Transform data into information.
- Support the expansion of clinical services.
- Expand e-business opportunities.
- Realize the benefits of innovation.
- Maximize the value of IT.
- Improve project outcomes.
- Prepare for the unexpected.
- Deploy a robust and agile technical architecture.
- Digitally enable new facilities, including the new hospital.

Information Systems Challenge

LMH has implemented Phase 1—an enterprise-wide EHR system developed by Cerner Corporation in 2008 at a cost of $20 million. Phase 2 of the project is to implement computerized provider order entry (CPOE) with decision-support capabilities. This phase was to have been completed in 2010, but has been delayed due to the many challenges associated with Phase 1, which still must be stabilized and optimized. LMH does have a fully automated pharmacy information system, albeit older technology, and Pyxis medication-dispensing systems on all units in the acute care hospitals. Computerized discharge prescriptions and instructions are available only for patients seen and discharged from the LMH emergency departments.

Currently, the pharmacy and nursing staff at LMH have been working closely on the selection of a smart IV pump to replace all of the health system's aging pumps and have put forth a proposal to spend $4.9 million in the fiscal year beginning July 2012. Smart pumps have been shown to significantly reduce medication administration errors, thus reducing patient harm. This expenditure would consume roughly half of all of the available capital dollars for that fiscal year.

The chief information officer, Marilyn Moore, PhD, understands the pharmacists' and nurses' desire to purchase smart IV pumps but believes the implementation of this technology should not be considered in isolation. She sees the smart pumps as one facet of an overall medication management capital purchase and patient safety strategic plan. Dr. Moore suggests that the pharmacy and nursing leadership team lead a medication management strategic planning process and evaluate a suite of available technologies that taken together could optimize medication safety (for example, CPOE, electronic medication administration records [e-mar], robots, automated pharmacy systems, bar coding, computerized discharge prescriptions and instructions, and smart IV pumps), the costs associated with implementing these technologies, and the organization's readiness to embrace these technologies. Paul Robinson, PharmD, the director of pharmacy, appreciates Dr. Moore's suggestion but feels that smart IV pumps are critical to patient safety and that LMH doesn't have time to go through a long, drawn-out planning process that could take years to implement and the process of gaining board support. Others argue that all new proposals should be placed on hold until CPOE is up and running. They argue there are too many other pressing issues at hand to invest in yet another new technology.

Discussion Questions

1. Describe the current situation as you see it. What are the major issues in this case?

2. Marilyn Moore, CIO, and Paul Robinson, director of pharmacy, have different views of how LMH should proceed. What are the pros and cons of their respective approaches? Which approach, if either, seems like an appropriate course of action to you? Explain your rationale.

3. Assume you are to mediate a discussion on this issue and that participants are to come to consensus on how best to proceed. What would you do?

CASE 4: STRATEGIC IS PLANNING FOR THE HOSPITAL ED

Major themes: strategic planning and IT alignment

Background Information

Founded in 1900, Newcastle Hospital today is a 375-bed, not-for-profit community hospital that serves over 200,000 residents of Newcastle County, New York. The hospital is approximately thirty miles from midtown Manhattan. It provides a full range of both primary and secondary medical and surgical services and is an affiliate of one of the large New York City hospital systems for both tertiary referrals and select residency programs. Newcastle Hospital has an independent governing body with 25 trustees; 604 active physicians; and 1,121 full-time equivalent (FTE) staff. Revenues of approximately $130 million per year come from 15,600 inpatient admissions; 71,000 outpatient visits; and 65,000 home care visits. Newcastle Hospital operates in a difficult environment characterized by relatively poor reimbursement and severe competition. There is one other acute care hospital in the county and a total of thirty-five others within a twenty-mile radius.

The sentinel event in the hospital's recent history occurred four years ago—a six-month nursing strike that alienated the workforce, decimated public confidence, and directly cost at least $19.5 million, effectively eradicating the hospital's capital reserves. Most of the senior management was replaced after the strike. When hired, the new CEO and CFO uncovered extensive inaccuracies that resulted in a reduction of reported net assets by almost $30 million and the near-bankruptcy of the hospital. The new management restated financial statements; began resolving extensive litigation; and set out to reestablish immediate operations, future finances, and long-term strategy. The new CEO states that "years of board and management neglect, plus the ravages of the strike complicated recovery, because standards, systems, and middle managers were universally absent or ineffective."

Among its many challenges, the challenges within the hospital's emergency department (ED) are particularly important to the overall recovery effort. The ED is described by the hospital CEO as the organization's "financial, clinical and public relations backbone." The ED sees 34,000 patients per year and admits 24 percent of them, constituting 51 percent of all inpatient admissions. In addition, the ED is a clinically distinguished Level II trauma center, with a long legacy of outcomes that compare favorably against regional, state, and national benchmarks. Finally, most community members have experience with the ED and consider it a proxy for the hospital as a whole, whether or not they have experienced an inpatient stay.

Currently, Newcastle ED patient satisfaction compared to patient satisfaction among peer organizations ranks at the 14th percentile in the Press Ganey New York State survey and the 5th percentile in national surveys. Since 1997, three organized initiatives to improve these results (especially regarding walkouts and waiting times) have failed, even though two involved prestigious consultants. After the management change, the new CEO diagnosed two core barriers to overcoming the ED problems: first, inflexibility and unwillingness to change among the ED physician management group that had been in place since 1987 and, second, an almost complete absence of the data required to define, measure, and improve the ED's service performance. The first barrier was addressed via an RFP process that resulted in engaging a new physician management group two years ago.

Information Systems Challenge

The present IS challenge follows directly from Newcastle Hospital's overarching strategic objectives: "satisfying patients and staff," "supporting ourselves," and "getting better every day" (that is, improving performance). The ED as presently structured has ill-defined manual processes and no information system. The challenge is selecting an ED information system with an emphasis on informing, not just automating, key ED processes, in order to support the overall strategic initiatives of the organization.

Several organizational and IT system factors that affect this IT challenge have been identified by the hospital CEO.

Organizational Factors

- *Undefined strategy.* Newcastle Hospital operated without a formal strategic action plan and corresponding tactics until two years ago. As a result, systematic prioritization and measurement of institutional imperatives such as improving the ED did not occur.

- *Data integrity.* Data throughout the hospital were undefined and unreliable. For example, two irreconcilable daily census reports made timely bed placement from the ED impossible.

- *Culture.* "Looking good," that is, escaping accountability, was valued more highly than "doing good," that is, substantively improving performance. Serious problems in the ED were often masked or dismissed as anecdotes, even in the face of regulatory citations and six- to eight-hour waiting times. The previous ED contract had contained no quality standards, and the ED physicians claimed to be busy "saving lives" whenever their poor service performance was questioned.

IT System Factors

- *IT strategy.* Paralleling the hospital, the IS department had no defined strategies, objectives, or processes. Alignment with hospital strategy and IT performance measurement were not considered. Although some progress has been made, this remains an area needing attention.

- *IT governance.* There is no IT steering committee at either the board or management levels. IT policies, service-level agreements, decision criteria, and user roles and responsibilities do not exist.

- *Functionality.* The IT applications portfolio is missing critical elements (for example, order entry, case management, nursing documentation, radiology) that would greatly benefit the ED, even without a dedicated ED system. The hospital's core information system is three versions out of date and certain functions have been bypassed by users altogether.

- *IT infrastructure and architecture.* The data center and most IT staff are located twelve miles away from the hospital, isolating IT both physically and culturally from users and patients. Software and networks have been arbitrarily and extensively customized over the years, without documentation, and inadequate hardware capacity has often been given as an excuse for not pursuing an ED system.

- *IT organization and resources.* IT spending has been, on average, less than 1 percent of the hospital's budget and IT staff have lacked essential training in critical applications and tools. Newcastle Hospital has been dependent on multiple IT vendors for a variety of implementation and operations support activities.

Discussion Questions

1. Outline the steps you would take to initiate a strategic planning process for improving the ED information system. How will you ensure that this plan is in alignment with the hospital's and department's overall strategic plans?

2. Multiple factors have contributed to the current state of the ED at Newcastle Hospital and are listed in the case. Which of these do you think will be the most difficult to overcome? Why?

3. The new CEO has good insight into the ED issues. Assuming that his assessment of the situation is accurate, discuss how his continued support could affect the outcome of any ED IS strategic plan.

4. Assume the CEO has appointed you to spearhead the ED IS strategic planning effort. What are the first steps you will take? Outline a general plan of action for the next three months. Indicate, by title, whom you would involve in the process. Explain your choices.

CASE 5: PLANNING AN EHR IMPLEMENTATION

Major themes: IT strategy; system implementation

Background Information

The Leonard Williams Medical Center (LWMC) is a 240-bed, community acute care hospital operating in a small urban area in upstate New York. The medical center offers tertiary services and has a captive professional corporation, Williams Medical Services (WMS). WMS is a multispecialty group employing approximately fifty primary care and specialty physicians.

WMS has its own board, made up of representatives of the employed physicians. The WMS board nominations for members and officers are subject to the approval of the medical center board. The capital and operating budgets of WMS are reviewed and approved during the LWMC budget process. The WMS board is responsible for governing the day-to-day operations of the group.

LWMC serves a population of approximately 215,000. There are five other hospitals in the region. One of these, aligned with a large clinic, is viewed as the primary competitor.

In its most recent fiscal year, LWMC had an operating margin of 0.4 percent. LWMC has $40 million in investments and has a long-term debt to equity ratio of 25 percent.

Information Systems Challenge

LWMC has been very effective in its IT efforts. It was the first hospital in its region to have a clinical information system. Bedside computing has been available on the inpatient units since the 1990s. The CIO and IT department are highly regarded. LWMC has received several industry recognitions for its efforts.

The LWMC information systems steering committee recently approved the acquisition and implementation of a CPOE system. This decision followed a thorough analysis of organizational strategies, the efforts of other hospitals, and the vendor offerings. LWMC is poised to begin this major initiative.

During a recent steering committee meeting, it was learned that the WMS physicians were anxious to acquire an electronic health record (EHR) system.

Two years ago a rival physician group had purchased an EHR system. WMS, concerned about a competitive threat, obtained approval of $300,000 to acquire its own EHR. The rival group has since encountered serious difficulties with implementation and has deinstalled the system. This troubled path caused WMS to slow down its efforts.

Now WMS has decided to return to its plans to implement a certified EHR. The physicians have begun to look at vendor offerings but have not involved the LWMC CIO and IT staff. The physicians have ignored the CIO's technical and integration advice and requirements during their EHR search.

The CEO is concerned about the EHR process and its disconnect from the medical center's IT plans.

Discussion Questions

1. What is your assessment of this situation? What are the physician group's possible reasons for deciding to proceed on an independent path?

2. If you were the CEO, what steps would you take to bring the hospital and physician group IT plans back into alignment? Should the EHR effort proceed or wait until the CPOE initiative is complete? Should you require that both systems come from the same vendor? Explain your rationale.

3. The LWMC board is concerned that the physicians are being naive about the challenges of EHR implementation, have established no measurable goals for the system, and have only weak incentives to make the implementation successful. How would you address these concerns?

CASE 6: IMPLEMENTING A CAPACITY MANAGEMENT INFORMATION SYSTEM

Major theme: system acquisition

Background Information

Doctors' Hospital is a 162-bed, acute care facility located in a small city in the southeastern United States. The organization had a major financial upheaval six years ago that resulted in the establishment of a new governing structure. The new governing body consists of an eleven-member authority board. The senior management of Doctors' Hospital includes the chief executive officer (CEO), three senior vice presidents, and one vice president. During the restructuring, the chief information officer (CIO) was changed from a full-time staff position to a part-time contract position. The CIO spends two days every two weeks at Doctors' Hospital.

Doctors' Hospital is currently in Phase 1 of a three-phase construction project. In Phase 2 the hospital will build a new emergency department (ED) and surgical pavilion, which are scheduled to be completed in eleven months.

Information Systems Challenge

The current ED and outpatient surgery department have experienced tremendous growth in the past several years. ED visits have increased by 50 percent, and similar increases have been seen in outpatient surgery. Management has identified that inefficient patient flow processes, particularly patient transfers and discharges, have resulted in backlogs in both the ED and outpatient areas. The new construction will only exacerbate the current problem.

Nearly one year ago Doctors' Hospital made a commitment to purchase a capacity management software suite to reduce the inefficiencies that have been identified in patient flow processes. The original timeline was to have the new system pilot-tested prior to the opening of the new ED and surgical pavilion. However, with the competing priorities its members face as they deal with major construction, the original project steering committee has stalled. At its last meeting nearly six months ago, the steering committee identified the vendor and product suite. Budgets and timelines for implementation were proposed but not finalized. No other steps have been taken.

Discussion Questions

1. Do you think the absence of a full-time CIO has had an impact on this acquisition project? Why or why not?

2. What steps should the CIO take to ensure that the capacity management system will be purchased and implemented? What do you see as the critical first step in this process? Why?

3. Discuss who you think should serve on the project steering committee. Who should serve as chair? Why?

4. At this point, what do you think is a realistic time frame for implementation of the capacity management system? What steps can be taken to ensure the new timeline is met despite competing priorities?

CASE 7: IMPLEMENTING A TELEMEDICINE SOLUTION

Major themes: system acquisition; use of emerging technologies

Background Information

Grand Hospital is located in a somewhat rural area of a midwestern state. It is a 209-bed, community, not-for-profit entity offering a broad range of inpatient and outpatient services. Employing approximately 1,600 individuals (1,250 full-time equivalent personnel), and having a medical staff of more than 225 practitioners, Grand has an annual operating budget that exceeds $130 million, possesses net assets of more than $150 million, and is one of only a small number of organizations in this market with an A credit rating from Moody's, Standard & Poor's, and Fitch Ratings. Operating in a remarkably competitive market (there are roughly 100 hospitals within seventy-five minutes' driving time of Grand), the organization is one of the few in the region—proprietary or not-for-profit—that have consistently realized positive operating margins. Grand attends on an annual basis to the health care needs of more than 11,000 inpatients and 160,000 outpatients, addressing more than 36 percent of its primary service area's consumption of hospital services. In expansion mode and currently in the midst of $57 million in construction and renovation projects, the hospital is struggling to recruit physicians, both to meet the health care needs of the expanding population of the service area and to succeed retiring physicians.

Grand has been an early adopter of health care information systems and currently employs a proprietary health care information system that provides (among other components)

- Patient registration and revenue management
- Electronic health records with computerized physician order entry
- Imaging via a PACS
- Laboratory management
- Pharmacy management

Information Systems Challenge

Since 1995, Grand Hospital has transitioned from being an institution that consistently received many more inquiries than could be accommodated concerning physician practice opportunities, to a hospital at which the average age of the medical staff has increased by eight years. There is a widespread perception among physicians that because of such factors as high malpractice insurance costs, an absence of substantive tort reform, and the comparatively unfavorable rates of reimbursement being paid physician specialists by the region's major health insurer, this region constitutes a "physician unfriendly" venue in which to establish a practice. Consequently, a need exists for Grand to investigate and evaluate creative approaches to enhancing its physician coverage for certain specialty services. These potential approaches include the effective implementation of information technology solutions.

The findings and conclusions of a medical staff development plan, which has been endorsed and accepted by Grand's medical executive committee and board of trustees, have indicated that because of needs and circumstances specific to the institution, the first areas of medical practice on which Grand should focus in approaching this challenge are radiology, behavioral health crisis intervention services, and intensivist physician services. In the area of radiology, Grand needs qualified and appropriately credentialed radiologists available to interpret studies 24 hours per day, 7 days per week. Similarly, it needs qualified and appropriately credentialed psychiatrists available on a 24/7 basis to assess whether behavioral health patients who present in the hospital's emergency room are a danger to themselves or to others, as defined by state statute, and whether these patients should be released or committed against their will for further assessment on an inpatient basis. Finally, inasmuch as Grand is a community hospital that relies on its voluntary medical staff to attend to the needs of patients admitted by staff members such as some ED personnel, it also needs to have intensivist physicians available around the clock to assist in assessing and treating patients during times when members of the voluntary attending staff are not present within or immediately available to the intensive care unit.

The leadership at Grand Hospital is investigating the potential application of telemedicine technologies to address the organization's need for enhanced physician coverage in radiology, behavioral health, and critical care medicine.

Discussion Questions

1. What are the ways in which Grand's early adoption of other health care information system technologies might affect its adoption of telemedicine solutions?

2. What do you see as the most likely barriers to the success of telemedicine in the areas of radiology, behavioral health, and intensive care? Which of these areas do you think would be the easiest to transition into telemedicine? Which would be the hardest? Why?

3. If you were charged by Grand to bring telemedicine to the facility within eighteen months, what are the first steps you would take? Whom would you involve in the planning process? Defend your response.

CASE 8: REPLACING A PRACTICE MANAGEMENT SYSTEM

Major themes: IT governance; system implementation

Background Information

University Physician Group (UPG) is a multispecialty group practice plan associated with the College of Osteopathic Medicine (COM). UPG employs 90 physicians and 340 clinical and business support personnel.

UPG has recently been profitable (with revenue from operations this fiscal year of $32 million and a retained profit of $500,000 from operations). However, prior year losses make UPG a breakeven organization.

Management and the physicians are focusing on strengthening the fiscal position of the organization. This focus has led to plans to restructure physician compensation, establish a self-insurance trust for professional liability, and improve the financial budgeting and reporting processes.

UPG has entered into a preliminary agreement to merge with Northern Affiliated Medical Group (NAMG). NAMG is a 150-physician multispecialty group located in the same city as UPG. NAMG holds a contract with the local county hospital to provide indigent care and serve as the faculty for the graduate medical education programs in family medicine.

Both organizations believe that the merged organization would be able to reduce expenses through the elimination of redundant functions and, because of greater geographical coverage and size, would improve their ability to obtain more favorable payer contracts.

Information Systems Challenge

For many years UPG has obtained practice management systems from Gleason Solutions (GS). The applications are hosted in a GS data center, reducing the UPG's need for IT staff.

Prior to the merger, UPG was in the process of examining replacements for GS. UPG had become displeased because of the GS applications' failure to incorporate new technologies and application features, limited ability to generate reports, and inflexible integration approaches to other applications.

Despite its displeasure, UPG now appears to be on the path to renewing the GS contract. GS executives have effectively lobbied several important physicians and administrators, and UPG's limited cash position makes the GS low-cost financial proposal attractive.

NAMG uses the GS applications and has also been examining replacing the system. NAMG has a strong IT department and will be providing IT support to the newly merged organization. After examining the market, NAMG has identified four potential vendors, including GS.

Discussion Questions

1. Would you suspend both organizations' pursuit of a new system until an IT strategic plan for the merged organization has been developed? Why? *Yes*

2. What steps would you take to integrate the system selection processes of the two organizations? *Plan , System analytics*

3. Implementing a practice management system is always challenging. What additional implementation risks are introduced by the merger? ⬅

4. Both organizations expect the result of the merger to be lower costs, improved patient service, and increased market power. What steps would you take to make sure that the new practice management system furthers these objectives? *– Plan Strategic – Management*

CASE 9: CONVERSION TO AN EHR MESSAGING SYSTEM

Major themes: system implementation; project management

Background Information

Goodwill Health Care Clinic is the clinical arm of Jefferson Health Sciences Center in a large southern city. The clinic was founded in the early 1950s as a place for faculty physicians to engage in clinical practice. Over the years the clinic has grown to 900 faculty physicians and 2,000 employees, with over one million patient visits per year. Clinic services are spread across eleven primary care and specialty care units. Each unit operates somewhat independently but shares a common medical record numbering system that allows consolidation of all documentation across units. Paper charts were used until two years ago, when the clinic adopted an electronic health record (EHR) system.

Goodwill Health Care Clinic uses a centralized call center to receive all patient calls. Patients call a central switchboard to schedule appointments, request medication refills, or speak to anyone in any of the eleven units. Call center staff are responsible for tracking all calls to ensure that each is dealt with appropriately. Currently the call center uses a customized Lotus Notes system that can be accessed by anyone in the system who needs to process messages. Messages can be tracked and then *closed* when the appropriate action has been taken. Notes created from closed messages are printed and filed in the appropriate patients' paper records. These notes cannot be accessed via the EHR.

Clinic staff are very comfortable with the current Lotus Notes system and it is used routinely by all units.

Information Systems Challenge

Goodwill Health Care Clinic requires all medication lists and refill information to be kept up to date in the EHR. Therefore, the existence of the current Lotus

Notes system means that the same information must be documented in two locations—first in the call center note and then in the EHR. This leads to duplication of effort and documentation errors. The potential for serious error is present. Physicians and other health care providers look in the EHR for the most up-to-date medication information.

Although the adoption of the EHR has been fairly successful, not all units use all of the available components of the EHR. A companion paper record is needed for miscellaneous notes, messages, and so forth. All units are recording office visits into the EHR, but not all have activated the lab results or the prescription writing features. Several units have been experiencing physician resistance to adding more EHR functions.

The EHR system has a messaging component that works like a closed e-mail system. Messages can be sent, received, and stored by EHR authenticated users. Pertinent patient care messages are automatically stored in the correct patient record. In addition, the EHR messaging system works seamlessly with the prescription writing module, which includes patient safety checks such as allergy checks and drug interactions.

The challenge for Goodwill Health Care Clinic is to implement the messaging feature and prescription writing component (where it is not currently being used) of their current EHR in the call center and the clinical units, replacing the existing Lotus Notes system and improving the quality of the documentation, not only of medication refills but of all patient-related calls. The long-term goal is to add a patient portal feature where patients can schedule appointments, send messages to their providers, and refill prescriptions electronically.

Discussion Questions

1. Outline the steps that you would take to ensure a successful conversion from the existing call center system to the new EHR compatible system. Defend your response.

2. Who should be involved in the conversion planning and implementation? Discuss the roles of the people on your list and your reasons for selecting them.

3. What are some strategies that you would employ to minimize physicians' and other users' resistance to the conversion?

4. Do you think that making sure all units are running the same EHR functions is a necessary precursor to the conversion to the messaging and prescription writing components? What information would be helpful in making this determination?

5. How might the implementation of the patient portal feature address some of the current issues? What workflow considerations will need to be made?

CASE 10: CONCERNS AND WORKAROUNDS WITH A CLINICAL DOCUMENTATION SYSTEM

Major themes: system implementation; project management

Background Information

Garrison Children's Hospital is a 225-bed hospital. Its 77-bed neonatal intensive care unit (NICU) provides care to the most fragile patients, premature and critically ill neonates. The 28-bed pediatric intensive care unit (PICU) cares for critically ill children from birth to eighteen years of age. Patients in this unit include those with life-threatening conditions that are acquired (trauma, child abuse, burns, surgical complications, and so forth) or congenital (congenital heart defects, craniofacial malformations, genetic disorders, inborn errors of metabolism, and so forth).

Garrison is part of Premier Health Care, an academic medical center complex located in the Southeast. Premier Health Care also includes an adult hospital, a psychiatric hospital, and a full spectrum of adult and pediatric outpatient clinics. Within the past six months or so, Premier has implemented an electronic clinical documentation system in its adult hospital. More recently the same clinical documentation system has been implemented at Garrison in both pediatric medical and surgery units and intensive care units. Electronic scheduling is to be implemented next.

The adult hospital drives the decisions for the pediatric hospital, a circumstance that led to the adult hospital's CPOE vendor being chosen as the documentation vendor for both hospitals. A CPOE system was implemented at Garrison Children's Hospital several years prior to implementation of the electronic clinical documentation system, which began in 2010.

Information Systems Challenge

A pressing challenge facing Garrison Children's Hospital is that nurses are very concerned and dissatisfied with the new clinical documentation system. They have voiced concerns formally to several nurse managers, and one nurse went directly to the chief nursing officer (CNO) stating that the "flow sheets" on the new system are grossly inadequate and she fears using them could lead to patient safety issues. Lunchroom conversations among nurses tend to center on their having no clear understanding of why the organization is automating clinical documentation or what it hopes to achieve. Nurses in the NICU and PICU seem to be most vocal about their concerns. They claim there is inconsistency in what is being documented and lack of standardization of content. The computer workstations are located outside the patients' rooms, so nurses generally document their notes on paper and then enter the data at the end of the shift or when they have time.

The system support team, consisting of nurses as well as technology specialists, began the workflow analysis, system installation, staff training, and go-live first with a small number of units in both the adult hospital and the children's hospital, beginning in January 2010. The NICU and PICU did not implement the system until May and June 2010. System support personnel moved rapidly through each unit, working to train and to manage questions. The timeline for each unit implementation was based on the number of beds in the unit and the number of staff to be trained. No consideration was given to staff members' prior experience with computers and keyboarding skills or to complexity of documentation and existing work processes.

Although there are similarities between the adult and pediatric settings, there are also many differences in terms of unit design, computer resources (hardware), level of computer literacy, information documented, and work processes, not to mention patient populations. Little time was spent evaluating or planning for these differences and completing a thorough workflow analysis. After the initial units went live, less and less time was spent on training and addressing unit-specific needs, due to the demands placed upon training staff to stay on the timeline in preparation for the next system implementation involving electronic scheduling.

The clinical documentation system was implemented to the great consternation and dissatisfaction of the end users (physicians, nurses, social workers, and so forth) at Garrison, yet the Premier clinicians are happy with it. Many Garrison physicians and nurses initially refused to use the system, stating it was "unsafe," "added to workload," and was not intuitive. A decision to stop using the system and return to the paper documentation process was not then and is not now an option. Physician "champions" were encouraged to work with those who were recalcitrant and nursing staff were encouraged to "stick it out," in hopes that system use would "get easier."

As a result, with their concerns and complaints essentially forced underground, Garrison clinical staff developed *workarounds*, morale was negatively affected, and the expectation that everyone would eventually "get it" and adapt has not become a reality. Instead, staff are writing on a self-created paper system and then translating those notes to the computer system; physicians are unable to retrieve important, timely patient information; and the time team members spend trying to retrieve pertinent patient information has increased. There have been clear instances where patient safety has been affected due to the problems with the appropriate use of this system.

Discussion Questions

1. What is the major problem in this case? What factors seem to have contributed to the current situation?

2. The nurses at Garrison argue that pediatric hospitals and intensive care units, in particular, are different from adult hospitals and that these differences should be clearly addressed in the implementation of a new clinical documentation system. Do you agree with this argument? Why or why not? Give examples from the literature to support your views.

3. How might the workflow issues and concerns mentioned in this case have been detected earlier?

4. Assume you are part of the leadership team at Garrison. How would you assess the current situation? What would you do first? Next? Explain the steps you would take and why you feel your approach is necessary.

5. What lessons can be learned from this case and applied to other settings?

CASE 11: STRATEGIES FOR IMPLEMENTING CPOE

Major themes: *system implementation; project management*

Background

Health Matters is a newly formed nonprofit health system comprising two community hospitals (Cooper Memorial Hospital and Ashley Valley Hospital), nine ambulatory care clinics, and three imaging centers. Since its inception two years ago, the information services department has merged and consolidated all computer systems under one umbrella. Each of the facilities within the health system is connected electronically with the others through a fiberoptic network. The organizational structure of the two hospitals is such that each has its own executive leadership team and board.

Seven years ago, the leadership team at Cooper Memorial Hospital made the strategic decision to choose Meditech as the vendor of choice for its clinical and financial applications. The philosophy of the leadership team was to solicit a single vendor solution so that the hospital could minimize the number of disparate systems and interfaces. Since then, Meditech has been deployed throughout the health system and applications have been kept current with the latest releases. Most nursing and clinical ancillary documentation is electronic, as is the medication administration record. Health Matters does have several ancillary systems that interface with Meditech; these include a picture archiving and communication system (PACS), a fully automated laboratory system, an emergency department tracking board, and an electronic bed board system. The leadership team at Ashley Valley Hospital chose to select non-Meditech products, because at the time Meditech did not offer these applications or its products were considered inadequate by clinicians. However, the current sentiment among the leadership team is to continue to go with one predominant vendor, in this case, Meditech, for any upgrades, new functionality, or new products.

The information system (IS) group at Health Matters consists of a director of information systems (who reports to the chief financial officer) and fifteen staff members. The IS staff are highly skilled in networking and computer operations but have only moderate skill as program analysts and project managers. The CEO, Steve Forthright, plans to hire a chief information officer (CIO) to provide senior-level leadership in developing and implementing a strategic IS plan that is congruent with the strategic goals of Health Matters.

Currently, the senior leadership team at Health Matters has identified the following as the organization's top three IS challenges. The current director of information systems has been somewhat involved in discussions related to the establishment of these priorities.

- To implement successfully computerized provider order entry (CPOE)
- To increase the variety and availability of computing devices (workstations or handheld devices) at each nursing station
- To implement successfully medication administration using bar-coding technology

Information Systems Challenge

The most pressing IS challenge is to move forward with the implementation of CPOE. The decision has already been made to implement the Meditech CPOE application. Several internal and external driving forces are at play. Internally, the physician leaders believe that CPOE will further reduce medication errors and promote patient safety. The board has established patient safety as a strategic goal for the organization. Externally, groups such as Leapfrog and the

Pacific Business Group on Health have strongly encouraged CPOE implementation. The CEO Steve Forthright has concerns, however, because Health Matters does not yet have a CIO on board and he feels the CIO should play a pivotal role. Much of Steve's concern stems from his experience with CPOE implementation at another institution, with a different vendor and product. Steve had organized a project implementation committee, established an appropriate governance structure, and the senior leadership team thought it had "covered the bases." However, according to Steve, "The surgeons embraced the new CPOE system, largely because they felt the postoperative order sets were easy to use, but the internists and hospitalists rebelled. The CPOE project stalled and the system was never fully implemented." Steve is not the only person reeling from a failed implementation. The clinical information committee at Health Matters is chaired by Mary White, who was involved in a failed CPOE rollout at another hospital several years ago. She was a strong supporter of the system at the time, but now speaks of the risks and challenges associated with getting physician buy-in and support throughout the health system.

Members of the medical staff at Cooper Memorial Hospital have access to laboratory and radiology results electronically. They have access through workstations in the hospital; most physicians also access clinical results remotely through smart phones. An estimated 35 percent of the physicians take full advantage of the system's capabilities. Almost all active physicians use the PACS to view images, and most use a computer to look up lab values. Fewer than half of the physicians use electronic signatures to sign transcribed reports.

Discussion Questions

1. Assume you are part of a team charged with leading the implementation of CPOE within Health Matters. How would you approach the task? What would you do first? Next? Who should be involved in the team? Lead the team?

2. The CIO hasn't been hired yet. Do you see that as a problem? Why or why not? What role, if any, might the CIO have in the CPOE implementation project?

3. To what extent does the fact that Health Matters is a relatively new health system simplify or complicate the CPOE implementation project? How do other health systems typically implement CPOE or other clinical information system projects of this magnitude?

4. How might you solicit the wisdom and expertise of others who may have undergone CPOE projects like this one? Or who have used Meditech's CPOE application? How might Steve Forthright's and

Mary White's prior experiences with partially and fully failed implementations affect their views in this case?

5. Develop a high-level implementation plan of key tasks and activities that will need to be done. How will you estimate the time frame? The resources needed? What role does the vendor have in establishing this plan?

CASE 12: IMPLEMENTING A SYNDROMIC SURVEILLANCE SYSTEM

Major themes: IT strategy; system implementation

Background Information

Syndromic surveillance systems collect and analyze prediagnostic and non-clinical disease indicators, drawing on preexisting electronic data that can be found in systems such as electronic health records, school absenteeism records, and pharmacy systems. These surveillance systems are intended to identify specific symptoms within a population that may indicate a public health event or emergency. For example, the data being collected by a surveillance system might reveal a sharp increase in diarrhea in a community and that could signal an outbreak of an infectious disease.

The infectious disease epidemiology section of a state's public health agency has been given the task of implementing the Early Aberration Reporting System of the Centers for Disease Control and Prevention. The agency views this system as significantly improving its ability to monitor and respond to potentially problematic bioterrorism, food poisoning, and infectious disease outbreaks.

The implementation of the system is also seen as a vehicle for improving collaboration between the agency, health care providers, information technology vendors, researchers, and the business community.

Information Systems Challenge

The agency and its infectious disease epidemiology section face several major challenges.

First, the necessary data must be collected largely from hospitals and in particular emergency rooms. Developing and supporting necessary interfaces to the applications in a large number of hospitals is very challenging. These hospitals have different application vendors, diverse data standards, and uneven willingness to divert IT staff and budget to the implementation of these interfaces.

To help address this challenge, the section will acquire a commercial package or build the needed software to ease the integration challenge. In addition, the section will provide each hospital with information it can use to assess its own mix of patients and their presenting problems.

The agency is also contemplating the development of regulations that would require the hospitals to report the necessary data.

Second, the system must be designed so that patient privacy is protected and the system is secure.

Third, the implementation and support of the system will be funded initially through federal grants. The agency will need to develop strategies for ensuring the financial sustainability of the application and related analysis capabilities should federal funding end.

Fourth, the agency needs to ensure that the section has the staff and tools necessary to appropriately analyze the data. Distinguishing true problems from the "noise" of a normal increase in colds during the winter, for example, can be very difficult. The agency could damage the public's confidence in the system if it overreacts or underreacts to the data it collects.

Discussion Questions

1. If you were the head of the agency's epidemiology section, how would you address the four challenges described here?

2. Which of the challenges is the most important to address? Why?

3. If you were a hospital CEO being asked to redirect IT resources for this project, what would you want in return from the agency to ensure that this system provided value to your organization and clinicians?

4. A strong privacy advocacy group has expressed alarm about the potential problems that the system could create. How would you respond to those concerns?

CASE 13: THE ADMITTING SYSTEM CRASHES

Major theme: disaster recovery

Background Information

Jones Regional Medical Center is a large academic health center. With 900 beds, Jones had 47,000 admissions in 2010. Jones frequently has occupancy in excess of 100 percent, requiring diversion of ambulances. In addition, Jones had 1,300,000 ambulatory and emergency room visits in 2007.

Jones is internationally renowned for its research and teaching programs.

The IT staff at Jones are highly regarded. They support over 300 applications and 12,000 workstations.

The admitting system at Jones is provided by the vendor Technology Med (TechMed). The TechMed system supports the master patient index; registration; inpatient charge and payment entry; medical records abstracting and coding; hospital billing and patient accounting; reporting; and admission, discharge, and transfer capabilities.

The TechMed system was implemented in 1998 and uses now obsolete technology, including a rudimentary database management system. The organization is concerned about the fragility of the application and has begun plans to replace the TechMed system two years from now.

Information Systems Challenge

On December 20, the link between the main data center (where the TechMed servers were housed) and the disaster recovery center was taken down to conduct performance testing.

On December 21, power was lost to the disaster recovery center, but emergency power was instantly put in place. However, as a precaution, a backup of the TechMed database was performed.

During the afternoon of December 21, the TechMed system became sluggish and then unresponsive. Database corruption was discovered. The backup performed earlier in the day was also corrupt. The link to the disaster recovery data center had not been restored following the performance testing.

Because there was no viable backup copy of the database, the Jones IT and hospital staff began the arduous process of a full database recovery from journaled transactions. This process was completed the evening of December 22.

The loss of the TechMed system for over thirty-six hours and the failure during that time of registration transactions to update patient care and ancillary department systems resulted in a wide variety of operational problems. The patient census had to be maintained manually. Reports of results were delayed. Paper orders were needed for patients who were admitted on December 21 and 22. Charge collection lagged.

Once the TechMed system was restored, additional hospital staff were brought in to enter, into multiple systems, the data that had been manually captured during the outage. By December 25, normal hospital operations were restored. No patient care incidents are believed to have resulted.

Discussion Questions

1. If you were the CIO of Jones Regional Medical Center during this system failure, what steps would you take during the outage? What steps would you take after the outage to reduce the likelihood of a reoccurrence of this problem?

2. The root cause analysis of the outage showed that process, technology, and staffing factors all contributed to the problem. What are some of the likely factors? Which of these factors do you believe are likely to have been the most important?

3. If you were a member of the audit committee of the Jones board of trustees, what questions would you ask the CIO?

4. What issues and problems should a disaster recovery plan prepare for? How does an organization determine how much to spend to reduce the occurrence and severity of such episodes?

CASE 14: BREACHING THE SECURITY OF AN INTERNET PATIENT PORTAL

Major theme: IT security

Background Information

Kaiser Permanente is an integrated health delivery system that serves over eight million members in nine states and the District of Columbia.[1] In the late 1990s, Kaiser Permanente introduced an Internet patient portal, Kaiser Permanente Online (also known as KP Online). Members can use KP Online to request appointments, request prescription refills, obtain health care service information, seek clinical advice, and participate in patient forums.

Information Systems Challenge

In August 2000, there was a serious breach in the security of the KP Online pharmacy refill application. Programmers wrote a flawed script that actually concatenated over eight hundred individual e-mail messages containing individually identifiable patient information, instead of separating them as intended. As a result, nineteen members received e-mail messages with private information about multiple other members. Kaiser became aware of the problem when two members notified the organization that they had received the concatenated e-mail messages. Kaiser leadership considered this incident a significant breach of confidentiality and security. The organization immediately took steps to investigate and to offer apologies to those affected.

On the same day the first member notified Kaiser about receiving the problem e-mail, a crisis team was formed. The crisis team began a root cause analysis and a *mitigation assessment* process. Three days later Kaiser began notifying its members and issued a press release.

The investigation of the cause of the breach uncovered issues at the technical, individual, group, and organizational levels. At the technical level, Kaiser was using new web-based tools, applications, and processes. The pharmacy module had been evaluated in a test environment that was not equivalent to the production environment. At the individual level, two programmers, one from the e-mail group and one from the development group, working together for the first time in a new environment and working under intense pressure to quickly fix a serious problem, failed to adequately test code they produced as a patch for the pharmacy application. Three groups within Kaiser had responsibilities for KP Online: operations, e-mail, and development. Traditionally these groups worked independently and had distinct missions and organizational cultures. The breach revealed the differences in the way groups approached priorities. For example, the development group often let meeting deadlines dictate priorities. At the organizational level, Kaiser IT had a very complex organizational structure, leading to what Collmann and Cooper (2007, p. 239) call "compartmentalized sensemaking." Each IT group "developed highly localized definitions of a situation, which created the possibility for failure when integrated in a common infrastructure."

Discussion Questions

1. How serious was this e-mail security breach? Why did the Kaiser Permanente leadership react so quickly to mitigate the possible damage done by the breach?

2. Assume that you were appointed as the administrative member of the crisis team created the day the breach was uncovered. After the initial apologies, what recommendations would you make for investigating the root cause(s) of the breach? Outline your suggested investigative steps.

3. How likely do you think future security breaches would be if Kaiser Permanente did not take steps to resolve underlying group and organizational issues? Why?

4. What role should the administrative leadership of Kaiser Permanente take in ensuring that KP Online is secure? Apart from security and

HIPAA training for all personnel, what steps can be taken at the organizational level to improve the security of KP Online?

CASE 15: ASSESSING THE VALUE AND IMPACT OF CPOE

Major theme: assessing the value of an HIT investment

Background Information

The University Health Care System is an academic medical center with over 1,200 licensed beds and over 9,000 employees. The system comprises the University Hospital, Winston Geriatric Hospital, Jefferson Rehabilitation Hospital, and two outpatient centers in the metropolitan area. The system has a history of being a patriarchal, physician-driven organization. When University Health Care first started taking patients, it was viewed as a mecca to which community physicians throughout the South referred difficult-to-treat patients. That referral mentality persisted for decades, so physicians within the system had a difficult time making the transition to an organization that had to compete for patients with other health care entities in the region.

In recent years, University Health Care System has evolved and given physicians proportionately more clout in decision making, in part because the health care leadership team has not stepped forward. Creating a balance between clinician providers and administrative leadership is a real issue. In the midst of the difficulty, both groups have agreed to embark on the electronic health record (EHR) journey. Currently about 55 percent of the system's patient record is electronic; the remainder is on paper. The physicians as a whole, however, have embraced technology and view the EHR as the "right road" to take in achieving the organization's goal of providing high-quality, safe, cost-effective patient care.

Information Systems Challenge

Currently, the University Health Care System is in the midst of rolling out the CPOE portion of the EHR project. A multidisciplinary decision-making project was established before beginning the initiative, and leaders and clinicians tried to educate themselves on what the CPOE project would entail. They were familiar with cases such as one at Cedars-Sinai where CPOE was halted after a physician uproar over the time it took to use and patient safety concerns. To help ensure this did not happen at the University Health Care System, the leadership team decided to take a slower, phased-in approach. Team members visited similar organizations that had implemented CPOE, attended vendor user-group conferences, consulted with colleagues from across the nation, and articulated the following project goals:

- Optimize patient safety
- Improve quality outcomes and reduce variation in practice through the use of evidence-based practice guidelines
- Reduce risk for errors
- Accommodate regulatory standards expectations
- Enhance patient satisfaction
- Standardize processes
- Improve efficiency

The board has made it very clear that it wants regular updates on the progress of the project and expects to see what the return on the investment has been.

Discussion Questions

1. How might you evaluate the CPOE implementation process at University Health Care System? Give examples of different methods or strategies you might employ.

2. How would you respond to the board's desire for a "return on investment" from this initiative? Is it a reasonable request? Why or why not?

3. Assume you are to lead the evaluation component of this project. You have reviewed the goals for the project. What *process* would you use to develop a plan for assessing the value of CPOE? Who would be involved? What roles would they play? How would you decide on the best metrics to use? What baseline data would you want to collect or review?

CASE 16: SELECTING AN EHR FOR DERMATOLOGY PRACTICE

Major theme: System acquisition

Background Information

Suppose you've just been hired as the practice administrator of an eight-physician dermatology practice. After several years of contemplation and serious deliberations, the physicians have made the strategic decision to invest in the selection and implementation of a facility-wide electronic health record (EHR) system. They also want to replace their practice management system (which includes patient scheduling and billing). It's an older system that is rather clunky. Ideally, they'd like to find an integrated practice management system that has an EHR component.

Dr. Dan Brown, the current CEO of the physician organization, has very little knowledge of information systems technology. He has been reluctant to move toward an electronic health record system for many years, primarily because he heard stories from a few his colleagues in other specialty areas who have implemented EHRs in their practices and have found the systems to be highly cumbersome and disruptive to the patient care process. One of his best friends claims he "spends an extra hour or two a night in the office because of the additional time demands of the EHR. He claims the system never seemed to work right." Dr. Brown is convinced that there are not any great dermatology-related EHR products on the market, but with the EHR incentive dollars available, and the opportunity to improve quality of patient care, he's open to taking another look. In addition, one of their newest partners, Dr. Pam Martin, just finished her residency program, where EHRs were an integral part of her training. She doesn't want to go back to a paper environment and is a big champion of the effort to select and implement an EHR. She has offered to help lead the effort. One of the other partners, Dr. John Harris, came back from a conference impressed with the vendor presentation from Allscripts and convinced it's the way the practice ought to go. The other physicians are nearing retirement and a little nervous about the possible disruption to the office.

Information Systems Challenge

Even though the patient records at the dermatology practice are paper-based, the practice has been using computerized practice management systems for patient scheduling and billing for years. Six months ago, they started to have a nurse enter physician-dictated notes into the paper record while in the examination room with the patient. The physician then reviews the notes at the end of the visit or day and signs off on them. This is in an effort to decrease the dictation and transcription that the practice had historically done, and to get the nurses and physicians "ready" for the EHR. The expectation is that nurses will do the bulk of the data entry in the exam room while the physicians are seeing the patients. However, the physicians will have to review the documentation and sign off on all entries.

The practice currently has approximately 4,000 patient visits per month, including 40 percent Medicare and 10 percent Medicaid. They hope to participate in the EHR incentive program and demonstrate meaningful use.

Discussion Questions

You are tasked with leading the team charged with the selection of the new practice management system, including EHR, for the practice.

1. You begin by convening a Practice Management-EHR Selection Team. Who would serve on the team? Who would serve as executive sponsor? Explain your rationale.

2. How might you conduct an EHR readiness assessment for this practice? What factors will be important to consider? Why?

3. Develop a draft system selection plan for this practice. What do you envision will be the practice's greatest challenges in selecting a replacement practice management system and a new EHR? Explain your rationale.

CASE 17: WATSON'S AMBULATORY EHR TRANSITION

Major theme: System acquisition
Primary care physicians play a key role in the U.S. health care delivery system. These providers integrate internal and external information with their clinical knowledge to determine the patient's treatment options. An effective ambulatory electronic health record (EHR) is critical to supply physicians with the information they need to provide quality care and maximize their efficiency. This case involves the decision-making process to replace an inadequate EHR system in a primary care network owned by a community hospital. The IT challenge reviewed in this case will be the decision-making process that optimizes provider support for the new EHR while addressing the strategic plan requirements of data integration, clinical application, and practice management functionality.

Background Information

Watson Community Association is a private, not-for-profit corporation that operates Watson Community Hospital (WCH), a 200-bed acute care facility located in Arizona. WCH has pursued a strategy of employing primary care physicians in their primary service area to provide convenient points of access for patients and to secure a primary care base for the specialists who utilize the hospital. WCH employs thirty-six physicians and seven midlevel providers in eight clinics, specializing in internal medicine, family practice, infectious disease, and gynecology.

In 2011, the WCH board of directors adopted a plan to implement a systemwide EHR to, among other things, improve patient safety, integrate information from ancillary systems, and provide access to patient information for all WCH caregivers. In addition, the plan calls for an evaluation of the effectiveness of the WCH physician clinic organization's EHR.

The WCH clinics currently use the XYZ Data Systems Integrated EHR and Practice Management System. This system has been operational for four years. The XYZ system was chosen because of its compatibility with the hospital's Meditech platform. Physician needs and application functionality were secondary considerations. As a result, physician system adoption and support has been poor. Under prior leadership, the hospital information technology (IT) department provided limited support for the XYZ EHR. The clinic organization was left to develop its own internal IT capabilities to manage the XYZ system and, as a result, the system has not been routinely updated.

The hospital has decided to stay with the Meditech platform to address the IT strategic plan for an integrated EHR. The clinic organization must now evaluate whether it is in their best interest to stay with the XYZ system, with strong Meditech compatibility, or move to a different EHR platform. The path of least resistance from the IT perspective would be to upgrade the XYZ system. This option offers the greatest integration and could be implemented much sooner. A new platform would require an evaluation and selection process and a significant conversion. With either scenario, physician support will be critical to a successful transition.

EHR Project Plan

Next is a description of the planning process developed by the leadership team to transition to a replacement EHR. Read and critique the plan by answering the questions that follow it.

Project Organization

The organizational phase of the project will involve establishing a project steering committee and identifying the leadership members who will ensure the project's success. WCH operates eight separate clinics, each with their unique teams and EHR experience. By necessity, the steering committee will need representation from each of these clinics. The project steering committee will likely have twenty to twenty-five members. In addition to provider representatives, the steering committee will also include nurses, medical assistants, and office managers from each clinic. IT representation is critical to the success of the project, and since the department provided poor IT support in the past, the chief information officer (CIO) will play an active role on the steering committee. A representative from finance should also participate on the committee, given the importance of billing and collections and other practice management issues.

The leadership of the steering committee will ensure the committee addresses key steps in the process and does so in a timely fashion. Ideally, the committee would be chaired by a provider who is respected within the group, is objective, and is a supporter of EHR technology. Although the clinic organization does not have a provider who meets all of these criteria, a physician with strong peer support and credibility will be selected to cochair the steering committee. To complement the clinical leadership, the CIO will serve as a cochair for the committee, providing technical expertise. This individual has implemented other EHR systems and will bring a structured process to the committee to ensure a thorough evaluation process.

Committee Development

Organizations often overlook the importance of understanding the emotional climate of a medical practice when implementing an EHR. Therefore, although the first task of the steering committee will be to define the project objectives, the existing concerns about an EHR transition require that a fair amount of time be devoted to addressing the emotional needs of the participants. Listening to practitioners and empathizing with their concerns will be critical to establish trust and overcome resistance during the EHR conversion.

To address this important issue, a series of discussion exercises will be used to encourage open dialogue and participant engagement. The first exercise will break the large group into teams of four to five members, and each team will discuss the lessons learned from the XYZ implementation that took place four years earlier. Team leaders will be handpicked for their facilitation skills and ability to listen. The group discussions will address the "change readiness" and will surface the major issues associated with the implementation. It will also allow the group members to get to know each other in a less formal setting than the large group. The larger committee will reconvene to discuss their findings and prepare a master list of implementation lessons learned.

While this exercise may raise a number of issues related to implementation, it is also important to openly discuss the current issues with the existing

EHR. Once again, small groups will be asked to discuss these issues to ensure participation by all members of the steering committee. Small groups will report out to the large group, and a summary of issues will be developed. This list, as well as the list of implementation issues, will set the stage for a later discussion regarding the scope of the project.

Project Scope and Objectives

Once the group has had the opportunity to express personal concerns and key issues have been identified, the group can turn their attention to defining the project objectives. Anxious committee members are often tempted to begin discussing whether the steering committee should upgrade this system or consider alternatives. When this occurs, discussions and conclusions are usually based on the emotional attachment to or disappointment with the current system. A more systematic review process will help frame this discussion to ensure the conclusion is based on facts and the needs of the clinic organization.

The leadership must guide the committee in developing project objectives that are based on the needs of the organization, not individuals. Returning to the list of implementation and current issues, the group will be asked to prioritize the concerns that were raised. This prioritization will focus the committee on the most pressing issues that must be addressed. With this background work, the committee will be positioned to articulate the goals of the committee. It will also define the scope of the project by determining what the project is and isn't intended to address. Invariably, users will raise issues that may not be solved by an EHR application. It is important that the end users review all issues, even though some of those issues may not prove to be within the scope of the project. Users with unrealistic expectations can end up frustrated and disengaged as the process unfolds. Defining the scope and the objectives clarifies expectations before options are considered.

Communication

The steering committee will need to establish plans to communicate with the larger audience of clinic users and stakeholders. A plan will be developed that provides this audience with regular updates. The plan must also address how the committee can solicit feedback from stakeholders during the evaluation and selection process. Regular minutes establish the record of the committee's work and provide a means for communicating with stakeholders. Special meetings with individual clinic groups will also be necessary to address rumors or provide more detailed information regarding the process. The steering committee must communicate regularly to ensure information is flowing to individuals.

Plan of Work

Once project objectives are established, the committee will prepare a plan of work. This plan will outline the specific action steps required to achieve the project objectives and the timeline for their completion. The plan of work focuses on the decision to upgrade the existing XYZ application and remain with a Meditech platform or move to a different software solution. The plan of work provides the steering committee with the road map to achieve their goals.

The key steps in the plan of work are identifying possible vendors, establishing system requirements, and completing a request for proposal (RFP) process. Vendor identification can occur simultaneously with establishing the project goals. This is a reasonable assertion as it will save time and will engage the clinic representatives in the process. The steering committee will select individuals to attend trade shows to maximize exposure to EHR products. IT staff will also participate in this review process to address technical requirements and issues.

Establishing system requirements is a critical step in the EHR decision-making process. The system requirements identify the needs of the organization and are the basis for the vendor evaluation process. The implementation and current issues lists developed by the committee will be used to develop the system requirements. Each clinic employee will receive a summary of these lists, and staff will be asked to provide additional input to steering committee representatives. In addition, the IT department will conduct a thorough evaluation of new advancements in EHRs and regulatory requirements that may impact the EMR choice. The first draft of the system requirements will be preliminary. As the steering committee begins to interact with vendors and complete site visits, additional functionality may be added to the requirements. It would not be prudent to submit RFPs to all vendors who claim to have a functional EHR. The steering committee will need to determine the top five to seven vendors, judging by the initial survey of qualified vendors, trade shows, and market information.

Well-defined system requirements will need to be established and included in the request for proposals. Packaging the system requirements in a format that provides structure for vendor responses and steering committee evaluations of vendor responses will be important, as will establishing a record of documentation throughout the acquisition process. The RFP document will provide the following:

1. Instructions for vendors
2. Organizational objectives
3. Organization background information
4. System goals and requirements

The vendors will be required to submit the following:

1. Vendor qualifications
2. Proposed solutions
3. Criteria for evaluating proposals
4. Contractual requirements
5. Pricing and support

The vendor review process will also encompass technical calls, vendor fairs, reference checks, site visits, and vendor presentations. These elements of the review process are designed to ensure that sufficient information is gathered to augment the proposals submitted by the vendors. It will not be feasible for all steering committee members to participate in these activities; therefore, individuals will be appointed to participate on their behalf.

Prior to reviewing the vendor proposals, the steering committee will develop vendor criteria that can be used to evaluate the proposals. Each member of the steering committee will be asked to score the proposals based on the criteria, and a summary score report will be developed. The Watson Community Hospital CEO will give the final approval to proceed with the conversion based on the report and recommendation from the steering committee. However, the final recommendation of the committee will not be based solely on the score report. Ideally, the final deliberations will involve a robust dialogue based on the mutual trust that has developed over time. Ultimately, the committee will balance their objective assessment of options with their intuition and their considerable knowledge of the clinic organization.

Conclusion

The WCH clinic organization will undergo a significant EHR transition if they upgrade the XYZ system or purchase another product. The process that is outlined in this plan provides the organization the best opportunity to make the right decision for the organization and establish support with key stakeholders for an EHR conversion. A good IT decision-making process requires discipline and objectivity. The structural elements of the process involve leadership, committee structure, system requirements, and a thorough RFP and evaluation process.

Discussion Questions

1. What are the strengths of this plan? What aspects do you think are particularly important?

2. How could the plan be improved? What, if anything, might you do differently if you were leading the effort? Explain your rationale.

3. What factors should the leadership team consider when deciding whether to stay with a single vendor for supporting both the hospital and primary care settings?

CASE 18: ASSESSING THE VALUE OF HEALTH IT INVESTMENT

Major theme: Value assessment

Background Information

Five years ago, senior leadership at the Southeast Medical Center made the decision to embark on the implementation of a host of new clinical applications in the inpatient units enterprise-wide. The four hospitals that comprise Southeast Medical Center include the Main Adult Hospital, the Children's Hospital, McKinsey Hospital, and the Institute of Psychiatry. They contracted with McKesson to implement the following applications:

- ED tracking system
- Replacement pharmacy information system
- Clinical documentation system (for all nurses and ancillary personnel; does not include physician notes)
- Medication administration using bar-coding technology
- Computerized provider order entry (CPOE)

In addition, several administrative applications were implemented, including a new operative scheduling system and materials management system. They also upgraded their clinical data repository viewer (referred to as Oacis). All applications are now operational.

Most recently, the board of trustees has approved replacement of Southeast's ambulatory care EHR. A system known as EasyDoc (a McKesson product) has been in use for years. However, the system was viewed by clinicians and

IT staff as antiquated and cumbersome to navigate. It is also very difficult to retrieve aggregate data from the system. Much of this is apparently due to its underlying database architecture and structure. EasyDoc also did not interface with the hospital clinical applications, and leaders were concerned that the system was not going to enable Southeast to achieve meaningful use criteria.

Clinicians have also been frustrated that Southeast has been using two different EHR systems, one for inpatient, and another for outpatient, and the two don't interface or give a complete picture of the patient's health record. With payment reform and the need to be able to more effectively manage patient care quality and outcomes, senior leaders recommended, and the board approved, replacement of the EasyDoc EHR with Epic ambulatory care EHR. The patient registration and billing system used in ambulatory care will also be replaced with Epic's practice management application. Long-term plans are to eventually replace the McKesson clinical applications with Epic in the inpatient sector as well.

The total cost of ownership for the replacement ambulatory EHR and practice management system is approximately $30 million. Included in this estimate are not only the software and hardware upgrades but also staff needed to implement and support the new applications. Replacing the McKesson clinical products with Epic inpatient EHR will be an additional $90 million. Again, this is an estimated total cost of ownership.

The primary purpose of the Epic EHR project is to provide clinicians access to a single, complete electronic health record that spans the patient's continuum of care and improves collaboration and coordination of care. Community providers and patients will have access to the system. Community partners (such as primary care providers) will be able to retrieve important patient information. Currently a local HIE exists that provides ED visit information to all local hospitals. This is to be expanded to include continuity of care documents (CCDs) and other relevant health information. Patients will be given access to their health information such as lab tests, X-ray results, and medications. They will also be able to schedule appointments and pay their bills online through a patient portal known as MyChart. Southeast physician leaders view patients as partners in their own care and are pleased to provide them access to information electronically.

Southeast providers treat a large population of patients with multiple chronic conditions. Managing chronic diseases using evidence-based, real-time support is considered essential. In addition, Southeast Medical Center has available a secure data warehouse of patient data that researchers and clinicians will be using more fully in the future to ensure that clinical research drives best care.

Discussion Questions

Assume you've been tasked with developing a plan to assess the value of Southeast's investment in the Epic outpatient and inpatient systems and expansion of its use of the data warehouse. The board is interested in knowing how these new and replacement systems have affected or will affect Southeast's ability to offer coordinated, collaborative care in a cost-effective manner. The facility fully intends to meet meaningful use criteria and report on quality outcomes. They realize that the traditional fee-for-service system in which providers are paid on volume will be a thing of the past.

1. How would you determine which metrics to use? Who would be involved in the process?

2. How would you know that a change is attributable to the EHR or data warehouse system and not something else?

3. Do you think traditional return on investment methods are useful in this case? Why or why not?

SUGGESTED LISTING OF PUBLISHED HEALTH IT-RELATED CASES

Information Technology and Clinical Operations at Beth Israel Deaconess Medical Center

by Richard Bohmer, F. Warren McFarlan

Source: Harvard Business School. 24 pages. Publication date: June 4, 2007. Prod. #: 607150-PDF-ENG

Describes the history of clinical computing at Boston's Beth Israel Hospital and the development, since the 1996 merger to form the Beth Israel Deaconess Medical Center, of an information system designed to support the delivery of patient care. The hospitals' CIO, John Halamka, MD, has overseen the development of an information system that places physicians at its center. Describes the design and function of five major components of the system: the online medical record, e-prescribing, physician order entry, the emergency department "dashboard," and the performance manager. Provides students with an opportunity to identify key design principles for health care information systems, and to discuss the unique implementation challenges that the health care delivery setting raises for CIOs and CEOs.

Partners Healthcare System: Transforming Health Care Services Delivery through Information Management

by Richard M. Kesner

Source: Richard Ivey School of Business Foundation. 15 pages. Publication date: Feb. 26, 2010. Prod. #: 909E23-PDF-ENG

This case considers the process of organizational transformation under-taken by Partners Healthcare System (PHS) since the 1990s as their hospital and affiliated ambulatory medical practices have adopted both EMR and CPOE systems. Encompassing a strategic investment in information technologies, widespread process change, and the pervasive use of institutional clinical decision-support and knowledge management systems, this story has been fifteen years in the making, culminating in 2009 with the networkwide use of EMR and CPOE by all PHS doctors. These developments in turn opened the door to the redefinition of services delivery and to the replacement of estab-lished therapies through the leveraging of the knowledge residing in 4.6 million now-digitized PHS patient records. As such, the PHS experience serves as a window into how one organization strove to address the daunting challenges of twenty-first-century health care services information management, as a template for success in the implementation of large-scale information systems among research-based hospitals across the United States, and more broadly as a learning platform for industry executives in their efforts to transform health care delivery through data and knowledge management.

Mount Auburn Hospital: Physician Order Entry

by Andrew McAfee, Sarah MacGregor, Michael Benari

Source: Harvard Business School. 18 pages. Publication date: Dec. 17, 2002. Prod. #: 603060-PDF-ENG

Mount Auburn Hospital is preparing to introduce a physician order entry (POE) system throughout the hospital, starting with the labor and delivery ward. POE systems replace paper-based and oral medication ordering processes with an information system; the physician uses the system to enter medication orders, which are then transferred to the hospital's pharmacy. This is Mount Auburn's first experience with POE systems, and the implementation team must determine how best to introduce the technology to the physicians and other personnel who will use it.

Moore Medical Corporation

by Andrew McAfee, Gregory Bounds

Source: Harvard Business School. 21 pages. Publication date: Apr. 23, 2001. Prod. #: 601142-PDF-ENG

Moore Medical is a medium-sized distributor of medical supplies to practitioners such as podiatrists and emergency medical technicians. At the time of the case, it has relied on traditional customer channels such as catalogues, phones, and faxes to communicate product offerings, promotions, and availability, and to take orders. It is now attempting to shift to a "bricks and clicks" distributor with a strong Internet presence. It has already made substantial investments in an e-commerce web site and in "back office" ERP software to improve the fulfillment performance of its four distribution centers. The ERP software has not lived up to expectations in all areas, and the company must decide whether to invest in more modules for this system that might address its shortcomings. It must also decide whether to make a significant additional investment in customer relationship management software.

CareGroup

by F. Warren McFarlan, Robert D. Austin

Source: HBS Premier Case Collection. 22 pages. Publication date: Jan. 29, 2003. Prod. #: 303097-PDF-ENG

Describes the circumstances leading to the three-and-a-half-day collapse of a major hospital group's IS capabilities. Identifies the technical reasons for the failure, management steps in dealing with the problem short-term, and the long-term lessons they believe they learned from the incident. This case is accompanied by a short video for educators to show in class.

University Health Network: The MOE-MAR Initiative

by Darren Meister, Ken Mark

Source: Richard Ivey School of Business Foundation. 22 pages. Publication date: Feb. 9, 2010. Prod. #: 906E13-PDF-ENG

The director of acute care information management at University Health Network is thinking about how to form a steering committee and several working groups to manage the implementation and ongoing operation of the medication order entry and medication administration record module. This initiative would be the most challenging and complex the IT department had ever undertaken. She would need to address the concerns of administration, physicians, and nurses.

STARS Air Ambulance: An Information Systems Challenge

by Malcolm Munro, Sid L. Huff

Source: Richard Ivey School of Business Foundation. 12 pages.
   Publication date: Feb. 26, 2008. Prod. #: 908E04-PDF-ENG

Shock Trauma Air Rescue Society (STARS) in Calgary, Canada, provides a safe, rapid, highly specialized, emergency medical transport system for the critically ill and injured by dispatching helicopters and air medical crew at any time. STARS operates a sophisticated communication system that links together hospitals, ground ambulance services, police, firefighters, search and rescue organizations, and park wardens. The recently appointed chief information officer (CIO) expected to inherit a sound information systems (IS) operation but soon discovered a number of problems that seriously impeded his ability to manage progress. These included a poorly organized department, excessive and undisciplined use of consultants, inadequate project management, independent IS operations and IS staff in other departments, other managers possibly resistant to change, and an IS department with no clearly organized role or mission. The basic issue in this case concerns what action the new CIO must undertake to ensure that the IS department can fully support the organization's mission.

Secrets of HIE Success Revealed: Lessons from the Leaders

by National eHealth Collaborative

Source: http://www.nationalehealth.org/ckfinder/userfiles/files
   /REPORT%20SecretsofHIESuccessRevealed.pdf

Publication Date: July 2011

This report features twelve case studies of health information exchange (HIE) organizations that are leaders in achieving sustainable enterprises built on the value created by efficiently exchanging health information and mobilizing its effective use at the point of care. These organizations have focused on building a successful HIE through innovation, continuous learning, and business discipline with the end goal of improving quality, care coordination, and cost-effectiveness of health care. Although each organization's business model and strategy is unique, reflecting the local, community-based nature of health care, each profile offers a rich source of ideas and guidance to help HIE organizations that are at earlier stages of their life cycle succeed.

NOTE

1. Information for this case was taken from J. C. Collmann and T. Cooper, "Breaching the Security of the Kaiser Permanente Internet Patient Portal: The Organizational Foundations of Information Security," *Journal of the American Medical Informatics Association*, 2007, *14*(2), 239–243.

Overview of the Health Care IT Industry

There is a health care information technology (IT) industry. This industry is composed of companies that provide hardware, software, and a wide range of services, including consulting and outsourcing, to health care organizations. The industry also includes associations that support the professional advancement of the health care IT professional, organizations that put on industry conferences, and publications that cover current topics and issues in the industry.

It is not possible to develop an IT strategy and implement that strategy without engaging this industry.

This appendix provides an overview of this industry. It will discuss

- The size, structure, and composition of the health care IT industry and characteristics of health care that affect the application of IT products and services
- Sources of information about that industry
- Health care IT associations

THE HEALTH CARE IT INDUSTRY

Health care is the largest sector of the U.S. economy ($2.8 trillion in 2012). It is not surprising that a large, diverse, and robust industry has developed to provide IT products and services to that sector. The health care IT industry is generally viewed as having three major markets; health care providers, health care insurance companies, and health care suppliers: for example, pharmaceutical companies, medical supply distribution companies, and health care device manufacturers. Some industry analyses cover the global health care IT market, and others focus on the market in the United States. We will focus on the health care provider market in the United States. (Appendix C provides a discussion of the international health care provider IT market.)

Size of the Industry

The health care IT market is expected to grow at a compound annual rate of 16 percent, reaching $53.8 billion worldwide by 2014 (MarketResearch.com, 2009). In general, growth in IT spending among health care providers is attributed to providers' pursuing IT "answers" to a range of challenges and issues facing them:

- Concerns over patient safety can lead to investments in computerized provider order entry (CPOE) and medication administration record systems.
- Cost pressures can lead to the use of IT to improve organizational efficiency.
- Problems with shortages of health care professionals and cost pressures can result in efforts to use IT to improve operational efficiency and reduce staff workloads.
- Compliance with new health care regulations, such as rules designed to improve the security of information systems or reduce fraudulent billing, often requires an IT response.
- Desires to improve patient service can lead to new systems designed to improve the process of obtaining an appointment or to reduce test result turnaround time.
- Initiatives designed to prepare the organization for payment reform will need a diverse supporting IT agenda.

Such answers are identified during the IT strategy and alignment process that was discussed in Chapter Thirteen.

The typical health care provider's IT spending is proportioned across the categories listed in Table A.1.

IT Spending Relative to Other Industries

Health care organizations will spend, on average, about 2.7 percent of their revenues on IT. This spending includes the cost of internal IT staff and the

Table A.1. Typical provider distribution of IT spending

Expenditure Category	Percentage of IT Spending
Hardware	10
Internal services	22
Software	7
Telecommunications[a]	28
IT services[b]	33

[a]Networks, Internet connections, and telephone costs.
[b]Implementation, consulting, and product maintenance services.
Source: Gartner, 2007.

cost of purchasing products and services from the market. Other industries spend more: for example, banks will spend 5.1 percent of their revenues on IT (Gartner, 2008).

Why does health care have this apparently lower level of IT spending than other information-intensive industries? To some degree the percentages reflect the cost structure of health care. Being a health care provider is a very labor- and capital-intensive business. Provider organizations must have a large number of relatively expensive staff such as physicians, nurses, and other health care professionals. Few other industries have this density of expensive workers. Health care providers, particularly hospitals, must invest large sums of money in buildings, supplies, and equipment. Manufacturers are also capital intensive; they must invest in plants and manufacturing equipment. However, most service organizations—for example, law firms, consulting organizations, and financial institutions—do not have the same levels of demand for buildings and equipment.

Hence, the relatively low percentages result from the need to make significant investments and bear significant ongoing costs in other aspects of the organization. The salaries of health care professionals and the costs of buildings, supplies, and equipment overshadow health care IT costs.

Other factors also play a role in producing relatively low levels of health care investment in IT:

- For many years health care organizations viewed IT as important for supporting day-to-day operations but not important strategically. An organization might believe that it was strategically more important to establish a new imaging center than it was to invest in an electronic health record system. To a degree, this orientation is changing as health care organizations realize that they cannot accomplish care improvement (and many other) goals without substantial IT investments. However, it can also be argued that IT is indeed less important in health care than in other industries. If a bank's computer systems stop working, the bank immediately stops working. No checks can be cashed. Taking deposits becomes difficult. In contrast, if a hospital's systems stop working, surgery can go on, medications can be given, and phlebotomists can draw blood.

- Health care organizations have fewer ways than other types of organizations do to obtain capital. Publicly traded organizations can issue stock. Health care organizations often have small operating margins that make it difficult for them to obtain debt from the bond market. This often-limited ability to obtain capital hinders these organizations' ability to make large IT investments.

- Many health care organizations are very small, having revenues of less than $40 million. Small organizations face a very difficult time hiring and retaining talented IT staff. This problem can make an organization hesitant to pursue IT investments because it is not sure that it can support the systems.

- IT investments often have their most significant impact when the operations that they are to support are complex and have large volumes of activity. For a small health care organization, the volume and complexity of activity may be sufficiently limited that an IT investment would not result in enough gain to justify that investment.

Structure of the Health Care Market

Table A.2 displays the taxonomy of the health care industry as defined by the North American Industry Classification System (NAICS). The NAICS outlines three major industry segments: payers, providers, and government health care. Each of the sectors in this classification (with each sector having a different NAICS code) represents a different submarket in health care. Some IT companies focus on the federal health care system, others on nursing homes, and yet others on physician offices. Some focus even more narrowly. Within the hospital sector (NAICS code 6222), for example, some IT companies focus on large academic medical centers and others focus on small community hospitals.

The health care IT market is not homogeneous. Different companies serve different segments. Some companies serve multiple segments by carrying diverse product lines or offering systems that will work in multiple sectors: for example, a clinical laboratory system is of interest to civilian and federal hospitals, large physician groups, and freestanding clinical laboratories.

Table A.2. Health care vertical market: NAICS taxonomy

Health care providers	Ambulatory services	Physician offices Dentist offices Other health Outpatient centers Laboratories Home health
	Hospitals	General medical and surgical Psychiatric and substance abuse Specialty hospitals
	Nursing and residential care	Nursing care Mental care Elderly care
Insurance	Health	Accident and health insurance Hospital and medical Service plans
Government health		Federal hospitals Local hospitals Government psychiatric and long-term care

Source: Gartner, 2008.

A rough taxonomy of companies that serve health care can be constructed:

- Some companies strive to have a product and service line that covers the full spectrum of health care settings. Hence, these companies will offer hospital information systems, physician office systems, nursing home applications, and applications for ancillary departments, such as radiology.
- Several companies focus on a specific setting: for example, hospitals or the physician's office, but not both.
- Some companies offer products that support an application needed by multiple sectors: for example, pharmacy systems or systems that support claims electronic data interchange between providers and payers.
- Some companies offer infrastructure: for example, workstations, networks, and servers that are used by all sectors. These companies usually do not offer applications.
- Several companies offer services used by multiple sectors: for example, IT strategic planning, application implementation, and consulting services.
- Some companies focus their service offerings on a specific type of organization—for example, improving the operations of physician

practices—or a specific type of service—for example, improving collections of overdue payments for a provider billing office.

There are literally thousands of companies that support the IT needs of the health care industry. In any given year, hundreds of companies may go out of business and hundreds of new companies may emerge. You can gain an appreciation of the diversity of health care IT companies by attending a large health care IT conference, such as the annual conference of the Healthcare Information and Management Systems Society (HIMSS), and visiting the exhibit hall.

Later in this appendix, we will present sources of IT information. These sources often discuss the products and services of health care IT companies.

Major Suppliers of Health Care IT Products and Services

Table A.3 provides a summary of the top vendors in the industry. These data, collected by the publication *Healthcare Informatics* (2011), rank companies according to their health information technology (HIT) revenue. Use such lists with caution, of course. In any given year, some companies will be acquired, and others will experience dramatic upturns and downturns in financial performance. Companies will disappear from the list, and companies will arrive on the list over the course of time. The products and services listed in Table A.3 are illustrative but do not make up a comprehensive list. Moreover, the fact that a company is large does not mean that it has the best solution for a particular need of a particular organization.

Table A.3. Major health care IT vendors, ranked by revenue

Company	HIT Revenue	Types of Products and Services
McKesson	$3.0 B	Applications, consulting services
Dell	$2.5 B	Hosting and infrastructure services
Care Fusion	$2.4 B	Medication safety technologies
GE	$1.9 B	Applications, consulting services
Cerner	$1.7 B	Applications, infrastructure services
CSC	$1.6 B	Consulting and integration services
Siemens	$1.4 B	Applications, infrastructure services
Emdeon	$900 M	Revenue cycle and clinical applications
Cognizant	$860 M	Integration and development services
Phillips	$780 M	Applications

Source: Company and revenue data from *Healthcare Informatics*, 2011.

Nonetheless, the data in Table A.3 are interesting for several reasons:

- Health care leadership should know the names and have a reasonable understanding of the major IT vendors that serve their type of organization; sooner or later the organization will be doing business with some of these vendors.
- The size of some of these companies is apparent, with several companies taking in over $1 billion in revenue.
- The diversity of products and services is also apparent. Some companies focus on applications, whereas others focus on consulting, outsourcing, data analysis, or transcription services.

When an organization needs to turn to the market for applications, infrastructure, or services, its leadership would be well served by reviewing several of the sources of information described in this appendix, talking to colleagues who may have recently pursued similar IT products and services, and engaging the services of consultants who keep close tabs on the health care IT industry.

SOURCES OF INDUSTRY INFORMATION

It is essential for the health care professional to identify sources that he or she can trust for current information on health care IT. This textbook cannot examine all the terrain covered by this industry. Moreover, the face of the industry can change quickly. New companies arrive as others disappear. New technologies emerge, and people's understanding of current technologies improves. Federal legislation that affects what health care IT is expected to do can surface rapidly.

These sources of information should be diverse: colleagues, consultants, vendors, conferences, and trade press. It takes time and some effort to identify your best sources. You will find some consultants helpful and others not so helpful. You will note that some publications are insightful and others are not.

The following sections provide a brief overview of publications you may find useful.

Periodicals

Among the high-quality health care information technology periodicals (journals and magazines) are

- *Health Data Management*
- *Health Management Technology*

- *Healthcare Informatics*
- *Healthcare IT News*

All the associations discussed later in this appendix also publish journals, magazines, or newsletters.

These publications can be supplemented with periodicals that cover the overall IT industry. They include

- *CIO*
- *CIO Insight*
- *Computerworld*
- *Information Week*

Several periodicals focus on vertical segments of technology; *Network World* and *eWeek* are examples.

Several periodicals address cross-industry management issues, including IT. These publications are

- *BusinessWeek*
- *The Economist*
- *The Harvard Business Review*
- *MIT Sloan Management Review*

In addition, there are magazines and journals that cover health care broadly. They often publish articles and stories on IT issues:

- *Health Affairs*
- *Hospitals & Health Networks*
- *Modern Healthcare*

You can obtain subscription information for these publications by visiting their web sites. An afternoon at a university library, medical library, or large public library spent perusing these publications would be worthwhile.

Books

In any given year, several books that cover various aspects of health care IT are published. Publishers that routinely produce such books and publish conference proceedings include

- Elsevier
- Healthcare Information and Management Systems Society
- John Wiley & Sons
- Jossey-Bass
- Springer-Verlag

Industry Research Firms

Finally, there are industry research firms that routinely cover IT generally and health care specifically. Such firms include Forrester, KLAS, Gartner, the Advisory Board, and HIMSS Analytics. These firms, and others, do a nice job of analyzing industry trends, critiquing the products and services of major vendors, and assessing emerging technologies and technology issues. They provide written analyses, conferences, and access to their analysts.

HEALTH CARE IT ASSOCIATIONS

All health care professionals should join associations that are dedicated to advancing and educating their profession. Health care chief financial officers (CFOs) often join the Healthcare Financial Management Association, and health care executives routinely join the American College of Healthcare Executives.

These associations serve several useful purposes for the person who joins. They provide

- Publications on topics of interest to the profession
- Conferences, symposiums, and other educational programs
- Information on careers and career development opportunities
- Data that can be used to compare performance across organizations
- Opportunities to meet colleagues who share similar jobs and hence have similar challenges and interests
- Staff who work with legislators and regulators on issues that affect the profession

These association products and services can be invaluable sources of information and experience for any organization or individual.

The health care IT industry has several associations that serve the needs of the health care IT professional. People who are not health care IT professionals will find that their own profession's association also routinely provides periodical articles and conference sessions that cover IT issues. For example, the Healthcare Financial Management Association may present conference sessions on IT advances in analyzing the costs of care or in streamlining patient accounting and billing processes.

The health care IT industry associations are discussed in the following sections. Additional information on these associations can be obtained through each association's web site.

American Health Information Management Association (AHIMA)

AHIMA is an association of health information management professionals. AHIMA serves largely what has historically been known as the medical records professional. AHIMA's members confront a diverse range of issues associated with both the paper and the electronic medical record, including privacy, data standards and coding, management of the record, appropriate uses of medical record information, and state and federal regulations that govern the medical record.

AHIMA sponsors an annual conference, produces publications, makes a series of knowledge resources available (news, practice guidelines, and competency tests), posts job opportunities, supports distance learning opportunities, and engages in federal and state policy lobbying. AHIMA also offers local and state chapters, which have their own conferences and resources.

The health information management profession has a process for certifying the skill levels of its professionals. AHIMA manages that certification process.

American Medical Informatics Association (AMIA)

AMIA is an association of individuals and organizations "dedicated to developing and using information technologies to improve health care." AMIA focuses on clinical information systems, and a large portion of its membership has an interest and training in the academic discipline of medical informatics. AMIA brings together an interesting mix of practitioners and academics.

AMIA offers an annual symposium, a spring congress, a journal, a series of working groups and special interest groups, and a resource center with job opportunities, publications, and news. AMIA carries out initiatives designed to influence federal policy on health care IT issues.

College of Healthcare Information Management Executives (CHIME)

CHIME is an association dedicated to advancing the health care chief information officer (CIO) profession and improving the strategic use of IT in health care (CIOs were discussed in Chapter Twelve). CHIME provides two annual forums, a newsletter, employment information, a data warehouse of information contributed by its members and vendors, distance learning sessions, and classroom-style training. CHIME is partially supported by the CHIME Foundation, established as a nonprofit organization by a group of vendors and consultants committed to advancing the CIO profession.

Healthcare Information and Management Systems Society (HIMSS)

HIMSS is an association dedicated to "providing leadership for the optimal use of health care information technology and management systems for the betterment of human health." HIMSS members are diverse, covering all segments and professions in the health care IT industry.

HIMSS sponsors an annual conference and series of symposiums and smaller conferences. It publishes books, a journal, and newsletters. HIMSS member services include employment information, industry and vendor information, certification programs, distance learning, and white papers. The association has special interest groups and local chapters, and it is actively working with the federal government to develop policy.

Other Industry Groups and Associations

Within the health care IT industry, organizations also exist that serve the needs of health care organizations (in contrast to the individual professional). This section will not attempt to list and describe them. However, examples include the University HealthSystem Consortium, which serves academic health centers; Voluntary Hospitals of America, which provides services to hospitals; and the Scottsdale Institute, whose members are large integrated delivery systems. These and other similar organizations have a partial or dedicated focus on health care IT.

All the associations and groups mentioned in this discussion provide publications and conferences. In addition, companies whose business is putting on conferences sometimes offer health care IT events. Quality publications in addition to those listed previously are available. The reader who is interested in developing a deeper appreciation of the wealth of conference and publication opportunities can type "healthcare IT publications" and "healthcare IT conferences" into a web search engine to locate many online sources of information.

SUMMARY

The health care IT industry is large and growing. The many pressures on health care organizations to perform and comply are leading them to invest in IT. The industry is served by a multitude of companies that provide products and services. These companies are diverse, both in revenue and in their choice of focus within the submarkets that compose the health care industry.

Professionals in the health care IT industry have formed associations that serve their information and development needs. These associations and industry publications are terrific sources of information on industry issues, emerging technologies, and the strengths and weaknesses of companies serving the industry. The industry faces a core challenge in its application of IT to improve health care; the complexities of care processes, medical data, and health care are often proving to have no boundaries.

LEARNING ACTIVITIES

1. Identify two companies that serve the health care IT market. Write a summary that lists each company's products, services, market focus, and size. Compare the two companies.

2. Pick one of the health care IT associations listed in this appendix. Develop a summary that describes the association's membership, activities, products, and services.

3. Select two periodicals that serve the health care IT industry and review an issue of each one. Comment on the types of topics and issues that these publications address.

REFERENCES

Gartner, Inc. (2007). Gartner identifies the top 10 strategic technologies for 2011. Retrieved November 2011 from http://www.gartner.com/it/page.jsp?id=1454221

Gartner, Inc. (2008). Forecast: Healthcare IT spending worldwide, 2006–2011. Stamford, CT: Author.

Healthcare Informatics. (2011). 2010 Healthcare Informatics 100 list. http://www .healthcare-informatics.com/ME2/dirsect.asp?nm=The+2010+HCI+100+List&sid=3F D926E0A2884506947FD7451869716C

MarketResearch.com. (2009). Global healthcare information technology (2009–2114). Rockville, MD: Author. http://www.marketresearch.com/MarketsandMarkets -v3719

APPENDIX B

Sample Project Charter

Information Systems

Mobile Mammography Van

Project Charter

Version 1.0

Created: 08/01/2012

Printed:

Prepared by: Sam Smith

Presented to: Karen Zimmerman

Project Charter Table of Contents

VISION OF THE SOLUTION
    Vision Statement
    Major Features
    Assumptions and Dependencies
    Related Projects
SCOPE AND LIMITATIONS
    Scope of Initial Release
    Scope of Subsequent Releases
    Out of Scope
PROJECT SUCCESS FACTORS
BUDGET HIGHLIGHTS
TIMELINE
PROJECT ORGANIZATION
PROJECT MANAGEMENT STRATEGIES
    Project Meetings
    Issue Management
    Scope Change Management
    Training Strategy
    Documentation Development Strategy
    Project Work Paper Organization and Coordination

FOREWORD

The purpose of a Project Charter is to document what the Project Team is committed to deliver. It specifies the project timeline, resources, and implementation standards. The Project Charter is the cornerstone of the project and is used for managing the expectations of all project stakeholders.

A Project Charter represents a formal commitment among Business Sponsors, Business Owners, Steering Committees, the Project Manager, and the Project Team. Therefore, it is the professional responsibility of all project members to treat this agreement seriously and make every effort to meet the commitment it represents.

Table B.1. Revision history

Name	Date	Reason for Changes	Ver./Rev.

BUSINESS REQUIREMENTS

Background

Sponsored by the Ogilvey Cancer Institute in partnership with the Boston Public Health Commission, neighborhood health centers, and community groups, Boston's Mammography Van provides mammography screening and breast health education throughout the City of Boston to all women, regardless of ability to pay, with a priority on serving uninsured and underserved women right in their neighborhoods. The Mammography Van program began in April of 2012, using GE software for registration, scheduling, and billing. All clinical documentation of the mammography screening has been performed manually since April 2012. Statistical reports generated to maintain state and federal guidelines are all done manually.

Project Overview

The project has two major objectives:

- Implementation of Mammography Patient Manager software to allow for online documentation of the clinical encounter with the patient.
- Implementation of a wireless solution on the van at the time of the new software implementation. This will allow real-time updating of the patient appointment information as well as registering walk-on patients on the spot. Online documentation will allow ease of reporting to the state and federal agencies.

The products evaluated for implementation are specific to the needs of a mobile program and will meet most, if not all, of the needs of the program.

Project Objectives

Boston's Mobile Mammography Van program will benefit monetarily with a software system because of the reporting capabilities available with online documentation. Grant money, as well as state and federal money, is available to the program if evidence is produced to support the needs of the grant and/ or the state and federal guidelines of mammography programs. The program will be more easily able to report on the information required by grants and governments to receive funding. There is also the current possibility that we are losing funding as a result of our current manual reporting practice.

The current program's resources spend valuable time manually calculating statistics. A software system will automate these processes, thus freeing the resources to perform more valuable functions. The van's mammography technician spends a lot of time manually updating and calculating which clients require additional follow-up. A software system will allow real-time reporting of which clients require which type of follow-up. This will decrease the amount of time the technician will spend manually determining which patient requires which follow-up letter. The program will be secure in its adherence to state and federal reporting guidelines for the van program as well as for the technicians working in the program.

Value Provided to Customers

- Improved productivity and reduced rework
- Streamlined business processes
- Automation of previously manual tasks
- Ability to perform entirely new tasks or functions
- Conformance to current standards or regulations
- Improved access to patient clinical and demographic information via remote access
- Reduced frustration level compared to current process

Business Risks

The major risk associated with the implementation is the selection of an incompatible vendor. There is always the concern that with a program that is new to the institution, the understanding needed to fully anticipate the needs of the program is incomplete. In addition, there is the risk that the software solution will increase workload as it offers more functions than are currently available to the user in a manual system.

Risk mitigation action items include this charter, which should clearly state the "in scope" objectives of the implementation. This should address both risks identified here.

VISION OF THE SOLUTION

Vision Statement

The Mobile Mammography Van program will be a more efficient and safe environment. The current lack of a software system introduces risks due to potential regulatory issues, patient safety issues due to potential missed follow-up, as well as program risks due to potential loss of funding. The proposed implementation of a software system alleviates these risks as well as introduces the prospect of future expansion of the program that is not easily achieved in the current environment.

The program should be able to handle more patients with the new software. The registration and scheduling process will stay the same, but the introduction of remote access will increase efficiency. Changes to appointments or patient demographic data can now occur on the van. An interface with the GE scheduling and registration software to the mobile mammography software will ensure no duplicate entry of patient data. The ability to document patient history online on the van will decrease the amount of paperwork filled out at the end of the day by the technician. There will also be the opportunity to track patients better by entering data during the day rather than at the end of the day.

The current transcription process is not expected to change. Films will still be read in the current manner, but reports will be saved to a common database. This will allow the technician or program staff to access the reports online. Entry of the BIRAD result (mammography result) will occur much more quickly and efficiently. Patient follow-up based on the BIRAD will be done more quickly as well. Letters can be automatically generated based on the results and printed in batches. All patient follow-up, including phone calls, letters, and certified letters can be captured in the system with a complete audit trail. This ensures the program's compliance with regulations concerning patient follow-up.

The film-tracking functions will also allow more accurate tracking of the patient's films. Accurate film tracking will increase the turnaround time for film comparisons and patient follow-up.

The ability to customize the software will increase the grant funding possibilities for the program. The program can introduce new variables or queries to the clients in order to produce statistical reports based on the gathered information. Increases in funding can lead to increases in the program's expansion. The increased expansion will increase the availability of free mammography to underprivileged women.

Major Features

- Interface can be implemented from GE system to OmniCare system (OmniCare supports clinical documentation) for registration information.
- Mammography history questionnaires can be preprinted and brought on the van for the patient to fill out.
- OmniCare will allow entry of BIRAD results.

- Transcribed reports can be uploaded or cut and pasted into OmniCare from the common database.
- Patient letters are generated from and maintained in OmniCare.
- Follow-up, including pathology results, will be maintained in OmniCare.
- Communication management functions will be maintained with full audit trail.
- Film tracking will be done in OmniCare.
- Statistical reporting will be facilitated.

Assumptions and Dependencies

The assumptions and dependencies for this project are few, but all are crucial to the success of the implementation. The software and hardware to be purchased for this implementation are key aspects of the project. The project is dependent on the remote access satellite hardware working as expected. The software vendor chosen during the vendor selection project is assumed to be the best fit for this program. The GE interface is a crucial assumption in this project. This working interface is key to the efficiencies this program is looking to achieve with the implementation. Resources are an assumption inherent in the budget. Appropriate resources to effectively implement the solution are important to the success of the implementation.

Related Projects

There are no related projects for this project. All needed work is included in this implementation project.

SCOPE AND LIMITATIONS
Scope of Initial Release

- GE interface for patient demographic and registration information
- Film tracking (possible bar coding for film tracking)
- Mammography history questionnaires
- BIRAD result entry
- Patient follow-up management
- Communications management
- Statistical reporting

- Custom fields management
- Remote access satellite installation

Interface Scope

- GE registration data

Organizational Scope

The OmniCare implementation will focus on the implementation of the software with the Ogilvey Cancer Institute program of the Boston Mobile Mammography Van. No other partner institutions are involved for the rollout. The film reads done at Metro Hospital are not included in this scope.

Conversion Scope

No data conversion is planned for this project.

Scope of Subsequent Releases

Future releases may try to include the Metro Hospital radiologists. Currently, as Metro reads the film, the radiologist dictates and the text is transcribed. It would be more efficient in future if the readings were automatically part of OmniCare.

Out of Scope

- Billing functions are not within the scope of this implementation. Billing is currently done via the GE system and will continue this way.
- A results interface is not within the scope of this implementation. The results of the mammograms will be available only on paper in the medical record or within the OmniCare solution. There will be no integration with the Results application.
- Scheduling and registration functions are not in scope for this implementation. These functions are currently done via the GE system. An interface from GE to provide this information in the OmniCare solution is planned.
- Entry of radiologists' data is not in scope for this implementation. It is listed as a possible scope of subsequent releases.

PROJECT SUCCESS FACTORS

- Increased turnaround time for patient follow-up
- Decreased turnaround time with films by film tracking
- Decreased time creating and managing reports
- Increased numbers of mammographies taken
- Decreased time spent by staff on administrative tasks

BUDGET HIGHLIGHTS

Capital budget	$52,550
Hardware	$10,000
Software	$30,000
Remote access	$6,200
First year remote service	$1,350
Contingency	$5,000

Project Staff Resources

IS analyst = .50 FTE for 6 months

Network services = .25 for 3–6 months

Karen = 40 hr./wk. for 4 months

Program asst. (Sarah) = 40 hr./wk. for 4 months

New person to be hired

Temp to do data entry conversion

TIMELINE

Project will commence on November 1, 2012, and be completed July 1, 2013. Approximate date of completion of major phases:

Analysis	January 1, 2013
Satellite installation	February 1, 2013
Registration interface	March 1, 2013
Film tracking	March 1, 2013
History questionnaires	May 1, 2013
Result entry	June 1, 2013
Communications management	June 1, 2013
Patient follow-up	June 1, 2013
Reporting	June 15, 2013

PROJECT ORGANIZATION

Business Sponsor(s)	Anne Jones, VP of External Affairs
Business Owner(s)	Karen Ruderman, Program Director
Steering Committee	Karen Zimmerman, Program Director
	Anne Johnson, Director of Planning
	Jerry Melini, Technical Director of Radiology
Project Manager	Charles Leoman
Project Team	IS analysts TBD
	Network Services IS staff TBD
	Karen Zimmerman, Program Director
	Sarah Smithson, Program Assistant
	Data Entry temporary staff

PROJECT MANAGEMENT STRATEGIES

Project Meetings

In order to maintain effective communication with Project Team members and the Mobile Mammography Van community, a series of standing meetings will be conducted. Meeting minutes will be documented and stored on the shared core team directory. The following meetings and facilitated sessions will be held.

Issue Management

Issue identification, management, and resolution are important project management activities. The Project Manager is responsible for the issue management process and works with the Project Team and Steering Committee (if needed) to agree on the resolution of issues.

Effective issue management enables

- A visible decision-making process
- A means for resolving questions concerning the project
- A project issue audit trail

The standard IS project issue management process and forms will be used and attached to this charter as needed.

Scope Change Management

Scope change management is essential to ensure that the project is managed to the original scope, as defined in this charter. The purpose of a scope management process is to constructively manage the pressure to expand scope.

Table B.2. Issue management

Decision-Making Level	Steering Committee	Project Team
Role	Resolves show-stopper issues and changes in scope. Acts as a sounding board for decisions and actions that affect user acceptance of the project. This includes anything that affects project milestones and outcomes. Reviews decisions, recommendations, and requests that are high in integration and complexity and that are not resolved at the Project Team level. Scope management and planning. Chaired by Business Sponsor.	Governs the actual work and the progress of the project. Reviews project work and status: —Resource issues —Vendor issues —Project risks Serves as working or focus group to report daily progress. Responsible for implementation decisions that have integration impact and that are of medium or high complexity. Cochaired by IS Project Manager and Business Owner.
Participants	Key stakeholders on business and IS sides.	All resources assigned to the project.
Meeting frequency	Meets regularly to ensure steady project progress.	Meets, as needed, weekly to monthly, for project status and updates.

Scope expansion is acceptable as long as

- Users agree that the new requirements are justified
- Impact to the project is analyzed and understood
- Resulting changes to project (cost, timing, resources, quality) are approved and properly implemented

Any member of the Project Team or other member of the Mobile Mammography Van community may propose a change to the scope of the project. The requester will initiate the process by completing a Change Request Definition Form. When necessary, the Project Manager will review and seek advice from the Steering Committee on scope changes that affect the project schedule or budget, or both.

The standard IS project scope management process and forms will be used and attached as appendixes to this charter, as needed.

Training Strategy
Training Scope

The program personnel consist of a program administrator, one mammography technician, one assistant to the administrator, and one patient educator and administration person. All of the employees will receive training for their specific role related to the process. The program administrator will learn all of the roles in order to fill in when needed. Additional training will be given to the other employees for backup purposes.

Training Approach

The vendor will provide the training during the initial implementation. The employees of the program will then train new employees.

Training Material Development

The vendor will provide training materials.

Documentation Development Strategy

The team will develop the following documentation:

- Technical operations procedure manual
- Policies and procedures related to the use and management of the system
- Application manuals, if needed
- OmniCare technical and application maintenance and support manuals, if needed

Project Work Paper Organization and Coordination

In order to keep the project documentation, meeting minutes, and deliverables organized and accessible to the core team, a project folder on the shared network will be established and maintained.

International Adoption and Use of Health Information Technology

Throughout the world, many countries are embracing health information technology (HIT) as a tool to more effectively deliver high-quality, cost-effective care while improving patient outcomes, increasing access, and engaging patients in their own care. Although the focus of this textbook has been primarily on the adoption and use of health care information systems in the United States, we believe that it is critically important for health care leaders to examine issues such as the adoption and use of HIT from a global perspective. Not only can we learn from other countries, but we live in a global society where the goal of electronic health record should be one that promotes health and spans an individual's lifetime, regardless of where an individual resides. Many other countries share the same challenges as those of the United States in meeting the needs of a growing number of patients with chronic conditions and serious illnesses and the need to reduce unnecessary or inappropriate care. Care systems are often fragmented and poorly coordinated (Schoen, Osborn, Doty, Squires, Peugh, & Applebaum, 2009). By studying health care reform efforts in other countries and examining the strategies they have used to promote the widespread use and adoption of health information technology, we have the opportunity to improve the quality and effectiveness of global health.

Countries such as Sweden and Denmark are well ahead of the United States and other developed countries in their use of health IT (Bernstein,

Bruun-Rasmussen, Vingtoft, Andersen, & Nøhr, 2005; Castro, 2009). Strong national-level leadership has played a key role in widespread adoption and use of electronic health record (EHR) systems. In this appendix, we describe the adoption and use of health IT in selected countries representing various regions of the world, with a focus on countries that are leaders in health IT adoption. We provide a brief description of how health IT is being used in each country. We found little information published on the use of health IT in South America or Africa, so these two regions of the world are not included in our analysis. Our focus is on the adoption and use of EHR systems, CPOE, e-prescribing, and the factors that have led to their deployment and use. We also discuss unique characteristics of the various health care systems and the incentives that may influence health IT adoption and use. We conclude with a discussion of the key factors that appear to have contributed to the successful deployment of health IT among countries leading the world in health IT adoption and use based upon work that Castro (2009) has done. (The Commonwealth Fund has collected data about the adoption and use of health IT among a number of countries since 2006. The most recent report, *International Profiles of Health Care Systems, 2011*, is an excellent source for additional information: Thomson, Osborn, Squires, & Reed, 2011.)

THE ADOPTION AND USE OF HEALTH IT FROM VARIOUS REGIONS OF THE WORLD

Studies that have examined the adoption and use of health IT internationally tend to focus on electronic health records (EHRs) and categorize them by use in primary care practice (Castro, 2009; Schoen, Osborn, Doty, Squires, Peugh, & Applebaum, 2009) and in hospitals (Castro, 2009). In most countries, primary care physicians provide the foundation for health care systems and serve as the hub in connecting care, providing continuity for patients and families, and ensuring access (Schoen et al., 2009). Among primary care practices, Northern European countries such as Sweden, Denmark, and Finland emerge as the global leaders in the use of EHR systems, with adoption rates ranging from 95 to 100 percent. Among hospital settings, both Sweden and Finland have nearly widespread EHR adoption. Rates of EHR adoption in primary care practices tend to be much higher than EHR adoption rates in hospitals. For example, in the South Pacific, the rates of EHR adoption in primary care practices in Australia and New Zealand are 95 percent and 97 percent, respectively, yet less than 10 percent of hospitals have adopted EHR systems in Australia and less than 1 percent in New Zealand. Jha, Doolan, Grandt, Scott, and Bates (2008) studied the use of EHRs in both primary care settings and hospitals in these countries and hypothesized that policymakers pay little attention to hospital

EHR adoption because there have been no clear financial incentives for hospitals to significantly improve the care they provide. Second, because hospital EHR systems are a huge financial investment, often disruptive, and require integration with legacy systems, without clear incentives, most hospitals see little reason to adopt EHR systems (Jha et al., 2008; Schoen et al., 2009).

Table C.1. shows adoption rates of health IT among the various countries, as well as data on country size, health care spending, and use of magnetic resonance imaging, as one measure of medical technology usage.

Following is a more detailed description of each country or region's use of HIT.

In Northern Europe: Norway, Sweden, Finland, and Denmark

Northern European countries such as Norway, Sweden, Finland, and Denmark spend between 9.6 percent and 11.5 percent of their GDP on health care. The population ranges from 4.3 million in Norway to 9.3 million in Sweden. All four countries have implemented national-level strategies to drive and coordinate EHR adoption. In Denmark, for example, physicians receive faster payments if they use EHR systems, and primary care physicians receive financial incentives for phone and e-mail consultations. Adoption of EHRs in Denmark is near universal. Adherence to interoperability standards is required, and all primary care physician EHR systems connect electronically to a national health information exchange network that is operated by a nonprofit organization known as MedCom (Gray, Bowden, Johansen, & Koch, 2011). This national network facilitates the electronic exchange of clinical data between primary care providers, specialists, hospitals, pharmacies, laboratories, and other health providers. MedCom also developed the national infrastructure, set standards, and provided technical assistance to health care providers and organizations as needed. Additionally, in 2004, the Denmark government mandated that general practitioners use health IT. The mandate included being able to receive electronically lab and X-ray results and discharge summaries from hospitals, as well as e-prescribing and referrals (Doupi, Renko, & Giest, 2010; Gray et al., 2011).

Sweden took a somewhat different approach to EHR adoption, but was still quite successful. In Sweden, twenty-one county councils or regions are primarily responsible for providing hospital and primary care services (Gray, Bowden, Johansen, & Koch, 2011). These same councils or regions have been responsible for the introduction of the EHR systems. When some of the systems were first introduced by local champions in the early 1990s, each region had a different system. Today, however, most of Sweden is covered by one of four

Table C.1. Health care IT usage and characteristics of system by country

		Australia	Canada	Denmark	Finland	Germany	Japan	Netherlands	New Zealand	Norway	Sweden	United Kingdom	United States
Health Care IT Usage	EHR Adoption Primary Care	95%	37%	95%	99%	68%	10%	99%	97%	97%	100%	89%	46%
	EHR in Hospitals	<10%	<10%	35%	100%	<5%	10%	<5%	<1%	n/a	88%	3%	8%
	CPOE Adoption in Hospitals	<5%	n/a	n/a	100%	<5%	n/a	20%	n/a	n/a	n/a	<5%	15%
Population, 2009	E-prescribing	81%	11%	100%	100%	59%	n/a	85%	78%	n/a	100%	55%	20%
	Total Population (1,000,000s of People)	29.9	33.4	5.5	5.2	81.9	127.5	16.4	4.3	4.8	9.3	62.2	306.6
	Percentage of Population over Age 65	13.3%	13.9%	16.1%		20.5%	22.7%	15.2%	12.8%	14.8%	17.9%		13.0%
Spending, 2009	Percentage of GDP Spent on Health Care	8.7%	11.4%	11.5%	9.2%	11.6%	8.5%	12.0%	10.3%	9.6%	10.0%	9.8%	17.4%
	Health Care Spending per Capita[d]	$3,445	$4,363	$4,348	$3,236	$4,218	$2,878	$4,914	$2,983	$5,352	$3,722	$3,487	$7,960
Medical Technology 2009	Magnetic Resonance Imaging (MRI) Machines per Million Population	5.9	8.0	15.4	19.4	n/a	43.1	11.0	9.7	n/a	n/a	5.9	25.9
	MRI Exams per 100,000 Population	23.3	43.0	37.8	n/a	n/a	n/a	43.9	n/a	n/a	n/a	n/a	91.2

[a] 2009.
[b] 2007.
[c] 1998–2008.
[d] Adjusted for differences in the cost of living.
[e] *Source:* Commonwealth Fund International Health Policy Survey of Primary Care Physicians, 2009.
[f] Self-reported as opposed to measured data.
Source: ORGANISATION FOR ECONOMIC CO-OPERATION AND DEVELOPMENT, 2011, unless otherwise noted.

EHR systems, and half of the county councils have adopted a single EHR system for both hospitals and primary care (Gray et al., 2011). EHRs are used for documentation by all physicians, most hospitals, and most ambulances. In emergency situations, patient information is automatically transferred from the ambulance to the hospital. Most Swedish EHRs contain clinical documentation, e-prescribing, and CPOE. Laboratories are entirely computerized, and computerized order entry for laboratory, radiology, and pathology services range from 20 percent to 70 percent, depending on the county council region (Gray et al., 2011). Most county councils provide for electronic exchange of hospital discharge summaries and enable patients to schedule appointments and refill prescriptions online.

Sweden implemented a National e-Health Strategy in 2006 in an effort to improve safety, accessibility, and quality of care, as well as facilitate patient mobility and meet growing demands from patients and health professionals. By 2009, the Center for eHealth of Sweden was established to provide a common infrastructure for supporting the widespread exchange of health information. Furthermore, each citizen has a unique identifier that is used to coordinate health care and social care across the continuum (Gray et al., 2011). The Patient Data Act of 2008 allows health care providers, with patients' consent, to access electronically information available from other providers. Citizens of Sweden also have the right to access their own health information, but systems for easily accessing data are not yet readily available nationally.

Like Denmark and Sweden, both Finland and Norway have been early adopters of HIT. Finland has widespread use of EHRs, CPOE, and e-prescribing in both ambulatory care and hospital settings. In 1996, Finland's Ministry of Social Affairs and Health established the first strategy on using IT to create a more integrated, patient-focused health care system. Two years later, the government revised the strategy to target specific goals for health IT, including ensuring that every citizen have a safe, secure EHR so that patient data could be shared with others (Castro, 2009). Finland launched several initiatives to further the adoption of EHRs, first for providers, and second in developing e-health services for citizens.

Ninety-seven percent of Norwegian general practitioners use an EHR in the practice, and 74 percent of them have broadband access (Doupi et al., 2010). The country has been engaged in activities promoting the adoption and use of EHRs for over fifteen years. Electronic exchange of patient data is also fairly common; 35 percent of practices exchange health care data with other care providers, and 88 percent of general practitioners in Norway receive laboratory results electronically. In 2010, Norway began requiring physicians to file for reimbursement electronically, thus significantly increasing their usage of information systems for administrative purposes (Doupi et al., 2010).

In Western Europe: United Kingdom and Germany

In Western Europe, the United Kingdom has invested a great deal in health IT over the past four decades. EHRs have been adopted by nearly 90 percent of general practitioners. General practice has been central to the U.K. health care system for years, and the country is viewed as a leader in providing primary care, although this was not always the case (Doran & Roland, 2010). In the late 1990s, the government introduced a range of clinical governance measures to stimulate quality improvement. Included in these measures were national guidelines for managing chronic diseases, mandatory clinical audits, financial incentives, public reports on quality, and annual reviews of physician performance (Doran & Roland, 2010). Physicians in the United Kingdom are now paid based on performance measures. One lesson the United Kingdom learned in transitioning to this new payment system was the importance of implementing the necessary infrastructure, such as the health IT system, as part of the process. They found a stable health IT infrastructure was essential to supporting the change in reimbursement practice.

Beyond the use of EHR, the U.K. National Health Service (NHS) has a national e-health portal called NHS Direct. It was designed to direct individuals to the most appropriate form of treatment, and it provides health advice and options. The NHS Direct portal provides a 24/7 telephone number for health information, and individuals residing in the United Kingdom can submit health care questions online and receive an e-mail response via a secure web site (http://www.nhsdirect.nhs.uk/en/About). NHS Direct also hosts the web site NHS Choices, which provides information on health conditions, treatment options, and drug regimens, as well as a list of providers in each patient's area. They also offer an online service called Choose and Book, which allows patients to schedule appointments with specialists at registered hospitals and clinics (http://www.chooseandbook.nhs.uk).

Clinical information exchange activities have also increased in recent years. One study found that clinical information exchange in the United Kingdom has been made possible by establishing appropriate policy (such as privacy protections), infrastructure (such as coding, authentication, standards), and systems of care, and by creating and selecting clinical applications with strong use of financial and clinical incentives (Payne, Detmer, Wyatt, & Buchan, 2011). Health IT vendors have played a critical role in this effort by participating in a national framework created by the NHS. General practitioners (GPs) are provided with incentives to use EHR systems, as the NHS reimburses GPs for hardware, software, and maintenance for using EHR systems that are certified and meet industry standards (much like the CMS

Medicare and Medicaid EHR incentive programs in the United States). Furthermore, when a patient is discharged from the hospital, the discharge summary is to be made available to the patient's GP within forty-eight hours or the hospital incurs a financial penalty at the end of the year (Payne et al., 2011). These incentives are intended to encourage health information exchange among providers.

In Germany, citizens are being issued electronic health insurance cards. These cards contain the same administrative data as Germany's existing health insurance card, such as name, date of birth, address, and insurance company. They have been designed to store health-related data such as emergency data, medications, allergies, drug intolerance, or indication of pregnancy (Global Centre for ICT in Parliament, 2011). The health cards and the underlying infrastructure were developed by Gematik (Jahn, Gartig-Daug, & Nagel, 2005). Beyond the electronic health insurance cards, the use of health IT in Germany is primarily in private physician practices. Hospitals have implemented EHRs to a much less extent (less than 5 percent). Incompatibility between systems remains a major challenge within many hospitals in Germany (Busse, Blumel, & Stock, 2011). Germany is also much larger than the other European countries studied, with a population of 81.9 million.

South Pacific: Australia and New Zealand

In the South Pacific, EHR adoption rates are high among primary care providers in Australia, with 95 percent using EHR systems, yet less than 10 percent of hospitals having them. The national strategy for health IT is managed primarily by the Australian Health Ministers' Advisory Committee, an intergovernmental committee of senior health administrators (Healy & Hall, 2011). Agreements are in place between government and other key agencies on developing, collecting, and exchanging data in an effort to improve health and delivery of health care services. One major initiative is to develop interoperable systems between health care providers, health care identifiers, secure messaging and authentication, and a clinical terminology and information service.

Similar to Australia, New Zealand has high EHR adoption rates in primary care (97 percent), but less than 1 percent of hospitals use them. Most physician practices are private, as are some hospitals, and all are expected to finance health IT investments from their operating budgets and to conform to national standards and guidelines (Gray et al., 2011). Today, all of New Zealand's 1,100 general practices use an EHR that supports a range of functions including primary care records, problem lists, progress notes, ordering of tests and medications, managing medications, issuing preventive reminders, and using decision-support capabilities (Gray et al., 2011). Health information exchange among providers is possible, and electronic communication with patients is beginning to occur through the use of patient portals. Similar to Denmark, New Zealand uses a private organization known as HealthLink to facilitate electronic communication between physician practices and other providers (such as laboratories), provide electronic messaging services, and assist with technical support.

Asia: Japan

The picture in Asia is quite different from that in Europe. Japan is perhaps the furthest behind in its adoption and use of HIT among the countries studied, but that may change in the years to come. HIT is not widely developed except for billing purposes. Approximately 10 percent of physicians and hospitals in Japan use EHR systems. Among large hospitals with four hundred beds or more, however, EHR adoption rates are approximately 25 percent (Tanaka, 2007). Health administrators in Japan have been historically reluctant to introduce EHR systems because of high acquisition and support costs (Tanaka, 2007). Demographic trends in Japan indicate a movement toward a "super-aged" society, whereby the percentage of the population sixty-five years or older exceeded 20 percent in 2005 and is projected to exceed 30 percent by 2030 (Onaya, Kaneda, & Fujii, 2011). Ninety percent of all municipal hospitals are operating in the red, causing hospitals in some regions to close or merge. In the face of these challenges, the Japanese government is looking to health care as a priority field in its national IT strategy. For example, by 2020, the Japan New Growth Strategy seeks to expand the economy by creating 100 trillion yen in new demand and generating employment for four million people. A major part of the strategy is a program called My Hospital Anywhere, which aims to use IT to improve health by electronically managing and using personal medical health data by linking emergency department data with personal health record data (Onaya, Kaneda, & Fujii, 2011).

The Japanese government has defined the national IT strategy and is establishing budgets. The strategy has four parts: (1) develop EHR that can be accessed by all providers, (2) develop health IT and telehealth platforms to link patients with health care providers in underserved areas, (3) create a platform that can monitor prescription drugs and adverse drug events in real time, and (4) create a claims database of all conditions and interventions to facilitate assessment of community needs and development of interventions (Squires, 2011). There are still a number of system-related issues, including operational and technological issues, that need to be addressed before EHRs are more widely used in Japan.

North America: Canada and the United States

In North America, both Canada and the United States have lagged behind many European and South Pacific countries in their widespread adoption and use of HIT, particularly EHR systems. Estimates indicate that approximately 37 percent of physicians and 54 percent of hospitals in Canada have adopted EHR systems (Urowitz et al., 2008). In 2001, Canada Health Infoway, Inc., known as Infoway, was established as a nonprofit corporation whose goal was that of a "strategic investor" to help make focused investments that would foster and accelerate the development of EHRs throughout Canada (Office of the Auditor General of Canada, 2010). Infoway works with the provinces and territories in Canada that are responsible for delivering health care services to set national direction and ensure that provincial and territorial strategies are aligned with national priorities. Infoway also funds projects within the provinces and territories, participates in project planning, and monitors the implementation of projects as well as the quality of deliverables. The federal government in Canada has granted Infoway $1.6 billion since it was established in 2001 to use in funding health IT-related projects. Although each province and territory may have an EHR system adapted to its needs, it is important that provincial and territorial systems are based on an agreed-upon set of principles and characteristics. To this end, Infoway, in consultation with the provinces, territories, and other stakeholders, identified the key requirements and core components of the EHR and developed the EHR Solution Blueprint to guide the national development of EHRs. First published in 2003, and revised in 2006, the Blueprint details how standards support the sharing of information securely and appropriately throughout Canada ("EHRs in Canada, Audit Report," 2010). Similar to Germany, Canada has a national agreement to use a distributed model approach, with patient data coming from different operational applications and all fourteen of its federal, provincial, and territorial governments participating (Arnold, Wagner, Hyatt, & Klein, 2007). Federal funding freezes and cuts have slowed or curtailed EHR adoption efforts in Canada in recent years (Webster, 2010).

In the United States, EHR adoption rates vary considerably, depending on the source used. Hospital EHR adoption has been appropriately 12 percent, while the adoption rates in physician practices range from an estimated 17 percent (DesRoches et al., 2008) to 56.9 percent (Hsiao, Hing, Socey, & Cai, 2011), depending on the source and definitions used. We expect these rates to increase significantly in the next five years, with the influx of CMS EHR Incentive dollars and the number of providers who have applied for, or have expressed interest in demonstrating, meaningful use. Coupled with health care reform including payment reform, health care providers are looking to manage populations of patients in a more patient-centered, cost-effective manner.

Quality outcomes and managing patient care across a continuum will be increasingly important.

LESSONS FROM GLOBAL LEADERS

What can we learn from these countries—particularly from those that are global leaders in health IT adoption? Daniel Castro (2009) conducted an extensive review of the literature to identify the countries that are leading the world in the adoption and use of health IT and to draw lessons that may be useful for other countries. From his analysis, he concluded that the degree of success or failure a country experiences with health IT depends upon a number of factors. No single approach will work in all countries, yet lessons can be learned from global leaders. The factors identified that have the potential to affect health IT adoption can be categorized as

- Organizational factors (such as leadership, health care system organization, and financing)
- Political factors (such as incentives and mandates)
- Institutional factors (such as size of country, structure of health care, cultural factors, and privacy issues)
- Technological factors (such as common infrastructure, standards, and unique patient identifiers) [Castro, 2009, p. 24].

Examples of each of these factors are provided next.

Organizational Factors

- *National leadership to promote HIT adoption and use.* National-level leadership is important to define national health IT goals and strategies, establish priorities, coordinate efforts to overcome barriers to health IT adoption, and identify incentives for adoption and use. National-level leadership is likely the *single largest* factor driving successful adoption (Castro, 2009). One could argue that until the passage of the HITECH Act, the U.S. government role has been to encourage, rather than lead, the health IT strategy. With the passage of HITECH, the federal government took a strong national-level leadership role in furthering the health IT agenda.
- *Health care system organization and financing.* The nation's health care system and the way in which it is financed can have a significant impact on health IT adoption. Countries with single-payer health care systems tend to be more likely to invest in health IT because the

benefits will accrue to those systems, unlike the United States, where the health care providers (hospitals and physicians) incur the vast majority of the costs, yet the majority of benefits are realized by patients, insurers, and purchasers of care.

Political Factors

- *Financial incentives for health information technology.* The initial high cost of purchasing and implementing an EHR system is a known barrier to adoption. Financial incentives can help spur adoption. Different countries may use different financial incentives. Examples include offering financial rewards to providers for meeting quality standards (United Kingdom), rewarding primary care providers that implement certain quality improvements (Australia), making HIT purchases tax-deductible (the Netherlands), and providing incentive payments for demonstrating meaningful use of EHR systems based on defined measures (United States). Japan, which has a low rate of EHR adoption, provides few financial incentives.

- *Government mandates.* Governments may either mandate the use of specific functionality or the use of specific technology. For example, Denmark requires primary care providers to use e-prescribing. Denmark also requires primary care providers to issue referrals electronically, schedule appointments online, and e-mail consultations. The government in Finland requires that all health care providers use the national patient record system.

- *Policies to support telemedicine and telehealth.* Countries such as Finland and Denmark have implemented policies that have promoted the use of telemedicine, such as providing reimbursement to physicians for remote consultations and paying for e-mail consultations. Besides reimbursement, licensing standards and laws can also affect the use of telemedicine across states and borders.

Institutional Factors

- *Size of country.* Smaller countries seem to be able to collaborate and coordinate with their various stakeholders more easily than larger countries with a diverse group of stakeholders. Countries with a more centralized health care system also seem to be able to achieve a higher level of coordination in the deployment of health IT.

- *Structural issues.* The size of the practice or organization can influence HIT adoption, as well as the number of HIT vendors and the number of competing pharmacies. In the United States, EHR adoption rates are much higher in larger physician practices and among larger hospitals. Larger practices are better equipped to share the costs across multiple providers, and larger hospitals typically have access to greater capital and HIT personnel and resources. In Germany, 75 percent of primary care physicians work in solo practices; in the Netherlands, the level is even greater, at 80 percent. Consequently, providers in these countries are forming cooperatives to gain benefits from working in a larger group, such as sharing IT services. Countries with fewer vendors and fewer competing pharmacies also seem to have an easier time adopting HIT.

- *Societal and cultural factors.* Factors such as the technological sophistication of the population, peer influences, and cultural norms may influence health IT adoption. Countries such as Denmark, Sweden, and the Netherlands consistently rank among the top nations in broadband adoption, and 95 percent of residents of Denmark have access to the Internet at home. Use of computers has been the norm for many years among primary care physicians. In fact, as early as 1998, patients in Denmark considered their physician second-rate if he or she didn't have a personal computer in the office. Peer pressure has also proven to be a major factor in the adoption and use of EHRs in Denmark and Sweden (Castro, 2009).

- *Privacy issues.* Many countries have implemented health information security legislation to protect patient privacy. For example, Sweden enacted the Patient Data Act in 2008, to allow data exchange between health care providers, while ensuring privacy and security of patient data. Patients in the Netherlands can opt out of electronic exchange of their data; however, only about 2 percent of patients have done so. New Zealand has fairly extensive privacy laws and security laws, yet consumers remain concerned about who has access to their information and how it is used (Naylor, 2010). The implication is that those countries that successfully address the privacy question have higher adoption rates than those that do not.

Technological Factors

- *Common HIT infrastructure.* One factor common to countries leading in HIT adoption is that they each have a national health IT strategy for developing a shared IT infrastructure whereby technology can be used by multiple stakeholders. For example, the Danish Health Data Network, managed by MedCom, allows health care providers and organizations to securely exchange patient data. In the Netherlands, the national coordinating body for HIT is the National IT Institute for Healthcare (NICTIZ), a nonprofit organization. NICTIZ has worked to develop a national HIT infrastructure known as AORTA. AORTA includes a national registration system for patients, workers, and insurers; and a system for authenticating and authorizing access to health records. Unlike the United Kingdom, which has historically had a centralized national EHR system, the Netherlands uses a decentralized system with a record locator service to point to patient data stored in regional databases (Castro, 2009). Development and adherence to interoperability standards must also be coordinated and enforced.

- *Use of unique patient identifiers.* Many countries have a unique national identifier that is issued to each citizen. The unique identifiers are used for a variety of purposes. Germany, for example, has not only a unique patient identifier, but also issues each citizen an electronic health insurance card. In the United States, we have not adopted a system of unique patient identifiers primarily because of privacy and security concerns and political oppositions. Instead, statistical or probabilistic matching is used in combination with various algorithms in an effort to correctly identify and match patient information. Such matching is not without problems (Castro, 2009).

CONCLUSION

Achieving widespread health IT adoption and use requires bringing together multiple stakeholders with competing interests toward a common goal. A central theme among countries leading in this arena is the need for national-level leadership, whether it takes the form of a government entity or a public-private partnership, responsible for establishing goals, determining strategies, measuring progress, and overcoming barriers to adoption. Alignment of incentives is also important. Reducing the financial barriers, shifting or sharing the financial risk, and providing incentives for HIT use are all important factors. Not surprisingly, in our analysis of the literature we found that in countries with high adoption rates government is intervening to promote the adoption of HIT either through direct regulation, financial incentives, or persuasive measures (including support measures such as providing education and training for change management). Governments of developed countries are evidently using their leverage as purchasers and payers to drive health IT adoption, which reflects the growing consensus about the vital "public good" to be expected from EHRs and improved health information exchange (Organisation for Economic Co-operation and Development, 2010). Grants and subsidies are the most common form of financial incentives. Bonuses or add-on payments that reward providers for adopting and diffusing HIT are also often used, particularly in countries where physicians are remunerated on the basis of fee for service.

Interoperability of systems is a challenge worldwide, and as countries look to exchange health information across the continuum of care, the challenges can seem daunting. The more stakeholders involved, the more complex the exchange can be. Policymakers need to address the technical challenges posed by health IT, as well as the privacy and security concerns. Interoperability issues can be addressed by bringing together various stakeholders to agree on standards, data definitions, and coding schemes. Coordination of efforts, however, is not an easy task and one that takes strong leadership, collaboration, and communication.

Widespread adoption and use of health IT is not the end-all, but *a tool* to better equip patients, providers, and other health care stakeholders in improving each nation's health care system and global health. Future research is needed to examine further the value gained to the individual, the health care organization or provider, and the health care system as a whole by having ready access to health information whenever and wherever it is needed.

REFERENCES

Arnold, S., Wagner, J., Hyatt, S. J., & Klein, G. M. (2007). *Electronic health records: A global perspective.* Healthcare Information and Management Systems Society (HIMSS). Retrieved February 2013 at http://himss.files.cms-plus.com/HIMSSorg /Content/files/DrArnold%20011207EISPresentationWhitePaper.pdf

Bernstein, K., Bruun-Rasmussen, M., Vingtoft, S., Andersen, S. K., & Nøhr, C. (2005). Modelling and implementing electronic health records in Denmark. *International Journal of Medical Informatics, 74*(2–4), 213–220.

Busse, R., Blumel, M., & Stock, S. (2011). The German health care system. *International Profiles of Health Care Systems* (pp. 57–64). New York: The Commonwealth Fund.

Castro, D. (2009). *Explaining international IT application leadership: Health IT.* Washington, DC: Information Technology and Innovation Foundation.

Commonwealth Fund. (2009). *2009 Commonwealth Fund international health policy survey.* New York: Author. Retrieved February 2013 from http://www .commonwealthfund.org/Surveys/2009/Nov/2009-Commonwealth-Fund -International-Health-Policy-Survey.aspx

DesRoches, C. M., Campbell, E. G., Rao, S. R., Donelan, K., Ferris, T. G., Jha, A., ... & Blumenthal, D. (2008). Electronic health records in ambulatory care: A national survey of physicians. *New England Journal of Medicine, 359*(1), 50–60.

Doran, T., & Roland, M. (2010). Lessons from major initiatives to improve primary care in the United Kingdom. *Health Affairs, 29*(5), 1023–1029.

Doupi, P., Renko, E., & Giest, S. (2010). Country brief: Norway. *Ehealth Strategies*. European Commission, DG Information Society and Media, ICT for Health Unit.

Global Centre for ICT in Parliament. (2011). Rollout of electronic health cards in Germany has started.

Gray, B. H., Bowden, T., Johansen, I., & Koch, S. (2011). Electronic health records: An international perspective on "meaningful use." *Issues in International Health Policy*. Publication 1565, Volume 28. New York: The Commonwealth Fund.

Healy, J., & Hall, J. (2011). The Austrian health care system. *International Profiles of Health Care Systems*. New York: The Commonwealth Fund. Retrieved February 2013 from http://www.commonwealthfund.org/~/media/Files/Publications/Fund%20Report/2011/Nov/1562_Squires_Intl_Profiles_2011_11_10.pdf

Hsiao, C., Hing, E., Socey, T. C., & Cai, B. (2011). *Electronic health record systems and intent to apply for meaningful user incentives among office-based physician practices: United States, 2001–2011*. NCHS Data Brief. Retrieved February 2013 from www.nchs/data/databriefs/DB79

Jahn, K., Gartig-Daug, A., & Nagel, E. (2005). Electronic health records within integrated care in Germany. *Telemedicine Journal and e-Health, 11*(2), 146–150.

Jha, A. K., Doolan, D., Grandt, D., Scott, T., & Bates, D. W. (2008). The use of health information technology in seven nations. *International Journal of Medical Informatics, 77*, 848–854.

Naylor, W. (2010). *Sharing patient health information: A review of health information privacy and electronic health records in New Zealand*. The Palliative Care Council of New Zealand, Cancer Control New Zealand. Retrieved February 2013 from http://www.cancercontrolnz.govt.nz

Office of the Auditor General of Canada. (2010). *Electronic health records in Canada: An overview of federal and provincial audit reports*. Retrieved February 2013 from www.oag-bvg.gc.ca

Onaya, T., Kaneda, N., & Fujii, H. (2011). Trends in national information technology strategy for healthcare. *FUJITSU Scientific and Technical Journal, 47*(1), 10–18.

Organisation for Economic Co-Operation and Development. (2010). *Improving health sector efficiency: The role of information and communication technologies*. Paris: Author.

Payne, T. H., Detmer, D. E., Wyatt, J. C., & Buchan, I. E. (2011). National-scale clinical information exchange in the United Kingdom: Lessons for the U.S. *Journal of the American Medical Association, 18*, 91–98.

Schoen, C., Osborn, R., Doty, M. M., Squires, D., Peugh, J., & Applebaum, S. (2009). A survey of primary care physicians in eleven countries, 2009: Perspectives on care, costs and experiences. *Health Affairs Web Exclusive*, w1171–w1183.

Squires, D. (2011). The Japanese health care system. *International Profiles of Health Care Systems* (pp. 73–77). New York: The Commonwealth Fund.

Tanaka, H. (2007). Current status of electronic health record dissemination in Japan. *Japan Medical Association Journal, 50*(5), 399–404.

Thomson, S., Osborn, R., Squires, D., & Reed, S. J. (Eds.) (2011). *International profiles of health care systems, 2011*. New York: The Commonwealth Fund. Retrieved February 2013 from http://www.commonwealthfund.org/~/media/Files/Publications/Fund%20Report/2011/Nov/1562_Squires_Intl_Profiles_2011_11_10.pdf

Urowitz, S., Wiljer, D., Apatu, E., Eysebach, G., DeLanardo, C., Harth, T., Pai, H., & Leonard, K. (2008). Is Canada ready for patient accessible electronic health records? A national scan. *BMC Medical Informatics and Decision Making, 8*(33), 1–7.

Webster, P. C. (2010). Canada's electronic health records initiative stalled by federal funding freeze. *Canadian Medical Association Journal News, 182*(5), E247–E248.

Index